A Bibliography
of Internal Medicine

COMMUNICABLE DISEASES

BY ARTHUR L. BLOOMFIELD, M.D.

THE UNIVERSITY OF CHICAGO PRESS

Library of Congress Catalog Number: 58-11470

THE UNIVERSITY OF CHICAGO PRESS, CHICAGO 37
Cambridge University Press, London, N.W. 1, England
The University of Toronto Press, Toronto 5, Canada

ⓒ *1958 by The University of Chicago. Published 1958*
Composed and printed by THE UNIVERSITY OF CHICAGO
PRESS, *Chicago, Illinois, U.S.A.*

THE surge of new knowledge in medicine has created a tremendous problem both for the student and for the practitioner. The periodical literature, for a long time unwieldy, has now become impossible to handle. The student with the shadow of the Specialty Board examinations always hovering over him tends to keep up on the new, the curious, and the esoteric at the expense of the fundamental and the historical. In current medical writing what is referred to as the "older literature" often turns out to be that of the previous decade. Few medical students nowadays (1957) remember Sir Thomas Lewis, George Minot, or F. G. Banting; most of them have never heard of Von Mering and Minkowski. In brief, there is real danger that we shall become completely cut off from our medical past and relapse into a sort of modern Dark Age.

Furthermore, after many years of teaching, I am convinced that some sort of historical approach, some understanding of the *development* of ideas, is essential for critical comprehension of a subject or of a disease. What a tragic world of ignorance was revealed by the medical student who wrote in an examination that the parasite of malaria was discovered by a man called "Vivax"!

How can this situation be corrected or at least helped? It was my thought, twenty-five years ago, that a selected bibliography which listed the important contributions of modern medicine (nineteenth and twentieth centuries) with critical comments might be useful and might stimulate both students and doctors to further reading and arouse their interest in the events which led up to modern knowledge. A start, made with typhoid fever (Arthur L. Bloomfield, "A student's bibliography of internal medicine: typhoid fever," Bull. Johns Hopkins Hosp., **51**:234, 1932), was enthusiastically received by my colleagues, but I was unable to go on with the project until the present time. My plan was to work through the domain of internal medicine in this fashion, dealing especially with those disorders whose past is long and which carry interesting historical implications: the present volume is concerned with communicable disease. In order to keep the mass of material within bounds, I have tried to include every reference of fundamental importance but to exclude those which add nothing essentially new. It will often happen, therefore, that the earliest article on a certain phase of the subject may be listed rather than the "best" or the most comprehensive. References to the vast very recent literature, the ultimate importance of which is not yet appraisable, are also necessarily limited. But the attempt has been made to make this bibliography, within these limits, definitive.

It has been a problem how far to pursue a subject into the literature of the basic sciences or of collateral branches of knowledge. Here the judgment of the compiler must be paramount, and I make no apology for my selections. The thought has always been, however, that this is a bibliography primarily for clinicians and for those with a general interest in the subject rather than for specialists.

Since many of the articles and books to which reference is made are in French and German as well as in English and since many articles were published in obscure or inaccessible journals, I have appended abstracts containing the substance of the material. The translations from foreign languages are my own.

Nearly every item has been seen by me and in most cases has been read and collated; the carelessness with which bibliographies are compiled has astonished me over and over again during this work; the reviewer had obviously not checked the original but had copied the errors of others. In older works especially, many references are incompletely given, thus creating endless labor for those looking up the original article.

The order in which to place the sections on various diseases has been a problem. I finally decided to put typhoid fever first as a small tribute to Sir William Osler's textbook, where, through many editions, discussion of this disease came first.

My thanks are due to the publishers of the various journals in which some sections of this bibliography have already appeared: the Stanford Medical Bulletin, the Bulletin of the Johns Hopkins Hospital, the Bulletin of the History of Medicine, the A.M.A. Archives of Internal Medicine, and the Journal of Chronic Diseases, for permission to reprint them.[1]

I am deeply grateful for the endless kindness and interest of Miss Clara Manson, librarian of the Lane Library of Stanford Medical School, who allowed me to set up an office in the library building, practically within the stacks. Had it not been for this and for the extraordinarily complete files of the Lane Library, my task would have been impossible. I am also in debt to all of the library staff for their unfailing co-operation; Mrs. A. Hoen especially pursued many an obscure reference with skill and tenacity.

Thanks are due to the National Library of Medicine, formerly the Armed Forces Medical Library, for the loan of a number of items.

Without the generous support and encouragement of the California Foundation for Medical Research, especially that of Dr. Jessie Marmorston, I should have had even greater difficulties in pursuing the work.

Finally, I have to thank my secretary, Miss Jean Mackenzie, for her tireless and skilful assistance at every point.

ARTHUR L. BLOOMFIELD

LANE LIBRARY
STANFORD UNIVERSITY MEDICAL SCHOOL
SAN FRANCISCO, CALIFORNIA
December 1957

[1] Bull. Johns Hopkins Hosp.: typhoid fever—51:234, 1932.
Stanford M. Bull.: scarlet fever—10:114, May, 1952. influenza—10:293, November, 1952. poliomyelitis—11:79, May, 1953. tuberculosis—12:217, November, 1954. pneumococcal pneumonia—13:493, November, 1955. syphilis, Part I—14:1, February, 1956. syphilis, Part II—14:77, May, 1956. smallpox and vaccination—14:137, August, 1956. diphtheria—14:205, November, 1956. plague—15:3; February, 1957, rabies—15:61, May, 1957.
J. Chron. Dis.: malaria—1:665, June, 1955. brucellosis—3:203, February, 1956. amebic dysentery—5:235, February, 1957. gonorrhea and gonococcal infection—5:592, May, 1957.
Arch. Int. Med.: cholera—96:734, December, 1955. meningococcus infection—97:79, January, 1956. rheumatic fever—98:288, September, 1956.
Bull. Hist. Med.: yellow fever—30:213, May–June, 1956.

TYPHOID FEVER

Artificial immunization	Refs. 20, 23, 24, 28
Bacteriology	Refs. 14, 15, 16, 17, 18, 21, 40
Blood count	Ref. 19
Carriers	Refs. 32, 33, 39
Contagiousness	Refs. 6, 7, 11, 12
Definition	Refs. 1, 2, 3, 4, 5, 7, 8, 9
Diagnosis	Refs. 25, 26, 27
Differentiation from typhus	Refs. 8, 9
Epidemiology	Refs. 13, 32, 33, 39
Etiology	Ref. 14
General articles and texts	Refs. 1, 2, 3, 4, 5, 7, 10, 12, 30, 31, 34, 37
Immunity	Refs. 6, 7, 20, 23, 41
Mode of transmission	Refs. 11, 12, 32
Paratyphoid	Ref. 22
Pathology	Refs. 1, 2, 3, 4, 5, 29, 44
Treatment	Refs. 35, 36, 38, 42, 45

Section 1

TYPHOID FEVER

FOR a good review of the early literature on typhoid fever see Gay (Ref. 43). It should be remembered that, up to the nineteenth century, clinical medicine was dominated largely by the Galenic point of view and that fevers were thought of in terms of vague influences, alterations of humors, and so on. Even keen clinical observers such as Huxham were so influenced by fantastic ideas of pathological physiology that their clinical descriptions, while objective, are largely meaningless. For the most part, it is impossible to determine with just what conditions the observer was dealing.

1. HUXHAM, John. An essay on fevers, to which is now added a dissertation on the malignant, ulcerous sore-throat. London: S. A. Cumberlege, 1782.

The essay is of importance partly because it represents the contemporary point of view on fevers in general and partly because Huxham is credited with being one of the first to differentiate, under the names of "slow nervous fever" and "putrid malignant fever," typhus and typhoid fevers. The accounts are, however, largely unintelligible and contain nothing definitive except, perhaps, the following passage from the account of putrid fever (p. 96): "The Stools, especially near the State, or in the Decline of the Fever, are for the most Part intolerably stinking, green, livid, or black, frequently with severe Gripes and Blood. When they are more yellow, or brown, the less Danger; but the highest, when they run off insensibly, of whatever Colour. It is likewise a very bad Symptom when the Belly continues hard, swoln, and tense after profuse Stools; for this is generally the Consequence of an Inflammation, or Mortification of the Intestines."

2. CHOMEL, A. F. Des fièvres et des maladies pestilentielles. Paris: Crochard, 1821.

During the early part of the nineteenth century there arose the remarkable school of French clinician-pathologists typified in the present instance by Chomel and Louis. Emancipated entirely from the domination of Galenic fantasy, they described what they saw in the clinic and at post mortem with amazing clarity and exactness. As examples of simple but nice use of language, these works remain unsurpassed in medical writing. Under the heading "La fièvre entéro-mesentérique" Chomel describes briefly what was undoubtedly typhoid fever and went a step ahead of his contemporaries, who had already observed intestinal ulceration in association with fevers, by regarding the ulcers as a feature of the disease rather than its cause. His ideas on epidemiology and contagion were indefinite, and he merely emphasizes the observed fact that "entéro-mesentérique" affected young people especially and, furthermore, those who were relative newcomers in Paris and who found themselves under altered conditions as regarded "air, food, drink, and occupation."

"The progress of the disease does not differ much from that of ordinary adynamic fever, unless it be in respect of the following symptoms: There is, in the second period, pain or tenderness on pressure in the right flank, diarrhoea, meteorism, and on opening the body one regularly finds ulcers of the intestines.

2

It has been alleged that the intestinal ulcers precede the febrile movement, but the facts upon which this opinion is based do not seem to us sufficient to support it" (p. 187). "If one opens the intestine throughout its extent with a scissors, and examines with care the alterations of which it is the seat, one encounters this remarkable fact: the internal surface presents ulcers, the more abundant, larger, and deeper, the nearer they are to the cecum and its valve . . ." (p. 192). "In some cases the serous membrane is the only one which is not destroyed; in others, even it is perforated, and the intestinal canal communicates with the cavity of the peritoneum; fecal material has in this way been able to escape and give rise to an inflammation which has precipitated the end of the subject" (p. 193).

Despite this admirable description, Chomel was not entirely clear or complete in his definition of the disease, and it remained for Louis (see Ref. 5) to give a definitive description. As regards differentiation from typhus, Chomel states (p. 189): "We will expose the distinctive signs of these two affections later." However, the only subsequent passage bearing on this point deals with it indirectly and occurs in a discussion of the significance of intestinal ulcers in fevers: "One cannot, then, reasonably conclude that the disturbance of general function which one observes in this disease be the effect of the lesion of the digestive tube. The intestinal ulcers are to putrid fever [typhoid and perhaps some other disorders] what buboes are to plague and to anthrax, *and what its proper eruption is to typhus,* namely, one of the phenomena of the disease and not the entire disease" (p. 234).

3. De la maladie à laquelle M. Bretonneau, médecin de l'hôpital à Tours, a donné le nom de dothinentérie, ou dothinentérite; par M. Trousseau, D.M.P. ancien interne du même hôpital, Arch. gén. de méd., **10**:67, 169, 1826.

The recognition of typhoid as a definite entity was in the air for some years before the definitive descriptions of Louis (see Ref. 5) and others. The idea of considering fevers as manifestations of a morbid state caused by miasm, atmospheric or telluric conditions, was being questioned, and various entities were being separated. While local and diffuse intestinal lesions were found and described in certain fevers, their relation to the disease in question and to dysentery in general was not yet clear. Trousseau's paper is of importance in the history of typhoid for two reasons: first, because it includes an analysis (somewhat polemic in style) of the contradictory views on fevers which agitated the physicians of the time (Prost, Petit and Serres, Broussais, Andral, and others) and, second, because it champions the priority of Trousseau's chief, Bretonneau, who is claimed to have clearly defined the clinical and anatomical features of typhoid under the name of "dothinentérite" as early as 1813. "He had been led to define a disease the seat of which seems to be exclusively in the glands of Peyer and of Brunner, which one encounters in the jejunum, ileum, and large intestine. He has . . . outlined the symptoms, has described precisely the manifestations of the malady on successive days, and has summarized the diagnostic points so clearly that there are few of his pupils who do not clearly distinguish this form of 'entérite' from all others" (p. 67). There follow excellent case reports with pathological notes especially on the intestinal ulcers.

4. HEWETT, Cornwallis. Cases showing the frequency of the occurrence of follicular ulceration in the mucous membrane of the intestines, during the progress of idiopathic fevers; with dissections, and observations on its pathology. London M. & Phys. J., **56**:97, 1826.

This is the first English account of typhoid which approaches completeness. The clinical features are well described, as are the pathological changes. However, the subject still remained confused, and Hewett distinctly follows the French observers and does not take the lead. It is not clear from his account as to how far he was convinced that typhoid was actually a specific disease; rather, one gets the impression that he regarded it as a reaction type of fevers in general. The descriptions of cases by Richard Bright in the following year (*Reports of Medical Cases* [London, 1827], I, 178) certainly refer to typhoid but are also noncommittal as to the implications of the disease.

5. LOUIS, P. Ch. A. Recherches anatomiques, pathologiques et thérapeutiques sur la maladie connue sous les noms de gastro-entérite, fièvre putride, adynamique, ataxique, typhoïde, etc., etc., comparée avec les maladies aïgües les plus ordinaires. 2 vols. Paris: J.-B. Baillière, 1829.

"In order to know how to proceed with a problem which could not be properly clarified by simple discussion, I collected, from 1822 to 1827, the histories of all the patients taken with acute diseases who were admitted to the Charité in the wards Saint-Jean and Saint-Joseph at that time in charge of M. Chomel. I assembled . . . one hundred and thirty-eight observations of 'typhoid' fever, of which fifty pertained to individuals who died. I have analyzed them all in order to find out which among the numerous lesions were proper to the 'typhoid affection,' and I have compared them to the alterations found as a consequence of other acute disorders in eighty-three subjects whose histories I had also collected. I made the same study with reference to symptoms in the patients both with typhoid and with other acute affections, whether they recovered or died; in brief, I analyzed the visceral alterations in one hundred and thirty-three subjects and the symptoms in nearly nine hundred.

"I have discarded from the material the facts which seemed to lack exactness, and when I drew my conclusions from the rest I had ever in mind this thought of the author of *Émile*: 'I know that truth lies in things and not in my mind which judges them, and the less of myself I put into the conclusions which I draw the more certain I am of approaching the truth'" (Introduction, p. ix).

Upon these observations Louis based his description of typhoid (which he separated clearly from other fevers) and to which no important clinical or gross anatomical fact has since been added. While the way had been prepared by others, to Louis belongs the credit of the first complete analysis of the disease. He recognized fully that the essential lesions were those of the intestine, mesenteric lymph nodes, and spleen and separated from them secondary and incidental findings. The clinical picture is admirably drawn, including discussions of rose spots, intestinal hemorrhage, and perforation. With regard to etiology, Louis maintains a conservative attitude and admits frankly that the cause of typhoid is unknown. His statistics, however, confirm the impressions current at the time that most of the cases occurred in young people recently come to Paris. No comments are made on the question of contagion. A point of special interest is the obvious severity of the typhoid fever of Louis in contrast to that of today.

The onset was usually abrupt and stormy, often with chills and with the early appearance of diarrhea and stupor. In almost one-fourth of Louis's fatal cases death occurred as early as the second week, of "toxemia" or secondary infection, and the general mortality was nearly 30 per cent. Septic complications, partly the result of neglect and poor hygiene doubtless, were frequent, including erysipelas, suppurative angina, and abscesses following the application of blisters.

Louis departed deliberately from the mystic traditions of ancient medicine: "It is not inappropriate to remark at this point that one cannot depend upon the authority of the ancients in questions relative to the seats of disease, since these questions can be cleared up only by comparison of symptoms with lesions and the ancients were ignorant of pathological anatomy. Neither is it true, as is often said, that facts do not grow old. Without doubt some well-observed facts do not grow old and cannot grow old, but the immense majority have grown old, and those which we gather today will grow old in their turn, for they carry more or less the imprint of the time, of its methods, more exact than those of previous periods and less rigorous than those which will follow us. It behooves those who devote themselves to observation to be impressed by this truth and to realize that the best work is only good in relation to its time and that it awaits another, more exact and more complete" (Preface, p. vii, n. 2).

6. [BRETONNEAU]. Notice sur la contagion de la dothinentérie; lue à l'Académie royale de Médecine, le 7 juillet 1829, par M. Bretonneau, médecin de l'hôpital de Tours, Arch. gén. de méd., **21**:57, 1829.

While the question of the contagiousness of typhoid had been raised and supported by the observation of scattered outbreaks in rural districts, it was generally held by urban physicians that the disease was not transmissible. Bretonneau was one of the first to attract serious attention to the probability of contagion in a spirited address before the Academy. He opens: "Typhoid fever is contagious; it is contagious in Paris, and nowhere is it more often contagious." "Often imported into a village, one sees it spread from the patient to some of the attendants. It then spreads from the affected family to another, and one generally observes that it is not to the nearest family but to those whose contacts have been most intimate and frequent." He proceeds to assemble many unassailable instances of spread of the disease by contagion and answers the main arguments to the contrary. Bretonneau was also one of the first to insist on the immunity produced by an attack.

7. SMITH, Nathan. A practical essay on typhous fever. New York: E. Bliss & E. White, 1824.

The essay is of special importance, first, because it is one of the earliest accessible accounts of typhoid fever in America and, second, because of Smith's clear recognition of the contagiousness of the disease. One regrets that the writer's hint of a subsequent enlargement of the work was never fulfilled. However, all the essential features are described. "The Typhous Fever . . . is a disease sui generis, exhibiting as little variety in the different individuals affected by it as some of the diseases which are acknowledged always to arise from contagion" (p. 15). "There is another marked point of analogy between Typhus[1] and the common contagious maladies, which is, that it rarely affects

[1] Probably a misprint; Smith evidently meant Typhous (Typhoid).

the same individual twice" (p. 16). ". . . For during the twenty-five years since I first attended patients in this disease, and in that time I have visited many hundreds, and have witnessed its prevalence several times in the same village, I have never known or heard of its recurrence in the same person" (p. 17). "That the Typhous Fever is contagious, is a fact so evident to those who have seen much of the disease, and who have paid attention to the subject, that I should have spared myself the trouble of saying anything with regard to it, did I not know that there are some physicians in this country, who still dispute the point; one, which I think can be as fully demonstrated, as that the measles, small-pox, and other diseases universally allowed to be contagious, are so" (p. 11). This assertion is elaborated and supported by specific instances.

8. Observations suggested by a comparison of the post-mortem appearances produced by typhous fever in Dublin, Paris, and Geneva. By H. C. Lombard, Physician to the Geneva Hospital; (communicated in a letter to Dr. Graves), Dublin J.M. Sc., **10**:17, 1836. Second letter from Doctor Lombard to Doctor Graves on the subject of typhous fever, Dublin J.M. Sc., **10**:101, 1836.

Lombard was thoroughly familiar with typhoid on the Continent and believed the intestinal lesion to be a constant one, although the English physicians did not at this time agree with the claims of the French in regard to a specific ulceration of Peyer's patches. On visiting Ireland, Lombard saw cases which seemed to be the same disease, but, to his surprise, no intestinal lesions were present at autopsy. The two letters are a summary of Lombard's reflections on his curious experience; he hit on the correct solution and concludes the second letter as follows: "You have two different fevers, one highly contagious, which I may call the *Irish Typhus,* and in which the cephalic symptoms predominate, to the exclusion of abdominal alterations; the other which is *sporadic,* and most likely not so infectious, and in which the abdominal symptoms are more prominent. . . ."

These letters had a great influence in stimulating accurate differentiation of typhoid from other fevers.

9. GERHARD, W. W. Art. 1: On the typhus fever which occurred at Philadelphia in the spring and summer of 1836; illustrated by clinical observations at the Philadelphia Hospital; showing the distinction between this form of disease and dothinenteritis or the typhoid fever with alteration of the follicles of the small intestine, Am. J.M. Sc., **19**:289, 1836; *ibid.,* **20**:289, 1837.

Although typhoid was being recognized by many as a distinct entity, there was still considerable confusion with other fevers, especially typhus. To Gerhard belongs the credit for definitive differentiation of typhoid from typhus on the basis of the cases which he studied in the wards of the Pennsylvania Hospital. Gerhard had been in Paris with Louis and, like other Americans who had studied abroad, recognized the identity of the disease in the two continents. He points out, however, that the British, while familiar with the intestinal lesions, regarded them as "a mere complication of ordinary typhus." An epidemic of typhus in Philadelphia gave him the chance to compare the two fevers. The anatomical lesions "were as different . . . as the pustules of smallpox are unlike the eruption of measles" and in both were different from those found in remittent fever (malaria). In regard to the clinical features: "When the disease is completely formed, the characters on which the distinctions between the two forms of fever rest are: 1. The suffusion of the eyes which occurs in every case, or nearly every case of typhus fever, with the dusky red aspect of the countenance. 2. The extreme stupor and inactivity of the mind even when positive delirium does not exist. 3. We also observe in typhus no constant abdominal symptoms. . . . 4. If to these symptoms be added the peculiar eruption of petechiae, which is scarcely ever absent in whites, there remains hardly a possibility of error. In typhoid fever we consider as distinctive characters, the prostration, the somnolence, the slow development of nervous symptoms, which are not so strongly marked as in typhus. The abdominal symptoms are tympanites, pains in the abdomen, and diarrhoea. The sibilant rhonchus is heard in the chest; and lastly, there is an eruption of rose-coloured papulae and sudamina upon the skin." He was sure that typhus was contagious but was not certain about typhoid.

10. BARTLETT, Elisha. The history, diagnosis and treatment of typhoid and of typhus fever, etc. Philadelphia: Lea & Blanchard, 1842.

While Smith (see Ref. 7), Jackson, and others had written briefly or incompletely on typhoid, Bartlett's book contains the first complete account of the disease in English. The article of 180 pages is a masterpiece of clinical writing and includes a careful analysis of current ideas, with temperate and well-reasoned conclusions. Bartlett accepted the idea of the contagiousness of typhoid, recognized that the cause was unknown but felt that the disease was specific, and concluded his work with this remark: "which disease, thus characterized and defined, differs essentially from all others, in its causes, in its symptoms, in its lesions; and is, in the present state of our knowledge, only to a limited extent under the influence of control of art" (p. 180).

11. BUDD, William. On the fever at the clergy orphan asylum, Lancet, 2:617, 1856.
BUDD, William. On intestinal fever: its mode of propagation, *ibid.*, p. 694.

While various writers such as Gendron and Bretonneau, in France, and Nathan Smith, in America, had already insisted on the contagiousness of typhoid, it remained for Budd to give such an impetus to the idea that it was soon accepted by many physicians. His papers are convincing examples of keen observation and clear logic. Budd stressed the importance of the bowel discharges in the transmission of the disease and sensed the existence of carriers (see below). "This species of fever has two characteristics: the first is that it is an essentially contagious disorder; the second that by far the most virulent part of the specific poison by which the contagion takes effect is contained in the diarrhoeal discharges which issue from the diseased and exanthematous bowel. The first case in the series may either be casual and imported or may be due to the local rekindling, through atmospheric or other changes, of poison which had remained as the dormant legacy of some previous attack." He went wrong in thinking the poison might diffuse from the excreta through the air, but he suggested the following prophylaxis: "These measures are founded on the power of chemical agents to destroy the infectious properties of contagious poisons. If it be certain that the intestinal discharges in this fever are the principal means of propagating the disease, it is no less certain that by subjecting the discharges on their issue from the body to the action of powerful disinfectants, they may be entirely deprived of this property." He used chloride of zinc.

Budd lamented the attitude of the Metropolitan Board of Health and of the Royal College of Physicians, who, like the Paris academicians in Bretonneau's day, opposed the idea of contagion and believed that the disease was generated by filth. In describing the epidemic at North Tawton, a town in which there had been no typhoid for years, he points out that the lack of sanitation could not alone be held responsible for the outbreak. He describes the dirty privies near the houses, the dung-heaps, and the pigs. "Nevertheless, these things existed for many years without leading to any of the results which it is the fashion to ascribe to them. Much there was, as I can myself testify, that was offensive to the nose, but fever there was none. In the course of time—as, was indeed, sure to happen—this element was at length added, and it was then found that the conditions which had been without power to *generate* fever, had but too great power in promoting its spread, when once the germ of fever had been introduced."

Budd sustained his thesis in subsequent articles and finally gathered all his data into a book (see Ref. 13).

12. MURCHISON, Charles. A treatise on the continued fevers of Great Britain. London: Parker, Son & Bourn, 1862.

To Murchison belongs credit for the first encyclopedic treatise on typhoid fever. The section on this disease which comprises some two hundred pages has influenced practically every succeeding account up to the present time. Points of especial importance are the elaborate catalogue of the nomenclature of the disease; a masterly, well-documented historical sketch with special attention to the distribution of typhoid and typhus fevers in England; the elaborate statistics as to geographical distribution, age, sex, season, etc.; the mortality statistics; and the vivid and accurate clinical descriptions. There are several exquisite colored plates depicting the distribution of rose spots. The discussion on contagion is of especial interest, since Murchison held out against the idea that typhoid was communicable and insisted on its origin from the emanations of sewage. In fact, he described the disease under the name of "pythogenic" fever (arising from putrescence). Most of Murchison's arguments against contagion can be explained by the doctrine of "carriers."

13. BUDD, William. Typhoid fever: its nature, mode of spreading, and prevention. London: Longmans, Green & Co., 1873.

In this book, already referred to above (see Ref. 11), the writer collects in a definitive manner his observations on the spread of typhoid fever. He levels his batteries, masked by the most delicate satire, at the anticontagionists and attacks especially the pythogenic theory, which carried the authority of Murchison's support. His final devastating argument against the spontaneous generation of typhoid from putrescent matter was based on the epidemiological facts of "the hot months of 1858 and 1859, when the Thames stank so badly." "The occasion, indeed, as already hinted, was no common one. An extreme case, a gigantic scale in the phenomena, and perfect accuracy in the registration of the results—three of the best of all guarantees against fallacy—were all combined to make the induction sure. For the first time in the history of man, the sewage of nearly three millions of people had been brought to seethe and ferment under a burning sun in one vast open cloaca lying in their midst. The result we all know. Stench so foul, we may well believe, had never before ascended to pollute this lower air. Never before, at least, had a stink risen to the height of an historic event. Even ancient fable failed to furnish figures adequate to convey a conception of its thrice Augean foulness. . . . At home and abroad, the state of the chief river was felt to be a national reproach. 'India is in revolt, and the Thames stinks' were the two great facts coupled together by a distinguished foreign writer, to mark the climax of a national humiliation. . . . Meanwhile the hot weather passed away; the returns of sickness and mortality were made up, and, strange to relate, the result showed, not only a death rate below the average, but, *as the leading peculiarity of the season,* a remarkable diminution in the prevalence of fever, diarrhoea, and the other forms of disease commonly ascribed to putrid emanations. . . . So that while pythogenic compounds were poisoning the air with what may be called a forty-thousand fever power the so-called pythogenic fever, so far from rising in proportion, fell much below its average" (p. 148).

The more important parts of the book, however, are those which deal systematically with the modes of transmission. Budd showed by well-documented studies of numerous outbreaks that the bowel discharges were the main source of infection; that the disease was water-borne; and that milk, food, contaminated linen, and fomites in general were sources of dissemination. He erred in insisting that the contagion might be air-borne and that the emanations from a sewer or water closet contaminated with the discharges from typhoid patients were dangerous. He insisted, however, on a specific virus as the *sine qua non* of typhoid and recognized the minute size of the "germ" and its capacity for multiplication.

The work is a masterpiece of exposition, argument, and fine rhetoric.

14. EBERTH, C. J. Die Organismen in den Organen bei Typhus abdominalis, Virchows Arch. f. path. Anat., **81**:58, 1880.

The discovery of the typhoid bacillus is generally ascribed to Eberth. His were, however, by no means the first attempts to find a microbic cause, and the present paper was preceded by numerous reports describing the presence of various bacteria in the tissues of patients dead of typhoid. These were, for the most part, obvious saprophytes or secondary invaders. The technical difficulties of studies of this sort eighty years ago must be kept in mind; modern methods of fixing, cutting, and staining had not yet been devised. Eberth treated alcohol-hardened tissues with acetic acid and in some cases stained with methyl violet and Bismarck brown. Masses of bacteria were found in a good many cases, especially in the spleen and mesenteric lymph nodes. They are described as tiny rods, at times with one or more sporelike bodies. The description seems far from conclusive; however, it is likely that Eberth was dealing with typhoid bacilli, at least in a good many instances. The article concludes: "These findings make it highly likely that the organisms found in the organs in typhoid fever stand in a [causal] relationship to the process."

Priority has been claimed for the observations of E. Klebs, which appeared in April, 1880 ("Der Ileotyphus eine Schistomycose," Arch. f. exper. Path. u. Pharmakol., **12**:231, 1880); but, while Klebs may well have seen typhoid bacilli, the description is not very satisfying, especially the reference to thread-like forms 80 μ in length.

R. Koch ("Zur Untersuchung von pathogenen Organismen," Mitt. a. d. k. Gsndhtsamte, **1:1**, 1881) reports the finding in tissues of typhoid patients of bacteria which seem to correspond to those described by Eberth; he suggested that Klebs's organisms were secondary invaders, as he found them only on the surface of necrotic ulcers.

15. GAFFKY. Zur Aetiologie des abdominal Typhus, Mitt. a. d. k. Gsndhts-amte, **2**:372, 1884.

Gaffky's paper is a landmark in the bacteriological study of typhoid. By better methods of staining bacteria in tissues, he confirmed the observations of Eberth and of Koch and showed beyond question that bacillary forms were almost always present in the tissues of typhoid-fever patients, especially in the spleen, liver, intestinal lymphoid tissue, and, to a lesser extent, the kidney. He pointed out clearly that the great variety of bacteria found in the superficial parts of the ulcers were probably secondary and unessential and that such organisms were not found in the depths of the diseased tissues. But, most important, he cultivated the bacilli from the spleen on slides coated with gelatin, isolated them in pure culture, and described accurately various characteristics, including motility. He was unable to grow the organisms from stools or blood and failed to produce anything resembling typhoid fever in animals by inoculation of pure cultures in various ways, although others had claimed that they had produced the disease with material from typhoid cases. The review of the literature is definitive to date and analyzes the whole problem of the bacteriology of typhoid fever in a sound and temperate manner at a time when bitter struggles for priority were likely to color medical writing. Gaffky was disappointed at being unable to produce the disease in animals, but he wisely concluded that this did not exclude the bacillus as the cause of typhoid and that further observations would be necessary to settle the question.

During the next few years typhoid bacilli were cultivated from blood, urine, stools, and other material *intra vitam*. For detailed references see Gay (Ref. 43).

16. PFEIFFER, A. Ueber den Nachweis der Typhus Bacillen im Darminhalt und Stuhlgang, Deutsche med. Wchnschr., **11**:500, 1885.

Credit for first isolating typhoid bacilli from the stools is usually given to Pfeiffer. The paper is of great interest because of the technical difficulties. Colonies were fished from plain agar plates and identified by appearance of the growth on potato. No fermentation or agglutination tests were available at that time, nor had differential plates been developed. It is questionable, however, whether Pfeiffer's criteria were altogether adequate and whether his diagnosis of typhoid bacilli was invariably correct.

Pfeiffer is apparently the first to have cultivated the bacillus from material outside the human body.

17. HUEPPE. Fortschr. d. Med., **4**:447, 1886.

In reviewing an article by Von Fodor on bacteremia, Hueppe states that he was able to cultivate typhoid bacilli from the urine in one of eighteen cases. This is apparently the first record of a successful attempt.

18. NEUHAUSS, R. Nachweis der Typhus Bacillen am Lebenden, Berl. klin. Wchnschr., **23**:89, 1886.

Many attempts to demonstrate typhoid bacilli in the blood during life were reported at about this time. Some of them consisted of direct microscopic study of the blood, others involved cultures of drops of blood obtained by incising rose spots or other areas of skin. Neuhauss, by the latter procedure, was apparently the first to obtain a positive culture. It was not until years later, when larger amounts of blood drawn from the vein were used, that the procedure became of practical diagnostic value (Schottmüller).

19. TUMAS, L. J. Ueber die Schwankungen der Blutkörperzahl und des Hämoglobingehalts des Blutes im Verlaufe einiger Infectionskrankheiten, Deutsches Arch. f. klin. Med., **41**:323, 1887.

Tumas was the first to report fairly complete studies of the blood count in typhoid fever. He observed that leukopenia was almost invariably present. W. S. Thayer (Johns Hopkins Hosp. Reps., **4**:83, 1894) made the first careful American studies and emphasized the diagnostic value of the blood count.

20. BEUMER and PEIPER. Bacteriologische Studien über die ätiologische Bedeutung der Typhus Bacillen, Ztschr. f. Hyg. u. Infectionskr., **2**:110, 1887.

In the course of attempts to produce typhoid fever experimentally, it was found that mice which had survived an initial small dose of typhoid bacilli later survived a much larger injection. The writers clearly recognized the possible application of such immunization to man, although they did not pursue the subject further at the time.

21. ANTON, B., and FÜTTERER, G. Untersuchungen über Typhus abdominalis, München. med. Wchnschr., **35**:315, 1888.

Fütterer first cultivated typhoid bacilli from the contents of the gall bladder at autopsy in typhoid cases. The identification was probably correct. He points out that the bile does not seem to have an inhibiting action on these bacteria. This work was the precursor of a host of studies which proved that the gall bladder was readily infected by way of the blood stream and that it was a common situation for persistence of bacilli during the "carrier state." For further references see Gay (Ref. 43).

22. ACHARD, Ch., and BENSAUDE, R. Infections paratyphoïdiques, Bull. et mém. Soc. méd. hôp. Paris, **13**:820, 1896.

The fact that there were a variety of organisms which resembled the typhoid bacillus was already known. Achard and Bensaude were the first, however, to report cases resembling typhoid from which "paratyphoid" bacilli were isolated.

They used the term "paratyphoid" in the sense of "resembling typhoid" rather than in the strict modern technical sense. The bacteriological distinction was made mainly on the basis of agglutination tests with specific sera.

23. PFEIFFER, R., and KOLLE, W. Ueber die specifische Immunitäts-reaction der Typhusbacillen, Ztschr. f. Hyg. u. Infectionskr., **21**:203, 1895–96.

The development of immunization was a logical sequel to preliminary studies. Of these, some of the most important were those of Pfeiffer and Kolle. In a series of clean-cut experiments they showed that the serum of typhoid convalescents contained substances which protected guinea pigs specifically against lethal doses of typhoid bacilli and that similar protective substances could be developed in the serum of goats, following repeated injections of culture. These observations, together with practical results already obtained in cholera, suggested attempts at human prophylaxis.

24. PFEIFFER, R., and KOLLE, W. Experimentelle Untersuchungen zur Frage de Schutzimpfung des Menschen gegen Typhus abdominalis, Deutsche med. Wchnschr., **22**:735, 1896.

Pfeiffer's attempts at prophylactic vaccination were stimulated by encouraging results which had been obtained in cholera. Pfeiffer injected subcutaneously about 2 mg. of fresh culture scraped from agar slants suspended in broth and sterilized at 56° C. There was usually a chill within 2 or 3 hours, followed by a rise in temperature to about 38.5° C. Only one injection was given. Serum drawn from the subjects about 11 days after the treatment was found to have as high a titer of protective bodies against experimental guinea-pig infection as did the serum of typhoid convalescents. On this basis Pfeiffer hoped that the prophylaxis would convey as complete a protection as a spontaneous attack of typhoid fever, since at that time the humoral bactericidal antibodies were regarded as entirely, or almost entirely, responsible for recovery from the disease.

25. GRUBER, Max, and DURHAM, Herbert E. Eine neue Methode zur raschen Erkennung des Cholera vibrio und des Typhus Bacillus, München. med. Wchnschr., **4**:285, 1896.

It was found that serum from guinea pigs immunized against cholera or typhoid developed the remarkable property when mixed with the bacteria in question under proper conditions of causing them to "stick together in large balls, and to lose their motility. We therefore have named these specific substances . . . agglutinins." In discussing the implications of this finding, Gruber and Durham laid special stress on the identification of unknown strains of bacteria by known immune sera. The alternative procedure of detecting specific immune bodies by testing against known cultures was, however, obvious and was later described from Gruber's laboratory by Grünbaum (see Ref. 27).

26. WIDAL, F. Sérodiagnostic de la fièvre typhoïde, Semaine méd., **16**:259, 1896.

While Widal's name has been attached to the agglutination test in typhoid, the original communication seems brief and inadequate and gives no credit to Gruber and Durham, who had already clearly described the phenomenon of agglutination. Widal added the patient's serum to broth cultures of typhoid bacilli in a proportion of 1 to 10 or 15 and incubated for 24 hours. Gross flocculation was observed at the end of this time.

27. GRÜNBAUM, Albert S. Preliminary note on the use of the agglutinative action of human serum for the diagnosis of enteric fever, Lancet, **2**:806, 1896.

Although Widal's paper appeared first, Grünbaum undoubtedly shares the credit for the development of this test, as his work was carried on in Gruber's laboratory during the preceding year and was the direct outcome of Gruber and Durham's work on agglutination. Grünbaum describes the microscopic method essentially as it is used today. "It is only in cases of enteric fever that the serum shows a distinct agglutinative action within thirty minutes when diluted sixteen times, and hence this reaction can be used as a diagnostic sign."

28. WRIGHT, A. E., and SEMPLE, D. Remarks on vaccination against typhoid fever, Brit. M.J., **1**:256, 1897.

Wright and Semple's paper appeared shortly after that of Pfeiffer and Kolle. They imply, however, that Pfeiffer plagiarized the idea from a paper of Wright's which appeared in the Lancet, **21**:807 (September 19), 1896, in which he claims to have put on record his first attempts at antityphoid inoculation. An inspection of this paper makes the implication seem unfair to Pfeiffer, since, as the title would suggest ("On the association of serous hemorrhages with conditions of defective blood coagulability"), the observations concern themselves with other matters. While it is mentioned incidentally that a horse and two men received injections of typhoid bacilli in connection with the experiments on blood coagulablity, there is not the slightest suggestion that the writer contemplated purposeful antityphoid prophylaxis. Pfeiffer's previous experimental work, furthermore, makes it evident that he already had the possibility of human immunization in mind.

Wright and Semple used essentially the same procedure as Pfeiffer, but they measured the result in terms of agglutinative titer of the serum of the subjects. They found that such serum, even if rich in agglutinins, did not have any material bactericidal effect in vitro, and hence they were more conservative than Pfeiffer in their conclusions as to the probable degree of protection which was to be expected. Wright later described his results and those of others (Lancet, **2**:651, 1902).

29. MALLORY, F. B. A histological study of typhoid fever, J. Exper. Med., **3**:611, 1898.

Important studies of the finer histological changes.

30. KEEN, William W. The surgical complications and sequels of typhoid fever. Philadelphia: W. B. Saunders, 1898.

A definitive monograph based on a careful analysis of reported cases and enriched by the author's wide experience. It remains a storehouse of information on the (from the clinical standpoint) all-important problem of typhoid complications.

31. CURSCHMANN, H. Der Unterleibstyphus. Vienna: Alfred Hölder, 1898.

The most comprehensive modern clinical treatise, with important literature to date arranged with the subject matter.

32. KOCH, Robert. Die Bekämpfung der Typhus. (Vortrag, gehalten in der Sitzung des wissenschaftlichen Senats bei der Kaiser Wilhelms Akademie am 28 November, 1902.) Veröffentlichungen aus dem Gebiete des Militär-Sanitätswesens, Vol. 21. Berlin: A. Hirschwald, 1903.

The control of typhoid epidemics was the outstanding problem of the disease at the end of the nineteenth century. While it was recognized that water and milk supplies contaminated by typhoid excreta were major factors, it had not been clearly appreciated that the most adequate way to check the spread of the disease was by disinfection of excreta at their source and isolation of the convalescents until they became bacillus-free. In this famous lecture Koch clearly outlined the logical methods of typhoid control: "There are therefore two conditions which must be fulfilled. In the first place we must be in a position to recognize the infectious agent with ease and certainty, and in the second place to dispose of it." To this end, special methods of readily identifying the typhoid bacillus in the stools were developed (Von Drigalski and H. Conradi, "Ueber ein Verfahren zum Nachweis der Typhusbacillen," Ztschr. f. Hyg. u. Infectionskr., 39:283, 1902), and stations were set up in typhoid districts for the control of carriers. These measures, together with improvement in sewage conditions, soon led to a great decrease in typhoid incidence in Germany.

33. VON DRIGALSKI. Ueber Ergebnisse bei der Bekämpfung des Typhus nach Robert Koch, Centralbl. f. Bakt., 35:776, 1904.

Drigalski's work amplified and extended that of Koch (see Ref. 32) especially with reference to carriers who had never had clinical typhoid fever. Drigalski stressed the carrier as the main cause of continuous endemic typhoid in distinction to extensive outbreaks due to contaminated water. He insisted on negative stool and urine cultures from convalescents before they were released from supervision.

34. McCRAE, T. Typhoid fever, in OSLER and McCRAE, Modern medicine, 2:70. Philadelphia and New York: Lea Bros., 1907. Also 3d ed., 1:63. Philadelphia and New York; Lea & Febiger, 1925.

The best modern English article, based largely on the Johns Hopkins case.

35. COLEMAN, Warren. Diet in typhoid fever, J.A.M.A., 53:1145, 1909.

One of the most important contributions to the treatment of typhoid fever was the proof that a liberal diet could be taken with beneficial results. While various clinicians from Robert Graves (1835) on had empirically advised the feeding of typhoid patients, it remained for Coleman and his associates (see Refs. 36, 38, 42) to establish by accurate scientific methods that food could actually be digested and absorbed and that nitrogen equilibrium could be maintained and weight loss prevented by high-caloric diets. This was a radical departure from previous practice. Until the high-calorie diet was introduced, stress was placed on intensive hydrotherapy (see E. Brand, *Die Hydrotherapie des Typhus* [Stettin, 1861]). One of the most notable results of the liberal diet is shortening of the period of convalescence, formerly so long and tedious. This series of studies is of great importance not only in relation to typhoid but because the principles which were established apply to other prolonged fevers as well.

36. SHAFFER, Philip A., and COLEMAN, Warren. Protein metabolism in typhoid fever, Arch. Int. Med., 4:538, 1909.

In carefully controlled metabolism studies of typhoid patients it is shown that the destruction of body protein (and loss of weight) which had been ascribed not only to fever but to obscure "toxic effects" could be prevented by feeding 10–15 gm. of nitrogen (60–90 gm. of protein) daily, together with an adequate carbohydrate ration. W. Coleman and E. F. DuBois showed later, however ("Calorimetric observations on the metabolism of typhoid patients with and without food," Arch. Int. Med., 15:887, 1915), that there was a "toxic" destruction of protein in typhoid, since patients might have a distinctly negative nitrogen balance on a diet which contained more than enough calories to cover heat production.

37. SCHOTTMÜLLER, H. Die Typhosen Erkrankheiten, *in* Mohr and Staehelin, Handbuch der inneren Medizin, 1:371. Berlin: Julius Springer, 1911.

Excellent summary with literature.

38. DuBOIS, Eugene F. The absorption of food in typhoid fever, Arch. Int. Med., 10:177, 1912.

One of the principal arguments against liberal feeding in typhoid was disposed of by these experiments, which showed that protein and carbohydrate could be absorbed as well as during health and that the absorption of fat was only moderately diminished.

39. LEDINGHAM, J. C. G., and ARKWRIGHT, J. A. The carrier problem in infectious diseases. New York: Longmans, Green & Co., 1912.

An authoritative summary of the carrier problem.

40. KUTSCHER, K. H. Abdominal typhus, *in* Kolle and Wassermann, Handbuch der pathogenen Micro-organismen, 3:717. 2d ed. Jena: Gustav Fischer, 1913.

Comprehensive review of the bacteriology of typhoid.

41. FORNET, W. Immunität bei Typhus, *in* Kolle and Wassermann, Handbuch der pathogenen Micro-organismen, 3:837. 2d ed. Jena: Gustav Fischer, 1913.

Comprehensive review of immunological aspects of typhoid fever.

42. COLEMAN, Warren. The influence of the high calorie diet on the course of typhoid fever. J.A.M.A., 69:329, 1917.

A summary of the end-results of the treatment.

43. GAY, F. P. Typhoid fever. New York: Macmillan Co., 1918.

A comprehensive summary of knowledge of the disease from the biological and epidemiological standpoint. The Bibliography is especially well selected and complete.

44. CHRISTELLER, E. Der Typhus abdominalis, *in* HENKE and LUBARSCH, Handbuch der speciellen pathologischen Anatomie und Histologie, 4:500. Berlin: Julius Springer, 1924.

Special emphasis on pathological changes. Extensive bibliography. Good colored plates of lesions, gross and histological.

45. WOODWARD, T. E., SMADEL, J. E., LEY, H. L., Jr., GREEN, R., and MANKIKAR, D. S. Preliminary report on the beneficial effect of chloromycetin in the treatment of typhoid fever, Ann. Int. Med., 29:131, 1948.

For nearly one hundred years typhoid fever remained refractory to every available drug, and the mortality was essentially unchanged. Woodward and his associates were engaged in testing a new antibiotic, chloromycetin (J. Ehrlich, Q. R. Bartz, R. M. Smith, D. A. Joslyn, and P. R. Burkholder, "Chloromycetin, a new antibiotic from a soil actinomycete," Science, 106:417, 1947) in cases of scrub typhus in Malaya, when it occurred to them to use the drug in the severe cases of typhoid fever which were present in the area. Ten cases were treated. Fever as a rule dropped rapidly, and the patients felt much better in a few days. Blood cultures promptly became sterile. Two of the ten patients (20 per cent) developed relapses with bacteremia after afebrile periods of 10 and 16 days. In one case intestinal perforation occurred on the second day of normal temperature, and in another a large intestinal bleeding took place on the fourth day of normal temperature. Woodward ("Chloromycetin and aureomycin: therapeutic results," Ann. Int. Med., 31:53, 1949) soon reported further experiences. Woodward, Smadel, and Ley ("Chloroamphenicol and other antibiotics in the treatment of typhoid fever and typhoid carriers," J. Clin. Investigation, 29:87, 1950) analyzed the treatment of 24 patients with chloramphenicol without a death. Again the relapse rate was about 20 per cent. The drug also failed to eliminate typhoid bacilli permanently from chronic carriers.

Meanwhile, Vernon Knight and his associates (V. Knight, F. Ruiz Sanchez, A. Ruiz Sanchez, S. Schultz, and W. McDermott, "Antimicrobial therapy in typhoid," Arch. Int. Med., 85:44, 1950), working with the severe typhoid fevers of Mexico, reported 13 cases treated with chloramphenicol without a death. J. E. Smadel, C. A. Bailey, and R. Lewthwaite ("Synthetic and fermentation type chloramphenicol [chloromycetin] in typhoid fever: prevention of relapses by adequate treatment," Ann. Int. Med., 33:1, 1950), alive to the frequency of relapses, prolonged the use of the drug to 14 days, which they found adequate to prevent relapse in their series.

Thus typhoid fever at long last has been to a large extent mastered by medical science.

CHOLERA

Section 2

CHOLERA

W E HAVE found no really comprehensive modern bibliography of cholera. Much of the early literature deals with descriptions of outbreaks of epidemics, and this phase of the subject is comprehensively dealt with by Hirsch (Ref. 10), as well as by C. Macnamara in *A History of Asiatic Cholera* (London: Macmillan & Co., 1876). A good general account of the disease is that of H. Harold Scott in his *History of Tropical Medicine* (Baltimore: Williams & Wilkins Co., 1939), 2:694. C. Liebermeister's *Cholera Asiatica und Cholera Nostras* (Vienna: Alfred Hölder, 1896) has appended to it a fairly comprehensive bibliography of the older literature. Finally, J. S. Chambers in his book *The Conquest of Cholera* (New York: Macmillan Co., 1938) gives in interesting detail the story of cholera, especially in the United States.

1. BRIGHAM, A. Treatise on epidemic cholera, including an historical account of its origin and progress to the present period. Hartford, Conn.: H. & F. J. Huntington, 1832.

Although epidemics of what was pretty clearly cholera had been described at various times (Ref. 10), the modern history of the disease dates from the outbreak at Jessore, in India, in 1817. Brigham's book opens with a year-by-year description of the progress of this epidemic, which spread over India during the ensuing years but did not reach Asia Minor and China until 1823. In 1829 the disease crossed the Urals and in 1830 spread along the Volga, reaching Moscow. In 1831 it appeared in many parts of Europe, including Berlin. In this year it also reached England (for detailed accounts of the various epidemics see Ref. 10). Next come accounts of the disease from various parts of the world. In the cases seen by the writer in New York he describes the symptoms as follows: "First, diarrhoea, though often of only short duration, then nausea and vomiting, though in some instances the vomiting was slight, to which succeeded a sinking of the circulation, coldness and blueness of surface, burning thirst, spasms and death. In most of the cases that I have seen, the discharges from the stomach and bowels were light colored, resembling arrow root and water or starch and water, and were without odor" (p. 104). In another account (p. 102) the stools are described as being "like rice water." "Besides the intestinal canal and skin all other organs furnished no secretion. Tears, pituita, saliva, and urine, the secretion of which is totally suspended; as to tears, the greatest anguish of dying, in full possession of the intellect, surrounded by all that is at once endearing and afflicting, could not produce them." The thickness of the blood is remarked, and it is stated that leeches could procure none. "The accounts of this disease, from Asia, Persia, Russia, Poland, England, Canada and the United States, all agree" (p. 105). The descriptions of "Appearances on Dissection" follow; aside from the evidence of desiccation, there is disagreement as to the significance of the findings. In some cases the gastrointestinal tract is said to show little; in others there were extensive lesions of the superficial layers.

As to treatment, it is hard to see how physicians could have failed to note the obvious evidences of dehydration; instead, bleeding and leeching and the usual variety of meaningless drugs were advised. In one account (p. 168) it is stated: "Let two tablespoons full of common kitchen salt, dissolved in six ounces of warm water, be given immediately." That the writer had no rational basis for this prescription becomes clear when he adds: "energetic complete vomiting will probably be produced by the salt." However, he adds later (p. 176): "The patients treated in this manner, that is, with a solution of common salt, were often very soon restored to health, and could hardly be recognized after a few hours." On page 243, however, a most interesting statement appears: "A few have been cured in New York by the injection of saline solutions into the veins. Dr. Rhinelander stated to the Board of Health of New York the case of Margaret Mehan, who was cured at Crosby Street hospital by injecting into the veins twenty-four ounces of a solution composed of one dram of carb. soda, and two drams of muriate of soda [common salt] dissolved in six pints of water. The operation was performed at 7 p.m. on July 21st [1832?]. Several other cases of cholera have been cured in a similar manner, both in this country and also in England, where the practice I believe originated. This practice is undoubtedly founded upon the fact, said to have been discovered by analysis; that the blood drawn from a patient affected with cholera, has lost a portion of its watery and albuminous parts, and also most of its natural saline ingredients."

There are introduced at this point two lectures by J. F. V. Broussais, of which the most interesting part is the discussion of contagion. The fact that several members of a household often had the disease "gives rise to the suspicion that there is a species of infection by which the patient communicates the disease to those who have charge of him." But, by their number and vociferousness, the anticontagionists vastly predominated at this time.

2. BELL, G. H. Treatise on cholera asphyxia or epidemic cholera. 2d ed. Edinburgh: William Blackwood, 1832.

Cholera went under a variety of descriptions: cholera asphyxia, blue cholera, epidemic cholera, Asiatic cholera, cholera morbus, etc.; many used the term "cholera morbus" for sporadic cases in distinction to the epidemic. This book, like many others at the time, deals with the whole subject. Worthy of mention, however, is the discussion on contagion: "Much stress has been laid on the fact that the Cholera has travelled along the banks of rivers. Undoubtedly it has done so; but in so far as regards India, the writers who rely so confidently on this fact, have not adverted to the peculiarity, that the progress of the disease along the banks of rivers, has not been confined, as they seem to suppose to navigable rivers. It has extended itself along the banks of rivers whether navigable or not" (p. 84). No one sensed the fact that the disease might be conveyed by contamination of the river water.

3. Documents communicated by the Central Board of Health, London, relative to the treatment of cholera by the copious injection of aqueous and saline fluids into the veins, Lancet, 2:274, 1832.

The first approach to a rational therapy for cholera was by W. B. O'Shaughnessy ("Proposal of a new method of treating the blue cholera epidemic by the injection of highly-oxygenated salts into the venous system," Lancet, 1:366,

1831–32), who was impressed by the thick black blood and recognized the need of restoring it to an oxygenated or arterial state. This he proposed to do by injection into the vein of "oxygenated salts," such as potassium nitrate and potassium chlorate. Nothing came of this, but a little later ("Experiments on the blood in cholera," Lancet, 1:490, 1831–32) O'Shaughnessy reported analyses of blood from cholera patients which gave him a lead in the right direction. He found the blood "has lost a large proportion of its water, it has lost also a great proportion of its *neutral* saline ingredients," and that "of the free alkali contained in healthy serum, not a particle is present." He also found that "urea exists in the cases where suppression of urine has been a marked symptom" and that "all the salts deficient in the blood, especially the carbonate of soda are present in large quantities in the peculiar white dejected matters." O'Shaughnessy issued a larger report on these findings with therapeutic suggestions which was reviewed in critical, if not hostile, fashion later in the year ("Report on the chemical pathology of the malignant cholera" (review) Lancet, 1:929, 1831–32). He says: "When absorption is entirely suspended as in those desperate cases which are unhappily now of daily occurrence in this metropolis, the author recommends the injection into the veins of tepid water holding a solution of normal salts of the blood." Meanwhile, W. Reid Clanny ("Case of cholera at Sunderland with an analysis of the blood taken from the patient," Lancet, 1:505, 1831–32) found that "in Elliot Todd [the patient] water, colouring matter and muriates of soda and potassa and carbonate of soda were respectively 644, 253, and 0 parts as against the findings in The Sailor [control] 756, 59, and 14 parts." The matter was soon pressed further. (W. B. O'Shaughnessy, "Chemical pathology of cholera," Lancet, 2:225, 1831–32; Clanny, "Composition of healthy and cholera blood," Lancet, 2:232, 1831–32). However, the first practical application of the method seems to have been made by Thomas Latta, as reported in the above-mentioned "Documents." Latta was stimulated by reading O'Shaughnessy's report on the blood in cholera. "The first subject of experiment was an aged female. She had apparently reached the last moments of her earthly existence, and now nothing could injure her. Having inserted a tube in the basilic vein, cautiously—anxiously, I watched the effects; ounce after ounce was injected, but no visible change was produced. Still persevering, I thought she began to breathe less laboriously, soon the sharpened features and sunken eyes, and fallen jaw, pale and cold, bearing the manifest imprint of death's signet, began to glow with returning animation, the pulse which had long ceased returned to the wrist; and in the short space of half an hour when six pints had been injected, she expressed in a firm voice that she was free of all uneasiness, actually became jocular, and fancied all she needed was a little sleep; her extremities were warm, and every feature bore the aspect of comfort and health." The patient soon became worse again and died; no further salt solution was injected.

Latta later worked out a formula—2 or 3 drams of muriate of soda and two scruples of the subcarbonate in 6 pints of water, injected at temperature of 112° F. He believed that larger amounts must often be given and attributed failure mainly to "too little and too late." A moribund woman was restored by injection of 330 ounces (9,900 cc.); "in 48 hours she smoked her pipe free from distemper" and proceeded to get well. "The apparatus I have used is Read's patent syringe, having a small silver tube attached to the extremity of the flexible injecting tube. The syringe must be quite perfect so as to avoid the risk of injecting air."

The report continues with abstracts of cases in which the saline therapy was used by Drs. Lewin, Craigie, Macintosh, and Racy. All agreed on the undoubted benefits of this form of treatment. We learn incidentally of the impunity with which unsterile solutions may be injected into the vein.

During the ensuing year there are more case reports in the Lancet, some favorable, some unfavorable, but, with the subsidence of the epidemic, this mode of therapy seems to have been neglected, although scattered case reports and notes are found through the years. The procedure never became standardized, and as late as 1873 A. Netter ("Des injections qui se pratiquent dans les veines des cholériques, et de la causes des variations des résultats obtenus jusqu'ici avec ce moyen thérapeutique," Gaz. hôp. Paris, **46**:1107, 1873) analyzes the difficulties and uncertainties of the method, pointing out that, while the immediate results are almost uniformly promising, the later effects are variable. He analyzed the situation more at length in a little monograph (A. Netter, *Vues nouvelles sur le choléra avec une étude sur les injections faites dans les veines* [Paris: J.-B. Baillière et fils, 1874]). The whole subject was later reviewed by Rogers (Ref. 19).

4. History of the rise, progress, ravages, etc. of the blue cholera of India (editorial), Lancet, **1**:241, 1831–32.

With the recent outbreak of cholera in England, the weekly medical journals for 1831–32 are filled with notes, suggestions, and case reports of the disease. The present article of 43 pages gives an authoritative review of current knowledge. After a section on the origin and spread of epidemic cholera, there is a vivid description of the symptomatology, emphasizing the vomiting and purging followed by muscle cramps, anuria, pulselessness, and the bluish shrunken appearance of the skin. As to pathology, emphasis is placed on the huge quantity of turbid fluid in the bowel with the deposit of immense amounts of "an argilaceous substance." Changes in the mucous membrane are also mentioned. "Every character of the cholera authorizes us in concluding, that it arises from failure of a portion of the *nervous system* [Bell]." The writers did, however, feel that cholera was communicable and quote the conclusions of Drs. Russell and Barry: "1. That the poison of cholera may be conveyed and communicated by man to man. 2. That like the poison of typhus, it is regenerated in great quantities by those who suffer its influence." The arguments against contagion are next summarized, and then there is a discussion of the confused irrational ideas on treatment which existed at the time.[1] It is of interest to read the arguments whereby almost everyone agreed on bleeding as the backbone of therapy.

[1] "The whole of Europe is little more than a vast advertisement, in which are announced, in colossal letters, the admirable recipes for the preservation against and the cure for this disorder. Here cincture is advised, there an elixer is lauded, and everywhere we meet abundant proof, that if this is the age of intelligence, knavery is not less on the increase. But even among men of the utmost science and purest intentions, equal diversity of sentiment prevails. One advocates venesection, while another as energetically cries it down. Sedatives and stimulants, emetics, cathartics and specifics, each have their strenuous supporters. It is worthy of remembrance too that these discussions are the fiercest among the actual witnesses of the disease."

The article concludes with a discussion of sanitary measures, especially the quarantining of ships. There is no mention of contaminated water playing a part in contagion.

5. TARDIEU, A. Du choléra épidémique. Paris: Germer Baillière, 1849.

These interesting lectures make clear that there had been no advance in understanding of the disease since the studies made in the epidemic of 1832. The usual atmospheric and telluric causes are discussed, and, as to the contagion, "we have seen the most ingenious theories, the most appealing, even for keen minds fall before an examination of the facts" (p. 148). As to treatment, there are mentioned ipecac, Dover's powder, calomel, bismuth subnitrate, cubebs, ammonia, camphor, ether, oil of Cajeput, guaco, hashish, chloroform, as well as "the barbarous attempts at transfusion of blood or injection of water into the veins." One can see that intravenous therapy was making no progress.

The clinical descriptions are vivid, and there is an excellent section, as one might expect from the French, on the pathology of cholera.

6. Report of the [Boston] Committee of Internal Health on the Asiatic cholera. Boston: I. H. Eastburn, 1849.

This careful report was issued as a result of the Boston epidemic of cholera in 1849. The major part of the book consists of detailed autopsy reports of 33 cases. No general conclusions are drawn, but in most of the cases the fluid material in the bowel, and the changes in mucous membranes are stressed. "Examined by the microscope [the bowel contents] the flocculi, suspended in the rice-water fluid, invariably consisted of columnar epithelium. The epithelium-cells were so abundant and well-defined as to leave no doubt that they constituted nineteen-twentieths of the mass of the flocculi. If maceration, however, is the only cause of the separation of such an enormous quantity of epithelium, how shall we explain it in the situations where no increased amount of fluid has existed? The mucous surfaces of the vagina, and of the urinary bladder are invariably smeared with a thick, whitish, pasty or creamy secretion, which on microscopic examination is seen to consist entirely of detached epithelium cells" (p. 47). Under "Treatment," it is stated that narcotics "totally failed of any beneficial effect." The same was true of stimulants, emetics, calomel, quinia, tannic acid, ginger, cinnamon, and elaterium. Ether by inhalation relieved the cramps, but no one recovered who used it in this way. As to venous injection: "In one or two cases there was temporary relief, but death invariably followed shortly after. We were not inclined to make new trials of this mode of treatment after the first six weeks of the epidemic." The time was not yet ripe to use the method properly.

7. SNOW, J. On the mode of communication of cholera. London: J. Churchill, 1849.

Snow advanced the view that cholera was disseminated by something in the fecal discharges of patients which was later ingested by healthy people, who thus acquired the disease. He stressed contaminated water supplies as the chief source. This was not a "study-chair" piece of reasoning, but Snow was indefatigable in field work which seemed to support his views. However, he could not at first gain any attention. In the monumental *Report of Epidemic Cholera, Drawn up at the Desire of the Cholera Committee of the Royal College of*

Surgeons by William Baly and William W. Gull (London: John Churchill, 1854), for example, six theories of causation are mentioned as possibilities. "The *Third* theory—that propounded by Dr. Snow—gives a more specific form to the doctrine of contagion. It supposes that the poison of cholera is swallowed, and acts directly on the mucous membrane of the intestines, is at the same time reproduced in the intestinal canal, and passes out, much increased with the discharges; and that these discharges afterwards, in various ways, but chiefly by becoming mixed with the drinking water in rivers or wells, reach the alimentary canals of other persons, and produce the like disease in them" (p. 5). But after several hundred pages of analysis the experts reject Snow's views: "Of the six theories, then, that alone is supported by a large amount of evidence which regards the cause of Cholera as a matter increasing by some process, whether chemical or organic, in impure or damp air, and assumes that, although, of course, diffused with the air, it is also distributed and diffused by means of human intercourse" (p. 223). But Snow fought on, and on January 21, 1854, for example, he spoke at the Medical Society of London as reported in the Lancet (1:109, 1854). There he laid out a rational method of therapy, emphasizing "medicines which have the effect of destroying low forms of organized beings," to be given for their local effect and that "it was useless to attempt to bring the patient out of the state of collapse by stimulants and the application of heat, and they should be given watery drinks, unless in desperate cases, in which it might be desirable to inject into the blood vessels a weak saline solution, resembling that portion of the blood which has been lost." The reporter continues: "Indeed, if a layman had been present at the meeting, he might have witnessed a remarkable illustration in the way in which 'doctors differ,' and surely his faith in physic would have been scarcely increased in strength. Every speaker seemed to have an opinion of his own on the subject of the nature and cause of the disease. The treatment was no less contradictory." Snow continued, however, to collect evidence in support of his views and in 1855 published a "Second Edition, much Enlarged" of his book, which embodies the contents of numerous papers published in the contemporary medical journals. This second edition has been reproduced as a belated tribute to Dr. Snow, in facsimile (*Snow on Cholera, Being a Reprint of Two Papers by John Snow, M.D.* [New York: Commonwealth Fund, 1936]). Snow did for cholera what Budd did for typhoid fever, and his work is required reading for all interested in the subject.

8. PETTENKOFFER, M. Untersuchungen und Beobachtungen über die Verbreitungsart der Cholera nebst Betrachtungen über Massregeln derselben ein Halt zu thun. Munich: J. G. Cotta, 1855.

This book, the work of Pettenkoffer, the famous hygienist, is based on meticulous observations on the cholera outbreak in Bavaria in 1854–55. Pettenkoffer's work consisted of careful study of the details of the epidemic and is definitely modern in tone. By studying spot maps of the location of cases in Munich and elsewhere, he convinced himself that contaminated water had nothing to do with the spread of cholera. He was sure, however, that the disease was communicable; he believed that the agent was present in urine and stools, and he consequently developed an elaborate system of disinfection. By 1875, Pettenkoffer had not changed his views a great deal (*Künftige Prophylaxis gegen Cholera, besprochen von Max v. Pettenkoffer* [Munich: Th. Riedel, 1875]). He believed that there was a specific cholera germ which occurred principally in the stools but that its transmission was bound up with certain special conditions of the soil and ground water. He still laid stress on disinfection of stools and everything else the cholera patient came in contact with.

9. FAUVEL, A. Le choléra, étiologie et prophylaxie etc., exposé des travaux de la Conférence Sanitaire Internationale de Constantinople. Paris: J.-B. Baillière et fils, 1868.

By the time of the epidemic of 1865–66, opinion had swung strongly to the view that cholera was contagious. As to the nature of the "materies morbi" and the mode of its propagation, there was, however, great dispute. Innumerable books and articles were published, of which we may mention as examples that of Bernard M. Byrne (*An Essay To Prove the Contagious Character of the Malignant Cholera* [2d ed.; Philadelphia: Childs & Peterson, 1855]) as well as *A Communication from the City Physician on the Asiatic Cholera: Is It a Contagious Disease?* [City of Boston, City Doc. No. 21] [1866]). Of great importance, however, is the "Report to the International Sanitary Conference." This body, consisting of 21 physicians representing various nations, was sent by the French government to Egypt at the start of the epidemic of 1865 "to study the progress of the disease, its march and its special character, with a view to arresting its onward movement." This valuable document of some 100 pages takes up the subject of cholera as a series of 33 questions which are discussed, analyzed, and voted on by the members of the commission for acceptance or rejection. The commission accepted unanimously the proposition that cholera is propagated by man and is transmissible. They concluded, however, that the principal mode of transmission was by emanation into the air, although water and certain ingesta might also serve as vehicles for the introduction into the organism of the generative principle of cholera through the respiratory passages and very probably also the digestive canal. The germ, however, was mainly in the dejecta and took its origin probably in the digestive canal. They thought that the "germ" could be transmitted only during the first few days of the disease. Many other questions are discussed. This document is especially important as representing the carefully considered views of a large group of top-flight physicians and scientists. An abstract of the report appeared in the Boston Medical and Surgical Journal ("Report of the cholera conference at Constantinople," **75**:42, 1866), and an English translation of part of the full report appeared in Boston in 1867.[2]

10. HIRSCH, A. Handbuch der historisch-geographischen Pathologie: Indische Cholera, **1**:279. 2d ed. Stuttgart: Ferdinand Enke, 1881. (HIRSCH, A., Handbook of Geographical and Historical Pathology, English translation by Charles Creighton, M.D., **1**:394. London: New Sydenham Society, 1883.)

Much of the literature on cholera is concerned with the epidemiology and with descriptions of outbreaks. Hirsch's book is the classical storehouse of informa-

---

[2] *Report to the International Sanitary Conference, of a Commission from That Body, to Which Were Referred the Questions Relative to the Origin, Endemicity, Transmissibility, and Propagation of Asiatic Cholera*, translated by Samuel L. Abbot, M.D. (Boston: Alfred Mudge & Son, 1867).

tion to date. Various epidemics all over the world are listed and documented. For more recent lists of outbreaks see Carl Mense, *Handbuch der Tropenkrankheiten* (2d ed.; Leipzig: Barth, 1914), **3**:243 ff.; H. Harold Scott, *A History of Tropical Medicine* (Baltimore: Williams & Wilkins Co., 1939), **2**:663 ff.; and Sir Leonard Rogers, *Bowel Disease in the Tropics* (London: Henry Frowde, 1921), chap. i, pp. 1 ff. C. Macnamara's *A History of Asiatic Cholera* (London: Macmillan & Co., 1876) may also be consulted.

11. Conferenz zur Erörterung der Cholerafrage. Verhandelt Berlin, im Reichsgesundheitsamt, am 26 Juli 1884. Abends 6 Uhr, Berl. klin. Wchnschr., **21**:477, 493, 1884. (English translation of Koch's remarks, Brit. M.J., **2**:403, 453, 1884.)

Koch tells how he went to Egypt to study cholera. After doing many autopsies, he convinced himself that the only plausible place to seek the germ was in the intestines. The changes varied from very slight lesions to reddening and swelling of Peyer's patches or even to a necrosis of the mucosa with a diphtheritic covering. On sections it was found that the space between the epithelium and the basement membrane of the glands was crowded with numerous comma-shaped bacilli. These were also found in the intestinal contents. The organisms and their cultural characteristics are described in detail. Koch found that the organism was short-lived and did not survive when dried on clothes or in soil. He found the comma bacillus in the dejecta of numerous cholera cases in almost pure culture. "In accordance with the cholera-material that I have so far examined, I think I can now assert that comma-bacilli are never found absent in cases of cholera; they are something that is specific to cholera." In patients with other diseases the comma bacilli were never found, nor were they obtained from two men who had had cholera, respectively, six weeks and eight days previously. Koch recognized, however, that further proof of the causal role of the bacillus was necessary, and he fed numerous small animals with fresh dejecta and with cultures. All remained well. He observed, however, that several laundresses who handled cholera linen came down with the disease; this he accepted as strong evidence. "If, therefore, an infection can be brought about by cholera-linen, then, as the comma-bacilli are the only micro-organisms in question, it can only be brought about by them." He asked how an organism confined to the intestine can make a person so ill and suggested that the germs produce soluble absorbable toxins. He recovered comma bacilli from a large tank in which a number of people did their washing and from which they also drank the water. He thought water and moist food the commonest ways of infection; dried material was a less likely source. Koch pointed out that the same person was rarely affected twice in the same epidemic; he concluded, therefore, that the disease was followed by a temporary immunity. Finally, he hoped that the discovery of the cholera bacillus would be of use in diagnosis and therapy.

The article, like Koch's work on the tubercle bacillus, seems complete and unassailable; it should be carefully studied by all interested in the subject.

In another paper ("I. Über die Cholerabacterien," Deutsche med. Wchnschr., **10**:725, 1884) Koch discussed the subject further and answered certain objections made by others. He did not mention dehydration and salt loss as a feature of this disease.

Koch went to India and confirmed the results he had obtained in Egypt.

As with every important bacteriological discovery, there were some who doubted and some who obtained contradictory results. In another communication ("Further researches on cholera," Brit. M.J., 1:6, 1886) Koch systematically answered (and demolished) his opponents. He also discussed animal experiments, and he thought that he had produced cholera in guinea pigs.

12. PFEIFFER, R. Untersuchungen über das Choleragift, Ztschr. f. Hyg. u. Infectionskr., 11:393, 1892.

The cholera bacillus was discovered during the lush flourishing of the bacteriological era. Everyone looked to immunological methods of diagnosis, protection, and therapy. There was an immediate debate as to whether cholera bacilli remained in the intestine and secreted a soluble exotoxin or whether, in process of disintegration, they yielded poisonous endotoxin. Pfeiffer made pioneer experiments to try to answer this problem; he injected small animals with broth cultures, with bacteria-free filtrates, and with living and dead bacteria. "In young aerobic cholera cultures there is a specific poison which displays extraordinary intense toxic action. This primary cholera poison is very closely related to the bacterial bodies and is perhaps an integral part of them." Pfeiffer later ("Studien zur Choleraätiologie," Ztschr. f. Hyg. u. Infectionskr., 16:268, 1894) elaborated these ideas. He produced immune sera of which "very small amounts are adequate to confer on guinea pigs pronounced protection against intraperitoneal injection of cholera virus." Issaeff ("Untersuchungen über die künstliche Immunität gegen Cholera," Ztschr. f. Hyg. u. Infectionskr., 16:287, 1894) confirmed Pfeiffer's work and showed that serum of human convalescents from cholera had high protective qualities against the bacteria but not against the endotoxins of the vibrios.

13. WASSERMANN, A. Untersuchungen über Immunität gegen Cholera asiatica, Ztschr. f. Hyg. u. Infectionskr., 14:35, 1893.

Although empirical attempts at human immunization against cholera had already been made by Ferrán (Ref. 16), it remained for the German workers to lay the experimental background. In the present paper the writer showed that "it is definitely possible to protect guinea pigs against the intraperitoneal infection with living cholera bacilli. In order to achieve this, one must inject cholera vibrios or their body substance in such doses that a mild specific illness, a general reaction, follows." R. Pfeiffer and A. Wassermann ("Untersuchungen über das Wesen der Choleraimmunität," Ztschr. f. Hyg. u. Infectionskr., 14:46, 1893) continued this work and emphasized the need of a clear experimental foundation before human beings were treated.

14. KOCH, R. Wasserfiltration und Cholera, Ztschr. f. Hyg. u. Infectionskr., 14:393, 1893.

In 1892 occurred the famous cholera epidemic affecting especially Hamburg, which was supplied with unfiltered water from the River Elbe, whereas the adjacent cities of Altona and Wandsbeck, which differed only in having a filtered water supply, had practically no cases of the disease. Koch discusses this situation in detail and draws the inevitable conclusions as to the epidemiology of cholera. Koch pursues the matter further ("Die Cholera in Deutschland während des Winters 1892 bis 1893," Ztschr. f. Hyg. u. Infectionskr., 15:89, 1893) in a long and interesting article.

15. PFEIFFER, R., and ISSAEFF. Über die specifische Bedeutung der Choleraimmunität, Ztschr. f. Hyg. u. Infectionskr., **17**:355, 1894.

This is the classical paper in which was described what was later known in immunology as the "Pfeiffer phenomenon." The authors showed that cholera vibrios injected into the peritoneum of an immune guinea pig underwent rapid dissolution; if another organism was injected or if the guinea pig was non-immune, the injected bacteria were unaffected. Pfeiffer, therefore, made an important contribution to the knowledge of cholera and discovered a general immunological principle as well. The protection turned out to be purely anti-bacterial, as the animals were just as sensitive to cholera "toxin." Pfeiffer later ("Weitere Untersuchungen über Wesen der Choleraimmunität und über specifisch bactericide Processe," Ztschr. f. Hyg. u. Infectionskr., **18**:1, 1894) restated his principle that "serum of animals which are actively immunized against cholera only shows a specfic action against the vibrios, whereas against other bacteria it behaves no differently than the serum of normal animals." In this elaborate paper he gave the details of further studies with vibrios and "toxin" in rabbits and guinea pigs. Pfeiffer assumed that his reaction could take place only in the animal body, but Metchnikoff (E. Metchnikoff, "Études sur l'immunité: sixième mémoire: Sur la destruction extracellulaire des bactères dans organisme," Ann. Inst. Pasteur, **9**:369, 1895) soon demonstrated extracellular lysis in hanging-drop preparations.

16. HAFFKINE, W. M. Anti-cholera inoculation: report to the Government of India. Calcutta: Thacker & Spink, 1895. See also HAFFKINE, W. M., Protective inoculation against cholera. London: W. Thacker & Co., 1913.

Ferrán in 1885 (J. Ferrán, "Nota sobre una vacuna quinca contra el cólera asiático," Rec. cien. méd., Barcelona, **11**:515, 1885) was apparently the first worker who claimed to produce immunity against cholera by subcutaneous injection of cholera bacilli. In another note ("Sur la prophylaxie du choléra au moyen d'injections hypodermiques de cultures pures du bacille-virgule," Compt. rend. Acad. d. sc., **101**:147, 1885) Ferrán described his method, which consisted simply of subcutaneous injections at 5-day intervals of three doses of a living broth culture of the bacilli. "I affirm to the Academy that the manner of abruptly interrupting the curve of mortality of an epidemic of cholera has today been accomplished by science." Ferrán did not, however, give any actual protocols, and his work seems to have been questioned at the time. A little later W. M. Haffkine ("Le Choléra asiatique chez le cobaye," Compt. rend. Soc. de biol., **44**:635, 1892) succeeded with injections of attenuated live cholera bacilli in rendering guinea pigs immune. "An animal having been vaccinated first with attenuated and then with 'exalted' virus is protected against every infection with cholera, no matter how one tries to produce it." He soon ("Le Choléra asiatique chez le lapin et chez le pigeon," *ibid.*, p. 671) reported the same findings with rabbits, and finally he showed that man could be safely injected with living cholera bacilli ("Inoculations de vaccines anticholériques à l'homme," *ibid.*, p. 740). E. H. Hankin ("Remarks on Haffkine's method of protective inoculation against cholera," Brit. M.J., **2**:569, 1892) submitted himself to inoculation by Haffkine and describes his own febrile and local reactions: "The evidence shows that M. Haffkine's method of inoculation is not attended by any grave disturbance of health, and that it can be practiced on human beings with perfect safety." A little later A. E. Wright and D. Bruce ("On Haffkine's method of vaccination against asiatic cholera," Brit. M.J., 1:227, 1893) described in detail the method of preparing the attenuated form of vaccine by treatment with phenol and the exalted form by guinea-pig passage. Their carbolized vaccine contained no live bacilli. The seat of election is injection under the skin of the flank, the first (attenuated) vaccine being given 3–5 days before the second (exalted) preparation.

Haffkine later went to India, where he used his method extensively under the sponsorship of the British and wrote his elaborate report to the government. Haffkine believed that the vaccine was effective, although the detailed figures are not very impressive. He stated very conservatively, however: "The results obtained seem to indicate that in the inoculation we possess a means of effectively combating cholera epidemics. I am of the opinion that this experimental stage is not yet in the advanced condition to be completely closed" (p. 47).

W. Kolle ("Zur activen Immunisierung des Menschen gegen Cholera," Centralbl. f. Bakt., 19:97, 1896) was another pioneer in anticholera immunization. In this important article he gives a valuable review of the theoretical basis for anticholera vaccination and quotes the fundamental experiments on which this is based. In practice he injected, first, chloroform-killed bacteria and 5 and 10 days later live virulent vibrios. Later he seems to have changed the vaccine to a culture killed by heating to 58° C. for 1 hour and preserved with 0.5 per cent phenol (P. Krause and T. Rumpf, in Mense, C., Handbuch der Tropenkrankheiten [2d ed.; Leipzig: J. A. Barth, 1914], 3:299). This is essentially the type of vaccine used at present by the United States Army.

M. L. Ahuja and Gurkirpal Singh ("Observations on cholera vaccine," Indian J.M. Research, 36:1, 1948) give experimental support for the use of a mixture of Inaba and Ogawa strains in preparing the vaccine.

The results of anticholera inoculation have, however, been variously judged. Major Greenwood and G. Udney Yule ("The statistics of antityphoid and anticholera inoculations, and the interpretation of such statistics in general," Proc. Roy. Soc. Med., Sec. Epidemiol. & State Med., 8:113, 1915), for example, who are expert statisticians, give a careful mathematical analysis of published results. While somewhat reserved, Major Greenwood says in conclusion that "so far as the data went, the case in favour of anti-cholera inoculation seemed to them strong."

R. Adiseshan, C. G. Pandit, and K. V. Venkatraman ("Statistical evaluation of anti-cholera inoculation as a personal prophylactic against cholera and its efficiency in the prevention and control of cholera epidemics," Indian J.M. Research, 35:131, 1947) found that the case incidence in 709,977 vaccinated persons was 1.57 per cent; in 2,119,568 unvaccinated it was 16.20 per cent. They thought that protection lasted for a minimum period of 6 months. The vaccine contained both Inaba and Ogawa subtypes of Vibrio comma and was given in one dose of 8,000,000 organisms. Quite recently L. Kant ("An assessment of the value of cholera vaccine as used in a single dose mass inoculation [a field observation]," J. Trop. Med., 54:223, 1951), in an observation covering 30,683 persons in India, reaffirmed the protective action of the vaccine.

17. GOTSCHLICH, F. Über Cholera und choleraähnliche Vibrionen unter den aus Mekka zurückkehrenden Pilgern, Ztschr. f. Hyg. u. Infectionskr., **53**:281, 1906.

Sooner or later it was inevitable that vibrios resembling those specific for cholera would be found. Gotschlich, working at the quarantine station at El Tor, examined the intestinal content of 107 pilgrims dead of various forms of dysentery or colitis, but not of cholera, in which he found vibrios in 38 cases. Many of these strains were agglutinated in high titer in anticholera sera, but they were actively hemolytic and differed in certain other respects from true cholera vibrios. The problem is fully discussed by Linton (Ref. 22). At any rate, it is established that vibrios resembling those of cholera but harmless or causing other bowel disturbances exist not infrequently.

18. KOLLE, W. Zur Frage der Serumtherapie der Cholera asiatica, Deutsche med. Wchnschr., **35**: 2046, 1909.

Since serum therapy has in the end been abandoned in cholera, we shall not attempt any lengthy bibliography. However, serum therapy had an active vogue at the turn of the century, and so it should not be entirely ignored. Kolle's paper is a summary of the whole situation by an authority in the field. He points out that the great difficulty is that cholera patients die of "intoxication" and not of bacterial invasion, whereas immune serum is essentially antibacterial. He reports a death rate of 37.5 per cent in serum-treated cases of severe cholera and in general is conservative in his predictions of the future of cholera immunotherapy.

19. ROGERS, L. The treatment of cholera by injections of hypertonic saline solutions with a simple and rapid method of intraabdominal administration, Philippine J. Sc., **4**:99, 1909.

We have already reviewed the early efforts at intravenous saline therapy in cholera (Ref. 3). Even in modern times it was variously judged. Rogers (*Recent Advances in Tropical Medicine* [2d ed.; Philadelphia: P. Blakiston's Sons, 1929], p. 192) cites death rates of from 59 to 70 per cent. Henry J. Nichols and Vernon L. Andrews ("The treatment of Asiatic cholera during the recent epidemic," Philippine J. Sc., **4**:81, 1909), on the other hand, felt that they had reduced the death rate to 20–40 per cent by intravenous infusions of 0.85 per cent salt solution. Rogers, however, not having had good final results with isotonic saline, concluded that salt was lost out of proportion to fluid and therefore doubled the strength of his solution. "On rapidly increasing the strength to double that formerly used (2 drachms of sodium chloride to the pint, or 1.35 per cent to which 3 grams of calcium chloride may be added) a most gratifying degree of success was obtained."

The mortality was reduced from 61 to 32.5 per cent. He calculated the amount of solution to be given by "estimating the percentages of serum and corpuscles with the haemocrite." Rogers later ("A simple curative treatment of cholera," Brit. M.J., **2**:835, 1910) discussed the treatment further and added to the saline injections internal administration of potassium permanganate to destroy "the specific toxins within the alimentary tract." He felt that he had increased the recovery rate seven fold. The idea of using salt solution more concentrated than isotonic saline was not, however, new when Rogers applied it.

Much earlier, G. Gaertner and A. Beck ("Über den Einfluss der intravenösen Kochsalzeinspritzung auf die Resorption von Flussigkeiten," Wien. klin. Wchnschr., **6**:563, 1893) laid down the principles of the subject and advocated concentrated salt solution in cholera as rational to check the immense transudation of fluid into the bowel. A. W. Sellards ("Tolerance for alkalies in asiatic cholera," Philippine J. Sc., **5**:363, 1910) emphasized the acidosis (increased tolerance for alkali) in cholera patients, especially those who were anuric, and he pushed the intravenous injection of solutions of sodium bicarbonate with what he thought were good therapeutic results. In the light of modern studies of electrolytes and fluid balance, it is difficult to evaluate this procedure. Yet up to the present time intravenous fluids in some form remain the backbone of the treatment of cholera.

20. GOODPASTURE, E. W. Histopathology of the intestine in cholera, Philippine J. Sc., **22**:413, 1923.

Goodpasture made definitive studies of the histology of the intestine in cholera. He found that one must have absolutely fresh material to avoid rapid post-mortem changes. He concluded that desquamation of epithelium was, for the most part, a post-mortem change but that ante-mortem desquamation might occur, recognizable at autopsy by the presence of ulcers with acute inflammatory exudate. "Anatomical evidence indicates that the great mass of vibrios is confined to the intestinal lumen, and, if toxic substances are formed there directly or indirectly as a result of their growth, they are absorbed early in the disease through an anatomically intact mucosa."

21. [COUVY]. Rapport sur les porteurs de germes de choléra, Bull. mensuel, Office internat. d'hyg. publique, Paris, **25**:1149, 1933.

W. Kolle first showed years ago ("Über die Dauer des Vorkommens von Choleravibrionen in den Dejecten von Cholerareconvalescenten," Ztschr. f. Hyg. u. Infectionskr., **18**:42, 1894) with daily cultures in 50 convalescents that the vibrios in all but 1 case disappeared in from 3 to 28 days.

Couvy recognized the discharge of cholera vibrios by those in the incubation period or during convalescence but doubted the occurrence of chronic "healthy" carriers. Probably some of those incriminated did not carry true pathogenic cholera vibrios. At any rate, the "chronic carrier" seems to play an insignificant part in the epidemiology of the disease. This comprehensive report includes elaborate statistics from the literature. The rarity of the persistence of the vibrios in convalescents is also brought out by the report of Y. Y. Ying ("The persistence of vibrios in cholera patients," Chinese M.J., **58**:595, 1940), who found in 200 cases of proved cholera that "a large proportion of cases (76.5 per cent) show positive stool cultures during the first week followed by a rapid decline thereafter, being 21.5 per cent for the second, 1.5 per cent for the third, and 0.5 per cent for the fourth week. Not a single case showed a positive culture after the fourth week."

22. LINTON, R. W. The chemistry and serology of the vibrios, Bact. Rev., **4**:261, 1940.

As is usually the case, the simple ideas of the early investigators in bacteriology have been displaced by highly complicated chemical and physical studies. It is outside the scope of this bibliography to review the subject in detail, but this comprehensive summary goes into the chemical structure of vibrios, their growth products, their metabolism and chemical classification, their antigenic structure, etc. The problems raised years ago by Pfeiffer (Ref. 15) and others are not yet fully solved.

23. FELSENFELD, O., DADTRADAY, W. S., SACHEKO, J. I., THORN, W., and NORSEN, J. In vitro sensitivity of recently isolated cholera vibrios to 10 antibiotics, Proc. Soc. Exper. Biol. & Med., **77**:287, 1951. With the advent of the newer antibiotics, it was inevitable that they should be tried against cholera. The present writers tested the action of 10 commonly used antibiotics against 53 recently isolated strains of V. comma. "The results showed a wide variation in susceptibility to these drugs according to the geographical origin of the vibrios." In a preliminary trial S. C. Seal, S. C. Ghosal, and M. M. Ghosh ("A preliminary trial of aureomycin [I. V.] in the treatment of cholera," Indian M. Gaz., **86**:287, 1951) found that in clinical use "no therapeutic advantage has been demonstrated." A. Das, S. Ghosal, S. K. Gupta, and R. N. Chandhuri ("Terramycin in cholera," Indian M. Gaz., **86**:436, 1951), in a somewhat more extensive trial, found also that oxytetracycline (terramycin) made no significant difference in the effects of treatment. Similar results were obtained by N. R. Koner and A. N. Sengupta ("Terramycin in cholera," Indian M. Gaz., **83**:469, 1951), although they found that the first negative report of stool culture had been obtained earlier in oxytetracycline-treated cases. On the other hand, E. Olejnik and S. Davidovitch ("Action of terramycin and chloromycetin on cholera vibrio in mice," Nature, London, **168**:654, 1951) found that mice inoculated intraperitoneally with V. comma could be saved by both oxytetracycline and chloramphenicol, provided that the drug was given within 5 hours after infection. S. C. Lahin ("Chemotherapy in cholera," Brit. M.J., **1**:500, 1951) tried sulfaguanidine and other sulfonamides in cholera without reducing the mortality rate.

The subject of antibiotics in cholera is treated editorially in the Journal of the Indian Medical Association (**22**:291, 1953), and the writer concludes: "The failure of these vibriocidal drugs once more emphasizes the immense importance both of prophylaxis and of the early restoration of body fluids on sound biochemical principles."

Apparently cholera comes like a storm and is quickly over, and the main therapeutic measure remains the restoration of fluid and salts.

24. AHUJA, M. L., KRISHNAN, K. V., PANDIT, S. R., and VENKATRA-MAN, K. V. Laboratory diagnosis of cholera, Indian J.M. Research, **39**:135, 1951.
Koch (Ref. 11) laid the foundation of laboratory diagnosis of cholera. The present note is an up-to-date statement of the best bacteriological procedure for isolating and identifying the cholera vibrio.

BACILLARY DYSENTERY

BACILLARY DYSENTERY

THE history of dysentery is obscured by the confusion which existed between the bacillary and amebic types before the recognition of the causal agents. Various observers noted, however, with keen clinical insight that the types of dysentery seen in the tropics were often associated with liver abscess, whereas such a lesion was conspicuously absent in the dysenteries of temperate climates. However, one is not certain, with many of the early articles, whether the writer was dealing with amebic or bacillary dysentery.

The history of the subject is summarized by Leonard Rogers (*Dysenteries: Their Differentiation and Treatment* [London: Oxford University Press, 1913]) and by Philip Manson-Bahr (*The Dysenteric Disorders* [2d ed.; Baltimore: Williams & Wilkins Co., 1943]). The monograph by W. C. Davison ("A bacteriological and clinical consideration of bacillary dysentery in adults and children," Medicine, **1**:389, 1922) is a storehouse of information on the subject, with a definitive bibliography to date of over five hundred titles. Hirsch (Ref. 5) gives a full account of the older epidemics everywhere, whereas outbreaks in Great Britain are dealt with by Charles Creighton (*A History of Epidemics in Britain* [Cambridge: Cambridge University Press, 1894], **2**:747).

The article by F. S. Cheever, "Bacillary dysentery and the Shigella," in R. J. Dubos, *Bacterial and Mycotic Infections of Man* (2d ed.; Philadelphia: J. B. Lippincott Co., 1952), page 437, is specially strong on the bacteriological intricacies of the subject; an authoritative modern discussion of the whole problem is to be found in G. S. Wilson and A. A. Miles in Topley and Wilson's *Principles of Bacteriology and Immunity* (4th ed.; Baltimore: Williams & Wilkins Co., 1955), **2**:1760.

1. ABERCROMBIE, John. Pathological practical researches on diseases of the stomach, the intestinal canal, the liver, and other viscera of the abdomen. Philadelphia: Carey & Lea, 1830.[1]

This book contains Abercrombie's justly famous description of acute dysentery: "There is generally pain in the abdomen, in some cases permanent, in others occurring in paroxysms of tormina; and it is usually accompanied by considerable tenderness when rather severe pressure is made, but distinct from the acute sensibility which accompanies inflammation of the peritoneum. There is more or less irritability of the bowels, sometimes in the form of diarrhoea, with copious stools, and sometimes of painful tenesmus with frequent scanty discharges of bloody mucus. There is generally some degree of fever. . . . The evacuations vary exceedingly in their character; consisting in some cases, of small quantities of bloody mucus or almost pure blood" (p. 242). The general description is supported by autopsy reports, for example: "The whole tract of the colon appeared moderately and uniformly distended. . . . Internally, it showed most extensive disease of the mucous membrane. This consisted of portions of the membrane, of various forms and degrees of extent, being of a fungous appearance and bright red colour, and sensibly elevated above the

[1] The English edition (1827) was not available to us.

level of the more healthy portions that were interposed between them. . . .
The small intestine and all the other parts were entirely healthy" (p. 251).
There are numerous pathological reports which shade off into other conditions,
but there is no doubt that Abercrombie reported many cases of true dysentery.

2. BALY, William. Gulstonian lectures [on dysentery], London M. Gaz.,
   N.S. 4:441, 485, 529, 1847.

It is difficult to select proper examples of bacillary dysentery from early nine-
teenth-century descriptions of dysentery, and many justly famous accounts may
have dealt largely with the amebic form. Epidemics of non-tropical dysentery
were most frequent in armies, jails, and asylums, and Baly's account is based
on the disease as seen in "the great Government Prison of Milbank." The paper
opens with a discussion of the pathology, which pretty clearly deals with the
bacillary and not the amebic type. Baly describes lesions from cases of three
degrees of severity. "Dysentery, in its most severe degree, is frequently fatal
in a very few days. The inflammation affecting a large extent of the mucous
membrane [of the colon] reduces it with extreme rapidity to the state of
sphacelus." Baly reviews with great care the work of others. "When the close
relation subsisting between dysentery and suppurative disease of the liver in
India is considered, it cannot but appear remarkable that, amongst the many
hundreds of cases of dysentery which have occurred in the Milbank prison
during the last seven years, not one has been complicated with hepatic abscess."
Baly was not, of course, dealing with amebic dysentery. There follows an excellent clinical description, in which, however, the writer leans heavily on Sydenham. Baly was totally at sea as to the cause of the disease. The jail physicians
concluded that it was due to a "local noxious influence," and with this Baly
agreed: "Here, as in other instances where dysentery is endemic in prisons,
workhouses, or lunatic asylums, the cause really producing it is, I believe, a
malaria rising from the surface of the ground around the building. There are
other influences from which dysentery might be supposed to arise, namely, diet,
the water used as drink, defective ventilation, and defective sewage. None of
these, however, can have been the apparent cause of the disease in the Peni-
tentiary." The reasons for this view are then gone into at length and show how
a strong case can be erroneously built up. The lectures conclude with remarks
on treatment. Baly relied mainly on "bloodletting, the administration of calomel
with opium, and gentle aperients."

Such, then, was the state of knowledge on dysentery about a hundred years
ago.

3. WOODWARD, Joseph Janvier. Outlines of the chief camp diseases of the
   United States armies as observed during the present war. Philadelphia:
   J. B. Lippincott & Co., 1863.

This important book on "camp disease" in the Civil War is also of interest as
indicating the general philosophy of epidemic disorders at the time. Thus
Woodward divides disease into "1. Miasmatic diseases. 2. Enthetic diseases.
3. Dietic diseases." Most sickness which we now know to be infectious is placed
in the miasmatic group. "The word miasmatic is, therefore, used in its original
broad sense, to include all disease due to the influence of miasms, whether those
arising from telluric sources, such as vegetable decomposition (koino-miasmata)

or those produced by the decomposition of matters derived from the human body (idio-miasmata)." Further, under conditions determining the character of camp diseases, there are sections on "Malarial Influences," "Crowd Poisoning," and "The Scorbutic Taint." In spite of these primitive ideas on communicable disease, Woodward's objective descriptions are excellent. Camp diarrhea is divided into simple diarrhea, acute enteritis, and acute dysentery, mainly, it would seem, on a basis of severity of symptoms. But even very acute cases seemed less severe; "the malignant dysentery of European armies had not yet made its appearance among our troops." "Any of the causes capable of producing acute enteritis may give rise to dysentery with those who are susceptible. Indigestible food, unhealthy water, exposure to heat, sleeping on damp ground, changes of temperature, and other causes . . . may give rise to this disorder. Malarial influence is a potent predisposing cause . . . a scorbutic habit . . . is also an important predisposing cause" (p. 223). An excellent description of the clinical features and of the pathological changes follows. No liver abscesses were encountered. Treatment began with a purge, followed by Dover's powder and astringents, such as acetate of lead and sulfate of copper if simple treatment did not suffice. A limited plain diet is emphasized, such as boiled milk with rice, beef essence, and mucilaginous or acidulated drinks. "There can be no doubt, however, that in moderate doses ipecuanha is a valuable remedy in the early stages of the disease, both from its action upon the skin and from the astringent effect upon the bowels."

We can see, then, how slowly progress was being made in both the understanding and the treatment of dysentery. Woodward later contributed a monumental volume on the *Alvine Fluxes* to the "Medical and Surgical History of the War of the Rebellion (1861–'65), Part II, Vol. I, being the second medical volume." This tremendous folio of nearly nine hundred pages deals in intimate detail with every phase of the subject—statistical, clinical, pathological, and epidemiological. "These disorders occurred with more frequency and produced more sickness and mortality than any other form of disease. . . . Soon no army could move without leaving behind it a host of the victims. They crowded the ambulance trains, the railroad cars, the steamboats. In the general hospitals they were often more numerous than the sick from all other diseases, and rivalled the wounded in multitude." There was a total of 1,739,135 cases of dysentery during the war, with 44,558 deaths. With regard to the question "Is dysentery contagious?" Woodward (p. 646) gives a masterful analysis of the literature and the contradictory opinions of others. "For myself, I strongly incline to adopt the view of the contagion of the stools for at least a certain class of dysenteric cases, yet I frankly admit the recorded evidence on this head is by no means so conclusive as that which we possess with regard to typhoid fever." The volume concludes with a long section on therapy, in which the merits of every conceivable drug and agent are discussed.

4. NIEMEYER, Felix. Lehrbuch der speciellen Pathologie und Therapie, chap. xiv, p. 747, article "Dysentery." 7th ed. Berlin: August Hirschwald, 1868.

Bitter arguments went on for years as to whether dysentery was contagious, and "evidence" pro and con was assembled. Niemeyer seems to have been one of the first, however, to make a clear, modern, precise statement in favor of contagion. "Dysentery is an infectious disease; it is to be distinguished from typhoid and other infectious diseases, however, by the fact that the dysentery poison produces demonstrable pathological changes only in the large bowel. . . . The dysentery poison has, to be sure, not been directly demonstrated to be an organic living substance, but arguments already discussed in connection with Typhoid and Cholera influence us to regard dysentery also as an infection of the body by a specific species of lower vegetable organism and to speak of a 'dysentery germ' just as we have talked of a 'typhoid germ' and a 'cholera germ.' The dysentery germ grows, thrives, and multiplies outside of the human body, and persons exposed to its location are in danger of sickening with dysentery. Favorable conditions for growth and multiplication of the dysentery germ . . . are present in tropical and subtropical regions; there dysentery rages over large areas. . . . It appears that the dysentery germ under favorable conditions always reproduces itself in the body of an infected individual, and that the dejections of those ill with dysentery contain the contagion or a precursor of it, for while not proved it is more than probable that lavatories, bedpans, and klysters which dysentery patients have used can transmit the disease to healthy contacts." Cold, wet, and eating unripe fruit are merely incidents which may predispose to infection with the specific germ which is the only direct cause.

5. HIRSCH, August. Handbuch der historisch-geographischen Pathologie, **3**:195. 2d ed. Stuttgart: Ferdinand Enke, 1883.

This article on dysentery contains first a historical outline and next a comprehensive summary of the geography of the disease, both heavily documented. There then follows an elaborate enumeration of epidemics and, finally, a discussion of the influence of diet, temperature, etc. Hirsch, even as late as 1886, is still conservative about a bacterial cause, but the article is nonetheless of great value.

6. CHANTEMESSE and WIDAL, F. Le Microbe de la dysentérie épidémique, Semaine méd., **8**:153, 1888.

Among the early claims for isolation of the microbe of dysentery, the most plausible is that of Chantemesse and Widal. Although the description is not complete, all the features mentioned are compatible with dysentery bacilli. "The presence of the bacillus which we describe in the intestinal wall, the mesenteric glands, and the deep organs of a man dead of an acute relapse of dysentery, the finding of it in the stools of five patients with dysentery, its absence in healthy man, the lesions which it gives rise to in the intestines and viscera of guinea pigs, plead in favor of its specificity."

Years later, during the course of a polemic on priority of discovery of dysentery bacilli which was waged between Shiga and Kruse, Chantemesse and Widal ("Ueber die Priorität der Entdeckung des Ruhrbacillus," Deutsche med. Wchnschr., **29**:204, 1903) again took up the cudgels and claimed priority for themselves. While it is highly likely that they dealt with dysentery bacilli, an impartial reader must admit that their evidence was not fully conclusive.

7. SHIGA, Kiyoshi. Ueber den Erreger der Dysenterie in Japan, Centralbl. f. Bakt., **23**:599, 1898.

The seriousness of the dysentery problem in Japan, where there were ninety thousand cases with twenty thousand deaths in 6 months, impelled Shiga to look for the causal agent. Since animals were resistant to the production of dysentery, Shiga sought an organism in the dejecta of patients which would be agglutinated by their blood serum similarly to the Widal test in typhoid fever. He reports finding in the stools and internal organs of thirty-six cases of dysentery an organism which was agglutinable by the serum of dysentery patients. "The bacillus is short, rounded at both ends and sluggishly motile. Morphologically it resembles the typhoid bacillus and is gram negative." He then describes cultural reactions on various media and points out that dextrose was not fermented. The bacillus was uniformly found in the dejecta of thirty-four patients and in the bowel wall of two men dead of dysentery. He was unable to obtain the organism from healthy people or from those with other diseases. The agglutinative reaction was also found to be specific. Infiltration followed by suppuration resulted from subcutaneous injection of cultures into guinea pigs. Introduction of culture into the stomach of young dogs or cats was followed in 1 or 2 days by slimy stools. Subcutaneous injection into man of killed culture produced a general febrile reaction, with painful induration at the site of inoculation, and the serum developed agglutinins within 10 days. "From the above-mentioned grounds one must assume that this bacillus has the most intimate connection with dysentery, and, indeed, I feel that one may regard this bacillus as the cause of dysentery."

In another more detailed paper (K. Shiga, "Ueber der Dysenterie bacillus [Bacillus dysenteriae]," Centralbl. f. Bakt., **24**:817, 870, 913, 1898) Shiga opens with an analysis of previous attempts to isolate a living agent from cases of dysentery. He thought it probable that amebae "played a role" in tropical dysentery but questioned the significance of the numerous claims that had been made for one or another bacterium. He then describes in great detail the morphological and cultural characters already mentioned in the first paper. He laid great stress on the specific agglutination test. From the bodies of two patients dead of dysentery the bacilli were found in large numbers in the wall of the bowel, which was the seat of an acute process. Where the process was old, there were few colonies of dysentery bacilli but many of *B. coli* and strepococci. Small animals receiving large subcutaneous doses of dysentery bacilli died in a few days; a dog fed an entire agar slant of culture developed diarrhea with recovery of dysentery bacilli and died in 5 days. Chickens and pigeons seemed unaffected by injection or feeding of bacilli. Small animals who received injections of killed dysentery bacilli developed specific agglutinins in their blood; Shiga himself, after an injection of one-twelfth of an agar slant of heat-killed bacilli, developed chills and fever and a painful induration at the site of inoculation, which he concluded was due to toxin produced by the bacilli, since, on incision, no organisms were recovered. He predicted that protection would be achieved by the development of proper sera.

As in the history of so many infectious diseases, the worker who first isolated the correct causal organism "skimmed the cream" and left relatively little for his successors to prove.

8. FLEXNER, Simon. On the etiology of tropical dysentery, Philadelphia M.J., **6**:414, 1900; also in Bull. Johns Hopkins Hosp., **11**:231, 1900.

In this masterly lecture Flexner first reviews the confused medley of etiological claims—amebic and bacterial—of the cause of severe dysentery. Unfortunately, the observations to which he refers so freely are undocumented. Next come clinical and pathological descriptions of various types of dysentery; the pathological histology of the acute non-amebic disease is precisely delineated. Flexner worked in the Philippine Islands and dealt with soldiers in the American army of occupation. Stool cultures disclosed two bacillary types; Type I corresponded in all its features with the bacillus of Shiga (Ref. 7). "That the bacillus is identical with the organism obtained by Shiga in the epidemic of dysentery which prevailed in Japan there can be no reasonable doubt." Flexner also found often, as the predominating organism, one whose "properties vary somewhat, but agree well with those of group B coli communis." Agglutination tests and animal inoculations with the Type I organism correspond pretty well with those described by Shiga, including the fact that the dead cultures were "toxic." As to specific serotherapy, Flexner was optimistic but reported no details. He concluded: "It is only natural to ask whether the foregoing considerations justify a belief in a specific organism of dysentery. My own sense is against that belief although it must be conceded that the varieties of the disease are fewer than the clinical and pathological-anatomical conceptions of the time would lead one to suppose. . . . I think I have shown that tropical dysentery consists of a bacillary and an amoebic form. . . . It is important to know whether the epidemic disease is more uniform in its causation and pathological anatomy. The studies of the Japanese disease by Shiga are highly suggestive of this conclusion, but additional observations will be required before we can accept as final his conclusions." A more precise account of this work appeared simultaneously (Simon Flexner, "The etiology of tropical dysentery," Centralbl. f. Bakt., **28**:625, 1900).

Shortly after, E. B. Vedder and C. W. Duval ("The etiology of acute dysentery in the United States," J. Exper. Med., **6**:181, 1901), working at the instigation of Flexner, studied dysentery in the United States and concluded that the disease here was "due to a bacillus undistinguishable from that obtained from the epidemics of dysentery in several other parts of the world" and that sporadic and institutional outbreaks were caused by this same organism, which was, in fact, the *Bacillus dysenteriae* of Shiga.

9. KRUSE, W. Ueber die Ruhr als Volkskrankheit und ihren Erreger, Deutsche med. Wchnschr., **26**:637, 1900.

Kruse studied an outbreak of acute dysentery in the little industrial town of Laar. In fresh cases the colonies of dysentery bacilli "were so numerous that they impressed one as being in pure culture, and the coarser colonies of colon bacilli were practically displaced." The organism failed to produce gas and, in contrast to Shiga's, seemed to be less motile. Animal inoculations "were all negative." Although the organisms made small animals ill, "they cannot achieve a local lesion in the large bowel." The organisms were agglutinated by the sera of patients after the seventh day. It is evident that Kruse's organism was closely related to those of Shiga and of Flexner.

10. STRONG, R. P., and MUSGRAVE, W. E. The bacillus of Philippine dysentery, J.A.M.A., **35**:498, 1900.

Strong and Musgrave made important studies on dysentery in the American forces in the Philippines simultaneously with those of the Flexner commission.

They defined the disease as "an acute infectious disease characterized anatomically by an extensive superficial necrosis of the mucosa and by hyperplasia and hemorrhagic infiltration of the lymph follicles of the large intestine, with induration and thickening of its walls, by hemorrhagic swelling of the adjacent mesocolic glands, and often by parenchymatous changes in other organs. The Bacillus dysenteriae is present in the acute stage of the disease, both in the discharges and in the superficial necrotic layer of the intestinal mucosa. Clinically the disease is marked by an acute onset, by very frequent mucous bloody stools, accompanied by an intense tenesmus and by an abrupt termination either in death—usually in from four to fifteen days—or by a gradual improvement, from which an early recovery takes place, or the disease may apparently pass into a subacute stage." They thought that infection probably occurred through contaminated water and food. They described in detail the reactions of the bacillus which they isolated and which they regarded as similar to, if not identical with, that isolated by Shiga in Japan.

The paper concludes with an admirable clinical description: "The period of incubation probably lasts not over 48 hours. . . . In one case in which a pure culture of the organism was swallowed symptoms of dysentery began to appear after 24 hours. The onset of the disease is usually abrupt. . . . Often a patient goes to bed feeling perfectly well; during the night he is suddenly attacked with dysentery, and it is not infrequent for these cases to have from twenty to forty stools during the night . . . generally within forty-eight hours or a shorter time the stools consist of nothing but reddish bloody mucus. Microscopically these discharges consist . . . of many red blood cells, leukocytes, epithelial cells and large epithelioid cells. The temperature . . . may often reach 103 or 104 F. or it may not rise above 102 F."

11. FLEXNER, Simon. A comparative study of dysenteric bacilli, Centralbl. f. Bakt., **30**:449, 1901.

During the year after Flexner (Ref. 8) reported his work, a number of observers isolated bacilli from dysentery cases (Strong, Ref. 10; Kruse, Ref. 9). It occurred to Flexner to compare these various organisms and to see whether they were all of one type. Although some very minor differences were noted, Flexner concluded: "The results of this comparative study leaves [sic] no doubt of the identity of the several bacilli with which I have worked. They indicate, moreover, that the acute dysenteries . . . whether in the far East, Germany, or the West Indies are due to the same organism. The justification for the view of a specific organism of dysentery would, therefore, seem to be near at hand. . . . There is little doubt in my mind that the acute epidemic dysenteries of this country are caused by the same micro-organism." The same material appeared in England (Brit. M.J., **2**:786, 1901).

12. MARTINI, E., and LENTZ, O. Ueber die Differenzierung der Ruhrbacillen mittels der Agglutination, Ztschr. f. Hyg. u. Infectionskr., **41**:540, 1902.

Following the work reported above (Ref. 11), it was pretty generally accepted that dysentery strains the world over were identical. Further isolations by others, summarized by Martini and Lentz, seemed to confirm this view. However, Kruse pointed out that his strain was non-motile and had no flagellae, whereas those of Shiga and of Flexner were motile and flagella-bearing. Vedder and Duval (Ref. 8) also raised the question of whether there might not exist in various strains those "individual differences and peculiarities such as may readily exist within the limits of a single species." However, Martini and Lentz were the first to claim significant differences among the various dysentery bacilli. They pointed out that agglutination tests with convalescent sera were inadequate to answer the question, and they prepared hyperimmune sera by immunization of goats. They showed that the bacilli of Shiga, of Kruse, of Flexner (New Haven strain), and of some others fell into one group, whereas those of Flexner (Manila), of Strong, of Kruse (asylum strain), and others fell into another. Lentz ("Vergleichende culturelle Untersuchungen über die Ruhr-bacillen und ruhrähnliche Bacterien nebst einige Bemerkungen über den Lakmusfarbstoff," *ibid.*, p. 559) tried out growth of various strains on sugars and found definite differences. Marmite, for example, was unaffected by Shiga and Kruse's strains, whereas it was fermented by Flexner and Strong's. This work, therefore, changed the point of view about the identity of all dysentery strains and showed that there were important differences, which subsequent work has amply confirmed. Thus W. H. Park, K. R. Collins, and M. E. Goodwin ("The dysentery bacillus group and the varieties which should be included in it," J.M. Research., **11**:553, 1904) found by agglutination tests that most dysentery bacilli fell into three serologically different groups. The first type, isolated by Shiga, did not ferment marmite, the second fermented marmite but did not split maltose or saccharose. The third type fermented marmite but also maltose and saccharose. Park suggested the name "dysentery bacilli" for the type isolated by Shiga and "para-dysentery" for all others. P. H. Hiss, Jr. ("On fermentative and agglutinative characters of bacilli of the 'dysentery group,'" J.M. Research, **13**:1, 1904), found, using similar methods, that these organisms fell into four groups, one of which was represented by the organism he described. "The marked pathogenicity of the Shiga-Kruse organisms as compared with that of the marmite-fermenting organisms, and the differences in the specific reactions called forth in the animal body by these various organisms, make it not improbable that . . . detectable differences may exist in the clinical or pathological picture induced by them. . . ." This prediction has been amply fulfilled. This paper begins with a definitive critical analysis of all bacteriological claims from Shiga's original paper to date (1904).

To appreciate, however, the intense interest and the elaborate work which was stimulated by the questions of the etiology of dysentery, at the turn of the century a major disease both of adults and children, the original reports must be read.

13. DUVAL, C. W., and BASSETT, V. H. The etiology of the summer diarrhoea of infants: a preliminary report, Am. Med., **4**:417, 1902.

So-called summer complaint was a common affection of babies during the hot months on the Atlantic seaboard. Duval and Bassett were able to isolate dysentery bacilli which they considered identical with those of Shiga from 42 cases of typical "summer complaint." "The specific organism was secured, also, from scrapings of the intestinal mucosa at autopsy, and in one case from the mesenteric glands and liver." The organism was obtained, however, with difficulty from mild cases and those of long duration on account of its presence in small numbers among the normal intestinal bacteria. This was a most important study, however, since it linked the summer diarrheas of babies with acute epidemics of dysentery in adults. Shortly after, M. Wollstein ("The dysentery bacillus in a series of cases of infantile diarrhoea," J.M. Research, **10**:11, 1903), working in New York, found organisms of the Flexner (Manila) type in infants and young children. "The bacilli are present in the stools for a period of two to three weeks, but may remain for a longer time." These findings were confirmed by numerous other workers and are reviewed by W. C. Davison ("Bacillary dysentery in children," Bull. Johns Hopkins Hosp., **31**:225, 1920). Davison gives a fine clinical description of the disease in infants.

> 14. HISS, P. H., and RUSSELL, F. F. A study of a bacillus resembling the bacillus of Shiga, from a case of fatal diarrhoea, with remarks on the recognition of dysentery, typhoid and allied bacilli, M. Rec., **63**:357, 1903.

In this paper Hiss and Russell describe the isolation and characteristics of the dysentery bacillus, which has ever since been recognized as representing a definite type. The organism fermented marmite and was specifically agglutinated. The patient from whom this bacillus was isolated was a child of one year, with rather mild diarrheal symptoms, without gross blood in the stools. He failed progressively and died in two weeks.

From this point on, the isolation and differentiation of innumerable races of dysentery bacilli becomes a matter more of bacteriology than of medicine and cannot be pursued further in this bibliography. Those interested are referred to the reviews of Erwin Neter ("The genus Shigella," Bact. Rev., **6**:1, 1942) and of Wilson and Miles (*loc. cit.*).

> 15. KRUSE. Die Blutserumtherapie bei der Dysenterie, Deutsche med. Wchnschr., **29**:6, 49, 1903.

It is difficult for one to realize today how much confidence was placed in the efficacy of vaccine and serum therapy in infectious disease at the turn of the century. Almost immediately after the dysentery bacilli were isolated, attempts at specific immunotherapy were undertaken. Kruse tells of early efforts to produce potent sera, the difficulty of finding a suitable animal, the toxicity of cultures, etc. Nonetheless, he concludes that beneficial effects are obtained insofar as the severity of the disease is mitigated, duration and convalescence shortened, and mortality lowered. A little later Shiga ("Ueber die Priorität der Entdeckung des Ruhrbacillus und der Serumtherapie bei der Dysenterie," Deutsche med. Wchnschr., **29**:113, 1903) claimed priority and stated that for several years the mortality under serum therapy was cut to one-third that of the untreated disease. With regard to prophylactic vaccination with killed cultures, on the other hand, Shiga ("Ueber Versuche zur Schutzimpfung gegen die Ruhr," *ibid.*, p. 327) early obtained no conclusive proof of effectiveness. An immense amount of work on immunotherapy was subsequently done, with results which were variously judged. The final verdict however as summarized, for example, by Cheever (*loc. cit.*) is that these procedures are probably ineffective and useless. At any rate, they have not stood the test of time, and neither vaccines nor sera are any longer advised. Thus H. J. Shaughnessy, R. O. Olsson, K. Bass, F. Friewer, and S. O. Levinson ("Experimental human bacillary dysentery," J.A.M.A., **132**:362, 1946) devised a method of producing bacillary dysentery in man and then showed that "human volunteers vaccinated with heat killed and ultraviolet irradiated vaccine . . . showed no significant immunity against experimental infection," which was effectively controlled by sulfadiazine.

16. TODD, Charles. On a dysentery toxin and antitoxin, J. Hyg., **4**:480, 1904.

Although Shiga (Ref. 7) had already referred to the toxicity of dysentery bacilli, Todd ("On a dysentery antitoxin," Brit. M.J., **2**:1456, 1903) was one of the first to recognize clearly a soluble exotoxin in distinction to the poisonous effects of whole or ground-up bacterial bodies. Todd re-emphasized the essentially local growth of the bacilli in epidemic dysentery from which toxin is absorbed to produce severe symptoms. Todd was able to isolate the soluble toxin from old cultures of B. *dysenteriae* (Kruse), to which horse and rabbit were highly susceptible, whereas guinea pig, rat, and mouse were very resistant. He produced in horses antitoxic sera which seemed to have a high protective effect. The soluble toxin seemed to be produced only by the Shiga type of bacilli, since attempts to isolate it from other strains of dysentery bacilli were unsuccessful. Much more work was done, but P. K. Olitsky and I. J. Kligler ("Toxins and antitoxins of Bacillus dysenteriae Shiga," J. Exper. Med., **31**:19, 1920) appear to have been successful in separating an exotoxin which produced paralyses and central nervous system lesions in rabbits, as well as an endotoxin, which injured the bowel and caused dysenteric symptoms. Sera containing antitoxins against both varieties were produced in horses. A modern authoritative summary of the problems of antigenic structure, somatic antigens, and toxins and classification is to be found in Cheever's article (*loc. cit.*).

17. SELIGMAN, E. Zur Bacteriologie der Ruhr im Kriege, München. med. Wchnschr., **63**:68, 1916.

The question of how long dysentery bacilli persisted in the stools was one of obvious importance. Seligman in the German army made stool cultures from fresh material from dysentery patients. Although only 38 per cent of all cases were positive, dysentery bacilli were isolated in 70 per cent during the first week of the disease, in 53 per cent in the second week, in 18 per cent in the third, whereas no culture was positive in the fourth week. Others, such as C. J. Martin and F. E. Williams ("The chance of recovering dysentery bacilli from the stools according to the time elapsing since the onset of the disease," Brit. M.J., **1**:447, 1918) reported similar results. Whereas, of cultures made during the first 5 days, 68.0 per cent were positive, only 17.4 per cent yielded dysentery bacilli from the sixth to the tenth day. An occasional culture was positive up to the fiftieth day. Apparently, the dysentery bacilli are "overwhelmed by a host of intestinal organisms" as the acute dysenteric process subsides. J. Schürer ("Ueber die Pathogenese der Dauerausscheider und Bazillenträger," Berl. klin. Wchnschr., **57**:106, 1920) takes up the question of prolonged carriage and believes that when this occurs, there is a local focus of chronic inflammation in the bowel in which the bacilli grow and from which they are discharged. W. Fletcher and D. L. Mackinnon ("A contribution to the study of chronicity in dysentery carriers," M. Res. Council, Spec. Rep. Ser.,

No. 27, 1919) divide carriers into those harboring Shiga bacilli and those with Flexner bacilli. The former may continue to be carriers for months or years after the critical attack and are usually invalids with chronic or intermittent bowel symptoms. The Flexner carriers are likely to be intermittent, but carriage may persist for years, even after a very mild initial attack. The proportion of carriers among convalescents was small, but some were remarkably persistent. "In the group of 847 non-dysentery convalescents there were 9 carriers of dysentery bacilli (1.06 per cent) and 6 of these gave a history of dysentery." These nine were all Flexner carriers.

The point of all this is that, whereas dysentery bacilli usually disappear rapidly from the stools, they occasionally persist, at times without an evident lesion.

18. MARSHALL, E. K., Jr., BRATTON, A. C., EDWARDS, L. B., and WALKER, E. Sulfanilylguanidine in the treatment of acute bacillary dysentery in children, Bull. Johns Hopkins Hosp., **68**:94, 1941.

The development of the sulfonamides created a revolution in the therapy of bacillary dysentery. E. K. Marshall, Jr., A. C. Bratton, H. J. White, and J. T. Litchfield, Jr. ("Sulfanilylguanidine: a chemotherapeutic agent for intestinal infections," Bull. Johns Hopkins Hosp., **67**:163, 1940) studied the pharmacological qualities of sulfanilylguanidine and found it appropriate for intestinal infections, insofar as it was poorly absorbed from the intestinal tract. In a clinical study of the drug in cases of bacillary dysentery, promising results were obtained, especially if the drug was used early. Furthermore, L. A. Rantz and W. M. M. Kirby ("The use of sulfaguanidine in the treatment of dysentery carriers," J.A.M.A., **118**:1268, 1942) found that dysentery bacilli disappeared from the stools during treatment with this drug and did not return during periods of observation of from 30 to 90 days. C. J. Smith *et al.* ("Acute bacillary dysentery [Flexner], treatment with sulfaguanidine and succinylsulfathiazole," J.A.M.A., **121**:1325, 1943) considered succinylsulfathiazole an even safer and more effective drug. T. L. Roberts and W. B. Daniels ("Succinylsulfathiazole in the treatment of bacillary dysentery," J.A.M.A., **122**:651, 1943), on the contrary, found that "succinylsulfathiazole produced no amelioration of the illness nor did it shorten its duration. This would be expected in an illness of only four days' duration." But the carrier rate was only 2.6 per cent in the treated cases as against 18.2 per cent in a comparable untreated group. A. V. Hardy, W. Burns, and T. De Capito ("Studies of the acute diarrheal diseases: cultural observations on the relative efficacy of sulfonamides in Shigella dysenteriae infections," Pub. Health Rep., **58**:689, 1943) compared the efficacy of sulfaguanidine, sulfasuxidine, sulfadiazine, and sulfathiazole. "There were moderate variations only in the efficacy of the four sulfonamides." Later A. V. Hardy and J. Watt ("Newer procedures in laboratory diagnosis and therapy in the control of bacillary dysentery," Am. J. Pub. Health, **44**:503, 1944) summarized the whole question and concluded: "Well absorbed sulfonamides as well as poorly absorbed preparations are effective in Shigella infections, and are recommended." It is obvious, therefore, that variations in response occur with different strains of Shigella and in different outbreaks, so that no preparation is proved to be consistently the best.

19. HARDY, A. V., MASON, R. P., and MARTIN, G. A. The antibiotics in acute bacillary dysentery, Ann. New York Acad. Sc., 1952, p. 1070. The writers had an opportunity in Korea to treat large numbers of cases of bacillary dysentery under well-controlled conditions with various antibiotics. Aureomycin, terramycin, and chloromycetin, as well as sulfadiazine and nonspecific measures, were used in different patients. The three antibiotics all were about equally effective and, within 7 days, 95–98 per cent of the patients were convalescent, and dysentery bacilli were no longer isolated. The figures for sulfadiazine and non-specific therapy, on the other hand, were only 60 and 62 per cent. "The differences in sigmoidoscopic findings, at the fourth day, were particularly impressive. Most of those on nonspecific therapy still had the hyperemic edematous bowel, probably with bleeding points, a copious mucopurulent exudate microscopically loaded with pus cells. In patients on antibiotics the hyperemia, edema, bleeding and exudate were gone, and the mucous membrane was clear, except for fading submucosal hemorrhagic areas. Clinically it was evident that the three antibiotics were all highly effective." F. S. Cheever ("The treatment of Shigellosis with antibiotics," Ann. New York Acad. Sc., 1952, p. 1063) gives an authoritative review of the whole subject of drugs and antibiotics in bacillary dysentery.

PLAGUE

Bacteriology	Refs. 2, 3, 4, 7
Clinical	Refs. 1, 3, 4
Epidemiology	Ref. 11
General	Refs. 1, 3, 4
Immunity	Ref. 8
Pathology	Refs. 1, 4, 9
Pneumonic plague	Ref. 6
Rats (role in plague)	Refs. 7, 10
Sylvatic plague	Ref. 12
Transmission (fleas)	Refs. 7, 10
Treatment, antibiotics	Refs. 14, 15, 16
Treatment, serum	Ref. 5
Treatment, sulfonamide	Ref. 13
Vaccination	Refs. 5, 8

PLAGUE

THE bibliography of plague presents many difficulties. A disease of such striking clinical and epidemiological features and of such malignancy could hardly fail to strike the popular fancy and to call forth a colossal mass of writing from ancient times on. We shall not attempt to deal with the narrow historical aspects of plague but rather refer the reader to the monumental work by Georg Sticker (*Ablandlungen aus der Seuchengeschichte und Seuchenlehre* [Giessen: Alfred Töpelmann, 1908], Vol. 1, Parts 1 and 2), which contains a bibliography of some two thousand titles. B. M. Lersch's *Geschichte der Volksseuchen* (Berlin: S. Karger, 1896) contains much valuable material on plague epidemics. A dependable and authoritative account is given in August Hirsch's invaluable monograph, *Handbuch der historisch-geographischen Pathologie* (2d ed.; Stuttgart: Ferdinand Enke, 1881), 1:349 (English translation by Creighton [London: New Sydenham Society, 1883], 1:494). Epidemics of plague in England are also told about in an interesting fashion in Charles Creighton, *A History of Epidemics in Britain* (Cambridge: Cambridge University Press, 1891), 1:470. A semipopular but readable account is also to be found in H. Harold Scott's *A History of Tropical Medicine* (Baltimore: Williams & Wilkins Co., 1939), 2:702.

Authoritative modern reviews of the bacteriology and immunology of plague are those by G. F. Petrie in *A System of Bacteriology in Relation to Medicine* (London, 1929), Vol. 3, chap. viii, p. 137, and by G. S. Wilson and A. A. Miles in Topley and Wilson's *Principles of Bacteriology and Immunity* (Baltimore: Williams & Wilkins Co., 1946), Vol. 2, chap. 73, p. 1627. Among general books on the subject, there are to be mentioned especially *Plague* by Wu Lien-Teh, J. W. H. Chun, R. Pollitzer, and C. Y. Wu (Shanghai Station, China: National Quarantine Service, 1936) and *Plague* by R. Pollitzer (Geneva: World Health Organization, 1954). These two works deal with every phase of the subject and have comprehensive bibliographies.

In addition, invaluable and extensive material is to be found in the reports of the plague commissions sent to the site of outbreaks by various nations, to wit:

Austrian Commission, *Denkschriften d. k. Akad. d. Wissenschaften, Wien, 1898–1900* (3 vols.).

German Commission, "Bericht über die Thätigkeit der zur Erforschung der Pest im Jahre 1897 nach Indien entsandten Kommission erstattet von Dr. Gaffky, Dr. Pfeiffer, Dr. Sticker, Dr. Dieudonné," Arb. a. d. k. Gsndhtsamte, Berlin, Vol. 16, 1899.

British Commission, Special reports in the Journal of Hygiene in the form of extra "Plague numbers" and "Plague supplements," 1906–15.

International Commission (Chinese), *Report of the International Plague Conference, Held at Mukden, April, 1911* (Manila: Bureau of Printing, 1912).

There is an immense literature of books and articles on individual outbreaks of plague, ranging all the way from critical scientific accounts to popular stories. We cannot attempt to document this material. An example or two may, however, be given. The great plague in London in 1665, for instance, has been immortalized by Defoe in his *Journal of the Plague Year* (many editions), as well as by Pepys in the diary. The contemporary bills of mortality (*London's Dreadful Visitation; or a Collection of All the Bills of Mortality for This Present Year, Etc., by the Company of Parish Clerks of London* [1665]) bring vividly before one the course of this epidemic. Walter G. Bell's book, *The Great Plague in London, 1665* (London: John Lane, The Bodley Head, Ltd., 1924) is a classical study of every phase of this outbreak, well illustrated, with full bibliography. Along with this material, *The Plague in Shakespeare's London* by F. P. Wilson (Oxford: Clarendon Press, 1927) is of great interest.

When plague disappeared from Europe in the early eighteenth century, the Continent was left in a state of terror lest the scourge again gain a footing. Fear of the plague and the elaborate quarantine measures adopted are all illustrated by the events connected with Shelley's death and burial.

When Shelley and his companion, Edward Elleker Williams, were drowned and later were washed up on the Tuscan shore, the local officers simply covered the bodies with quicklime. Trelawney, the friend of Shelley, with Byron and Leigh Hunt, had to exercise the greatest efforts to gain permission even to approach the bodies and to cremate them. "After a variety of applications and correspondence with Mr. Dawkins, Secretary of Legation, the English consul Falkener, and the Governor of Leghorn—I obtained from the latter an order to the officer on the coast—commanding the lookout tower nearest to that part of the beach on which Williams had been found and buried—to deliver to me his body—and an officer of the Sanitair Office to accompany me and see that it was consumed to ashes. Mr. Dawkins likewise obtained me an order of the like purport and condition from the Lucchese government—for the body of Shelley found and interred on their coast. . . . I proceeded on shore, and after showing my bill of health I was allowed to land. The captain of the port with another officer received me on shore." They then proceeded to the spot where the body lay. "At equal distances along the coast stood high square towers . . . for the double purpose of preventing smuggling and enforcing the quarantine laws, the latter being here severer than in any part of the world. . . . We then with instruments made for the purpose of dragging wrecked seamen out of the sea—for you are on no account allowed to touch a body—we dragged the remains out of the grave. . . . The soldiers who appeared superstitiously fearful had withdrawn themselves as far as possible" (*Letters of Edward John Trelawney, ed. H. Buxton Forman* [Oxford: Oxford University Press, 1910], p. 4). One can picture the scene as Trelawney has so vividly described it—the hot yellow beach, the glittering sunshine, the blue sky, the pines in the background, and the colorful uniforms of the frightened soldiers shrinking back from the proceedings.

No better popular account of the plague and the reaction of the people to it can be found than that of Kinglake in his remarkable book, *Eothen, or Traces of Travel Brought Home from the East* (London: John Ollivier, 1844):

"I had come to the end of this wheel-gong Europe, and now my eyes would see the Splendour and Havoc of the East.

"The two frontier towns are less than a cannon-shot distant, and yet their people hold no communion. The Hungarian on the North, and the Turk and Servian on the southern side of the Save are as much asunder as though there were fifty broad provinces that lay in the path between them. Of the men that bustled around me in the streets of Semlin, there was not, perhaps, one who had ever gone down to look upon the stranger race which dwells under the walls of that opposite castle. It is the Plague, and dread of the Plague, which divide the one people from the other. All coming and going stands forbidden by the terrors of the yellow flag. If you dare to break the laws of the quarantine, you will be tried with military haste; the court will scream out your sentence to you from a tribunal some fifty yards off; the priest instead of whispering to you the sweet hopes of religion will console you at duelling distance, and after that you will find yourself carefully shot, and carelessly buried in the ground of the Lazaretto.

"When all was in order for our departure, we walked down to the precincts of the Quarantine Establishment, and here awaited us a 'compromised' [a 'compromised' person is one who has been in contact with people or things supposed to be capable of conveying infection] officer of the Austrian government, who lives in a state of perpetual excommunication. The boats, with their 'compromised' rowers, were also in readiness.

"After coming in contact with any creature or thing belonging to the Ottoman Empire, it would be impossible for us to return to the Austrian territory without undergoing an impressment of fourteen days in the odious Lazaretto" (chap. 1).

1. VIRCHOW, Rud. 1. Ueber die Pest, Berl. klin. Wchnschr., **16**:117, 1879.

Virchow gives an authoritative statement of the contemporary status of plague. There is emphasis, as one might expect, on the pathological lesions—buboes, hemorrhages, etc.—and their significance. Virchow considered the disease infectious and contagious: "It seems to me that the resemblance of plague and anthrax is so great that I consider it very likely that an organism will be found which is the cause of the affection [plague]." He therefore emphasized the importance of isolation of patients, disinfection, and quarantine. The views of those who did not regard plague as contagious are brought out in the study of E. H. Ackerknecht, "Anticontagionism between 1821 and 1867," Bull. Hist. Med., **22**:562, 1948.

2. YERSIN, [Alexandre]. Sur la peste de Hong Kong, Compt. rend. Acad. d. sc., **119**:356, 1894.

M. Duclaux communicated to the academy passages from a letter addressed to the Pasteur Institute by Dr. Yersin, who had been sent to Hong Kong to study plague during the great outbreak of 1894. After a brief clinical description he says: "The first bacteriological studies were made on living subjects. Examination of the blood drawn from the finger at various stages of the disease did not show any microbes, and cultures were sterile. The bubos, on the other hand, showed in abundance and in pure state a very small bacillus, short with rounded ends, not staining by the method of Gram." In two fatal cases the bacillus was found in the buboes and less abundantly in other glands and very rarely in the blood at the moment of death. The liver and spleen were enlarged and contained the specific bacillus. Mice inoculatd with a little material from a bubo died in 24 hours, with the bacilli in the glands, organs, and blood. Guinea pigs died in 3–6 days. The microbe was early grown on gelatin.

A little later Yersin ("La Peste bubonique à Hong Kong," Ann. Inst. Pasteur, **8**:662, 1894) wrote a more formal report: "When I arrived [at Hong Kong], more than 300 Chinese had already succumbed. . . . These are the symptoms . . . sudden onset after incubation of 4–6 days, shock, and prostration. Strong fever often with delirium. A bubo in the groin generally appears in the first day, reaching the size of a hen's egg. Death occurs usually by 48 hours, often sooner. If life is prolonged beyond 5 or 6 days, the outlook is better." In some cases the bubo does not have time to form, one then observes mucous membrane hemorrhages and petechiae in the skin. Mortality is high—about 95 per cent in the hospitals. "In the infected quarters many dead rats litter the ground. . . . The lodgings of the Chinese of the poor classes. . . . contain an unbelievable number of people. . . . Many are without windows and below the level of the ground. . . . The only remedy would be to burn up the Chinese town." It has been observed that plague, before striking human beings, acts with great intensity on mice, rats, buffaloes, and pigs.

He describes again in more detail the isolation of the organism. "The ends of the bacilli stain more intensely than the centers, sometimes they seem surrounded by a capsule." White, transparent colonies developed on gelatin. The bacillus also grew well on coagulated serum. The appearance in broth was characteristic: clear liquid with grumous deposits on the walls and bottom of the tube. Examined under the microscope, the cultures showed chains of short bacilli. If one opened the body of a guinea pig dead of plague, one found hemorrhages in the abdominal wall, pink edema at the site of inoculation and around the neighboring glands, which were large and filled with bacilli. The intestine was often hyperemic, the adrenals congested, the kidneys violaceous, the liver large and red, the spleen very large, frequently a sort of eruption of little miliary tubercles. Yersin noted in subcultures that, after several days, large colonies appeared which showed a great reduction in virulence on injection into animals. Dead rats found in the houses and streets always contained the microbe in immense numbers. "Plague is then a disease both contagious and inoculable. It is probable that rats constitute the principal vehicle, but I have shown that bats can also serve as agents of transmission." He thought that the avirulent strains which developed in cultures were capable of conferring immunity against plague on an animal and stated that he would report further on this point.[1] It is obvious that Yersin skimmed the cream of plague studies.

3. KITASATO, S. The bacillus of bubonic plague, Lancet, **2**:428, 1894.

Kitasato, who had been sent to Hong Kong to study the same epidemic as Yersin, began his work on June 14. His findings and Yersin's were not the same at all points (Ref. 2), and it is an interesting question whether they deserve equal credit as co-discoverers of the plague bacillus. "The bacilli are to be found in the blood, in the buboes, in the spleen, and in all other internal organs of the victims of plague. The bacilli are rods with rounded ends, which are readily stained by the ordinary aniline dyes, the poles being stained darker than the middle part, especially in blood preparations, and presenting a capsule

---

[1] An interesting study of Yersin and his discovery is found in *Yersin et la peste* (Lausanne: F. Rouges et Cie, 1944), which contains articles by various authors and reprints of Yersin's own reports.

sometimes well marked, sometimes indistinct." Cultural characteristics are then described. Mice, rats, guinea pigs, and rabbits were all highly susceptible to inoculation and died in from 2 to 5 days. Mice and guinea pigs could be infected by feeding. Kitasato reported the effects of desiccation, heat, and chemicals on the bacilli. The paper concludes with "a short review of the Plague generally." Kitasato obviously regarded the disease as communicable and urged rigid cleanliness, disinfection, and isolation. "Dead bodies covered with quicklime are either to be burned or buried. . . . Mice and rats which have died spontaneously in dwelling houses should be carried away with proper precautions." Kitasato, however, like Yersin, did not sense the true relationship between rats and plague; they were unaware of the vector.

4. AOYAMA, T. Ueber die Pestepidemie in Hong-Kong im Jahre 1894, Mitt. a. d. med. Facultät d. Kaiserlich-Japanesichen Universität, **3**:115, 1897.

Aoyama gives a most interesting and comprehensive report on every phase of the Hong Kong epidemic of 1894, but the most important section is that on the plague organism. He notes that both Yersin and Kitasato found "specific" bacteria in plague cases at about the same time, but he raises the question of whether the organisms of the two workers were not different. In summary: "Dr. Yersin has not stated that the bacilli in the blood and in the lymph nodes are morphologically different, whereas Kitasato says they differ and those from the blood possess a capsule. Furthermore, according to Yersin, the plague bacilli are Gram-negative, whereas Kitasato finds them sometimes positive. . . . According to Yersin, after animal inoculation, the regional lymph nodes are always swollen, whereas Kitasato found such swelling rare." Aoyama himself often found mixed infections, and he concluded that the organisms which Kitasato found in the blood were simply streptococci. He believed that suppuration of buboes was due to superinfection with some other organism than the bacillus of plague. Ogata (Ref. 7) also concluded that the organisms of Yersin and Kitasato were distinct, and he listed the differences in tabular form, although as distinguished a bacteriologist as W. Kolle ("Zur Bakteriologie der Beulenpest," Deutsche med. Wchnschr., **23**:146, 1897) disagreed. The whole question is analyzed by E. Lagrange ("Concerning the discovery of the plague bacillus," J. Trop. Med., **29**:299, 1926).

Aoyama also gave interesting clinical observations. He mentioned hyperacute (lightning-like, *blitzartige*) cases which died in 24 hours before buboes appeared, but he evidently did not recognize the pneumonic form. He stated that he saw only one instance of pneumonia in the Chinese hospital. The article concludes with a comprehensive description of the pathological changes. He emphasized especially the lesions in lymph nodes through the body and those of smaller patches of lymphoid tissue. The glandular swelling consisted of "hyperaemia, dilation of vessels, exudate, hemorrhage, cellular hyperplasia, and immense bacterial growth." He described blood leukocytes of up to 200,000. The spleen was usually large; otherwise no specific lesions were mentioned.

An immense literature on the bacteriology of plague promptly appeared. A comprehensive discussion of the plague bacillus is to be found in Pollitzer (*op. cit.*, p. 71) and in the article by Petrie (*loc. cit.*)

5. YERSIN, CALMETTE, and BORREL. La Peste bubonique, Ann. Inst. Pasteur, **9**:589, 1895.

No sooner had Yersin isolated the bacillus of plague than his associates at the Pasteur Institute in Paris began immunization and protection experiments in animals. A series of passages yielded organisms of "fixed" virulence. "The present note had for its object to show the possibility of immunizing animals against plague and to cure those who were fatally infected by this disease." Rabbits and guinea pigs were injected with organisms heated at 58° C. for 1 hour. "In general 3 or 4 injections . . . sufficed to vaccinate the rabbit against a subcutaneous injection of virulent bacilli." These workers also tried the preventive and curative action of serum of rabbits immunized against plague: "3 cc. of such serum sufficed to protect a rabbit against a subcutaneous injection of virulent plague bacilli. This same amount of serum injected 12 hours after inoculation stops growth of the microbe and cures the rabbit of the plague." They then immunized a horse, whose serum developed a marked preventive and curative action against plague in mice. Normal sera or sera prepared against other bacteria had no effect. These experiments from the hands of such outstanding observers attracted much attention, the more so when a letter from Yersin to the academy arrived from Canton, China, dated June 29, 1896, in which he reported the brilliant cure of a young man sick with plague by injection of "serum prepared at Nha-Tsang" ("Historique du premier cas de peste traité et guéri par l'emploi de sérum anti-pesteux," Bull. Acad. de méd., Paris, **36**:195, 1896). Yersin's letter was accompanied by a communication from the French consul-general at Canton confirming his claims: "Dr. Yersin has administered serum to a Chinese Catholic gravely ill with plague. Absolute success." Following the reading of this letter, M. Bruardel announced: "A recent telegram informs me that M. Yersin has already treated twenty-seven cases of plague by his method with success in every case." A little later, E. Roux ("Sur la peste bubonique: essais de traitement par le sérum antipesteux, à propos d'une note du Dr. Yersin, médecin de 2e classe des Colonies, directeur de l'Institut Pasteur de Nha-Tsang," Bull. Acad. de méd., Paris, **37**:91, 1897) reported to the academy on Yersin's work. It now appeared that Yersin had treated twenty-three cases of plague, of which two had died. Roux said that the serum was ineffective if the disease was too advanced but was very efficacious if used in the first phases. In conclusion, the president of the academy "thanks M. Roux for his important communication, and asks him to transmit to Dr. Yersin congratulations and encouragement" (*unanimous applause*).

Unfortunately, this early enthusiasm soon had to be tempered, and it would serve no purpose to attempt to review the huge literature on serum therapy. N. H. Choksy ("On recent progress in the serum therapy of plague," Brit. M.J., **1**:1282, 1908), an outstanding authority on the subject, in a review of the use of various early sera reported death rates of 60–80 per cent. He pointed out further that no effect was to be expected in septicemic patients. In appropriate cases there was a mortality of 63.5 per cent as against 74 per cent in the controls. "The whole secret of the treatment lies in applying the serum very early . . . if given between twenty-four and forty-eight hours its action is not so well marked and after forty-eight hours it does not appear to affect the course perceptibly." At best, therefore, the serum appeared of highly limited value. Furthermore, in reports on plague investigations in India issued by the advisory committee appointed by the Secretary of State for India, the Royal Society, and the Lister Institute ("The serum treatment of human plague," J. Hyg., Vol. **12,** Suppl., p. 326, 1912) it is concluded: "From the whole enquiry it appears that the administration of the available sera is not a practicable means of bringing about any material diminution in the mortality from plague in India." Many antiplague sera had been prepared by all sorts of methods, using various animals. They are enumerated in R. F. Platzner's review ("Evaluation of therapeutic agents in plague," U.S. Naval M. Bull., **46:**1674, 1946). For the most part, they have been variously judged by different observers in different outbreaks. The whole question of serum therapy of plague is concisely reviewed by Pollitzer (*op. cit.,* p. 454). Thus the story is much the same as with antipneumococcal and antimenigococcal sera—the effect of certain sera is possibly prophylactic or curative in the treatment of mild cases at the very onset.

6. CHILDE, L. F. The pneumonic type of plague, Indian M. Gaz., **32:**231, 1897.

Childe, working in India, noted that, as the epidemic progressed, "one observed that coincidently with the increased death-rate due to plague, there was a large and unexplained increase assigned to remittent fever and respiratory diseases" without superficial buboes. "And at the end of December I met with a case which had been diagnosed as broncho-pneumonia, but which turned out to be one of plague affecting the lungs, without causing any marked enlargement of the lymphatic glands—a case, in fact, of plague pneumonia." Anatomically, the lungs showed engorgement, edema, and pneumonic patches; the lymphatic glands were little, if at all, enlarged; the pneumonic patches showed, under the microscope, immense numbers of plague bacilli, which were grown in pure culture. Up to the time of this report Childe had made postmortem examinations on twelve such cases; the patients were all brought to the hospital with no suspicion of plague. The course was that of a fulminating bronchopneumonia, with death in a few days; the patients cough up watery seromucous fluid slightly blood-tinged. The physical signs were mainly those of bronchopneumonia—patches of râles. Childe considered pneumonic plague as highly communicable by air-borne transmission, in contrast to the low contagiousness of the bubonic form. "With regard to the literature I have not been able to find any published account of this form of plague but it was evidently recognized during the Pali epidemic of 1836 . . . and perhaps the 'black-death' of the middle ages . . . was really a severe type of this plague-pneumonia."

In 1911 the Chinese government appointed a commission (*Report of the International Plague Conference Held at Mukden, April, 1911* [Manila, 1912]) to study a tremendous epidemic of pneumonic plague in Manchuria. The commission collected evidence (p. 423) that rat infection played no part in this epidemic but that the disease was spread by dissemination of bacilli by cough. R. P. Strong, working with the commission, showed that the same strains of bacilli were involved in bubonic and pneumonic forms of plague and that organisms from pneumonic cases injected into animals produced the bubonic form (pp. 435, 438). The whole situation is summarized by W. G. Liston ("The epidemiological features of bubonic and pneumonic plague contrasted, XVIIth Internat. Cong. Medicine, London, 1913, Sec. XXI," Trop. Med. & Hyg., Part 1, p. 9, 1914).

R. P. Strong and O. Teague ("Studies on pneumonic plague and plague immunization. II. The method of transmission of infection in pneumonic plague and manner of spread of the disease during the epidemic," Philippine J. Sc., **7B**:137, 1912) studied in detail the transmission of pneumonic plague. *Bacillus pestis* was not expelled on quiet breathing, but on cough it was widely disseminated into the surrounding air, even when no gross droplets of sputum were visible. Strong and Teague emphasized the importance of masks and other protective measures in the presence of the pneumonic form of plague. They also ("IV. Portal of entry of infection and method of development of the lesions in pneumonic and primary septicemic plague; experimental pathology," *ibid.*, p. 173) believed that the primary point of infection in pneumonic plague was not the tonsil but some part of the respiratory passages. "Having reached the lung tissue, the bacilli rapidly multiply and produce at first pneumonic changes of the lobular type and shortly afterward more general lobar involvement of the lung tissue."

The whole subject of pneumonic plague is exhaustively covered in the monograph of Wu Lien-Teh (*A Treatise on Pneumonic Plague* [Geneva: League of Nations, Health Organization, 1926]).

7. OGATA, M. Ueber die Pestepidemie in Formosa, Centralbl. f. Bakt., **21**:769, 1897.

Ogata and a group of associates were sent to Formosa to study plague. He reported numerous bacteriological observations. He always found the bacilli in the blood and organs of infected small animals but did not find them constantly in the blood of human cases, even when severe. "Fleas on plague rats contain virulent plague bacilli, which, after the death of the rat, can convey the plague bacillus to man." "Plague may be primarily a disease of rats, and this animal may be the immediate cause of the spread of the disease in man." He therefore rated high the disposal of sick and dead rats in plague control. He also stated that in Formosa the inhabitants looked on plague as primarily a pest of rats and actually designated it "rat pest." This paper seems to give the first clear statement of the transmission of plague by the rat flea. A little later P.-L. Simond ("La Propagation de la peste," Ann. Inst. Pasteur, **12**:625, 1898) presented a beautiful epidemiological study of plague in India, from which he concluded that man is of little consequence in the transmission of bubonic plague and that transmission is not by air or water. "It is an animal which the observed facts denounce as the most active propagator of plague, it is the rat." He went on to condemn the rat flea as the agent which transmitted plague from rat to man. He pointed out the important and now well-recognized fact that the death of rats preceded the death of men from plague.

J. Constantin Gauthier and A. Raybaud ("Recherches expérimentales sur le rôle des parasites du rat dans la transmission de la peste," Rev. d'hyg., **25**:426, 1903) subjected the question to experimental study and concluded: "Transmission of plague by parasites is possible. We have seen it take place from rat to rat by the intermediation of the fleas of this animal. It does not occur by simple contact of animal with animal when all parasites are excluded from the experiment. Fleas gathered from rats bite man without difficulty, and this may be the cause of epidemics. This study seems to us, therefore, a full confirmation of the theory of Simond." Further proof of these early observations was reported by the British Plague Commission ("Experiments upon the transmission of plague by fleas. I. Historical introduction," J. Hyg., **6**:425, 1906, and "II. Transference of plague from rat to rat," *ibid.*, p. 435). In Part I is reviewed the literature to date, and in Part II definitive experiments are described which show that plague can be transferred from rat to rat by fleas without direct contact of the animals. The commission further showed ("Further observations on the transmission of plague by fleas with special reference to the fate of the plague bacillus in the body of the rat flea [*P. cheopis*]," *ibid.*, **7**:395, 1907) that the stomach of the flea could hold 0.5 cu. mm. of blood, that plague bacilli multiplied in the stomach and were passed out in the feces, and that a flea bite could serve as portal of entry for plague bacilli. A. W. Bacot and C. J. Martin ("Observations on the mechanism of the transmission of plague by fleas, XVIIth Internat. Cong. Medicine, London, 1913, Sec. XXI," Trop. med. & Hyg., Part II, p. 9, 1914) showed by ingenious experiments that rat fleas could transmit plague during the act of sucking; they also studied the distribution of plague bacilli in infected fleas.

The whole subject of the various insect vectors is documented in Pollitzer (*op. cit.*, chap. 7, p. 315).

8. HAFFKINE, W. M. Remarks on the plague prophylactic fluid, Brit. M.J., **1**:1461, 1897.

Following the previous observations on vaccination with killed cultures of plague bacilli (Ref. 5), the subject was taken up intensively by Haffkine at the request of the British government. In this paper Haffkine gave his directions for preparing the "prophylactic fluid." His rationale was as follows: "I decided to make an atteempt to effect both a reduction of the susceptibility and of the case mortality, by combining in the prophylactic substances large quantities of bodies of microbes together with intensified extracellular toxins." For this purpose he added to the nutritive media large quantities of "clarified butter." "When the fluid is filled with a rich jungle the growth is shaken off the drops of butter, and brought down to the bottom of the liquid." The microbes were killed by a temperature of 70° C. maintained for 1 hour. "In a quiet position in the test tubes two different substances are then obtained: a thick white sediment and a perfectly limpid fluid. Injected subcutaneously into animals they produce (1) the sediment, a local inflammation and a nodule at the seat of inoculation, with little fever or general effect; and (2) the fluid, a considerable rise of temperature and a general affection, with no noticeable local effects." Haffkine attributed to this mixture both prophylactic and therapeutic effects. A little later, editorial comment ("Haffkine's plague prophylactic," Brit. M.J., **1**:1492, 1897) was as follows: "On reading the description of his [Haffkine's] technique one cannot help being struck by the roughness of the methods employed, and by the wonderful success that attended them. That the introduction into the body of the mixture which results from the growth of the plague bacillus in a mass chemically so complicated as a mixture of native 'ghee' and bouillon should cause the inoculated to suffer to an extent about twenty times less than the non-inoculated . . . is indeed a remarkable fact." Haffkine covered essentially the same ground in another article ("The plague prophylactic," Indian M. Gaz., **32**:201, 1897). Through the years there has grown up a vast literature describing plague vaccines prepared in innumerable ways, always in the attempt to find something more effective. The subject is well reviewed, with literature, in Pollitzer (*op. cit.,* p. 138). Turning to recent times, K. F. Meyer, S. F. Quan, and A. Larson ("Prophylactic immunization and specific therapy of experimental pneumonic plague," Am. Rev. Tuberc., **57**:312, 1948) immunized mice with avirulent strains of *B. pestis* or with killed plague bacilli and found marked protection against a subsequent intranasal challenge. Finally, K. F. Meyer ("Immunity in plague: a critical consideration of some recent studies," J. Immunol., **64**:139, 1950) gave a masterful analysis of the mechanism of infection and immunity in plague, and Pollitzer (*op. cit.,* chap. 3, p. 115) comprehensively reviewed, with literature, the subject of immunology in plague, as well as (*ibid.,* chap. 10, p. 523) its control and prevention. "For several years the Armed Forces [see J. Love, J. F. Shaul, A. Margileth, and R. R. Martelle, 'The status of immunization in 1954,' M. Clin. North America, September, 1954, p. 1493] have used suspensions of P. pestis killed by formalin. The basic course consists of 2 subcutaneous injections of 1 ml. of this suspension at 7 to 10 day intervals. Each ml. contains 2000 million organisms. This yields partial protection for 4 to 6 months, so booster doses are advised every 4 to 6 months so long as one resides in an area where plague exists."

9. DÜRCK, Hermann. Beiträge zur pathologischen Anatomie der Pest, Beitr. z. path. Anat., 6 Supplementheft, p. 1, 1904.

Although the classical studies on the pathology of plague are those of H. Albrecht and A. Ghon ("Pathologisch-anatomische Untersuchungen mit Einschluss der pathologischen Histologie und Bakteriologie," Denkschriften k. Akad. Wissensch., Wien, Vol. **66**, Part II, p. 227, 1898), handsomely illustrated with photographs and reproductions of microscopic preparations, they are published in a rather inaccessible situation. Dürck, also, working in Bombay during the epidemic, reports autopsies on sixteen cases of bubonic plague in meticulous detail, both gross and microscopic, with beautiful illustrative plates. The pathology of plague both in experimental animals and in man is thoroughly reviewed, with references to the literature, by Pollitzer (*op. cit.,* p. 179). The special pathology of the pneumonic form was extensively studied in the Manchurian epidemic by R. P. Strong, B. C. Lowell, and O. Teague ("Studies on pneumonic plague and plague immunization. VII. Pathology," Philippine J. Sc., **7B**:203, 1912).

10. Reports on plague investigations in India: epidemiological observations in Bombay City, J. Hyg., **7**:724, 1907.

Outbreaks of disease in rats were generally observed to precede outbreaks of plague in man. According to A. Rennie ("The plague in the East," Brit. M.J., **2**:615, 1894), "In Canton rats were the only animals observed to suffer; an exceptional mortality was observed amongst them two or three weeks before cases of plague were noted, and this sequence of events persisted throughout the epidemic. A high mortality amongst rats in a district of the city quite free from sickness was most surely followed by an outbreak of plague, so much so that people came to regard these rodents as heralds of the coming evil, and when possible hastened removal to safer quarters. They would come out of their holes in broad daylight, run and tumble about in the streets in an aimless and dazed manner and die."

However, there was disagreement as to the exact circumstances and their significance, as brought out in a thorough review of the literature by the English Plague Commission ("Digest of recent observations on the epidemiology of plague," J. Hyg., **7:**694, 1907). The elaborate Bombay studies showed that *Mus decumanus*, typically "an out-of-door wandering rat," was chiefly responsible for the diffusion of plague among the rats throughout Bombay city and that the decumanus epizoötic preceded an epizoötic in *Mus rattus*, which is essentially a house rat. It is from the latter that the rat flea transmits the plague bacilli to man, leading finally to a human epidemic.

11. WHITE, F. Norman. Twenty years of plague in India with special reference to the outbreak of 1917–18, Indian J.M. Research, **6:**190, 1919.

The epidemiology of plague is of great interest. In this important paper White describes the situation in India, where from 1898 to 1918 at least ten million people died of the disease. Variations in intensity of plague outbreaks are related to rainfall, variations in resistance on the part of the rat population, efforts to eradicate rats, etc.

12. ELTON, C. S. Plague and the regulation of numbers in wild animals, J. Hyg., **24:**138, 1925.

Elton gives a comprehensive summary of the occurrence of plague in wild rodents. The list includes marmots in Transbaikalia; marmots in the Caucasus; squirrels, monkeys, and field mice in India; gerbils and wild mice in South Africa; muskrats in Senegal; wild rodents in England; and ground squirrels in California. He concluded that most rodents regulated their numbers by increasing to a point at which some sort of epizoötic such as plague occurred, which killed off a large proportion of them. This cycle recurred indefinitely, perhaps regulated by various factors such as climatic conditions. These epizoötics were quite different from plague in domestic rats, and it has been a question whether human plague results from them. Wu Lien-Teh ("A further note on natural and experimental plague in tarbagans," J. Hyg., **22:**329, 1924) considered it "as practically certain that the tarbagan gives rise to the outbreaks of plague which occur yearly in Transbaikalia and that it started the outbreaks in Manchuria in 1910–11 and 1920–21." Plague among the ground squirrels of California was first reported by G. W. McCoy ("Plague among ground squirrels," Am. J. Hyg., **10:**589, 1910), as well as a few human cases from this source. Karl F. Meyer ("The Sylvatic Plague Committee," Am. J. Pub. Health, **36:**961, 1936) takes up the problem of the Sylvatic plague in California, and the whole subject of hosts of the infection is exhaustively dealt with in Pollitzer (*op. cit.*, chap. 6, p. 251).

13. CARMAN, John A. Prontosil in the treatment of oriental plague, East African M.J., **14:**362, 1938.

Carman seems to have been the first to use a sulfonamide in the treatment of plague. In a small series the death rate was 50 per cent as against 100 per cent in the controls. H. Schütze ("Chemotherapy in plague infection," Lancet, **1:**266, 1939), shortly after, reported various sulfonamide derivatives as effective in experimental plague of rats and mice. From then on, the journals contained many reports of the use of sulfonamides in plague. An important paper, for example, was that of A. T. W. Simeons ("One thousand cases of bubonic plague treated in an emergency plague hospital," Indian M. Gaz., **81**:235, 1946). He stressed the early institution of treatment with sulfadiazine; when the drug was given within the first 24 hours, the mortality was only 6.61 per cent, whereas when its use was delayed 24 hours, the death rate rose to 19.67 per cent. In one thousand cases the mortality was 18 per cent. The whole subject is reviewed by J. M. Ruegsegger and H. Gilchrist ("Plague: a survey of recent developments in the prevention and treatment of the disease," Am. J. Trop. Med., **27**:683, 1947).

14. HORNIBROOK, J. W. Streptomycin in experimental plague, Pub. Health Rep., **61**:535, 1946.

Hornibrook first tested the value of streptomycin in experimental plague in mice. He found a definite prophylactic and curative effect; for example, when treatment (2 mg. per day) was started 2 days following inoculation and continued for 6 days, nine out of ten mice survived for 14 days, whereas 80 per cent of untreated controls died. A little later, N. E. Wayson and M. C. McMahon ("Plague: treatment of experimental animals with streptomycin, sulfadiazine, and sulfapyridine," J. Lab. & Clin. Med., **31**:323, 1946) also showed that streptomycin had a definite therapeutic effect in mice and guinea pigs with plague. The use of a combination of streptomycin and sulfadiazine did not seem to add to the effectiveness of either. Denis Herbert ("Streptomycin in experimental plague," Lancet, **1**:626, 1947) also made a thorough study of the subject. He found that in guinea pigs infected by subcutaneous injection, 3½-day courses of streptomycin injections (40,000 units/kg/day) gave 100 per cent survival, even when administration was delayed for 48 hours after infection. Streptomycin was more effective than sulfathiazole, and penicillin was only slightly effective. K. F. Meyer, S. F. Quan, and A. Larson ("Prophylactic immunization and specific therapy of experimental pneumonic plague," Am. Rev. Tuberc., **57**:312, 1948) also concluded that thus far the most effective therapeutic agent known for plague was streptomycin. "Over 90 per cent of experimentally infected mice, when in the septicemic state of lobular plague pneumonia, may be cured with 5 mg. of streptomycin. It is recommended that human pneumonic plague be treated early in the course of the infection with daily doses of 4 to 6 gms. of streptomycin, and that treatment should continue for not less than six to ten days."

15. KARAMCHANDI, P. V., and RAO, K. Sundar. Streptomycin in human plague, Lancet, **1**:22, 1948.

These writers were the first to report the use of streptomycin in human plague. They described five cases, all extremely ill, whose temperatures promptly became normal after about 4 gm. of streptomycin over a period of 36 hours. A little later Ch. Haddock and A. Valero ("Streptomycin in bubonic plague," Brit. M.J., **1**:1026, 1948), working in Haifa, treated with streptomycin three patients who did not respond to sulfonamides, with speedy recovery. The buboes appeared to be uninfluenced if treated late and required incision and drainage. C. H. Huang, C. Y. Huang, L. W. Chu, and T. F. Huang ("Pneumonic plague," Am. J. Trop. Med., **28**:361, 1948) report a case of proved primary pneumonic plague in which recovery took place following continued therapy with sulfonamides and streptomycin. P. Wagle ("Recent advances in the treatment of bubonic plague," Indian J.M. Sc., **2**:489, 1948) also found streptomycin the most effective drug. In cases with heavy blood-stream invasion, the mortality of patients treated with serum was 100 per cent, with sulfadiazine 50 per cent, and with streptomycin 27.2 per cent. From this time on, numerous confirmatory papers appeared. K. F. Meyer ("Modern therapy of plague," J.A.M.A., **144**:982, 1950) summarized the whole matter of therapy. Streptomycin is advised as the agent of choice, to be supplemented in very severe cases by oral use of aureomycin, chloramphenicol, or terramycin, as well as antiplague immune serum globulin. If antibiotics are not available, the sulfonamides (sulfadiazine or sulfamerazine) are advised.

16. SOKHEY, S. S., and HABBU, M. K. Aureomycin and chloromycetin in the treatment of experimental plague, Indian J.M. Research, **38**:197, 1950.

The writers found both these antibiotics highly effective in experimental plague in mice. Even when given after septicemia had developed, a suitable dose saved almost all the animals. These drugs had the advantage over streptomycin in being effective when given by mouth, and this was the first report on their use in plague. A little later K. Ramachandran ("Treatment of plague with aureomycin," J. Indian M.A., **21**:217, 1952) cured thirteen of fifteen cases of bubonic and septicemic plague by use of aureomycin. F. R. McCrumb and others ("Chloramphenicol and terramycin in the treatment of pneumonic plague," Am. J. Med., **14**:284, 1953) found in pneumonic plague that either chloramphenicol, terramycin, or streptomycin produced dramatic clinical response in those patients receiving therapy prior to the twentieth hour.

In summary, then, the position as to therapy seems at present (1957) as follows: "Immune" sera have had a checkered career for many years. None of them seems very effective. Perhaps used very early, they have slight protective and antitoxic effects in mild cases. Sulfonamides, especially sulfadiazine, have a definite therapeutic effect, especially when used early in mild cases. The antibiotics—streptomycin, aureomycin, terramycin, and chloramphenicol—seem by far the most potent weapons, since they have cured advanced, septicemic, and pneumonic cases. The question of modern therapy is discussed and documented by Pollitzer (*op. cit.*, chap. 8, p. 409, "Clinical aspects").

17. ONESTI, Silvio J. Plague, press, and politics, Stanford M. Bull., **13**:1, 1955.

It has happened repeatedly that public officials have refused to acknowledge the presence of plague when the disease had obviously appeared in their midst. Such was the case in San Francisco in the outbreak of 1900. The story of this incident is vividly told and fully documented by Onesti. "The account of the bubonic plague in San Francisco is one of the darkest pages in the history of North American medicine."

Section 5

BRUCELLA INFECTION

Bacteriology	Refs. 2, 3, 4, 9, 13, 14, 15, 19, 27, 29
Blood, in	Ref. 36
Cattle, relation to brucellosis	Refs. 9, 31
Chronic or ambulatory form	Refs. 8, 17
Clinical	Refs. 1, 2, 3, 4, 5, 8, 10, 20, 22, 31
Diagnosis	Ref. 44
Epidemiology	Ref. 20
General	Refs. 1, 2, 3, 4, 6, 12
Goats, relation to Malta fever	Refs. 16, 18
Immunology	Refs. 11, 25, 26, 28
Mode of infection	Refs. 21, 23, 32
Pathology	Refs. 24, 30, 34, 43
Serum diagnosis	Refs. 7, 8, 26
Treatment	Refs. 35, 37, 38, 39, 40, 41, 42

Section 5

BRUCELLA INFECTION

THE book by Surgeon-Captain Louis Hughes (Ref. 6) is generally accepted as the storehouse of information on the early knowledge of Malta fever. I. F. Huddleson's monograph, *Brucellosis in Man and Animals* (New York: Commonwealth Fund, 1943), contains much useful general, as well as bacteriological, information and has a comprehensive bibliography. The monograph by H. J. Harris, *Brucellosis (Undulant Fever), Clinical and Subclinical* (2d ed.; New York: Paul B. Hoeber, 1950), is also to be mentioned. This volume of some six hundred pages deals with every phase of the subject; under the heading of "Symptomatology," for example, all the rare clinical phenomena of brucellosis, such as endocarditis, ocular troubles, intermittent hydrarthrosis, and others, are described with references to the literature. However, the recent authoritative work of W. W. Spink, *The Nature of Brucellosis* (Minneapolis: University of Minnesota Press, 1956), with bibliography of some nine hundred titles, supersedes all previous books on the disease. With regard to the bacteriology of brucellosis, the article by J. T. Duncan, L. E. H. Whitby, and A. D. McEwen in *A System of Bacteriology in Relation to Medicine* (London: H.M. Stationery Office, 1930), ch. ix, p. 386) is authoritative and comprehensive, as is the section in Topley and Wilson's *Principles of Bacteriology and Immunity* (3d ed.; Baltimore: Williams & Wilkins Co., 1946), 2:1692. As to general bibliographies, Hughes's book contains a comprehensive list of references to the early literature (Ref. 6, p. 29) and is supplemented by a compilation of publications from 1897 to 1907 by J. W. H. Eyre in the British Commission *Reports* (Ref. 12), Part V, (1907), p. 66.

1. MARSTON, J. A. Report on fever (Malta), Army Medical Department, Statistical, Sanitary, and Medical Reports for the Year 1861, p. 486. London: Harrison & Sons, 1863.

Although it is probable that "Malta fever" had existed for a long time in the Mediterranean Basin, the early accounts of fevers in this location were too confused for intelligent classification.[1] Marston discussed the fevers seen at Malta and, after separating typhoid and some others, gives, we believe, the first recognizable account of Malta fever under the designation of "Mediterranean remittent." "By this is meant a fever characterized by the following symptoms and course: A preliminary stage of subacute dyspepsia, anorexia, nausea, headaches, feeling of weakness, lassitude, and inaptitude for exertion, mental or physical, chills, muscular pains; lastly a fever having a very long course—three to five, or ten weeks—marked by irregular exacerbations and remissions, great derangement of the assimilative organs, tenderness in epigastric region, splenic enlargement, slight jaundice, without any exanthem. Neither

---

[1] The book by William Burnett (*A Practical Account of the Mediterranean Fever, as It Appeared in the Ships and Hospitals of His Majesty's Fleet on That Station: With Cases and Dissections* [London: J. Callow, 1816]) is mentioned as giving an early account of Malta fever, but one searches through it in vain for anything that can be recognized as the disease in question.

bronchitis or diarrhoea as a rule. The patient is prone to relapses, and the disorder is followed by a protracted convalescence and chloroanaemic aspect; very frequently also by rheumatism of some form or other, but without any tendency to lesion of the peri- or endocardial membranes. Pathologically, it is marked by congestion or inflammation, with softening of the enteric mucous membrane, without any lesion of Peyerian follicles, but with hypertrophies of liver and spleen. There is no fever so irregular as this in its course and symptoms. . . . Convalescent stage. It is now that the anaemic, but puffy-looking face, and the dejaded [*sic*] look attract attention. Supposing that no relapses occur, the patient rarely recovers perfectly without suffering from rheumatism or some form of neuralgia." The cause of the disease Marston guessed to be filth and poor sanitation.

However, there was no clear general recognition of the disease until Bruce (Ref. 2) isolated the causal organism, as is shown by the confusion displayed in contemporary accounts (G. F. Duffey, "On rheumatic orchitis as a sequel to fever," Dublin J.M. Sc., **53**:97, 1872; W. C. McLean, "On 'Malta Fever'; with a suggestion," Brit. M.J., **2**:224, 1875; O. G. Wood, "Malta fever," Edinburgh M.J., **22**:40, 1876; J. Lane Notter, "On Malta fever," Edinburgh M.J., **22**:289, 1876).

2. BRUCE, David. Note on the discovery of a micro-organism in Malta fever, Practitioner, **39**:161, 1887.

Bruce, working in the army at the Station Hospital at Valletta, Malta, began his paper as follows: "This fever . . . has a wide distribution in the Mediterranean. It is identical with the Rock fever of Gibraltar, the Neapolitan fever of Naples, the Country fever of Constantinople, and the New fever of Crete. . . . On further investigation I have no doubt this list could be much enlarged. . . ." Although a good deal has been written on the clinical aspects, "there is, as far as I am aware, no notice regarding the presence of micro-organisms in the organs of fatal cases."

Bruce next sketched the clinical features: "It is a disease of long duration, ninety-one cases . . . having an average stay in hospital of 85.5 days. The fever which often runs high, is continued, remittent and intermittent in type. . . . An undulatory type of curve is frequently observed, the undulations being separated by a period of apyrexia. . . . Sometimes these undulations persist for a long time: in one case I observed two well-marked waves between the 120th and 160th days of the disease." Bruce also emphasized enlarged spleen, sweats, constipation, bronchitis, pains, swelling of joints, and orchitis. "The mortality is as a rule exceedingly small."

Five fatal cases were examined for micro-organisms, the first by means of stained sections, the remaining four by inoculation into tubes containing agaragar nutrient jelly. In the first case sections of spleen stained by Gram's method and also with methylene blue showed enormous numbers of single micrococci scattered through the tissues. Bruce next inoculated blood from severe cases, obtained by puncturing the fingertip, into tubes of agar; they remained sterile except for two which were obviously contaminated. Bits of spleen were also inoculated into the tubes. Growth was slow, but it appeared in all the tubes placed in the incubator at 37° C. after a period of 68 hours. "The growth appeared at first as minute pearly-white spots scattered around the point of puncture. Small round colonies could be seen along the needle track . . . examined under a high power, innumerable small micrococci are seen." Similar findings were obtained in three other fatal cases. "From a consideration of the above facts I think it will appear to be sufficiently proved: (*a*) that there exists in the spleen of cases of Malta fever a definite micro-organism; and (*b*) that this micro-organism can be cultivated outside of the human body. . . . I have already cultivated four successive generations. It remains now to be seen what effect, if any, this micro-organism has on healthy animals . . . where it is to be found; how it gains entrance to its human host; and many other points." Curiously enough, Bruce did not state whether the organism was Gram-positive or -negative. He did emphasize the absence of intestinal lesions, thus eliminating confusion with "enteric" fever.

In a second paper ("The micrococcus of Malta fever," *ibid.*, **40**:241, 1888) Bruce obtained the same organism from another fatal case and described it more in detail: "It is oval in form and measures from .0008 millimetres to .001 millimetres. . . . In sections they are seen to be scattered singly or in pairs throughout the substance of the tissue, and never occur in masses." "One fact to be noted is the rapidity with which the micrococci became wholly unstained by the addition of absolute alcohol." The organism showed no sign of growth at a temperature below 22° C. Bruce gave a frequency curve of case incidence; most cases occurred during May–August, but some were encountered even in winter. Bruce injected some culture into a monkey's arm; after a severe febrile illness the animal died, and the organism was recovered from spleen and liver. Small animals, on the whole, gave negative or doubtful results on inoculation.

3. BRUCE, David. Observations on Malta fever, Brit. M.J., **1**:1101, 1889. Bruce, no longer in Malta but now assistant professor of pathology at the Royal Victoria Hospital, Netley, writes a masterful systematic article on Malta fever. He begins with "Definition. An endemic disease of long duration, characterized by fever, continuous, remittent and intermittent in type, in most cases enlarged spleen, profuse perspiration, sudamina, constipation, relapses almost invariably, accompanied by pains of a rheumatic or neuralgic character, sometimes swelling of joints or orchitis, ending almost always in complete recovery; in fatal cases enlargement and softening of spleen, congestion of the duodenum and upper part of jejunum, no swelling or ulceration of Peyer's glands, and the constant occurrence in various organs of a species of micrococcus." These various features are next analyzed in detail; the prevalent view that this, like many other fevers, was due to sewage, "bad air," or bad smells is discussed. Bruce points out that young adults are most frequently affected; that Malta fever alternates with enteric fever, from which and from malaria it must be differentiated; that whether or not one attack conveys immunity is uncertain. The details of symptoms are analyzed in brilliant fashion as the differential diagnosis is discussed. As to pathologic changes, Bruce describes as the principal lesion proliferation of endothelial cells in lymph nodes, spleen, and other organs, together with congestion, cloudy swelling, and in certain situations infiltration of small round cells. The lesions of typhoid and malaria are definitely absent. He concludes: "1. Malta fever is a specific disease. . . . 2. It is caused by the entrance into the system of a minute parasite. 3. No drug at present known has any power of modifying the action of the bacteria in the system. 4. Treatment is to be principally directed to keeping up the patient's strength by fluid, easily digested

food, and, when required, by stimulants, and by attention to ordinary hygienic principles. Removal of the patient from the infective area does not cut short the course of the fever."

Bruce knew nothing of the chronic low-grade forms of infection; he thought of the disease as analogous to typhoid. In these papers there is also no mention of goats or any implication that they are concerned with the disease. The mode of entry of the organism was a complete mystery.

In still another paper ("Notes on Mediterranean or Malta fever. I. Its bacteriology," Brit. M.J., **2**:58, 1893) Bruce added still more observations, all confirmatory. He produced the disease in several monkeys, from which he again recovered the organism, which he now called *Micrococcus melitensis.*[2] A beautiful undulating temperature chart from Monkey VI is reproduced, extending over a period of 98 days. The bacteriologic features are redescribed, and Bruce now states that the organism is Gram-negative.

4. HUGHES, Louis. Investigations into the etiology of Mediterranean fevers, Lancet, **2**:1265, 1892.

A. G. P. Gipps ("On Malta fever," Tr. Epidemiol. Soc. London, N.S., **9**:76, 1891) isolated an organism similar to that of Bruce from two cases of Malta fever, but Hughes's work, also done in Malta, was much more extensive. Hughes again described the disease: "Clinically it has a peculiarly irregular temperature curve, consisting of intermittent waves of pyrexia of a distinctly remittent type, each wave lasting from one to three weeks, with generally an apyrexial interval of two or three days. . . . This pyrexial condition is usually very chronic, lasting even six months or more, and is not markedly affected by quinine or arsenic. It is usually accompanied by obstinate constipation, progressive anemia and debility, and is followed, in a large number of cases, by very chronic neuralgic and rheumatic complications from which the patient may not recover for perhaps two years. The death rate is very low; but as the average stay in hospital is 70 to 90 days the expense incurred by the State . . . has reached an enormous sum." Hughes recovered the organism from the spleens of five fatal cases; he carried it through six generations of pure culture. In two cases it was demonstrable microscopically in fresh splenic substance. The organism was not found in other disorders, such as enteric fever. Hughes produced the disease in series in monkeys. He gave a detailed description of the organism and its cultural characteristics. He emphasized the slow-growing, delicate character of its growth on the available media. He concluded that the presence of the organism was connected with human excrement, but he also believed "that the poison of this fever, when infecting the human body, is aerial in nature . . . and that in most cases it enters the human frame by way of the air passages." No mention was made of goats.

It is of interest that both Bruce and Hughes were so imbued with the current theories of miasms that they were reluctant to give up the idea of air-borne infection, even though they had produced Malta fever in monkeys by subcutaneous injection.

---

[2] "This morn we came near Malta, or, as 'twas called formerly Melita, from the abundance of honey they have there, gathered by the bees from the aniseeds and flowers thereof, which grow on this island abundantly" (*The Diary of Henry Teonge, Chaplain on Board H.M.'s Ships Assistance, British and Royal Oak, 1675–1679* [New York: Harper & Bros., 1927]).

Both Bruce ("Sur une nouvelle forme de fièvre rencontré sur les bords de la Méditerranée," Ann. Inst. Pasteur, 7:289, 1893) and Hughes ("Sur une forme de fièvre fréquent sur les côtes de la Méditerranée," Ann. Inst. Pasteur, 7:628, 1893) wrote systematic articles on the disease in 1893, using mainly their old material. Hughes concluded his paper in rather confused fashion: "It appears to be a contagious fever of a mobile type [*d'un type mobile*] characterized by an indefinite duration and an irregular course caused by a poisoning of the blood of fecal origin and capable of assuming an aerial organized form." Bruce, on the other hand, was more clear: "I believe I have shown that the *Micrococcus melitensis* is the cause of Mediterranean fever and that this is an absolutely specific disease distinct from typhoid and malaria. As to the important question of the mode of entry of the parasite into man whether by air, water or food one does not know yet, and the difficulty in growing the organism is an obstacle in answering this question."

5. HUGHES, M. Louis. Undulant (Malta) fever, Lancet, **2**:238, 1896.

Hughes first gives an immense list of the names which have been applied to the disease and, after criticizing them, suggests the designation "undulant fever." "It has occurred to me that the term 'Undulant Fever' by referring to the peculiar pyrexial curve so characteristic of the disease, might prove a serviceable name. The name appeals forcibly to the clinical observer, who standing in a ward surrounded by cases of this fever (as anyone may do in summer in any of the military hospitals of Malta) gazes at the temperature charts on the walls and notices the way in which the recorded pyrexial curves undulate across the paper in waves of varying degree."

6. HUGHES, M. Louis. Mediterranean, Malta or undulant fever. London: Macmillan & Co., 1897.

This book is a landmark in the history of the subject, as Hughes summarized in authoritative fashion all that was known to date about the disease. "When the writer arrived in Malta towards the end of the year 1890, for a six year tour of service in that place, he found that his medical work would chiefly consist, during the greater part of the year, of treating a fever about which no two medical officers appeared to agree, respecting its cause, treatment, or even name. Some even doubted its specific nature, calling it a variety of enteric or malarial fever, and until the writer had been present at a post-mortem examination on a fatal case, he was himself prejudiced in favour of all serious cases being of an enteric [typhoid] nature. The fallacy of this theory soon became apparent, and extended clinical and pathological experience showed how much there was to learn, and how little to guide anyone, in the study of this important fever." Hughes himself acquired Malta fever and learned first hand about it. (Preface.) He gave the following definition of the disease, on which he elaborated at length: "An endemic pyrexial disease, occasionally prevailing as an epidemic, having a long and indefinite duration, an irregular course with an almost invariable tendency to undulatory pyrexial relapses. It is usually characterized by constipation, profuse perspirations, and accompanied or followed by symptoms of a neuralgic character. Ofter accompanied by swelling and effusion of the joints and other rheumatoid symptoms. After death, the spleen is found to be enlarged and often softened, many of the organs congested, but Peyer's glands neither enlarged nor ulcerated, nor is ulceration present in other parts of the small intestine. There is a constant occurrence in certain tissues of a definite species of micro-organism" (p. 1). He insisted that undulant fever was a specific disease, to be clearly distinguished from typhoid fever and malaria; he discussed the differential diagnosis in detail. He gave arguments in favor of the name he had suggested—undulant fever. Then comes a historical sketch of the disease of the greatest value, followed by an invaluable bibliography through 1897, giving many references not to be found anywhere else. The next chapter deals with a description of the organism and the results of animal inoculation. As to predisposing causes Hughes went wrong, like all before him, and vaguely blamed the disease on lack of sanitation, which certainly was outstanding in Malta at the time and is graphically described. Goats are not mentioned anywhere in the book. While the disease occurred throughout the year, most cases were in July, August, and September. Apparently, one attack conferred immunity. Hughes distinguished malignant cases—very severe, although rarely fatal, the undulatory type ("finally the patient is reduced to an emaciated, anaemic, and bed-ridden condition"), an intermittent type, and irregular and mixed types. There is a brilliant section on symptoms—with illustrative temperature curves—in which every phase of the clinical features is analyzed. The overall mortality was about 2 per cent. The gross morbid changes at autopsy were not very striking; the spleen was invariably enlarged and congested. Microscopically the appearances "are not in any way specially characteristic of undulant fever, but rather those of severe and prolonged pyrexia acting on the tissues of the body." Neither Hughes nor Bruce apparently found the specific lesion described later (Refs. 24, 30). As to treatment: "There is no drug of a specific nature at present known which will cut short an attack of the fever by its action on the virus as does quinine in ague, and mercury in syphilis."

7. WRIGHT, A. E., and SMITH, F. On the application of the serum test to the differential diagnosis of typhoid and Malta fever, Lancet, 1:656, 1897.

Wright, who was an early pioneer in serodiagnosis of infections, described the technique of his method. Serum from the patient was mixed with young cultures of various bacteria in capillary tubes. A positive test was indicated by macroscopic clumping. Wright was able, by means of this test, to differentiate clinically doubtful cases of Malta fever and typhoid fever. In another paper (A. E. Wright and D. Semple, "On the employment of dead bacteria in the serum diagnosis of typhoid and Malta fever," Brit. M.J., 1:1214, 1897), the use of dead cultures was introduced and found to give just as definite results as live organisms. Wright and Semple spoke of the advantages of this method to the general practitioner: "It will obviously be possible for every medical man to obtain a supply of capsules of dead typhoid and Malta fever bacteria for serum diagnosis from a central laboratory. He will be able to carry about these cultures without risk."

8. MUSSER, J. H., and SAILER, Joseph. A case of Malta fever, Philadelphia M.J., 2:1408, 1898.

The writers report a typical case of "Malta fever" in an army officer, who had probably contracted the disease in Puerto Rico. A characteristic chart of prolonged undulating fever is shown, and the patient's serum agglutinated a culture of Bruce's organism in a dilution of about 1:50. In "Further notes on a case of Malta fever; a study in serum diagnosis," *ibid.*, **4**:89, 1899, they give a follow-up report on this patient, whose fever dragged along and whose serum repeatedly agglutinated *Micrococcus melitensis* but gave no Widal reaction for typhoid.

This is claimed to be the first case reported in the Western Hemisphere.[3] Charles F. Craig ("The symptomatology and diagnosis of Malta fever with the report of additional cases," Internat. Clin., **4**:89, 15th Ser., 1906) described instances from the army, including one of a nurse who had never been out of the country, apparently the first recorded indigenous case. Her serum aggluti-nated the organism in a dilution of 1:250. Craig also referred to chronic cases: "In many cases of Malta fever, however, after the initial attack, a chronic in-fection results and is characterized by symptoms so slight as to be almost un-recognizable unless watched for and understood." He pointed out that this form of the disease was often confused with chronic arthritis and muscular rheuma-tism, and he reported examples. Malaria, typhoid fever, tuberculosis, pneu-monia, septicemia, relapsing fever, Hodgkin's disease, and articular rheumatism are to be considered in the differential diagnosis. He also emphasized the lack of pathognomonic symptoms, postulated a wide unrecognized distribution of the disease and the importance of applying the "serum-test" in all undetermined cases of fever in all regions. Thus Craig definitely widened the concept of the disease from that of the early writers (see also Ref. 17).

    9. BANG, B. Die Aetiologie des seuchenhaften ("infectiösen") Ververfens, Ztschr. f. Thiermed., **1**:241, 1897.

Abortion of cattle had long been considered contagious. J. Penberthy ("Enzo-ötic abortion," J. Comp. Path. & Therap., **8**:100, 1895) quoted a statement in the *Complete Farmer* for 1807 as follows: "It is considered certainly contagious and when it happens the abortion should be immediately buried and the cow kept as widely apart as possible from the herd." As the bacteriologic era de-veloped, it was inevitable that an infectious agent should be sought. Nocard, for example ("Recherches sur l'avortement épizootique des vaches," Rec. de méd. vét., **3**:669, 1886), made cultures from the puriform material laid down be-tween the uterus and ovum and isolated two types of bacteria—micrococci and short, thick bacilli. Although he was not able to grow them in pure culture, it is highly probable that the "micrococci" were identical with *B. abortus*. Bang was able to obtain the generative organs fresh from a cow in which abortion was threatened. Cultures were made within 6 hours of death. When the uterus was opened under aseptic conditions, "we saw between the mucosa and the egg an abundant, non-odorous exudate . . . the examination of cover glass preparations of this material stained with methylene blue (Loeffler) immediately disclosed the presence of very small bacteria apparently in pure culture. . . . Infectious abortion is to be considered as the consequence of a specific uterine catarrh caused by a special bacterium." Bang was able to grow the organism in pure culture in deep tubes of serum gelatin agar, in which colonies appeared in a

---

[3] The cases of J. M. Da Costa ("Protracted continued fever," Am. J.M. Sc., **3**:629, 1896), sometimes mentioned in the literature as being instances of brucellosis, are too indefinite to allow any conclusions. Such cases at the time were often called typhoid-malaria, the designation used in the first run of the Surgeon-General's catalogue.

definite zone about 0.5 cm. under the surface and 1–1.5 cm. thick. No colonies grew above or below this zone, which indicated that the organism was sensitive to oxygen tension. The colonies were small and round and consisted of small bacilli of the same appearance as those found in the uterine exudate. Further cultural characteristics are given. Bang soon obtained material from twenty-one cases of contagious abortion and the *"Abortusbacilli"* were found in practically all. In two experiments, in which a pure culture of the bacillus was introduced into the vagina of the cow, abortion followed. "By these two observations we have brought full proof that the organisms discovered by us are the cause of epidemic abortion." "We have had no opportunity to experiment with goats," but "a colleague saw a goat abort living in a stable where cows had previously aborted. This makes it highly likely that our bacillus is also infectious for goats." Here, then, is the first hint of a relation between Malta fever of goats and contagious abortion of cattle.

Bang's work was soon confirmed by Hugo Preisz ("Der Bacillus des seuchenhaften Ververfens," Centralbl. f. Bakt., **33**:190, 1903) and subsequently by many other workers.

10. BIRT, C., and LAMB, G. Mediterranean or Malta fever, Lancet, **2**:701, 1899.

Final direct proof of the causal role of *M. melitensis* in Malta fever was brought by laboratory infections, two of which were reported by these authors. In one case a man accidentally scratched himself with the needle of a syringe with which he had just injected living growth into a horse. Fifteen days later he went through a typical attack of Malta fever. In a second case a man injected a small amount of agar culture into his arm. Sixteen days later, symptoms set in, and he pursued a characteristic course. K. F. Meyer and B. Eddie ("Laboratory infections due to Brucella," J. Infect. Dis., **68**:24, 1941) later reported and analyzed "74 histories of brucellosis observed among bacteriologists, pathologists and other workers who in the course of their duties were exposed to Brucella in the laboratories of the United States." They adduced evidence that "injections with dead vaccines fail to prevent laboratory infections."

11. LEISHMAN, W. B. Some experiments in connection with "stimulins," Tr. Path. Soc. London, **56**:344, 1905.

Leishman, working in the early days of studies on phagocytosis and opsonins ("stimulins"), showed that ingestion of *M. melitensis* by leukocytes was tremendously increased by adding a little Malta fever convalescent serum to the mixture. The average number of germs phagocyted by each polynuclear was increased, for example, from 17.6 to 70. I. F. Huddleson, H. W. Johnson, and E. E. Hamann ("A study of the opsono-cytophagic power of the blood and allergic skin reaction in Brucella infection and immunity in man," Am. J. Pub. Health, **23**:917, 1933) later elaborated and laid stress on this test, along with a skin test, as an indication of infection with Brucella. "Infection in an individual is indicated by a positive allergic skin test obtained with Brucella nucleoprotein in conjunction with negative or low opsono-cytophagic activity of the whole citrated blood for Brucella." The value of this test has been variously judged by others (Ref. 44).

12. Reports of the Commission appointed by the Admiralty, the War Office and the Civil Government of Malta, for the investigation of Mediterranean fever, under the supervision of an Advisory Committee of the Royal Society, Parts I–VII. London: Harrison & Sons, 1905–7.

"The Mediterranean Fever Commission had its origin in a letter from Mr. Secretary Lyttleton, dated January 25, 1904, addressed to the Royal Society, in which he states that his attention has recently been called to the prevalence of Mediterranean fever in Malta among th Naval and Military forces, as well as the civil population.

"It accordingly appeared to him to be desirable that the investigation of this fever should be taken in hand, and he addressed a despatch to the Governor of Malta proposing the appointment of a joint Commission representing the Army, the Navy and the Civil Government."

The Royal Society nominated a committee to direct the investigations, which were published in seven parts over a period of three years. Every phase of the subject was studied—bacteriology, epidemiology, relation of the disease to goats, transmission to animals, and clinical features. In the final section, practical recommendations for controlling Malta fever were made. The commission did monumental work and really "skimmed the cream" in the study of the disease. In subsequent sections we shall mention some of the most important individual studies; they will be listed under the heading "British Commission."

13. HORROCKS, W. H. Further studies on the saprophytic existence of Micrococcus melitensis, British Commission, Part I, p. 14, 1905.

The author concluded: "1. The M. melitensis retains its vitality in sterilized tap water for 37 days. 2. In a Maltese soil, allowed to dry naturally, the M. melitensis survives 43 days. . . . 3. The M. melitensis survives for 72 days in a damp soil. 4. Exposure to the sun for a few hours kills the M. melitensis. 5. The M. melitensis survives for 25 days in sterilized sea-water."

14. HORROCKS, W. H. On the recovery of the Micrococcus melitensis from the urine, faeces, and sweat of patients suffering from Mediterranean fever, British Commission, Part I, p. 21, 1905.

Horrocks isolated the organism from the urine of many patients from the fifteenth to the eighty-second day of disease; he was unable to isolate it from feces or sweat. J. Crawford Kennedy ("On the recovery of Micrococcus melitensis from the urine of Mediterranean fever patients," British Commission, Part III, p. 56, 1905) recovered the organism from 186 of 1,974 samples of urine examined. He found that excretion would appear to be of two kinds: (1) an enormous sudden gush or (2) a long-continued excretion of small quantities. Bacteremia continued in some cases after the patients had been discharged as clinically well.

15. GILMOUR, R. T. Description of a method of cultivating the Micrococcus melitensis from small quantities of peripheral blood and inoculation experiments with the micro-organisms isolated, British Commission, Part I, p. 73, 1905.

Gilmour drew blood by venipuncture and succeeded in isolating *M. melitensis* in broth culture. It is of interest that preparation for the procedure consisted of shaving the arm, scrubbing with brush and carbolic soap, with sterile nail brush and water, for 20 minutes, swabbing with ether for 10 minutes, and, finally, scrubbing with perchloride of mercury for ¼ hour. "A sterile dressing should then be applied, soaked in the same disinfectant, until the time of the operation [the venipuncture], about 24 hours afterwards." E. A. Shaw ("Interim report of experimental work, etc.," British Commission, Part I, p. 95, 1905) summarized the work of the commission to date and pointed out with reference to blood culture that the organism existed in the circulation "in relatively very small amount"; that it might be isolated at any stage of the disease, as early as the 7th day, as late as the 98th, and even after the temperature had been normal for several days, as in Keefer's case (Ref. 31); and that there was no regular relation between the number of organisms in the blood and its agglutinating power. In a still later paper, Shaw ("On the quantitative bacteriological examination of the blood of 103 Mediterranean fever patients," British Commission, Part III, p. 5, 1905) reported isolation of the organism in about two-thirds of the patients. "M. melitensis exists in the blood in relatively small amount, not having been found in association with a less quantity of blood than 4 cu. mm., and that only in two cases out of 103."

16. HORROCKS, W. H. Preliminary note on goats as a means of propagation of Mediterranean fever, Proc. Roy. Soc. London, **76**:378, 1905.

Horrocks wished to ascertain, by experimental inoculation, whether goats could be infected by *M. melitensis.* Preliminary examination of the animals showed, however, that their serum agglutinated the organism in dilutions up to 1:300 and that cultures of milk, even when the goat appeared well, often yielded *M. melitensis.* Horrocks concluded: "The results obtained show that some of the goats in every herd examined are suffering from Mediterranean fever. The M. melitensis is exuded in the milk in enormous numbers when the disease has been present sufficiently long. . . ." He also isolated the organism from the urine of goats "when the disease has existed for some time."

Associated in this work with Horrocks was Dr. T. Zammit, who actually carried out the first agglutination tests with the sera of six goats ("A preliminary note on the examination of the blood of goats suffering from Mediterranean fever," British Commission, Part III, p. 83, 1905). This was the first proof that goats were of importance in the transmission of Malta fever. Horrocks, with J. C. Kennedy ("Goats as a means of propagation of Mediterranean fever," British Commission, Part IV, p. 37, 1906), later elaborated his early studies. He found that 41 per cent of the goats in Malta were infected, judged by the serum reaction, and that 10 per cent of the goats supplying milk appeared to excrete *M. melitensis,* often with no change in the physical characteristics of the milk and without the animal's exhibiting signs of ill-health. Excretion was often intermittent. Monkeys and goats were infected by feeding cultures or by feeding infected milk, with an incubation period of 3–4 weeks. Goats also became infected by feeding on dust polluted with urine from patients. Finally, Horrocks found that pasteurization (68° C. for 10 minutes) destroyed the *M. melitensis* in infected goat's milk.

17. SHAW, E. A. The ambulatory type of case in Mediterranean or Malta fever, British Commission, Part IV, p. 8, 1906.

Shaw examined the blood of 525 dockyard workers, all apparently healthy. Among these a markedly positive reaction was given by the blood serum in 22 cases. On taking the temperatures, several had slight elevations of over 99°. From 3 of these cases *M. melitensis* was recovered from both blood and urine; from 1 it was obtained from the blood only, and from 6 from the urine only. The author concluded that the existence of ambulatory cases, previously uncertain, is now proved (see also Craig, Ref. 8).

Observations of this sort have been repeatedly made throughout the years, as, for example, by Parker Dooley ("Undulant fever, an epidemic of subclinical infection with Brucella," Arch. Int. Med., **50**:373, 1932), who found that in a group of 263 persons using infected raw milk, 41 per cent were found to have serum agglutinins against *Brucella abortus*, and 2 had clinical undulant fever.

This phase of the subject has recently been subjected to penetrating analysis by W. W. Spink ("What is chronic brucellosis?" Ann. Int. Med., **35**:358, 1951). He discusses the vague entity often diagnosed as chronic brucellosis and sets up criteria which justify a positive diagnosis.

18. SHAW, E. A. Mediterranean fever in goats, cows, and other animals, British Commission, Part IV, p. 16, 1906.

Shaw infected goats experimentally and also studied the incidence of natural infection. Of 96 goats in full milk, 30 were found to have sera which agglutinated *M. melitensis*. Organisms were recovered from the milk in 9 of these, and their infectivity was demonstrated on a monkey. Shaw thought that the most likely route of infection was via the gastrointestinal tract. It is of great interest that he found 10 of 33 *cows* infected; *M. melitensis* was recovered from the milk of 2 of them. No relation was sensed, however, between these findings and those of Bang (Ref. 9).

19. KENNEDY, J. Crawford. Bacteriological examination of cases of Mediterranean fever, British Commission, Part IV, p. 92, 1906.

In post-mortem material *M. melitensis* was frequently recovered from spleen, liver, kidney, lymph nodes, bone marrow, and bile but never from intestines, salivary glands, tonsils, pleural or cerebrospinal fluid.

20. DAVIES, A. M. Report on the prevalence of Mediterranean fever amongst British troops in Malta, 1905, British Commission, Part IV, p. 105, 1906.

It is of interest that at the end of this elaborate study the writer concluded that water and milk had nothing to do with transmission but that infection most likely occurred "by direct or semi-direct contagion or through the agency of mosquitos."

21. EYRE, J. W. H., McNAUGHT, J. G., KENNEDY, J. C., and ZAMMIT, T. Report upon the bacteriological and experimental investigations during the summer of 1906, British Commission, Part VI, p. 3, 1907.

This report contains, among other interesting material, an account of the famous incident of the outbreak of Mediterranean fever on board the S.S. "Joshua Nicholson," which was transporting 61 milch goats from Malta to Antwerp, where they were transferred to the S.S. "St. Andrew" bound for New York. During the voyage the personnel of the ship drank largely of goat's milk, and a considerable number acquired Malta fever. Thus there was carried out an "unpremeditated experiment" in transmission of the disease from goat to man.

A more complete history of this outbreak is given by F. H. A. Clayton (British Commission, Part VII, p. 107, 1907).

Among the conclusions of this report were the following: The most common method of acquiring the disease is by the ingestion of infected articles of food—mainly milk. The next common path of infection is by subcutaneous inoculation (see also Ref. 32) during the handling of contaminated material—usually milk. *Micrococcus melitensis* is not destroyed during the process incident upon the manufacture of the ordinary ice creams or of the native cheeses, and it may be present in the retail articles, living and unaltered in virulence.

As a result of these studies, the writers drew up "Recommendations as to preventive measures in connection with Mediterranean fever in Malta," of which the main points were the control of infected animals and the elimination of infection in foodstuffs.

22. FERENBAUGH, Thomas L. Endemic Mediterranean fever (Malta fever) in Southwest Texas," J.A.M.A., **57**:730, 1911.

Ferenbaugh first suspected that the "goat fever" which occurred in young men working in a "goat camp" in the Pecos River country was really Malta fever. He reported four patients with indeterminate prolonged fever whose sera all gave positive agglutination tests with *M. melitensis*. In a second paper with Gentry (E. R. Gentry and T. L. Ferenbaugh, "Endemic Malta [Mediterranean] fever in Texas with the isolation of the Micrococcus melitensis from two patients," J.A.M.A., **57**:889, 1911) he isolated the organism in broth cultures from two more patients. In a third paper, Gentry and Ferenbaugh ("Endemic Malta [Mediterranean] fever in Texas," *ibid.*, p. 1045) made an epidemiologic study, in which they demonstrated infection by means of agglutination tests in 34 per cent of the goats examined. "All cases of Malta fever found have occurred in territory devoted to goat-raising and all patients either gave a history of drinking unboiled goat's milk or were actively connected with the goat-raising industry." Finally, in a fourth paper ("Malta fever in Texas," *ibid.*, p. 1127), Gentry and Ferenbaugh reported more extensive observations on infection among the bands of goats, of which there were approximately 175,000, raised for the mohair which they produced. They suggested that infection arose from dust as well as from drinking milk. These studies were of great importance because they demonstrated endemic infection in a goat-raising area in the United States quite analogous to the situation in Malta.

23. SCHROEDER, E. C., and COTTON, W. E. II. The bacillus of infectious abortion found in milk: Twenty-eighth Annual Report of the Bureau of Animal Industry, U.S. Department of Agriculture, Washington, p. 139, 1911.

During routine tests for tubercle bacilli in milk by means of guinea-pig inoculation, curious lesions (see Ref. 24) resembling tuberculosis but lacking acid-fast bacilli were encountered in some animals. The disease was transmissible from guinea pig to guinea pig. Milk from perfectly healthy cows, tuberculin-negative, sometimes produced these lesions. A small organism, identified as *Bacillus abortus*, was found in the milk which caused the disease resembling tuberculosis. There is a detailed description and good pictures of the lesions in the guinea pig which correspond to those described by Smith and Fabyan (Ref. 24). The striking thing in this study was the frequent occurrence of *B. abortus* in the milk of perfectly healthy cows. The writers did not definitely link these milk-borne bacilli to any human disease, but they did think that "the germ forms another link in the long chain of facts that point unmistakably to the proper pasteurization of all milk . . . as a measure essentially necessary for the protection of public health." A few years later E. C. Fleischner and K. F. Meyer ("Observations on the presence of the Bacillus abortus bovinus in certified milk," Am. J. Dis. Child., **14**:157, 1917) carefully reviewed the whole subject and added observations of their own, from which they concluded: "B. abortus is, for practical purposes, always present in the certified milk produced in the San Francisco Bay regions."

24. SMITH, Theobald, and FABYAN, Marshall. Ueber die pathogene Wirkung des Bacillus abortus Bang, Centralbl. f. Bakt., **61**:549, 1912.

After the appearance of the report of the British Commission, it was assumed that all Malta fever resulted from drinking goat's milk or other contact with goats. Until the work of Smith and Fabyan, infection with *B. abortus* remained a strictly veterinary problem. No relation was suspected between the two in the causation of disease. With material from contagious abortion, Smith and Fabyan were able to produce a chronic disease in guinea pigs featured by enlarged and engorged spleen, enlarged lymph nodes, and small nodules in the liver. The disease was passed in series through guinea pigs, and *B. abortus* was isolated in pure culture from the lesions which were reproduced by it. The disease ran as long as eleven months without very drastic external appearances. Sometimes there were overt lesions of bones and joints. Smith and Fabyan found microscopically "a chronic inflammatory process closely resembling tuberculosis." There were foci of epithelial cells and lymphoid cells, occasionally with necrotic centers. The details must be read in the original communication. Bacilli were found especially in spleen but also in lymph nodes, bone marrow, liver, kidney, and lung and were grown from the lesions. Smith and Fabyan concluded, first, that contagious abortion was caused in America as in Europe by *B. abortus* Bang. Second, they suggested that the overt lesions of contagious abortion were not always primary but were secondary to slow general infection of the sort described in guinea pigs. "That the 'Abortbacillus' appears in milk is very probable." Conclusions: "(1) B. abortus Bang is most probably the only cause of contagious abortion. (2) B. abortus produces in guinea pigs a peculiar generalized diease which rarely leads to death. It resembles tuberculosis, and is characterized by chronic interstitial new growths, which, for the most part, consist of epithelial and lymphoid cells. (3) B. abortus can be present in milk, and it is therefore indicated to investigate whether it has any causal relationship with any chronic disease of man."

M. Fabyan ("A contribution to the pathogenesis of B. abortus Bang. II," J.M. Res., **26**:441, 1912) a little later wrote up much the same material in English. He described in great detail the pathology of the disease produced in guinea pigs.

25. NÈGRE, L., and RAYNAUD, M. Melitensis et paramelitensis, Compt. rend. Soc. de biol., **72**:791, 1912.

The authors had already shown ("Sur l'agglutination du 'Micrococcus melitensis' par les sérums humains," *ibid.*, **70**:472, 1911) that *M. melitensis* was agglutinated frequently not only by sera from patients with Malta fever but by many "normal" sera as well. The present study concerns a strain of *M. melitensis,* with all the typical cultural characteristics, which was agglutinated only feebly by convalescent Malta fever serum, whereas five other strains were agglutinated in titers of 1:1,000 to 1:5,000. An immune serum, however, prepared from this strain failed entirely to agglutinate the other five strains, whereas it agglutinated the homologous strain in a titer of 1:500. Thus they had separated an immuno-logically different strain of *M. melitensis,* which they designated "parameli-tensis" by analogy to parameningococci and paradysentery bacilli. This work was later extended ("Identification des paramelitenses, par l'épreuve de la saturation des agglutinins," *ibid.,* p. 1052) by agglutination and absorption tests.

26. LARSON, W. P., and SEDGWICK, J. P. The complement fixation reaction of the blood of children and infants, using the Bacillus abortus as antigen, Am. J. Dis. Child., **6**:326, 1913.

From the work of Cotton and Schroeder (Ref. 23) the writers knew that 10 per cent of market milk contains *B. abortus* and also that animals may be infected per os. They wondered, therefore, whether humans were ever infected; and they examined the blood of 425 children by complement fixation, using *B. abortus* as antigen. Of these 425, they found 73 positive. The antibodies could also be absorbed by suspensions of the bacilli. These investigators definitely raised the question of human infection with *B. abortus,* but they went no further and made no suggestion of the occurrence of undulant fever in man as a result of infection with it.

27. Report of the chief of the Bureau of Animal Industry. Annual Reports of the Department of Agriculture for the Year Ended June 30, 1914, p. 86. Washington: Government Printing Office, 1914.

The report includes reference to premature hairless pigs which were sent in to the Department of Agriculture for examination. "Cultures made from liver, stomach contents and kidneys revealed an organism resembling Bacillus abortus in cultural and morphological characteristics. These cultures when used as antigens in both agglutination and complement-fixation tests gave the same results with two known negative, two known positive and with unknown bovine sera, as were obtained with an antigen prepared from B. abortus of Bang from bovine origin." This seems to be the first report of a porcine strain. Whereas the finding is often attributed in the literature to J. Traum (see, for example, H. J. Harris, *Brucellosis* [2d ed.; New York: Paul B. Hoeber, 1950], p. 9), his name is not mentioned in the report which emanated from the Pathological Division under the direction of Dr. John R. Mohler. Actually, E. S. Good and W. V. Smith ("Bacillus abortus [Bang] as an etiological factor in infectious abortion of swine," J. Bact., **1**:415, 1916) seem to have first isolated, from the afterbirth of an aborting sow and from numerous other tissues, organisms which they were unable to distinguish from *B. abortus.*

C. P. Beattie and R. M. Rice ("Undulant fever due to Brucella of the porcine type—Brucella suis," J.A.M.A., **102**:1670, 1934) report a milk-borne epidemic of 30 cases of undulant fever due to *Brucella suis.* The organism was obtained by blood culture from 6 to 14 patients and from the milk of one cow. Infection with porcine strains seemed especially common in Iowa. A. V. Hardy, C. F.

Jordan, and I. H. Borts ("Undulant fever, further epidemiological and clinical observations in Iowa," J.A.M.A., **107**:559, 1936) found that 70 per cent of 124 cases were caused by this type. C. F. Jordan and I. Borts ("Brucellosis and infection caused by three species of Brucella," Am. J. Med., **2**:156, 1947) more recently reviewed the subject.

28. FLEISCHNER, E. C., and MEYER, K. F. The bearing of cutaneous hypersensitiveness on the pathogenicity of the Bacillus abortus bovinus, Am. J. Dis. Child., **16**:268, 1918.

The authors noted the resemblance between the experimental lesions of *B. abortus* in guinea pigs and those of tuberculosis (Ref. 24). Hence they did skin tests with extracts of *B. abortus* and with abortus bacilli. Guinea pigs with lesions invariably gave a positive skin reaction. Guinea pigs which had been injected with dead cultures or in which no disease developed always gave a negative skin test. The authors therefore drew analogies to tuberculin testing and concluded that a positive skin test to "abortin" indicated active infection. On the other hand: "In a series of seventy-five infants fed on a high bacillus abortus containing milk, cutaneous hypersensitiveness was not present," and the writers regarded this as suggestive evidence that *B. abortus bovinus* was not highly pathogenic for infants.

29. EVANS, Alice C. Further studies on Bacterium abortus and related bacteria. II. A comparison of Bacterium abortus with Bacterium bronchisepticus and with the organism which causes Malta fever, J. Infect. Dis., **22**:580, 1918.

Since it had been shown that the Malta fever organism commonly infected goat's milk on the island of Malta and that *B. abortus* commonly infected cow's milk in this country, it occurred to Evans to make a detailed comparison of the two. Using elaborate cultural and immunologic tests, she found that "the organism which causes Malta fever is unquestionably a rod form and should be called Bact. melitensis. But melitensis is very closely related to Bact. abortus. The only test which has been found to distinguish these two organisms is the agglutination of Bact. melitensis in higher dilutions of melitensis serum than will agglutinate Bact. abortus. The agglutination tests as they have been used to diagnose infections of Bact. melitensis in goats and human subjects cannot be relied on to dishinguish one from the other." This was pioneer work in pointing out the similarity of the bacteria which cause Malta fever and contagious abortion of cattle. Evans continued and elaborated her studies ("The serological classification of Brucella melitensis from human, bovine, caprine, porcine and equine sources," Pub. Health Rep., **38**:1948, 1923).

M. L. Fusier and K. F. Meyer confirmed and elaborated Evans' work ("Principles in serological grouping of B. abortus and B. melitensis: correlation between absorption and agglutination tests," J. Infect. Dis., **27**:185, 1920) and suggested that the "B. abortus and B. melitensis group be given generic rank in the Bacteriaceae family as the genus 'Brucella.'" Meyer also pursued these studies with E. B. Shaw ("A comparison of the morphological, cultural, and biochemical characteristics of Br. abortus and Br. melitensis: studies on the genus Brucella," J. Infect. Dis., **27**:173, 1920).

30. SMITH, Theobald. A characteristic localization of Bacillus abortus in the bovine fetal membranes, J. Exper. Med., **29**:451, 1919.

The elucidation of the pathologic histology of Brucella infection was opened by the observations of T. Smith, who found *B. abortus* in the epithelial covering of the chorion. He noted that the more or less specific localization and multiplication of bacteria within cells not having phagocytic functions had been demonstrated in leprosy and syphilis. E. W. Goodpasture and K. Anderson ("The problem of infection as presented by bacterial invasion of the chorioallantoic membrane of chick embryos," Am. J. Path., **13**:149, 1937) confirmed these findings in chick embryos inoculated with Brucella. They noted that the bacilli enter ectodermal epithelial cells and proliferate there, as they do in chorionic epithelium of the calf. G. F. Buddingh and F. C. Womack ("Observations on the infection of chick embryos with Bacterium tularense, Brucella, and Pasteurella pestis," J. Exper. Med., **74**:213, 1941) described the growth of Brucella in chick embryos more in detail, confirming the findings of Goodpasture and Anderson. They also described involvement of the endothelial cells lining the blood vessels. K. F. Meyer ("Observations on the pathogenesis of undulant fever: essays in biology [Berkeley and Los Angeles: University of California Press, 1943], p. 439) described the pathologic histology in a laboratory worker who died within eleven days of an acute septicemia with *Brucella suis:* "First and foremost is the intracytoplasmic multiplication of the bacteria in the epithelium of Bowman's capsule and the convoluted tubules. . . . This selective intracellular parasitism in mesenchyme cells of various organs is doubtless of greatest significance in the pathogenesis of Brucella infections. . . . There is no proof that the brucellas multiply in the blood stream. . . . Their presence in macrophages and polymorphonuclear leukocytes is justly attributed to phagocytosis. . . . Once in the cytoplasma, they find conditions favorable for multiplication and protection against phagocytosis." Meyer gives an interesting and detailed analysis of the problems of pathogenesis of Brucella infection.

Further studies along this line are those reported by W. W. Spink ("Pathogenesis of human brucellosis with respect to prevention and treatment," Ann. Int. Med., **29**:238, 1948); R. D. Sundberg and W. W. Spink ("Histopathology of lesions in bone marrow of patients having active brucellosis," Blood, Suppl. 1, p. 7, 1947); W. W. Spink, F. W. Hoffbauer, W. W. Walker, and R. A. Green ("Histopathology of the liver in human brucellosis," J. Lab. & Clin. Med., **34**:40, 1949); and M. Ruiz Castenada ("Studies on the pathogenesis of brucellosis," Proc. Soc. Exper. Biol. & Med., **64**:298, 1947).

31. KEEFER, Chester S. Report of a case of Malta fever originating in Baltimore, Maryland, Bull. Johns Hopkins Hosp., **35**:6, 1924.

Z. Khaled ("A comparative study of bovine abortion and undulant fever from the bacteriological point of view," J. Hyg., **20**:319, 1921) raised the question of "whether or not B. abortus being so closely related to B. melitensis is capable of producing an undulant or other form of fever in man." Without definite proof, he reported having seen cases in Egypt "which have never had a chance of ingesting goat's milk and yet suffered from typical melitensis fever confirmed by laboratory diagnosis." Still earlier, C. Kennedy ("Preliminary notes on the presence of agglutinins for the Micrococcus melitensis in the milk and blood serum of cows in London," J. Roy. Army M. Corps, **22**:9, 1914) referred to two cases of undulant fever in people who had never been out of England. It remained for Keefer, however, to report the first case of "a disease in man corresponding to Malta fever due to an organism belonging to the abortus group."[4] Keefer's patient, a laboratory worker, is of great interest. He ran a typical undulating fever, and between October 19 and January 10 yielded thirteen positive blood cultures with one to six colonies per cubic centimeter of Brucella. The infection was probably due to cow's milk, and, by appropriate serologic tests, Keefer showed that the organism was of the abortus type. Thus the melitensis and abortus types were finally brought together clinically as well as immunologically. Alice Evans was also hot on the trail ("Malta fever: cattle suggested as a possible source of infection, following a serological study of humans," Pub. Health Rep., **39**:501, 1924) as a result of comparative study of human sera, but she described no actual patients.

Other cases of "Malta fever" due to *B. abortus* were soon reported, such as those of C. M. Carpenter and H. E. Merriam ("Undulant fever from Brucella abortus," J.A.M.A., **87**:1269, 1926), who described two typical instances in which the organism was isolated from the blood and proved by agglutination absorption tests to be the abortus variety. "Contagious abortion and undulant fever" were also discussed at a meeting of the Royal Society (Brit. M.J., **1**:554, 1925).

32. HARDY, A. V., HUDSON, Margaret G., and JORDAN, C. F. The skin as a portal of entry in Br. melitensis infections, J. Infect. Dis., **45**:271, 1929.

The frequency of undulant fever in the employees of a meat-packing plant suggested to the writers that Brucella infection through the skin might be a common occurrence. Guinea pigs were readily infected by spreading culture on the shaved or clipped skin. That such infection was not due to organisms which entered via the digestive tract is made clear by the much lower occurrence of infections when culture material was actually fed by mouth. The significance of the skin route seemed to be confirmed by the frequency of infection in workers in the packing house, where those who actually killed and cut the animals had the disease much more frequently than those who worked in the offices or elevators or handled boxes, carried meat, etc.

The importance of infection through the skin had been recognized long before the present work by the British Commission (Ref. 21).

---

[4] In regard to Keefer's case, Huddleson (*op. cit.,* p. 68) says: "Duncan [J. T. Duncan, in discussion of "Contagious abortion and undulant fever," Brit. M.J., **1**:544, 1925] was the first to recognize and report cases of Brucellosis due to Br. abortus." Duncan reports a case in a brief paragraph in which he states conservatively that "the weight of the evidence pointed to B. abortus as the cause of Rhodesian undulant fever in man" but "experimental proof was still awaited; as also was a really trustworthy test to distinguish B. abortus from B. melitensis." As to Keefer's culture, Huddleson states: "Several years later the author had an opportunity to study this culture and it was then found to be Br. suis." At any rate, Keefer reported the first case of what was clinically Malta fever in which a member of the Brucella group other than melitensis was proved to be the cause.

33. KRISTENSEN, Martin, and HOLM, Per. Bakteriologische und statistische Untersuchungen über Febris undulans in Dänemark, Centralbl. f. Bakt., **112**:281, 1929.

The authors give a critical discussion of the relation of infection with *B. abortus* to abortion in women. They are skeptical about such an infection playing a significant part in human pathology, although they allude to the case of a woman who aborted in the seventh month, from whose placenta the abortus bacillus was grown, although none was recovered from the organs of the fetus. C. M. Carpenter and R. Boak ("Isolation of Brucella abortus from a human fetus," J.A.M.A., **96**:1212, 1931) later isolated *B. abortus* from the placenta and the fetal organs of an early abortion in a woman who did not have undulant fever. They given an exhaustive review of the literature on the finding of abortus in the generative organs of humans and of various animals but leave undecided the case for *B. abortus* playing an important role in human abortion.[5]

34. SHARP, William B. Pathology of undulant fever, Arch. Path., **18**:72, 1934.

The morbid anatomy of brucellosis is comprehensively reviewed with bibliography. The writer points out the scant material in the literature and the paucity of distinctive gross lesions. "The most essential item in the general pathologic alteration is a proliferation of cells belonging to the reticulo-endothelial system." H. J. Harris in his book, *Brucellosis* (*loc. cit.*), gives a long list of all the lesions which have been described in various organs (p. 91) and then a detailed discussion with references to the literature.

35. CARPENTER, Charles M., and BOAK, Ruth A. The treatment of human brucellosis: a review of current therapeutic methods, Medicine, **15**:103, 1936.

The writers give a comprehensive review, with literature, of the methods of treating brucellosis before the antibiotic era. They point out the difficulty of evaluating any therapeutic measure in a disease which runs such a variable course both as to time and as to severity. They discuss vaccine therapy, serum therapy, therapy with toxic filtrates, therapy with various chemicals such as dyes, arsphenamines, etc., foreign protein therapy, and therapy with induced fever. The conclusion from all of this is: "A successful method for the treatment of brucellosis still awaits development, for as yet no therapeutic agent has been found which has been proved to alter, to a significant degree, the natural course of the disease."

36. CALDER, R. M., STEEN, C., and BAKER, L. Blood studies in brucellosis, J.A.M.A., **112**:1893, 1939.

Careful studies of the blood counts were made in several hundred cases. The leukocytes were normal, diminished, or increased. Active lymphocytosis was the most striking feature encountered.

[5] Dr. Charles E. McLennan, professor of obstetrics and gynecology at Stanford University, tells me that, as of today (1956), local infection with *B. abortus* is not considered significant in human abortion.

37. JONES, D., METZGER, H. J., SCHATZ, A., and WAKSMAN, S. A. Control of Gram-negative bacteria in experimental animals by streptomycin, Science, **100**:103, 1944.

It was inevitable that streptomycin, an antibiotic potent against Gram-negative bacteria, would be tried against Brucella. Waksman, the discoverer of this antibiotic, himself here reports the protection of 15-day chick embryos against infection with Brucella by treatment with streptomycin, when untreated controls succumbed. A little later, I. Live, F. G. Sperling, and E. L. Stubbs ("Effect of streptomycin on experimental brucellosis in guinea pigs," Am. J.M. Sc., **211**:267, 1946) found that 2,000 units of streptomycin daily in six doses seemed to eliminate the infection from most guinea pigs when treatment was begun 1 week after infection.

W. H. Hall and W. W. Spink ("Therapy of experimental Brucella infection in the developing chick embryo. I. Infection and therapy via the allantoic sac," J. Immunol., **59**:379, 1948) later developed a method for testing therapeutic agents against Brucella by injecting them into the allantoic sac of the developing chick embryo. Sulfadiazine and streptomycin in combination were found to be more effective against *B. abortus* and *B. suis* than either drug alone. J. M. Shaffer and W. W. Spink ("III. The synergistic action of streptomycin and sulfadiazine," J. Immunol., **60**:405, 1948) with the same technique soon showed that such combined action represented a true synergism. R. Magoffin, D. Anderson, and W. W. Spink ("IV. Therapy with aureomycin," J. Immunol., **62**:125, 1949) explored aureomycin alone and in combination with other agents.

38. REIMANN, H. O., PRICE, A. H., and ELIAS, W. F. Streptomycin for certain systemic infections and its effect on the urinary and fecal flora, Arch. Inst. Med., **76**:269, 1945.

In contrast to its apparent effect in experimental brucellosis (Ref. 37), streptomycin has been reported of doubtful value in human infection. Thus Reimann states that treatment with streptomycin was inconclusive in three cases. D. E. Nichols and W. E. Herrell ("Streptomycin, its clinical use and limitations," J.A.M.A., **132**:200, 1946) also found the results of treatment of brucellosis disappointing in a number of cases, although in some it had a temporary suppressive effect. However, W. H. Hall and W. W. Spink ("In vitro sensitivity of Brucella to streptomycin: development of resistance during streptomycin treatment," Proc. Soc. Exper. Biol. & Med., **64**:403, 1947) found most strains of Brucella sensitive to streptomycin in the test tube, although one strain from a patient with Brucella endocarditis became resistant during therapy; and G. H. Finch ("Streptomycin therapy in undulant fever," Am. J. Med., **2**:485, 1947) thought that he had obtained favorable results in several cases.

39. PULASKI, E. J., and AMSPACHER, W. H. Streptomycin therapy for certain infections of intestinal origin, New England J. Med., **237**:419, 1947.

The authors treated two acute cases of brucellosis with a combination of streptomycin and sulfonamide therapy, which seemed to produce a cure. C. W. Eisele and N. B. McCullough independently tried the same device; the simultaneous use of streptomycin and sulfadiazine they thought was curative when either drug used separately failed. "A prolonged constant septicemia promptly ceased," and no relapse occurred in a seventeen-month period. W. W. Spink, W. H. Hall, J. M. Shaffer, and A. I. Braude ("Human brucellosis, its specific treatment with a combination of streptomycin and sulfadiazine," J.A.M.A., **136**:382, 1948), following successful trials in chick embryos (Ref. 37), treated nine patients with a combination of sulfadiazine and streptomycin with "more satisfactory results than any other therapy used to date." They advised streptomycin intramuscularly in doses of 0.5 gm. every 6 hours for 7 days and sulfadiazine with an initial oral dose of 4 gm. and then 1 gm. every 4 hours for at least 2 weeks. These writers later amplified their results ("Treatment of brucellosis with streptomycin and a sulfonamide drug," *ibid.*, **139**:352, 1949). Although not absolutely secure, this form of therapy is followed by fewer relapses, and the appearance of streptomycin-resistant Brucella has not occurred.

40. SPINK, W. W., BRAUDE, A. I., CASTENADA, M. R., and GOYTRA, R. S. Aureomycin therapy in human brucellosis due to Brucella melitensis, J.A.M.A., **138**:1145, 1948.

Working in Mexico with patients ill with undulant fever due to *B. melitensis,* in contrast to those seen in Iowa with disease due to *B. abortus,* the writers found aureomycin by mouth the most effective remedy. However, they have certain reservations, and in an addendum at the end of the paper there is some tempering of enthusiasm because of relapses. Enthusiastic reports also soon appeared from various sources, such as those of M. S. Boyer, E. B. Schoenbach, R. M. Wood, and P. H. Long ("The treatment of acute brucellosis with aureomycin," Bull. Johns Hopkins Hosp., **84**:444, 1949) and of V. Knight, F. Ruiz-Sanchez, A. Ruiz-Sanchez, and W. McDermott ("Aureomycin in typhus and brucellosis," Am. J. Med., **6**:407, 1949). Later W. W. Spink, W. H. Hall, and R. Magoffin ("Follow-up study of therapy in forty-eight culturally proved cases of brucellosis: streptomycin and sulfadiazine, aureomycin, and chloramphenicol [chloromycetin[(R)]]," Arch. Int. Med., **88**:419, 1951) reported follow-up studies of 48 patients treated with various combinations of antibiotics and sulfonamides. The results with streptomycin and sulfadiazine and with aureomycin seemed about equal, about one-half recovering promptly and remaining well; with chloramphenicol the results were not quite so good. So, too, in an elaborate study, E. M. Yow and W. W. Spink ("Experimental studies on the action of streptomycin, aureomycin and chloromycetin on Brucella," J. Clin. Investigation, **28**:871, 1949) found strains of *B. abortus, B. suis,* and *B. melitensis* all sensitive in vitro to the three antibiotics. The action of streptomycin was bactericidal, while aureomycin and chloromycetin were bacteriostatic. A little later, W. E. Herrell and T. E. Barber ("A new method for treatment of brucellosis," J.A.M.A., **144**:519, 1950) reported good results from treatment with a combination of aureomycin by mouth and streptomycin intramuscularly.

41. KNIGHT, V., SANCHEZ, F. R., and SANCHEZ, A. R. Terramycin in the treatment of human brucellosis, Arch. Int. Med., **87**:835, 1951.

In the hope of finding an antibiotic therapy for brucellosis which would not be followed by relapses, the authors used terramycin, which proved highly effective in the treatment of the acute manifestations. There were, however, a significant number of relapses.

42. ABERNETHY, Robert, and SPINK, Wesley W. The influence of cortisone and adrenocorticotrophic hormone on brucellosis. I. Cortisone in experimentally infected animals, J. Clin. Investigation, **31**:945, 1952.

In mice with acute brucellosis, steroids converted a relatively mild infection into a fulminating and fatal illness. In contrast, cortisone did not appear to alter the course of the disease or the tissue reactions in chronically infected animals. In contrast also, ACTH administered to a patient with acute brucellosis (W. W. Spink and W. H. Hall, "II. Adrenocorticotrophic hormone [ACTH] in acute and chronic human brucellosis," J. Clin. Investigation, **31**:958, 1952) was accompanied by prompt and remarkable improvement, although the blood cultures remained positive. "The only indication for cortisone or ACTH at the present time in acute or chronic brucellosis is in patients who are quite ill and toxic. And even then, treatment should be carried out only for a few days and simultaneously with antibiotic therapy."

43. SPINK, W. W. Some biological and clinical problems related to intracellular parasitism in brucellosis, New England J. Med., **247**:603, 1952.

In an important paper Spink puts his finger on the difficulty involved in all chemotherapy and antibiotic therapy of brucellosis, namely, the intracellular situation of the parasite which guards it against the action of chemicals, antibiotics, and sera which may be lethal in the test tube. He reviews and analyzes the whole subject with comprehensive bibliography. In another paper (J. M. Shaffer, C. J. Kucera, and W. W. Spink, "The protection of intracellular Brucella against therapeutic agents and the bactericidal action of serum," J. Exper. Med., **97**:77, 1953) Spink and his associates devised a method for the study of intracellular Brucella in vitro. Such Brucella were protected to a great extent against the action of antibiotics. Actually, no method of therapy so far devised has completely overcome this barrier; it is apparently bacteria protected against attack within cells which cause the frequent relapses in spite of therapy.

44. SPINK, W. W., McCULLOUGH, N. B., HUTCHINGS, L. M., and MINGLE, C. K. Diagnostic criteria for human brucellosis, J.A.M.A., **149**:805, 1952.

This paper is a critical appraisal by experts of the various diagnostic tests which have been used. They point out that the only unimpeachable proof of brucellosis is isolation of the organism. Agglutination in a titer of 1:320 or over allows a presumptive diagnosis. The skin test gives insecure results.

PNEUMOCOCCAL PNEUMONIA

Bacteremia	Ref. 49
Bacteriology	Refs. 8, 9, 13, 14, 15, 21, 23, 24, 48
Chlorides, suppression	Ref. 5
Circulation	Refs. 42, 43
Clinical description	Refs. 1, 2, 4, 5, 7, 38, 61
Complications	Refs. 10, 22, 38
Diagnosis, physical	Refs. 1, 4, 7
Epidemiology	Refs. 17, 19, 39
Etiology, bacterial	Refs. 8, 9, 13, 15, 16, 18, 21, 23, 24, 48
General	Refs. 7, 38, 59, 61
Immunity	Refs. 23, 25, 26, 28, 32, 34, 39, 47, 50, 51, 54, 57, 63
Pathology	Refs. 1, 2, 3, 5, 6, 55, 57
Penicillin therapy	Ref. 62

(*Continued on following page*)

PNEUMOCOCCAL PNEUMONIA

MODERN knowledge of lobar pneumonia begins clearly and precisely with Laënnec. Before Laënnec, all was vague and, indeed, almost medieval. At one stroke, the discoverer of auscultation, the leader of the great French school of clinician pathologists, brought order out of confusion and gave a description of the disease which is still reflected in the textbooks of today. However, Laënnec and his followers thought of pneumonia as they did of *a* pleurisy, or *a* fever, or *a* diarrhea, as a general entity; it was not until the second half of the nineteenth century that the concept of "croupous" or "lobar pneumonia" as a specific disease emerged, and this concept was confirmed and established in the last quarter of the century by the discovery of the pneumococcus. The early literature is immense, and no purpose is served by giving more than several illustrative references.

The invaluable volumes of White (Ref. 59) and of Heffron (Ref. 61) contain extensive bibliographies for which every student of pneumonia must feel grateful. Our own references try to cover the high spots of the development of knowledge through the early days of bacteriology, the era of serum therapy, and, finally, of the conquest of the disease by modern antibiotics. In making a selection from the vast literature on the biology of pneumococcus—types, somatic protein and capsular carbohydrate, behavior in the body—we have tried to pick out only those studies which have a fundamental bearing on clinical problems.

1. LAËNNEC, R. T. H. Traité de l'auscultation médiate et des maladies des poumons et du cœur, 1:393. 2d ed. Paris: J. S. Chaudé, 1826.

As in all his other descriptions, Laënnec is the supreme master. In simple, vivid language he gives a picture of pneumonia to which little can be added today. He enumerates three stages—engorgement, hepatization, and purulent infiltration (resolution)—with the auscultatory signs and with a brilliant discussion of the symptoms and course of the disease. It is obvious that Laënnec's account still influences modern textbooks. The character of the breathing, says Laënnec, depends on the functional disturbance in the lung; the sputa are described in detail. Although the term "purulent infiltration" was an unfortunate one and probably meant no more than normal resolution, actual abscess formation seems to have been common in Laënnec's day. Long exposure to cold is emphasized as a cause of the disease: "The Russian who leaves his stove to roll in the snow, the bakers who, practically naked, emerge from the torrid atmosphere of their ovens to expose themselves to a cold several degrees below zero are not usually taken with pneumonia; but the 'porte-faix,' who stand for a long time at street corners, are often attacked." Laënnec recognized epidemics of pneumonia of unknown cause.

Treatment, as in all contemporary accounts, was irrational: the diet of only sugar and mucilaginous substances, bleeding, tartar emetic, etc., are discussed at length.

The original account should be read by every student.

2. STOKES, William. A Treatise on the diagnosis and treatment of diseases of the chest. Part I. Diseases of the lung and windpipe. Dublin: Hodges & Smith, 1837.

Stokes probably represented the best British clinical practice of the day. His account of pneumonia is, however, "transitional" between the older vague descriptions and the new picture which was emerging as a result of Laënnec's work. Stokes leans heavily on Laënnec and constantly refers to him. He enumerates the usual stages of the disease—engorgement, solidification, and resolution—with related auscultatory signs; much stress is placed on postpneumonic abscess, and there is a separate section on typhoid pneumonia. Under treatment, bleeding, following Louis, is emphasized, along with antimony in the form of tartar emetic. Mercury is also mentioned. It is obvious that knowledge was still in a rather primitive stage.

3. ROKITANSKY, Carl. Handbuch der speziellen pathologischen Anatomie, 2:84. Vienna: Braumüller & Seidel, 1842.

The term "croupous pneumonia" was already in use. Rokitansky, following Laënnec (Ref. 1), recognized three stages: engorgement, hepatization, and purulent infiltration. The last seems to be simply normal resolution. The pathological changes are vividly described and easily recognized.

4. SKODA, Joseph L. Abhandlung über Perkussion und Auskultation, p. 243. 3d ed. Vienna: Braumüller & Seidel, 1844.

Skoda added to Laënnec's auscultatory findings those of percussion. One notes the intense interest in physical diagnosis at this time, so that a pneumonia was thought of more as an anatomical process than as a specific disease.

5. REDTENBACHER, Wilhelm. Beobachtungen am Harne bei Lungenentzündungen, Ztschr. d. k. k. Gesellsch. d. Ärtze Wien, 1:373, 1850.

Although Redtenbacher seems to have been the first to point out clearly the diminished excretion of chloride in pneumonia—a phenomenon universally recognized since then—a great deal of modern study has not fully elucidated the exact mechanism of this phenomenon (see Francis W. Peabody, "Studies of inorganic metabolism in pneumonia with especial reference to calcium and magnesium," J. Exper. Med., 17:71, 1913; F. William Sunderman, "Studies of serum electrolytes. IV. The chloride and nitrogen balances, and weight changes in pneumonia," J. Clin. Investigation, 7:313, 1929; T. S. Wilder and T. G. H. Drake, "Metabolism of chloride and total fixed base in pneumonia and the relation to salt and water retention," J. Clin. Investigation, 7:353, 1929).

6. FLINT, Austin. A treatise on the principles and practice of medicine, chap. iv, p. 152. Philadelphia: Henry C. Lea, 1866.

Flint represented the best medical practice of his time in America, and one is not surprised to find an excellent chapter on lobar pneumonia. The pathology is well described in relation to history and physical signs. There is no suggestion that Flint suspected the disease to be communicable. He mentioned death from pulmonary embolus but regarded the clots as having been formed in the right ventricle and pulmonary artery. Treatment was "symptomatic," but the rationale given for various procedures, such as the use of ammonia to prevent heart clots, has little meaning today.

7. JÜRGENSEN, Theodor. Kruppöse Pneumonie, *in* Handbuch der speziellen Pathologie und Therapie, ed. H. v. ZIEMSSEN, 5:3. Leipzig, 1874.

This article of 183 pages is a classic and deals with every phase of lobar pneumonia. Modern in tone, no better discussion of the subject appeared in the next thirty-five years. Jürgensen clearly defines lobar pneumonia as a specific disease. In contrast to the usual opinion of the time, he is convinced that it is an infection. "Croupous pneumonia is a general illness, not a local one. The inflammation of the lung is only a main symptom; the general phenomena are not to be explained by the local lesion. The assumption of a specific etiologic agent is necessary. Croupous pneumonia belongs, then, to the group of infectious diseases. . . . Not all inflammation-producing agents can cause croupous pneumonia. It takes a 'something' with specific characteristics—just as with typhoid."

There are comprehensive discussions of "etiology" (cold was just a predisposing factor, not the "frigus unica pneumoniae causa"), of epidemiology, and of vital statistics. The pathological description is complete, the clinical account lucid and objective. Legends such as that of "critical" days are disposed of. Treatment is essentially expectant. Jürgensen erred in believing that death was due to a specific cardiac weakness, and he directed his therapy toward "stimulating" the heart. He thought bleeding and antiphlogistics accomplished this. Interestingly enough, the doctrine that patients with lobar pneumonia died of circulatory failure dominated therapeutic thinking until dispelled many years later by Newburgh and his associates (Refs. 42, 43).

8. KLEBS, E. Beiträge zur Kenntnis der pathogenen Schistomyzeten. VII. Die Monadien, Arch. f. exper. Path. u. Pharmakol., 4:409, 1875.

Klebs reviews the evidence in favor of lobar pneumonia as an infection. Most important, he thinks, is the appearance in outbreaks or epidemics and that in such outbreaks cases occur without the usual alleged precipitating causes, such as exhaustion or exposure to cold. In a number of instances he attempted at autopsy to secure uncontaminated material. He found in lung and meninges little spheres about 0.8 μ in diameter which he was sure were organisms and not fat droplets. He was able to grow these in "egg white." It is not clear just what these "monads" were, but they showed a lively motility, which would seem to prove that they were not pneumococci. Although much quoted in the literature as the first isolation of pneumococcus, the paper is unconvincing.

9. EBERTH, C. J. Zur Kenntnis der mykotischen Prozesse, Deutches Arch. f. klin. Med., 28:1, 1880–81.

Eberth in the early years of the bacteriological era had made general studies of all sorts of infections. In this article he describes (with autopsy) a typical case of lobar pneumonia in which a purulent meningitis was present. In both lung and meninges, cocci were demonstrated, often in pairs or chains, different from the "cocci of pyemia." These organisms were almost surely pneumococci, although Eberth did not go so far as to claim a specific etiological agent. Koch, also, in a general discussion of clinical bacteriology (Robert Koch, "Zur Untersuchung von pathogenen Organismen," Mitt. a. d. k. Gsndhtsamte, **1**:46, 1881) described and pictured cocci, the nature of which is uncertain, in a pneumonic lung.

10. OSLER, William. Infectious (so-called ulcerative) endocarditis, Arch. Med., **5**:44, 1881.

"Under the terms *diphtheritic, ulcerative, malignant, septic* or *infectious* endocarditis, *arterial pyaemia, mycosis endocardii,* physicians now recognize one of the most formidable of cardiac affections, characterized by a peculiar morbid process on the valves, blood contaminations, constitutional symptoms of the typhoid or pyaemic types and usually associated with multiple emboli." In this classical article Osler clearly notes the association of endocarditis and meningitis with lobar pneumonia and describes masses of "micrococci" on the valves. Osler, in contrast to many contemporary bacteriologists, was himself uncertain as to the significance of these cocci.

11. PASTEUR, L., avec la collaboration de MM. CHAMBERLAND et ROUX. Sur une maladie nouvelle, provoquée par la salive d'un enfant mort de la rage, Compt. rend. Acad. de sc., **92**:159, 1881.

Pasteur inoculated a "little mucus" from the mouth of a child dead of rabies into rabbits, which died within a day or two. Saliva and blood from these rabbits was injected into others, which also died promptly. Pasteur passed the disease on through a number of generations. He soon noticed that "the blood of the animals was invaded by a microscopic organism of very curious properties." There follows a beautiful description of lance-shaped diplococci. "Each of these little bodies is surrounded by a sort of aureole . . . produced by a mucoid substance . . . resembling the cocoon of the silkworm." Pasteur did not believe this disease or organism had anything to do with rabies, "a different disease of long incubation period." He left the problem with the thought that further work was essential.

At the meeting of the Academy of Medicine of March 29, 1881, the secretary read a report for M. Vulpian (Bull. Acad. méd., Paris, 2d ser., **10**:394, 1881) in which he described the death of rabbits a day or two after subcutaneous injection of saliva from *healthy* men, with passage of the disease by injection of blood from the infected rabbits and the finding of organisms corresponding to Pasteur's in the blood. He thus furnished a link between the work of Pasteur and that of Sternberg (Ref. 12).

12. STERNBERG, George M. A fatal form of septicemia in the rabbit, produced by the subcutaneous injection of human saliva, Nat. Board Health, Ann. Rep., 1881, p. 87,

Sternberg, following Pasteur, found that 1 or 2 cc. of his own sputum injected subcutaneously into rabbits "infallibly produces death within 48 hours." Variable results were obtained with the saliva of others. However, the saliva of "Dr. S." always showed exceptional virulence. The "course of the disease and the post-mortem appearance indicate that it is a form of septicemia." The blood and other tissues contained a vast number of micrococci similar to the organism described by Pasteur. Sternberg was puzzled because other experimenters, such as Pasteur, had obtained their material from a disease source, whereas his was derived from the saliva of healthy people; he saw no reason, however, why the disease should not be the same. He speculated further on the presence in the mouth of pathogenic bacteria along with many harmless ones. From a modern standpoint the type and the virulence of pneumococci in different salivas would account for Sternberg's variable findings.

He also noted that the "virulence" of saliva was destroyed by boiling, that it was lost when kept for 24 hours at 37° C. or when carbolic acid was added or when the serum from a dead rabbit was filtered.

13. FRIEDLÄNDER, C. Ueber die Schizomyzeten bei der acuten fibrösen Pneumonie, Virchows Arch path. Anat., **28**:319, 1882.

Friedländer's report, the first of any real significance from the bacteriological standpoint, concerns eight cases of lobar pneumonia. The material was obtained at post mortem and consisted of stained sections. The same sort of micro-organisms were found in all—lance-shaped diplococci—often in tremendous numbers, especially in red hepatization. They were undoubtedly pneumococci. Friedländer clearly showed that the cocci were found in large numbers in the lymphatics of the edematous interstitial connective tissue which ran from the margin of the hepatized tissue toward the air-containing parenchyma, thus anticipating the modern work of Robertson (Ref. 57) and others. This finding was regarded as very important: "It brings unequivocal proof that the micro-cocci get into the tissue juices and actually grow in living tissue." Are these micrococci the cause of pneumonia? asked Friedländer. He felt that anatomical studies did not absolutely settle the question but thought that the fact that most pneumonias resulted from "cold" was not incompatible with a bacterial etiology; cold might predispose to invasion by "pneumococci." This was the standard concept for many years until pneumococci were separated into groups (Ref. 40).

14. [LEYDEN]. Ueber infektiöse Pneumonie, Verhandl. d. Ver. inn. Med. zu Berlin, November 20, 1882, *in* Deutsche med. Wchnschr., **9**:52, 1883.

The previous work had all been on post-mortem material. Leyden reported the finding of cocci corresponding to those described by Friedländer (Ref. 13) in lung puncture fluid from a patient. This was confirmed at autopsy. At the same meeting Günther reported finding diplococci by lung puncture in a patient very ill with pneumonia. Günther's drawing was said to show a capsule. These observations were taken as evidence of the infectious nature of lobar pneumonia. Maximilian Mátray ("Ueber Pneumoniecoccen," Wien. med. Presse, **24**:732, 766, 1883) made systematic studies of the sputa of patients with lobar pneumonia and found typical lance-shaped diplococci in smears, often in huge numbers. He regarded these, probably correctly, as identical with the pneumonia coccus described by Friedländer, another example of how confused the situation was at the time.

15. FRIEDLÄNDER, C. Die Mikrococcen der Pneumonie, Fortschr. d. Med., **1**:715, 1883.

Friedländer quickly extended the work discussed in his first paper (Ref. 13). The characteristic cocci were found in some fifty cases. Friedländer reported that one of his co-workers, Dr. Gram of Copenhagen, had succeeded in developing a method whereby the cocci were intensely blue-stained in contrast to a faintly counterstained background. He stated that Drs. Günther and Leyden were able to demonstrate the cocci in "pneumonia-juice" obtained by lung puncture, a procedure which was revived as a diagnostic measure many years later (Ref. 48). Dr. Günther also noted that the cocci were surrounded by an unstained capsule (Ref. 14). Friedländer studied the capsules extensively in material obtained by lung puncture at autopsy. He concluded that the capsule was mucinous, not an artifact but a product of the vital processes of the microorganism. Capsules were less evident in material from late cases (after the fifth day). He presumed that encapsulated cocci would be found in the blood of severely ill patients. Friedländer and his associates readily grew the organisms in pure culture on Koch's gelatin medium and subcultured them through many generations. Gram-positive diplococci were obtained in great quantity, but in these culture strains no capsule was demonstrated. However, when the bacteria were injected into mice, the animals all died within a day or so, with innumerable *capsulated* organisms in blood, lung, and pleura. Friedländer did not quite understand that he had produced a septicemia rather than simply a severe pneumonia with overflow into the blood stream, and he was unable to infect rabbits. He observed slight differences in size and shape and capsule formation in different animals under various circumstances. Friedländer considered his findings strongly in favor of the "infectious" theory of lobar pneumonia.

Anyone who studies this paper will be convinced that Friedländer saw and described the pneumococcus. There were two puzzling features, however. Friedländer's coccus, in distinction to true pneumococcus, did not produce disease in rabbits, and it grew profusely on almost any medium. Also, in some of his pictures rod-shaped organisms are shown. Fränkel (Ref. 23) promptly seized on these discrepancies to claim that Friedländer's organism was actually a bacillus and that it was quite different from the true pneumococcus which he, Fränkel, had described so well. Here is a mystery probably never to be solved. Friedländer clearly began with pneumococcus. All his many typical cases of lobar pneumonia could not possibly have been "Friedländer pneumonia." Somewhere along the line, however, things evidently became confused with another encapsulated organism—*Klebsiella pneumoniae*. Fränkel left no stone unturned to deprive Friedländer of any credit, although Friedländer's name clearly deserves mention in the discovery of pneumococcus, much more so than that of Weichselbaum (Ref. 21).

16. TALAMON, Ch. Note sur le coccus lancéole de la pneumonie lobaire fibrineuse, Progr. méd., Paris, **11**:1030, 1883.

Talamon had been working on the pneumonia problem when Friedländer's paper (Ref. 15) stimulated him to make a report. He concluded with an admirable summary: "Lobar pneumonia is an infectious disease produced by the multiplication in the lung of a special microbe. This microbe can be found in the pneumonic exudate from the living patient. It is not in the blood except in certain cases, probably very rare, in the agonal stage. It has a characteristic lanceolate form, like a grain of wheat. It can be isolated and grown in appropriate media. One can produce with it experimentally fibrinous lobar pneumonia in the rabbit." There can be no doubt that Talamon deserves credit for early accurate work on the subject, and one is not surprised that the French often speak of Fränkel's observations as a confirmation of those of Talamon. The paper was read at the November 30 meeting of the Société Anatomique of Paris.

17. EMMERICH, Rudolph. Pneumoniecoccen in der Zwischendeckenfüllung als Ursache einer Pneumonie-Epidemie, Fortsch. d. Med., **2**:153, 1884.

Pneumonia had been epidemic at the Amberg prison for several months. From dust in the floor crevices Emmerich was able to cultivate "pneumonia cocci" and to kill rabbits with culture material. No pneumonia cocci were recovered from dust of rooms where there had been no cases of pneumonia. A number of other contemporary workers published similar findings (for summary see Washbourn's Croonian lectures [Ref. 32]), some of which are not very convincing, although confirmed later by the comprehensive work of Stillman (Ernest G. Stillman, "Further studies on the epidemiology of lobar pneumonia," J. Exper. Med., **26**:513, 1917). Stillman found that, from the dust of houses in which cases of Types I and II lobar pneumonia had been ill, pneumococci of the same sort could be recovered. In dust from rooms in which there had been no cases of pneumonia, pneumococci were found in 29 per cent of sixty-two specimens. These were almost always of the types normally found in the mouth. The epidemiological implications are discussed.

18. FRÄNKEL, A. Die genuine Pneumonie, Verhandl. d. Kong. f. inn. Med., 3d Cong., p. 17. Wiesbaden: J. F. Bergmann, 1884.

Fränkel, speaking in a symposium on pneumonia on April 21, 1884, succeeded in thoroughly confusing things. First he reported, in contradiction of Friedländer's experience (Ref. 15), infection of *rabbits* by some, but not all, strains of the "pneumonia coccus." He referred to Friedländer's observations on capsule formation and declared that there was another organism which also was encapsulated and closely resembled the pneumonia coccus to be found in the mouths of normal people. This organism injected into rabbits often caused death in 24–48 hours, and Fränkel designated it the coccus of sputum septicemia (Refs. 11, 12). Fränkel had no idea that this organism could be related to the cocci found in cases of lobar pneumonia and came to the conclusion that, because similar organisms are found in normal saliva, "it is not possible to characterize the pneumonia micrococcus as such."

Friedländer, in discussion, had no direct rebuttal but stuck to his guns. Half-a-dozen other prominent physicians talked but added nothing.

19. MENDELSOHN, Martin. Die infektiöse Natur der Pneumonie, Ztschr. f. klin. Med., **7**:178, 1884.

This comprehensive article begins with a review of the reported epidemics and outbreaks of pneumonia in various localities, in military establishments, in jails, and in houses. Convincing instances of spread by contagion are described. The writer does not think that pneumonia is caused by bad weather, since most cases occur in the spring. He confirms previous bacteriological studies and agrees that there is a specific organism. Mendelsohn contributes little in regard to the mode of transmission but notes that pneumonia recurs frequently in the same person and that an attack apparently confers no lasting protection. He speculates at length about the immunity of pneumonia with no final conclusion.

This paper is especially valuable for its comprehensive review of contemporary ideas.

20. STERNBERG, George M. The pneumonia coccus of Friedländer (Micrococcus pasteuri, Sternberg), Am. J.M. Sc., **90**:106, 1885.

This important paper illustrates well the confusion which existed as to the definition of the pneumococcus. Sternberg wished to name the coccus of sputum septicemia (Refs. 11, 12) in honor of Pasteur; he also considered the organism obtained from sputa of healthy people identical with the "pneumonia-coccus" of Friedländer. He found that cocci obtained from lungs of lobar pneumonia patients corresponded to Friedländer's description. He concluded: "The pneumonia-coccus of Friedländer is identical specifically with the micrococcus previously described by me which is commonly found in normal human saliva." He thought that pneumonia was an autoinfection promoted by alcohol or "any other depressing agency."

21. WEICHSELBAUM, A. Ueber die Aetiologie der akuten Lungen- und Rippenfellentzündungen, Med. Jahrb., N.S., **1**:483, 1886.

In this article of nearly seventy-five pages, Weichselbaum gives a valuable review of the contemporary literature on the bacteriology and etiology of pneumonia, which is followed by his own studies. In typical lobar pneumonia the finding of *Diplococcus pneumoniae* was constant enough to make him feel, with Fränkel, that it was the usual organism, although in his conclusions Weichselbaum said: "The acute inflammations of the lung, including genuine croupous pneumonia, may be caused by a variety of bacteria." Streptococci, staphylococci, and the organism of Friedländer, which grew freely on all media at room temperature and was non-pathogenic for rabbits, were found in some cases. No precise statement was made as to the type of disease, although Weichselbaum isolated staphylococci from lobular rather than from lobar pneumonia. Weichselbaum found pneumococci not only in the lungs but in the loose connective tissue of the neck, in the paranasal sinuses, and in the meninges; there was evidently a bacteremia in these cases. On the whole, his work has been taken as a confirmation of Fränkel. An abbreviation of Weichselbaum's article appeared in the same year (Weichselbaum, "Ueber die Aetiologie und pathologische Anatomie der Lungenentzündungen," Wien. med. Presse, **27**:820, 1886). Later, in still another long paper, Weichselbaum ("Ueber seltenere Lokalization des pneumonischen Virus [Diplococcus pneumoniae]," Wien. klin. Wchnschr., **1**:573, 1888) reviewed the status of the pneumococcus and dwelt especially on lesions other than in the lung—meningitis, endocarditis, pericarditis, arthritis, etc. He definitely formulated pneumococcal infection as a disease not necessarily confined to the lungs but rather a general infection with variable localization. In reviewing Weichselbaum's work, one sees no special reason why his name should have become attached to the pneumococcus; Friedländer had a much better title.

Friedländer's organism still remains a mystery. It was pretty clearly not a true pneumococcus; how, then, was it found so often by Friedländer in cases with all the earmarks of ordinary acute lobar pneumonia? (See Refs. 13, 15.)

22. SENGER, Emil. Bakteriologische Untersuchungen über die Pneumonie und pneumonische Metastasen, Arch. f. exper. Path. u. Pharmakol., **20**:389, 1886.

Senger felt that infection might spread from a primary pneumonia to other situations (metastases). He described especially meningitis, endocarditis, and pericarditis with the finding of typical cocci in all situations. The concept of a bacteremia in association with many such metastases is not clearly brought out.

23. FRÄNKEL, A. Bakteriologische Mitteilungen, Ztschr. f. klin. Med., **10**:401, 1886.

The first part of this lengthy communication is essentially a confirmation and extension of the work of Pasteur and of Sternberg (Refs. 11, 12). There is a disagreeable and quarrelsome tone, and Friedländer especially seems to receive digs on every possible opportunity. Fränkel spoke of the organism obtained from saliva as the micrococcus of sputum septicemia. Part 2 is concerned with the isolation of bacteria from lobar pneumonia. Fränkel was a careful and skilled bacteriologist and clearly isolated, grew, and defined the pneumococcus. He insisted that the organism isolated by Friedländer was something quite different, partly because it did not kill rabbits and partly because of its profuse growth on gelatin. He concluded that the micrococci f sputum septicemia were ubiquitous and caused pneumonia if there was a precipitating cause, especially cold, and this doctrine of the genesis of pneumonia held sway until the discovery of pneumococcus types (Refs. 37, 40).

As to Friedländer, it seems clear that Fränkel crowded him out of the picture and really forced on him the bacillus which for so long has borne his name. Actually, the weight of evidence, as anyone who carefully studies Friedländer's papers will see (Refs. 13, 15), is that he clearly first saw and adequately described the pneumococcus. An authoritative and fair appraisal of the matter is to be found in White (Ref. 59, pp. 11 ff.).

In this paper, also, Fränkel makes perhaps the first observation on acquired pneumococcal immunity in rabbits. An animal, inoculated by scarification of the ear with culture material, which survives has become immune "and a second inoculation proceeds without reaction."

24. FRÄNKEL, A. Weitere Beiträge zur Lehre von den Mikrococcen der genuinen fibrinösen Pneumonie, Ztschr. f. klin. Med., **11**:437, 1886.

Fränkel describes a case of meningitis in association with lobar pneumonia; he was able to recover the pneumococcus from the meninges. The bacteriology of pneumococcus is further elaborated in this paper, and Fränkel notes the speed with which pathogenicity is lost in culture and that virulence can be restored by animal passage. Fränkel was an expert bacteriologist and undoubtedly deserves credit for clearly defining the characteristics of pneumococcus. He also raises the question of whether every case of true lobar pneumonia is caused by one specific organism or whether the disease may be a reaction to a variety of germs. He concludes that it is a specific disease, always caused by pneumococcus.

Fränkel loses no opportunity to be disagreeable to Friedländer, whom he pursues quite unreasonably, and sets himself up as the sole elucidator of the etiology of lobar pneumonia. It was in this paper also that the name "pneumococcus" first appeared.[1]

25. KLEMPERER, G., and KLEMPERER, F. Versuche über Immunisierung und Heilung bei der Pneumokokkeninfektion, Berl. klin. Wchnschr., 28:833, 1891.

The 1890's were the beginning of the golden age of serum therapy. Doctors, "like stout Cortez when with eagle eyes he stared at the Pacific," saw a vast ocean of opportunity and dreamed of curing all infections by appropriate sera. The Klemperers were among the first to attempt systematically to immunize animals against pneumococcal infection. As antigens they used culture filtrates treated in various ways and old pneumonic exudates apparently free of organisms. There was no standard procedure and no fixed challenge dose. An "immune" rabbit was said to resist 1 cc. of the most virulent culture intravenously, and its serum in turn was able to "cure pneumococcal septicemia." This serum also was capable of immunizing other rabbits against a challenge given as long as 4 weeks later. There are lengthy speculations as to the mechanism of this immunity which have little meaning in the light of modern knowledge. The Klemperers also made preliminary observations in man and found that a dose of pneumococci fatal for a rabbit could be injected subcutaneously into man with impunity. G. Klemperer later exposed his general ideas on immunization ("Die Beziehung verschiedener Bakteriengifte zur Immunisierung und Heilung," Ztschr. f. klin. Med., 20:165, 1892).

26. KRUSE, Walther, and PANSINI, Sergio. Untersuchungen über den Diplococcus pneumoniae und verwandte Streptococcen, Ztschr. f. Hyg. u. Infektionskr., 11:279, 1892.

This authoritative article of nearly one hundred pages summarizes to date views on the biology of pneumococcus and on pneumococcal infection and immunity. It is of special importance, since a phenomenon which is probably that of bacterial dissociation (Ref. 53) is described for the first time. Unfortunately, most of the contemporary observations have little meaning in terms of modern immunology; indeed, many statements are hard to accept, but they indicate the great surge of interest in preventing and curing infections by immunotherapy.

27. MOSNY, E. Recherches expérimentales sur la vaccination contre l'infection pneumonique, Arch. méd. expér. et anat. path., 4:195, 1892.

Mosny was unable, in elaborate studies, to confirm the work of the Klemperers and others at all points. Animals could be protected against only relatively avirulent strains of pneumococcus from which spontaneous recovery might take place. This shows how confused and unstandardized the subject was. Mosny also showed that pneumococcus could grow in immune serum (see Ref. 47).

---

[1] The chronology of the various names applied to the cocci of pneumonia is given in White (Ref. 59, p. 1). We have noted the principal contributions to the early bacteriological study of pneumonia. Many more of lesser importance are reviewed by White (Ref. 59, pp. 6–11).

28. WASHBOURN, J. W. Experiments with the pneumococcus, with special reference to immunity, J. Path. & Bact., **3**:214, 1896.

Washbourn tried to bring some order into the subject. He showed clearly that a fatal dose of pneumococci might be withstood if injected intraperitoneally in rabbits *along with* some serum from an "immune" animal. He raised the question of different strains or races of pneumococci. He showed that pneumococci grew well in immune serum but were clumped at the bottom of the tube instead of growing diffusely (Ref. 31).

29. EYRE, J. W., and WASHBOURN, J. W. Resistant forms of pneumococcus, J. Path. & Bact., **4**:394, 1897.

Bacterial dissociation is clearly described, and the forms probably correspond to what were later designated as "rough" and "smooth" variants (Ref. 53).

30. DENYS, [J.]. Recherches sur le sérum antipneumococcique, Ann. Soc. méd.-chir. d'Anvers, **2**:51, 1897.

Denys, in studying immunization of rabbits against pneumococci, emphasized the role of *phagocytosis:* "In summary, immunity of the rabbit against the pneumococcus has its root in a modification of its serum. It is true that the serum by itself is powerless, but without it the leukocytes find themselves disarmed." Immunization of rabbits was by this time well established, and doses of 1 cc. of serum could protect against 100,000 lethal doses of pneumococci. Denys turned his attention to the preparation of serum in horses and goats and found that immune horse serum "1. Prevents infection. 2. Cures infection when it is already under way. 3. Neutralizes the toxins of the pneumococcus." The subject was beginning to assume an orderly aspect.

31. BEZANÇON, F., and GRIFFON, V. Pouvoir agglutinatif du sérum dans les infections expérimentales et humaines à pneumocoques, Compt. rend. Soc. de biol., **49**:551, 579, 1897.

Bezançon and Griffon made a special study of agglutination and found that immune serum diluted fifty fold might still be potent. They also tried to develop a diagnostic test analogous to Widal's test for typhoid fever. Pneumococci grown in serum from pneumonia patients in several instances grew in clumps with clear supernatant, whereas there was a diffuse clouding of other sera. Here, then, were the rudiments of the diagnostic test which later was so essential in typing pneumococci (Ref. 40).

32. EYRE, J. W. H., and WASHBOURN, J. W. Further experiments with Pane's antipneumococcus serum, Brit. M.J., **2**:1247, 1899.

A number of workers had been preparing antipneumococcic serum in large animals, and a few cases of human pneumonia had been treated (Refs. 25, 30). Eyre and Washbourn seem to have been the first to raise the question whether such sera might not be effective against all strains of pneumococcus. They used a serum prepared by Pane of Naples, and they found that it had considerable protective power for rabbits against only four out of five strains which were all similar in culture, morphology, and virulence. They concluded: "There exist varieties of pneumococcus which at present can only be distinguished by the action of antipneumococcus serum." Work of this sort pointed inevitably to the necessity of systematically classifying pneumococcus types (Ref. 40).

The whole subject of pneumococcus infection and immunity is well summarized to date in the Croonian lectures by J. W. Washbourn ("The natural history and pathology of pneumonia," Brit. M.J., **2**:1301, 1378, 1440, 1528, 1902).

33. NEUFELD, F. Ueber eine spezifische bakteriolytische Wirkung der Galle, Ztschr. f. Hyg. u. Infektionskr., **34**:454, 1900.

Description of the lytic effect of bile on pneuococcus.

34. NEUFELD, F. Ueber die Agglutination der Pneumococcen und über die Theorien der Agglutination, Ztschr. f. Hyg. u. Infektionskr., **40**:54, 1902.

In the course of this scholarly article on agglutination of pneumococci, Neufeld describes the phenomenon of capsular swelling (quelling) when pneumococci are mixed with antiserum. Since the phenomenon later turned out to be type-specific, it was adopted as a quick method of identifying pneumococci in sputum (E. Beckler and P. MacLeod. "The Neufeld method of pneumococcus type determination as carried out in a public health laboratory: a study of 760 typings," J. Clin. Investigation, **13**:901, 1934; G. M. Cooper and A. W. Walter, "Application of Neufeld reaction to the identification of types of pneumococci," Am. J. Pub. Health, **38**:491, 1935).

35. ANDERS, J. M. Serum therapy of pneumonia, J.A.M.A., **43**:1777, 1904.

In a useful paper Anders analyzes all the reported cases of pneumonia treated with the early sera, which were, of course, not type-specific. He concludes that the reduction in mortality is so slight that general use of the sera is not warranted but that further efforts to devise an efficacious serum are strongly advisable.

36. NEUFELD, F., and HÄNDEL. Ueber Herstellung und Prüfung von Antipneumococcenserum und über die Aussichten einer spezifischen Behandlung der Pneumonie, Ztschr. f. Immunitätsforsch. u. exper. Therap., **3**:159, 1909.

The writers described methods of producing therapeutic immune serum from horses and of testing its efficacy. They recognized the necessity of using large amounts of serum, of isolating the organism from the patient, and of seeing whether the available serum was protective against it.

Neufeld and Händel summarized their views on the entire subject of serum therapy in pneumonia in a later paper ("Zur Frage der Serumtherapie der Pneumonie und der Wertbestimmung des Pneumococcenserums," Berl. klin. Wchnschr., **49**:680, 1912).

37. NEUFELD, F., and HÄNDEL. Weitere Untersuchungen über Pneumococcen-Heilsera, Arb. a. d. k. Gsndhtsamte, **34**:293, 1910.

In the preceding decade a vast amount of work on antipneumococcal sera had been done. This work is reviewed in White (Ref. 59, pp. 103 ff.). Neufeld and Händel, however, devised a standard mouse-protection test and with it were able to show that an immune horse serum which protected against many strains was totally ineffective with others. The writers made a start at investigating this phenomenon systematically, but it remained for Dochez and Gillespie so to extend pneumococcus typing that it became the basis for specific serum therapy (Ref. 40).

38. CHATARD, J. A. An analytical study of acute lobar pneumonia in the Johns Hopkins Hospital from May 15, 1889, to May 15, 1905, Johns Hopkins Hosp. Rep., **15**:55, 1910.

There was a great tradition in the Osler Clinic at Johns Hopkins of describing disease on the basis of careful firsthand observations. Studies of malaria and of typhoid fever had already been made. In this paper a very valuable clinical study of pneumonia is reported, based on analysis of actual case records. Subsequent papers by various authors in the same volume deal with the pathological anatomy of lobar pneumonia (p. 81), the leukocytes in lobar pneumonia (p. 89), terminal pneumonia (p. 99), termination in recovery (p. 103), pneumococcic endocarditis (p. 139), pericarditis (p. 155), empyema (p. 167), thrombosis (p. 189), arthritis (p. 229), meningitis (p. 247), and delayed resolution (p. 277).

39. COLE, Rufus. Pneumococcus infection and immunity, J.A.M.A., **69**:693, 1912.

At the turn of the century the death rate from lobar pneumonia, although it varied in different places and in different outbreaks, was, on the whole, of the order of 25 per cent. Furthermore, the doctor was really helpless and could do little more than see to it that the patient had good nursing. In the attempt to solve this colossal problem and develop effective methods of therapy, the Rockefeller Hospital for many years took the lead in this country. Rufus Cole, director of the hospital, from time to time wrote important and useful papers covering the progress of the work. The present one was one of the first. Other important summaries by Cole are: "Pneumococcus infection and immunity," Arch. Int. Med., **14**:56, 1914; "Pneumococcus infection and immunity," New York M.J., **101**:1, 59, 1915; "The nature of pneumonia," Proc. Inst. Med., Chicago, **9**:2, 1932; "The treatment of pneumonia," Ann. Int. Med., **10**:1, 1936. Further papers by Cole are listed in Heffron's bibliography (Ref. 61, pp. 961–62), and detailed reviews of the literature may be found in Heffron (Ref. 61, pp. 204 ff.) and in White (Ref. 59, pp. 427 ff.).

40. DOCHEZ, A. R., and GILLESPIE, L. J. A biological classification of pneumococci by means of immunity reactions, J.A.M.A., **61**:727, 1913.

Although much work on this subject, culminating in that of Neufeld and Händel (Refs. 36, 37), had been done abroad, this paper remains the classical study. Here it was clearly brought out by mouse-protection and agglutination tests that as many as 65 per cent of pneumococci from patients with pneumonia fell into two distinct immunological types; that 14 per cent more could be identified by cultural qualities as *Pneumococcus mucosus* (Type III), whereas only 22 per cent fell into a miscellaneous group. The differentiation of these types served for years as a basis for developing specific therapeutic sera.

Lister, working at the same time in South Africa (F. S. Lister, "Specific serological reactions with pneumococci from different sources," Publ. South African Inst. M. Res., **1**:1, 1913), came to essentially the same grouping of pneumococcus strains.

41. COLE, Rufus. The treatment of pneumonia by means of specific serums, J.A.M.A., **61**:663, 1913.

This is the earliest statement about serum therapy from the Rockefeller Hospital. Hyperimmune sera, prepared in horses, were of such a potency that 1 cc. protected animals against a million lethal doses *if injected with the bacteria.* If serum was given *after* the infection was well under way, even a huge amount was ineffective. On these facts Cole enunciated two principles in the serotherapy of pneumonia. First, treatment should be begun as early in the disease as possible; second, large doses of potent serum should be used. In practice, 100 cc. of serum were usually given intravenously once or twice daily. Bloomfield later showed that blood-stream invasion was the critical point and that, as long as the blood culture was negative, the effects of serum were good, whereas if the blood culture was positive, the results were poor regardless of day of disease. In other words, serum seemed to aid, up to a certain point, in preventing overwhelming infection, but beyond this, as in the mouse, it was impotent (A. L. Bloomfield, "The therapeutic value of Type I antipneumococcus serum," J.A.M.A., **81**:1437, 1923).

42. NEWBURGH, L. H., and MINOT, George R. The blood-pressure in pneumonia, Arch. Int. Med., **14**:48, 1914.

There was an old tradition in medicine that primary circulatory failure was the cause of death in lobar pneumonia. A drop in blood pressure in millimeters of mercury below the pulse rate expressed in beats per minute (Gibson's index) was regarded as a very bad prognostic sign, and every effort was made to combat this symptom. Newburgh and Minot's observations, showing that low systolic pressure was not "invariably of evil omen" and that systolic pressure was often higher in fatal cases than in those which recovered, disposed of the idea that blood-pressure measurements could be used as a basis for prognosis in pneumonia (see also Ref. 43).

43. NEWBURGH, L. H., and PORTER, W. T. The heart muscle in pneumonia, J. Exper. Med., **22**:123, 1915.

Newburgh and Porter perfused the hearts of dogs dead of pneumonia and concluded that the heart muscle was not functionally impaired in pneumonia, since the pneumonic ventricle beat normally as soon as it received normal blood. They concluded that circulatory failure was an incident in dying pneumonia patients but not a primary disturbance. This work did much to change the emphasis in treatment from the circulation to the infectious process (see also Ref. 42).

44. DOCHEZ, A. R., and AVERY, O. T. Varieties of pneumococcus and their relation to lobar pneumonia, J. Exper. Med., **21**:114, 1915.

Dochez and Avery extended the studies of Dochez and Gillespie (Ref. 40) and again found that about 75 per cent of the pneumococci from cases of pneumonia fell into three groups. If these highly pathogenic strains were the same as the pneumococci so constantly present in the mouths of healthy people, infection should soon become universal. A study was therefore made of the types of pneumococci in the salivas of healthy people, and, almost without exception, members of the three virulent groups which usually cause pneumonia were absent, while the pneumococci present were the relatively avirulent heterologous types. Furthermore, following acute lobar pneumonia, the types causing the disease almost always disappeared shortly and were replaced by the usual mouth varieties. Rarely was a carrier of fixed-type pneumococcus encountered. This important work at one stroke disposed of the long-held idea that pneumonia was always an autogenous infection with strains of essentially harmless pneumococci carried in the mouth and that some "resistance-lowering" factor allowed invasion to occur. It became clear that infection usually resulted from a virulent strain which was not indigenous to the patient's upper air passages.

45. DOCHEZ, A. R., and AVERY, O. T. The occurrence of carriers of disease-producing types of pneumococcus, J. Exper. Med., **22**:105, 1915. After Dochez and Gillespie had isolated special types of pneumococci (Ref. 40) from cases of pneumonia, it was natural to inquire whether these disease-producing organisms were the same as the pneumococci found in the mouths of so many healthy people. The question was partly answered in the preceding reference (Ref. 44). It now became necessary to find out more about the circumstances of the occasional carriage of virulent fixed types. It turned out that, for a time, "healthy persons intimately associated with cases of lobar pneumonia harbor the disease-producing types of pneumococcus. In every such instance the pneumococcus isolated has corresponded in type with that of the infected individual. . . . The existence of the carrier state [of virulent pneumococci] among healthy persons and among those recently recovered from pneumonia establishes a basis for understanding the mechanism by means of which lobar pneumonia spreads and maintains its high incidence from year to year." Virgil P. W. Sydenstricker and Alan C. Sutton ("An epidemiological study of lobar pneumonia," Bull. Johns Hopkins Hosp., **28**:312, 1917) found in a group of workmen living in very close contact, among whom there was a high incidence of fixed-type pneumonia, that the presence of Types I and II pneumococci in the salivas of healthy men showed the remarkably high figure of 22 per cent. Another extremely important study is that of E. G. Stillman, "Further studies on the epidemiology of lobar pneumonia," J. Exper. Med., **26**:513, 1917.

An immense amount of work was subsequently done on the incidence of carriers of various types in relation to disease, contact, season, climate, etc. This work is reviewed in detail with bibliography in Heffron (Ref. 61, pp. 342 ff.). The summary by Maxwell Finland ("Recent advances in the epidemiology of pneumococcal infections," Medicine, **21**:307, 1942) is also useful.

Even more recent interesting studies have been made, such as those of W. G. Smillie, Frank A. Calderone, and Jeane M. Onslow, "The epidemiology of the pneumococcus," Am. J. Hyg., **37**:156, 1943. They found in a group of 111 men who were followed through a season that pneumococci of many types were highly prevalent; one man harbored seven different pneumococcus types in his throat during the period of observation, whereas many were persistent carriers of the same strain. Carriage seemed to have no definite relation to clinical pneumonia.

46. AVERY, Oswald T. A further study on the biological classification of pneumococci, J. Exper. Med., **22**:804, 1915.

The original groups of pneumococci described by Dochez and Gillespie (Ref. 40) were eventually found to be divisible into many more types (Ref. 56). Avery's paper represented a start in this direction when he showed that at least three subgroups of pneumococcus Type II could be recognized by specific immune reactions.

47. STRYKER, Laura M. Variations in the pneumococus induced by growth in immune serum, J. Exper. Med., **24**:49, 1916.

Stryker made the important observation that pneumococci grown in immune serum did not become more virulent but lost their virulence. The bacteria at the same time lost their capsules and were phagocyted in normal serum. Virulence and capsule could then be restored by animal passage. These observations were a prelude to the discovery, so important in the mechanism of pneumococcus infection, that invasiveness was associated with the presence of the specific capsular substance (Ref. 50) and that recovery from infection was dependent on the neutralization of this capsular substance by naturally produced immune bodies or by foreign serum (Ref. 51).

48. AVERY, Oswald T., CHICKERING, H. T., COLE, Rufus, and DOCHEZ, A. R. Acute lobar pneumonia, prevention and serum treatment. Monogr. Rockefeller Inst. M. Research, No. 7, 1917.

In this important monograph the Rockefeller workers summarize their studies on pneumonia to date. The methods for isolating pneumococci and "typing them" by mouse inoculation and by agglutination are described. The details of preparing immune horse sera and the technique of serum therapy are given. One hundred and seven cases of Type I lobar pneumonia were treated, with a mortality of 7.5 per cent as against a mortality of 25–30 per cent in the same hospital before the era of serotherapy. Unfortunately, conditions vary so much in different places and different outbreaks that years went by without everyone being convinced of the efficacy of the serum under every circumstance. It is impossible to quote all the vast literature on the subject, but the material is critically analyzed in Heffron's book (Ref. 61, p. 880). Among 3,611 cases of Type I pneumonia, for example, treated in various localities, the mortality varied in different groups from 4.1 to 47 per cent, with over-all death rates of 16.5 per cent.

Since serum therapy has been entirely replaced by antibiotics, the controversy as to the value of the former becomes largely of historical interest. However, certain landmarks should be mentioned. One of the great difficulties with the early use of large quantities of unrefined horse serum was the high incidence of severe serum reactions. These were described in detail by A. L. Bloomfield ("Effects of serum therapy in lobar pneumonia," Bull. Johns Hopkins Hosp., **28**:301, 1917) and others. An advance was made by L. D. Felton ("Isolation and concentration of specific antibodies of antipneumococcic sera," Boston M. & S.J., **189**:136, 1923) when he succeeded in concentrating the crude serum. Later, concentrated rabbit antisera largely replaced horse serum (K. Goodner, F. L. Horsfall, Jr., and R. J. Dubos, "Type-specific antipneumococcic rabbit serum for therapeutic purposes; production, processing, and standardization," J. Immunol., **33**:279, 1937; see also Heffron, Ref. 61, p. 872). The whole subject is authoritatively reviewed by F. T. Lord and R. Heffron (*Pneumonia and Serum Therapy* [New York: Commonwealth Fund; London: Oxford University Press, 1938]).

49. SUTTON, Alan C., and SEVIER, Charles E. A study of the bacteremia in lobar pneumonia, Bull. Johns Hopkins Hosp., **23**:315, 1917.

The writers made daily quantitative blood cultures on a consecutive series of patients. "Ninety-three per cent of the patients with persistently negative blood cultures recovered without complication. Of the patients with positive blood cultures all with over five colonies per cc. at any period of the disease died, except one with twenty colonies on admission who received serum therapy." This work showed very clearly that bacteremia was not the cause of death but that bacteremia was an indication that the powers of resistance of the patient against infection were breaking down; his immunological status, in other words, came to resemble that of the mouse, which notably has little resistance against pneumococcus infection. From these observations Bloomfield drew conclusions as to the practical efficacy of serum therapy (Ref. 41), which has little curative value after increasing bacteremia is under way. However, it was shown later that patients even with progressive bacteremia could be saved by a powerful pneumococcidal agent such as penicillin (Ref. 62). Sutton and Sevier's observations were confirmed by others (Jesse G. M. Bullowa and Clare Wilcox, "Incidence of bacteremia in the pneumonias and its relation to mortality," Arch. Int. Med., **55**:558, 1935). Important recent studies on bacteremia in pneumonia are those of O. H. Robertson, Morton Hamburger, Jr., and Lucien A. Gregg, "On the nature of bacteremia in experimental pneumococcal pneumonia in the dog," J. Exper. Med., **97**:283, 1953; Lucien A. Gregg and O. H. Robertson, J. Exper. Med., **97**:297, 1953.

50. HEIDELBERGER, M., and AVERY, O. T. The soluble specific substance of pneumococcus, J. Exper. Med., **38**:73, 1923.

The writers showed that the soluble specific substance formed by pneumococci (A. R. Dochez and O. T. Avery, "The elaboration of specific soluble substance by pneumococcus during growth," J. Exper. Med., **26**:477, 1917) "consists mainly of a carbohydrate," which is type-specific. In another paper (O. T. Avery and M. Heidelberger "Immunological relationships of cell constituents of pneumococcus," J. Exper. Med., **38**:81, 1923) it was pointed out that the protein of pneumococcus exhibited only species-specificity, whereas the soluble substance was type-specific. These observations became of the greatest importance in practical work on immunity. The immense literature is reviewed by White (Ref. 59, pp. 238 ff.), but for a brief authoritative summary see Oswald T. Avery, "The role of specific carbohydrates in pneumococcus infection and immunity," Ann. Int. Med., **6**:1, 1932.

51. AVERY, Oswald T., and HEIDELBERGER, Michael. Immunological relationships of cell constituents of pneumococcus (second paper), J. Exper. Med., **42**:367, 1925.

In this paper the writers first hinted at the concept, so fundamental in practical immunology of pneumococcus infection, that the soluble capsular substance of the organisms had to do with the virulence of the infection and that specific immune bodies dissolved or neutralized such capsular substance, rendering the pneumococci vulnerable. "If final proof be brought for the conception that the capsular zone of the organism is largely composed of this carbohydrate substance, is part of the defense mechanism of the cell, and is the site of its initial contact with antibody, then these soluble bacterial polysaccharides acquire new significance not only in the serological reactions of the cell, but in the actual process of infection and immunity in the host."

It has recently been shown that highly virulent strains produce more soluble specific substance than do moderately virulent or avirulent strains (Colin M. MacLeod and Marjorie R. Krauss, "Relation of virulence of pneumococcal strains for mice to the quantity of capsular polysaccharide formed in vitro," J. Exper. Med., **92**:1, 1950; Barry Wood, Jr., and Mary Ruth Smith, "Host-parasite relationships in experimental pneumonia due to pneumococcus Type III," J. Exper. Med., **92**:85, 1950). This work was carried forward and elaborated by improved methods in subsequent papers (Michael Heidelberger and Oswald T. Avery, "The soluble specific substance of the pneumococcus (second paper)," J. Exper. Med., **40**:301, 1924; Michael Heidelberger, Walther F. Goebel, and Oswald T. Avery, "The soluble specific substance of pneumococcus (third paper)," J. Exper. Med., **42**:727, 1925).

52. BARACH, Alvan L. Methods and results of oxygen treatment of pneumonia, Arch. Int. Med., **37**:186, 1926.

Because of the obvious anoxemia which is so common in pneumonia (C. Lunsgaard, "Anoxemia in lobar pneumonia," Medicine, **4**:345, 1925), it was hoped that oxygen administration might be a fundamentally helpful measure in acute lobar pneumonia. Barach in this paper reviews the subject authoritatively and concludes: "The value of oxygen treatment is felt to be supportive and not curative." Carl A. L. Binger's paper is also of importance ("Anoxemia in pneumonia and its relief by oxygen inhalation," J. Clin. Investigation, **6**:203, 1928). The technique of oxygen administration is fully detailed in Alvan L. Barach, *Principles and Practice of Inhalational Therapy* (Philadelphia, 1944).

53. GRIFFITH, Fred. The significance of pneumococcal types; J. Hyg., **27**:113, 1928.

In this now classical paper Griffith presented an elaborate study on the interconversions of "rough" and "smooth" strains of pneumococci in relation to virulance and to epidemiological problems. A method of producing the "S" to "R" change is described. A great deal of work has subsequently been done on the transformation of pneumococcus types. The Rockefeller group found that a nucleic acid of the desoxyribose type was concerned with the transformation of pneumococcus Type III (Oswald T. Avery, Colin M. MacLeod, and Maclyn McCarty, "Studies on the chemical nature of the substance inducing transformation of pneumococcal types," J. Exper. Med., **79**:137, 1944). Recent work on this complex subject is illustrated by the work of Austrian (Robert Austrian and Colin M. MacLeod, "Acquisition of M protein by pneumococci through transformation reactions," J. Exper. Med., **89**:451, 1949; and Robert Austrian, "Morphological variation in pneumococcus," J. Exper. Med., **98**:21, 35, 1953).

54. TILLETT, William S., and FRANCIS, Thomas, Jr. Cutaneous reactions to the polysaccharides and proteins of pneumococcus in lobar pneumonia, J. Exper. Med., **50**:687, 1929.

Only a few of the vast number of papers on immunity reactions can be mentioned in this bibliography, but some of those having immediate clinical application should be discussed. Tillett and Francis found that an intradermal injection of pneumococcus polysaccharide caused a prompt reaction of the wheal type when the patient had recovered from infection. The reaction was type-specific and was associated with the presence of specific antibodies in the circulating blood. This skin test became an important practical guide to treatment because the development of a positive reaction indicated that recovery was under way (see also T. Francis, Jr., and W. S. Tillett, "Cutaneous reactions in pneumonia: development of antibodies following the intradermal injection of type-specific polysaccharide," J. Exper. Med., **52**:573, 1930; Thomas Francis, Jr., "The value of the skin test with type-specific capsular polysaccharide in the serum treatment of Type I pneumococcus pneumonia," J. Exper. Med., **57**:617, 1933; J. C. Edwards, C. L. Hoagland, and L. D. Thompson, "Type specific polysaccharide skin test in serum therapy of pneumonia," J.A.M.A., **113**:1876, 1939).

55. LÖSCHCKE, H. Untersuchungen über die kruppöse Pneumonie, Beitr. z. path. Anat., **86**:201, 1931.

Löschcke's important studies on pathogenesis were made on human material and really preceded the experimental observations of Robertson and his group (Ref. 57). Löschcke concluded that the infection of alveoli occurred not by the blood stream but by inhalation of pneumococci. He thought that a "hyperergic" reaction led to outpouring of edema fluid, in which pneumococci grew rapidly, and that infection spread from alveolus to alveolus through the pores of Kohn and by overflow from one bronchus into another.

56. COOPER, Georgia, ROSENSTEIN, Carolyn, WALTER, Annabel, and PEIZER, Lenore. The further separation of types among the pneumococci hitherto included in group IV and the development of therapeutic antisera for these types, J. Exper. Med., **55**:531, 1932.

From the first differentiation of types of pneumococci (Refs. 40, 44) emphasis had been placed on the development of specific antisera. Through the years the original serological groups were found to consist of more and more immunologically distinguishable types. This work went on all over the world, and the numerous papers are summarized in White (Ref. 59, p. 103). Cooper and her associates were able to describe thirty-two types, and antisera suitable for clinical trial were prepared for fourteen, while Eddy later found that the number had risen to seventy-five (B. F. Eddy, "Nomenclature of pneumococcus types," Pub. Health Rep., **59**:449, 1944). Certain clinical associations with various types were also pointed out.

As one sees, the typing and serotherapy of pneumococci were becoming exceedingly complex, when the discovery first of sulfonamides (Ref. 60) and later of penicillin (Ref. 62) made them obsolete in clinical practice after dominating the field for nearly thirty years.

An authoritative evaluation of the whole problem of pneumococcus types is that of Maxwell Finland, "The present status of the higher types of antipneumococcus serums," J.A.M.A., **120**:1294, 1942.

57. TERRELL, Edward E., ROBERTSON, Oswald H., and COGGE-SHALL, Lowell T. Experimental pneumococcus lobar pneumonia in the dog. I. Method of production and course of the disease, J. Clin. Investigation, **12**:393, 1933.
ROBERTSON, Oswald H., COGGESHALL, Lowell T., and TERRELL, Edward E. II. Pathology, *ibid.*, p. 433.
ROBERTSON, Oswald H., COGGESHALL, Lowell T., and TERRELL, Edward E. III. Pathogenesis, *ibid.*, p. 467.

There is a vast literature of speculation and experiment on the pathogenesis of lobar pneumonia which is reviewed by Heffron (Ref. 61, p. 232). These now classical observations of Robertson and his associates following Löschcke (Ref. 55) initiated a new era because they revealed the intimate details of the lesion and demonstrated that spread of infection was carried on a peripheral wave of bacteria-containing edema fluid. These findings were confirmed by many workers. C. Loosli ("The pathogenesis and pathology of experimental Type I pneumococcic pneumonia in the monkey," J. Exper. Med., **76**:79, 1942) reviewed the earlier work and presented observations of his own, which seem definitely to disprove former views that bacterial spread in the pneumonic lung is through the lymphatics. He supported the idea, now generally accepted, that the organisms enter new alveoli through the pores of Kohn and by the bronchi.

Robertson later presented an important summary of his work: "Newer knowledge concerning the inception of pneumonia and its bearing on prevention," Ann. Int. Med., **18**:1, 1943.

58. BLAKE, F. G., HOWARD, M. E., and HULL, W. S. Artificial pneumothorax in lobar pneumonia, Medicine, **15**:1, 1936.

Artificial pneumothorax had a brief but enthusiastic vogue in the therapy of lobar pneumonia. The subject is reviewed in this monograph.

59. WHITE, Benjamin. The biology of pneumococcus. New York: Commonwealth Fund; London: Oxford University Press, 1938.

This comprehensive book, with a bibliography of nearly sixteen hundred references, deals with every phase of the biology of pneumococcus and is an invaluable storehouse of information.

60. WHITBY, Lionel E. H. Chemotherapy of pneumococcal and other infections, with 2-(*p*-aminobenzenesulphonamido) pyridine, Lancet, **1**:1210, 1938.

The discovery of the sulfonamides initiated a new era in the chemotherapy of infections. Attempts at chemotherapy of pneumonia many years before with quinine derivatives seemed promising, but they were abandoned, because of toxic effects on the optic nerves, in favor of serotherapy, which held sway until 1938 (H. G. Moore and A. M. Chesney, "A further study of ethylhydrocuprein [Optochin] in the treatment of acute lobar pneumonia," Arch. Int. Med., **21**:659, 1918). Whitby found sulfapyridine much more effective than sulfanila-mide in experimental pneumococcus infection, and the clinical use of the drug was soon begun. The early work is reviewed in F. T. Lord, E. S. Robinson, and R. Heffron, *Chemotherapy and Serum Therapy of Pneumonia* (New York: Commonwealth Fund; London: Oxford University Press, 1940). The results were moderately satisfactory, but, just as in the early days of steam, ships still carried some sail, so sulfonamide therapy was often combined with serum. The frequency of empyema and of severe nausea and vomiting with sulfapyridine was found objectionable, and the whole subject was still under debate when the advent of penicillin made the drug obsolete. Other sulfonamides were also tried, and some of the useful papers on the whole subject are: S. M. Evans and Wilfred F. Gaisford, "Treatment of pneumonia with 2-(p-aminobenzene-sulphonamido) pyridine," Lancet, **2**:14, 1948; J. M. Ruegsegger, N. L. Brokers, M. Hamburger, and E. S. Grupen, "The treatment of pneumococcal pneumonia with sulfapyridine," Am. J.M. Sc., **206**:323, 1943; H. F. Flippin, L. Schwartz, and A. H. Domm, "Modern treatment of pneumococcic pneumonia," J.A.M.A., **121**:230, 1943; A. E. Price and G. B. Myers, "Treatment of pneumonia with sulfathiazole," Arch. Int. Med., **70**:558, 1942; W. S. Tillett, "Specific anti-pneumococcal immunity in relation to the chemotherapy of pneumonia," J. Clin. Investigation, **21**:511, 1942; F. T. Billings and W. B. Wood, Jr., "The use of sulfadiazine in the treatment of pneumococcal pneumonia," Bull. Johns Hopkins Hosp., **69**:314, 1941; M. Finland, F. C. Lowell, and E. Strauss, "Treatment of pneumococcic pneumonias with sulfapyridine, sulfathiazole, and serum," Ann. Int. Med., **14**:1184, 1941. Colin M. MacLeod ("Chemotherapy of pneu-mococcic pneumonia," J.A.M.A., **113**:1405, 1939) discussed the mechanism of sulfonamide action in pneumonia and pointed out that sulfonamides exert a strictly bacteriostatic effect until immune bodies and the phagocytic system are sufficiently effective to extirpate the infection. Thus sulfonamides and serum supplement each other, in contrast to the bactericidal effect of penicillin (Ref. 62). The important paper of D. D. Woods ("The relation of p-amino-benzoic acid to the mechanism of the action of sulphanilamide," Brit. J. Exper. Path., **21**:74, 1940) should also be mentioned.

61. HEFFRON, Roderick. Pneumonia, with general reference to pneumo-coccus lobar pneumonia. New York: Commonwealth Fund; London: Oxford University Press, 1939.

This monumental book supplements that of White (Ref. 59) and deals with every phase of lobar pneumonia. There is a bibliography of 1,471 references.

62. KEEFER, Chester S., BLAKE, Francis G., MARSHALL, E. Kennerly, Jr., LOCKWOOD, John S., and WOOD, W. Barry, Jr. Penicillin in the treatment of infections, J.A.M.A., **122**:1217, 1943.

Penicillin was soon tried in all sorts of infections. In this early report Keefer and his associates stated: "The pneumococcus is extremely sensitive to the action of penicillin. . . . It is plain . . . that penicillin is another potent weapon in the treatment of pneumococcic pneumonia." This statement was based on collected reports of forty-two patients, of whom only six died. However, the paper of Tillett and his associates (William S. Tillett, Margaret J. Cambier, and James E. McCormack, "The treatment of lobar pneumonia and pneumococcal empyema with penicillin," Bull. New York Acad. Med., **20**:142, 1944), giving details of management, showed clearly the superlative effect of penicillin. Among forty-six patients, only three (6.5 per cent) died. Above all, "bacteremia which occurred in 14 patients disappeared in every instance following injection of penicillin." Tillett also pointed out the value of intrapleural injections of penicillin in pneumococcic empyema. When penicillin first became available, supplies were scarce and uncertain, so that many cases were treated with serum, sulfonamides, and penicillin.

Colin M. MacLeod and Edna R. Stone ("Differences in the nature of antibacterial action of the sulfonamides and penicillin in their relation to therapy," Bull. New York Acad. Med., **21**:375, 1944) point out that, in contrast to sulfonamides (Ref. 60), penicillin exerts a direct bactericidal effect on pneumococcus both in the test tube and in the body. Thus penicillin cures without specific immunity being essential, although the development of immunity is, of course, desirable.

A recent summary of the practical use of antibiotics in pneumococcus pneumonia is that of Harry F. Dowling ("Pneumococcal and streptococcal infection," *in* Henry Welch, *Principles and Practice of Antibiotic Therapy* [New York: Medical Encyclopedia, Inc., 1954], p. 295).

63. WOOD, W. B., Jr. The mechanism of recovery in acute bacterial pneumonia, Ann. Int. Med., **27**:347, 1944.

From the early days of the subject there has been speculation and experiment on the mechanism of recovery from lobar pneumonia and of the dramatic phenomenon of the crisis. For the most part, the older work attempted to link recovery with the appearance of demonstrable antibodies. It has not been clear, however, whether all such antibodies were the cause of recovery or whether they were simply coincident (see White, Ref. 59, and Heffron, Ref. 61, for the early literature).

Wood summarizes newer views on the mechanism of recovery, especially with reference to surface phagocytosis, which may begin to operate in the absence of antibodies. This work was presented more in detail previously (W. Barry Wood, Jr., Mary Ruth Smith, and Barbara Watson, "Studies in the mechanism of recovery in pneumococcal pneumonia. IV. The mechanism of phagocytosis in the absence of antibody," J. Exper. Med., **84**:387, 1946) and was later summarized with full bibliography (W. Barry Wood, Jr., "Studies on the cellular immunology of acute bacterial infections," Harvey Lect. 1951–52 [New York: Academic Press, Inc., 1953], p. 72).

SCARLET FEVER

Bacteriology	Refs. 5, 6, 10, 11, 15, 16, 27, 28, 29
Clinical description	Refs. 1, 2
Immunity reactions	Refs. 14, 17, 20, 21, 22, 24, 25, 26, 30, 31
Lesions	Refs. 3, 4
Pathogenesis	Refs. 7, 12, 18, 19
Penicillin therapy	Ref. 32
Postscarlatinal disorders	Refs. 1, 13
Serum therapy	Refs. 8, 9, 23

Section 7

SCARLET FEVER

IN FOLLOWING the tangled thread of increasing knowledge through the vast literature on scarlet fever, the reader should remember that the main problems which have caused so much confusion in the past have now been solved. If the earlier students of the disease had stuck to their guns when they proposed, first, that the rash of scarlet fever is due to a soluble toxin produced in the throat by the causal organisms and, second, that a permanent immunity to the rash toxin is usually conferred by an attack without lessening susceptibility to subsequent infection with the same types of hemolytic streptococci, many of the puzzles which later perplexed the most astute observers would have been resolved.

It will not be profitable to attempt to define the origins of the obviously descriptive terms "scarlet fever" and "scarlatina." An excellent discussion of the problem is to be found in the book by J. D. Rolleston (*The History of the Acute Exanthemata* [London: William Heinemann, 1937], p. 47), who points out that these designations were already in common use in the seventeenth and eighteenth centuries. "My little girl, Susan, is fallen sick of the meazles, we fear, or at least, of a scarlett feavour," said Samuel Pepys in his diary under the entry for November 10, 1664.

Aside from the *Index Medicus* and the *Index Catalogue* of the Surgeon-General's Library, extensive bibliographies may be found in the following:

ESCHERICH, T., and SCHICK, B. *Der Scharlach.* (Vienna: Alfred Hölder, 1912), especially the older literature.

Annals of the Pickett-Thomson Research Laboratory (London: Baillière, Tindall & Cox, 1924–25), 1:115; v. 6 (1930).

WILLIAMS, ANNA W. *Streptococci in Relation to Man in Health and Disease* (Baltimore: Williams & Wilkins Co., 1932), chapter on scarlet fever, p. 125, and Bibliography, p. 221.

RANTZ, LOWELL A., *The Prevention of Rheumatic Fever* (Springfield, Ill.: Charles C Thomas, 1952), recent literature.

1. WELLS, William Charles. Observations on the dropsy which succeeds scarlet fever, Tr. Soc. Improvement M. & Chir. Knowledge, **3**:167, 1812. Although the dropsy following scarlet fever was mentioned in seventeenth- and eighteenth-century accounts, the first useful description in English was that of Wells: "Its first appearance is generally on the twenty-second or twenty-third day after the commencement of the preceding fever. If I can trust, however, to the report of a careful mother it may come as early as the sixteenth day; and I know from my own observations that its attack may be delayed to the twenty-fifth. When it has not appeared before the end of the fourth week, I have always ventured to affirm that its attack was no longer to be dreaded." "Contrary to what might have been expected, the dropsy often comes on after a very mild fever, and when the person, who had suffered it, appeared to have nearly or altogether recovered his former health." "In the beginning of the disease the

urine is scanty." "There is no doubt of the unusual colour being occasioned by the red matter of the blood." "There is another part of the blood which I have almost always found present in the urine of persons affected with this dropsy which is serum."

On the whole, however, this is a primitive account, and there is no speculation as to the cause or nature of the trouble. But by 1861 W. Hamburger ("Ein Beitrag zur Lehre und zur Therapie des Brightschen Scharlachhydrops," Vrtljschr. prakt. Heilk., 1:24, 1861) was thinking critically on the subject. He did not believe that nephritis was caused by the rash, because nephritis is absent after other exanthemata, such as measles or smallpox. He did not think exposure to cold an adequate explanation; nephritis might occur in the most carefully safeguarded children and not in those who "ran around barefooted." He pointed out the difference in frequency of nephritis in different epidemics, and he noted that nephritis might follow the mildest case and that, indeed, Bright's disease not preceded by recognized scarlet fever might still result from the same cause. He recognized, as other postscarlatinal effects, lymphadenopathy and acute articular rheumatism. His speculations on the exact cause are, however, meaningless to the modern reader, and it remained for Schick to introduce the concept of a hypersensitive reaction (Ref. 13).

2. TROUSSEAU, A. Clinique médicale de l'Hôtel-Dieu de Paris, 1:1, Scarlatine. Paris, 1861.

It is impossible to attribute to any one man the first adequate clinical description of scarlet fever. The pre-nineteenth-century accounts of Sydenham, of Fothergill, of Huxham, and of others are often referred to, but one finds them quite inadequate. What may have been scarlet fever was confused with throat infections, such as diphtheria, and possibly with various other "ulcerous" sore throats; the rashes of scarlet fever, of measles, and perhaps of pandemic influenza were not clearly distinguished. In some accounts sore throat is not mentioned at all; the classification of simple, anginose, and malignant forms of scarlet fever was for a long time popular. The severity of outbreaks varied, and the incidence of combined infections, such as scarlatina and diphtheria, and of violent, secondary, mixed infections must have been frequent. Furthermore, many accounts are diluted by lengthy dissertations on the weather, the winds, the prevalence of other disease, and all sorts of extraneous matter. Or the observer is distracted by lengthy discussions of the appearance of the urine, the character of the sweats, etc. Finally, the emotional overlay on the part of the physicians and parents, helpless in the face of what was often a disease terrifying in its malignancy, made unbiased reporting difficult.[1] It was only gradually, therefore, that adequate accounts, with good descriptions of the throat and of the rash and with clear definitions of the course of the disease and its complications, emerged.

---

[1] "So fatal have been the results, so fearful the ravages, so widespread the devastation of the disease, so interesting the period of life at which it commonly occurs, just as parental hopes are budding with promise, and the tendrils of affection entwining themselves most closely round the heart, that the very name is a signal of distress, and its introduction into the family circle is looked upon as the angel of death with an irreprievable warrant to destroy" (Casper Morris, *Lectures on Scarlet Fever* [Philadelphia: Lindsay & Blakiston, 1851], p. 1).

It is Trousseau, the master clinician, who gives the first account of scarlet fever in the modern sense, stripped of emotional overlay and inconsequential verbiage. He points out the great differences in severity of various outbreaks. "Scarlet fever may not appear on the skin; it is not less serious on this account." The complications are varied and unpredictable, in contrast to measles. He quotes a case to show that the incubation period may be as brief as 24 hours. There are minutely accurate descriptions of the character and course of the rash and of the sore throat. "From the first day of the disease, the palate is red like the skin, and the tonsils are swollen and violaceous. There appear on the tonsils little white spots. They are different from the false membrane of diphtheria. They are pultaceous and appear to be the secretions from the surface of the [tonsillar] ulcers. As the rash fades, the tonsils get rid of these [white] patches, although they remain reddened and sometimes ulcerated: the disease is cured." Trousseau clearly distinguishes the peeling of scarlet fever from the branlike desquamation of measles. In contrast to diphtheria, "scarlatina does not like the larynx." There is an accurate description of the postscarlatinal disorders: "I cannot repeat too emphatically that in scarlet fever one cannot consider the patients cured until a long time after the cessation of all morbid phenomena." He emphasizes anasarca: "This accident occurs in convalescents not only if they have been exposed to cold or have committed some imprudence but even when they have remained quiet with the best of care and the most constant solicitude." The associated hematuria and albuminuria are discussed. Trousseau differentiates the usual postscarlatinal "rheumatism," pleurisy, pericarditis, and endocarditis from the occasional suppurative lesions. He points out that it is rare for children who have had attacks of "acute articular rheumatism" to escape a later attack of the dance of Saint Guy (chorea).

Trousseau came very near to understanding the implications of scarlatina without rash. "I have seen members of the same family who, having had the sore throat without eruption, were then immune to scarlet fever even though the others around them were more or less violently attacked [with scarlet fever]." "A child returned from school where there was an outbreak of scarlet fever; she had sore throat and headache and could hardly swallow. The next day the tonsils were swollen, but there was no trace of skin rash. Before this child was well, scarlatina attacked her two sisters and father. The two sisters had the rash and later peeled; the father had only a few pink specks on his skin and did not peel." In another family three children were sick with scarlet fever. Two adult servants were attacked with violent tonsillitis, but there was no exanthem. Trousseau credits Graves with describing anasarca following subclinical scarlatina indicated only by overt attacks in other members of the family. "These passages prove, therefore, that under the skies of Dublin as under the skies of Paris the same things are manifest."

Trousseau's discussion of treatment is of less interest to the modern student, but, on the whole, little has been added to this admirable description, which occupies some thirty closely printed pages and should be read by every student of communicable disease, if possible in the original (translation: A. Trousseau, *Lectures on Clinical Medicine* [Philadelphia: Lindsay & Blakiston, 1869], **2**:183).

3. HEUBNER, Otto. Beobachtungen über Scharlachdiphtherie, Jahrb. f. Kinderh., **14**:1, 1879.

At a time when the throat lesions of scarlet fever and diphtheria were badly confused, Heubner made histological studies of the tonsils from patients with what appeared to be uncomplicated scarlet fever, who died in the first few days of the disease. "Scarlatinal 'diphtheria' is intimately bound up with the entire disease—scarlet fever—and is to be sharply differentiated both clinically and histologically from primary diphtheria."

4. NEUMANN, I. Ueber die histologischen Veränderungen der Haut bei Morbillen und Scharlach (Wiener) Med. Jahrb., p. 159, 1882.

This appears to have been the first attempt at a systematic biopsy study of the skin in scarlet fever. The main findings were hyperemia, edema, extravasations of blood cells, and some inflammatory cells. Details as to day of disease on which the specimens were obtained are lacking. P. G. Unna (*Die Histopathologie der Hautkrankheiten* [Berlin: A. Hirschwald, 1894], p. 628) also emphasized the immense dilation of the blood vessels with only a few inflammatory cells. E. Rach later (Beitr. path. Anat., **47**:455, 1910) amplified the earlier observations. He emphasized hyperemia, exudate, into the superficial skin layers, the collection of the exudate into tiny vesicles, and, finally, death of epithelium with desquamation. He regarded the process as toxic rather than inflammatory in the classical sense.

5. LOEFFLER, Friedrich. Untersuchungen über die Bedeutung der Mikro-Organismen für die Entstehung der Diphtherie beim Menschen, bei der Taube und beim Kalbe, Mitt. a. d. k. Gsndhtsamte, **2**:421, 1884.

The relationship of streptococci to disease, as well as the occurrence of these organisms in healthy people, was recognized early in the bacteriological era, so that in the 1880's there was already a huge literature on the subject. By that time streptococci had been isolated from erysipelas, puerperal fever, and scarlet fever. It is extremely difficult to assign priority. Those interested in pursuing details may scan the *Index Catalogue* of the Surgeon-General's Library, in which, up to 1910, there are some seventy closely printed pages of references to scarlet fever alone. Most of the findings in the early papers are confused by inadequate methods of isolation, mixed infection, difficulties in classification, etc. For example, Hallier ("Der pflanzliche Organismus im Blute der Scharlachkranken," Jahrb. f. Kinderh., **2**:169, 1869) has been credited with being the first to isolate streptococci from the blood of scarlet fever patients. An examination of his paper, however, shows that he was dealing with a mold; his drawings are quite conclusive; they show hyphae, conidia, etc.[2]

Loeffler, in a monumental paper primarily on diphtheria, seems to have been the first definitely to isolate pyogenic streptococci from cases of scarlet fever. In a number of cultures of "diphtheria" complicated by scarlet fever, he clearly describes chains of cocci which can be seen penetrating from the necrotic sur-

[2] To show how important is examination of original reports in establishing priority, Pohl-Pincus (Centralbl. f. d. med. Wissensch., **21**:640, 1883) has been spoken of in the literature as the first to describe streptococci in scarlet fever. Actually, he examined desquamated skin by direct smears and described cocci which in all probability were staphylococci. There is no evidence that he identified streptococci.

faces into the lymphatics of the tonsils. Cultures in meat infusion peptone gelatin yielded colonies of long-chained streptococci. From the internal organs of fatal cases these organisms were also readily obtained in pure cultures, which produced suppuration, especially in joints, when injected into rabbits and other animals. Loeffler's precise and convincing work is in sharp contrast to that of most contemporaneous observers; his success was due to his excellent methods and technique. The whole position was well summarized by Escherich (Centralbl. f. Bakt., **1**:381, 1887). From this time on, no competent observer doubted the frequent or constant occurrence of streptococci in scarlet fever. The questions debated were whether these organisms were the primary cause of the disease, secondary invaders, or incidental findings of no consequence at all. Obviously, these questions could not be finally answered until better methods of isolating and classifying streptococci were developed (see Refs. 15, 16, 28, 29), which showed that cultures properly made from the pharynx early in scarlet fever yield *hemolytic* streptococci in every case (Ref. 16).

6. The relation between milk-scarlatina in the human subject and disease in the cow. Report of Mr. W. H. Power and of Dr. Klein to the Local Government Board entitled "Milk scarlatina in London, 1885," Practitioner, **37**:61, 143, 1886.

Another important link in the chain of evidence incriminating streptococcal infection as a cause of scarlet fever came from observations on so-called milk scarlatina. The literature, especially from England, of the last quarter of the century is full of reports of outbreaks of the disease which seem clearly related to ingestion of milk. It was Power, however, who in this classical study definitely traced an outbreak in London through the retailer in South Marylebone to a particular cow in the dairy farm supplying the milk. This is a brilliant example of public health "detective work" and should rank as a classic with Budd's observations on typhoid fever. Study of the lesions of the diseased udders by Dr. Klein yielded in culture "micrococci, arranged as diplococci, and as shorter or longer chains—streptococcus—these latter sometimes of great length." "The milk, during the act of milking, is pretty sure to become contaminated. The organisms would find in the milk a good medium in which to multiply. Such milk would then practically correspond to an artificial culture of streptococcus such as we have found capable of setting up a general disease when inoculated subcutaneously into calves." The description of the animal lesions are of interest; it was noted, for example, that "sections through the kidney showed well marked glomerulonephritis."

7. BERGÉ, André. Sur la pathogénie de la scarlatine, Compt. rend. Soc. de biol., **5**:1012, 1893.

When Dochez and the Dicks thirty years later described the local growth of streptococci in the throat with production of a soluble toxin, not enough credit was given to the precise observations of Bergé, whose conclusions were as follows:

(1) "Scarlet fever is a local infection." (2) "The infectious agent which causes it is a streptococcus; in ordinary scarlatina the streptococcus grows in the crypts of the tonsils where it secretes an 'erythemogenic' toxin, the diffusion of which into the organism produces the exanthem and enanthem after the manner

of certain known toxins." (3) "In puerperal or in wound scarlatina the strepto-cocci grow in the uterus or in the wound."

Reasons supporting these statements are given, and the identity of acute streptococcal tonsillitis and scarlet fever, except for the rash, is pointed out. Bergé's final sentence shows him to have been many years ahead of his time: "As to the immunity conferred by scarlatina, it exists only against the rash because the tonsillitis, on the contrary, recurs frequently after scarlet fever."

Had later workers appreciated these findings, much useless labor would have been saved. Indeed, this point of view seems to have been "in the air" in the nineties. A. Baginsky, for example, raises the question of whether scarlet fever was not caused by cocci, "which had the ability when growing in a limited focus in the pharynx to flood the body with a toxin which by the hematogenous route brings out on the skin the scarlatinal exanthem" ("Zur Aetiologie der Diphtherie," Berl. klin. Wchnschr., **29**:183, 1892). Numerous other writers in the succeeding ten years came to similar conclusions, and the literature to date is summarized by G. Gabritschewsky ("Ueber Streptococcenerytheme und ihre Beziehung zum Scharlach," Berl. klin. Wchnschr., **44–1**:556, 1907). Many contemporary writers also stated their unequivocal belief that streptococci were the cause of scarlet fever on the basis of the constant presence of these bacteria in the throat in the disease, response to specific serum therapy, and production of a rash by scarlatinal streptococcal vaccine (Gabritschewsky, Centralbl. f. Bakt., **41**:844, 1906). It was Jochmann's influence (Ref. 12) which weighed against this view.

8. MARMOREK, Alexandre. Le Streptocoque et le sérum antistrepto-coccique, Ann. Inst. Pasteur, **9**:593, 1895.

Although work was already being done on the differentiation and virulence of streptococci, attempts at preparing immune sera against these bacteria had been rudimentary and had concerned mainly small laboratory animals. Marmorek made important observations on the growth and virulence of streptococci; he concluded that strains from human disease were all of one sort and that strepto-cocci of erysipelas, for example, were not the specific cause of the disease, to be sharply differentiated from pyogenic streptococci obtained from an abscess. He thought that the type of disease produced depended on portal of entry and virulence. All this is of interest in view of the claims made many years later that the streptococci of scarlet fever and of erysipelas were immunologically dis-tinct (Refs. 10, 16), which in the end (Ref. 29) turned out to be incorrect. Marmorek immunized large animals, including horses, with increasing amounts of living virulent streptococci. The procedure required six months to a year. A pony, for example, received thirteen injections, comprising about 195 cc. of cul-ture, over a period of five months. The serum was used therapeutically in all sorts of streptococcal infections, including scarlatina. The results were encour-aging but not conclusive. Temperature often fell quicky, toxic symptoms were abated, and in small animals definite protective effects were obtained. These results seem much like those described by Blake with Dochez's serum thirty years later (Ref. 23).

Marmorek concluded this pioneer paper as follows: "We are not unaware of how much caution is necessary in judging a new remedy. We must beware of hasty conclusions. We have exposed the facts, and doctors may be anxious to use this serum. This has not yet reached the point of efficiency we hope for. At any rate, let doctors not forget the necessity of a bacteriological diagnosis, without which they expose themselves to serious mistakes." These observations are amplified in another paper: "Traitement de la scarlatine par le sérum antistreptococcique," *ibid.*, **10**:47, 1896.

Marmorek immunized his animals with whole-broth cultures. It has been pointed out that his sera may, therefore, have had both antitoxic and antibacterial potency, which might explain the excellent prompt effects which he achieved in some cases.

Attempts at serum therapy have played such a great part in elucidating the problems of scarlet fever that this paper and those subsequently listed (Ref. 9) on the same subject are especially important.

9. MOSER, Paul. Ueber die Behandlung des Scharlachs mit einem Scharlach Streptococcenserum, Wien. klin. Wchnschr., **15**:1053, 1902.

Moser was unable to obtain good results with Marmorek's serum (Ref. 8). Thinking this might be due to differences in the infecting strains, he immunized horses with "many strains" of scarlatinal streptococci, using a mixture of living cultures. "Since clinical observation of scarlet fever revealed signs not only of infection but also of intoxication, we presumed that a specific streptococcus serum might influence both infection and intoxication." Moser gave 30–180 cc., usually in one dose, subcutaneously, apparently without much consequent serum sickness. He found that if the serum was given early in the disease, there was, especially in severe cases, remarkable improvement in well-being, suppression of rash or rapid fading, fall of temperature and pulse rate, and clearing of toxic symptoms. As one reads the results, they are certainly impressive. Moser was less sure that pyogenic or postscarlatinal complications were prevented or altered. On the basis of these results he raised the question of whether "streptococci are not the real cause of scarlet fever and not just a combination with an unknown agent." He also felt with Von Pirquet that scarlatinal streptococci were a special group and were agglutinated by immune sera in "an entirely different way from other streptococci."

Moser's work is just as impressive as that of Blake, using Dochez's serum, many years later (Ref. 23). Why, then, did antiscarlatinal sera, after extensive trials between 1895 and 1905, fall largely into disuse in subsequent years until revived by Dochez and the Dicks (Ref. 20)? First of all, it was difficult to standardize the sera, and, as the beneficial effect was undoubtedly due mainly to neutralization of soluble toxins, antisera against strains which were not good toxin-producers would be useless. Horses also vary in their response to immunization. In some cases, perhaps, too little serum was used. Hence the clinical results were so variable as not to be convincing to all. Furthermore, the influential paper of Jochmann (Ref. 12), in which he definitely concluded that streptococci were not the cause of scarlet fever, discouraged further attempts. Thus Osler in 1910 (*Principles and Practice of Medicine* [7th ed.; New York: D. Appleton & Co., 1910], p. 140) at the end of his article on scarlet fever has a brief paragraph on serum treatment, in which he simply states that it has been used in Europe but he does not advise it.

A critical and comprehensive review of the contemporary literature on the subject is that of Bela Schick ("Ueber die weiteren Erfolge der Serumbehandlung des Scharlach," Deutsche med. Wchnschr., **31**:2092, 1905), and later that of Escherich and Schick (*Der Scharlach* [Vienna: Alfred Hölder, 1912]).

10. MOSER, Paul, and VON PIRQUET, C. Agglutination von Streptococcen durch Pferdeserum, Wien. klin. Wchnschr., **15**:1086, 1902.

These were the first systematic attempts to define scarlatinal streptococci as a group. The authors found that antisera prepared against scarlatinal streptococci agglutinated any strain isolated from the blood of scarlet fever patients in as high titer as the homologous strain, but streptococci from other sources were agglutinated in no higher titer than with normal horse serum. Antisera prepared from non-scarlatinal strains did not agglutinate scarlatinal streptococci in high titer. Moser and Von Pirquet found, in brief, what Dochez observed nearly twenty years later (Ref. 15). F. Neufeld ("Ueber Immunität und Agglutination bei Streptococcen," Ztschr. f. Hyg. u. Infektionskr., **44**:161, 1903), a very reliable worker, was, however, unable to confirm Moser's work. He found that antistreptococcal rabbit sera had a specific agglutinating effect against the homologous scarlatinal strain but that they agglutinated streptococci from various sources equally well. G. H. Weaver ("Agglutination of streptococci, especially those cultivated from cases of scarlatina by human sera," J. Infect. Dis., **1**:91, 1904) also pointed out the technical difficulties in this sort of work and concluded: "The agglutination reaction between the streptococci cultivated from cases of scarlatina and the serum from cases of scarlet fever is in no way specific."

It is of interest that, years later, this whole dispute was repeated with the same outcome (Refs. 15, 16, 28, 29).

11. SCHOTTMÜLLER, H. Die Artunterscheidung der für den Menschen pathogenen Streptococcen durch Blutagar, München. med. Wchnschr., **50**:849, 1903.

Schottmüller had introduced the technique of blood culture in 1897 and soon found that the appearance of colonies on blood-agar plates might be of diagnostic value. He found that colonies of pathogenic streptococci showed a "characteristic circular light area around them. This light area, which results from the complete absorption of the hemoglobin, has an area of 2–3 mm." Schottmüller clearly distinguished the green-producing non-hemolytic streptococci and gave them the designation "*mitior seu viridans*." He never found the latter type in scarlet fever or in pyogenic processes. He did not realize, however, that *S. viridans* is the most important constituent of the normal basic flora of the upper air passages.

This work was of fundamental importance and really was the start of a useful subdivision of streptococci (Ref. 15). It was elaborated years later by J. Howard Brown in his monograph (*Use of Blood Agar for Study of Streptococci* [Monogr. No. 9] [New York: Rockefeller Institute for Medical Research, 1919]).

12. JOCHMANN, G. Die Bacterienbefunde bei Scharlach und ihre Bedeutung für den Krankheitsprocess, Ztschr. f. klin. Med., **56**:316, 1905.

This long and well-reasoned discussion by a recognized authority on infectious disease brought to a head the controversy as to whether streptococci were the

primary cause of scarlet fever. Jochmann critically reviewed the extensive literature pro and con and added observations of his own. His final conclusion was
that streptococcus was not the primary cause but was responsible for septic
complications. His reasons were that scarlet fever patients who died of septic
complications after a week or more of the disease almost all had streptococci
in the blood, whereas streptococci were conspicuously absent in the hyperacute
cases who died within one to three days after onset. "Here the scarlatinal poison
unfolds its pure effect before streptococci have become operative." He also
noted that streptococci are rarely cultivated from the blood during the first few
days of the disease, and he could not explain the immunity conferred by an
attack of scarlatina in contrast to the well-known susceptibility to repeated
streptococcal infections. He also believed that there was nothing specific about
the streptococci of scarlet fever but thought that they could produce ordinary
pyogenic infections in other situations.

Jochmann was an extraordinarily astute observer and thinker. Most of the
points which to him were evidence against a streptococcal etiology are now
readily explained. He was keen enough to see that scarlet fever in its early days
was a highly specific disease and not a suppurative process in the strict sense;
he concluded that, if the septic stage, obviously different, was due to streptococci, there must be some other cause for the primary disease. This is not far
from the truth, since the soluble toxin plays a prominent part in the early phenomena, while the later septic features are now known often to be due to a
different streptococcus from the original strain (Ref. 27). Jochmann could not
understand the surprising therapeutic effects sometimes achieved with Moser's
serum. "In hypertoxic cases with high fever, somnolence, green diarrhea, feeble
pulse, etc., temperature falls within 4–12 hours after injection, and the children
wake up as from a sleep. However, suppurative complications come later, so
that the serum has no effect on these or on the postscarlatinal after-illness." The
answer, of course, was that Moser's serum, prepared by injection of broth cultures of streptococci, had the same antitoxic effects which the Dicks demonstrated twenty-five years later (Ref. 20).

At any rate, on the strength of Jochmann's prestige, the idea that streptococcus did more than cause the complications of scarlet fever was pretty much
abandoned until the work of Dochez created a new impetus (Ref. 15).

13. SCHICK, B. Die Nachkrankheiten des Scharlach, Jahrb. f. Kinderh.,
    1907, Ergänzungsband, p. 132.

There is an immense late-nineteenth-century literature on postscarlatinal disorders. It remained for Schick, however, as a result of his work with Von Pirquet
on serum sickness (*Die Serumkrankheit* [Leipzig and Vienna: F. Deuticke,
1905]), to sense the resemblance to an allergic reaction and to suggest a hypersensitive state as an explanation of scarlatinal "after-sickness." Schick clearly
differentiated the renal lesions of early scarlet fever from postscarlatinal nephritis. He realized that in the asymptomatic interval lay the clue to the nature
of the process. He pointed out that the components of the postscarlatinal syndrome were probably all the results of some common cause. He included fever,
lymphadenitis, nephritis, "rheumatism," and endocarditis. He thought that
altered reactivity was associated with a flareup of the original "contagium." If
one reasoned in terms of serum sickness, it was necessary to assume the presence

of the original antigen which could participate in an antigen-antibody reaction to produce a toxic agent.

The most modern point of view is really only an elaboration of Schick's ideas. Some have invoked the notion that a reinfection with a different type of hemolytic streptococcus may furnish the antigen for a reaction as a result of sensitization in the original illness to products of streptococcal metabolism (see L. A. Rantz, P. J. Boisvert, and W. W. Spink, "Hemolytic streptococcus sore throat, the post-streptococcic state," Arch. Int. Med., **79**:401, 1947).

14. SCHULTZ, W., and CHARLTON, W. Serologische Beobachtungen am Scharlachexanthem, Ztschr. f. Kinderh., **17**:328, 1918.

The Schultz-Charlton rash extinction test became an invaluable tool in studying the immunology of scarlet fever. Schultz and Charlton showed that both convalescent scarlatinal serum and normal serum injected intradermally (1.0 cc.) blanched the rash. The blanching began in about 5–6 hours and persisted throughout the illness, in contrast to that produced by epinephrine, which began within a minute or two and disappeared in 5–6 hours. Schultz and Charlton concluded, therefore, that their reaction was not due to simple vasoconstriction. Furthermore, convalescent serum drawn on various days gave a negative test up to the fourteenth day, when positives began to appear; all sera from the nineteenth day on extinguished the rash. Schultz and Charlton had no idea as to the cause of this phenomenon, which was later shown to be due to neutralization of erythrogenic toxin by specific antitoxin (Refs. 17, 20, 26). K. Birkhaug (J. Clin. Investigation, **1**:273, 1925) reviews the contemporary literature on the Schultz-Charlton test and adds observations of his own. He found that neither convalescent nor normal sera blanched the rash if it had been present over 2–3 days. Dochez's antiscarlatinal horse serum was highly effective.

15. DOCHEZ, A. R., AVERY, O. T., and LANCEFIELD, R. C. Studies on the biology of streptococcus. I. Antigenic relationships between strains of Streptococcus hemolyticus, J. Exper. Med., **30**:179, 1919.

Dochez and Avery had concluded their work on pneumococcic types ("Monogr. Rockefeller Inst. M. Research," No. 7 [October 16, 1917]), and it was natural for them to embark on similar studies of streptococci. Hemolytic streptococci from human sources were shown, by agglutination reactions with immune sera prepared in animals and by protection tests, to fall into at least four biological types.

It was these observations which led Dochez and his associates to attempt to find out whether the streptococci of scarlet fever fell into a uniform immunological group; hence it must be regarded as an important landmark in the subject. The improved technique used by these workers seemed to promise more definite results than the inconclusive attempts previously made to answer this question (Ref. 10).

16. BLISS, Walter P. A biological study of hemolytic streptococci from the throats of patients suffering from scarlet fever. Preliminary report, Bull. Johns Hopkins Hosp., **31**:173, 1920.

Attempts at serological classification of streptococci from cases of scarlatina had been made years earlier with variable success (Ref. 10). Bliss, following Dochez's work (Ref. 15), found that about 80 per cent of strains of hemolytic streptococcus from the throats of scarlet fever patients in the first week of the disease were agglutinated by four different antistreptococcic sera made from similar organisms, but none were agglutinated by antistreptococcal sera of non-scarlatinal origin except in rare cases. Bliss later amplified these studies ("Studies on the biology of streptococcus," J. Exper. Med., 36:575, 1922). Although he noted various exceptions and differences in carbohydrate fermentation among the "scarlatinal" strains, he definitely concluded that the streptococci from scarlet fever comprised a specific type. Future work was to show his view to be incorrect, but it furnished a tremendous stimulus to studies of the etiology of scarlet fever, including the definitive human inoculation experiments of the Dicks.

Other workers at the same time, using similar methods, came to the conclusion that scarlatinal streptococci fell into a distinct group (cf. R. Tunnicliff, "Specific nature of the hemolytic streptococcus of scarlet fever," J.A.M.A., 74:1386, 1920; "Further studies on the specificity of streptococci," ibid., 75:1339, 1921; "Observations on the spread and persistence of the hemolytic streptococci peculiar to scarlet fever," J. Infect. Dis., 29:91, 1921). Tunnicliff observed that the strains obtained during convalescence and in complicating lesions were often different from those isolated during the acute phase. She also found that persons associated with scarlet fever patients may develop tonsillitis without an exanthem and may harbor streptococci which belong to the same biologic group as those isolated from typical cases of scarlet fever. M. H. Gordon ("A serological study of haemolytic streptococci," Brit. M.J., 1:632, 1921) also concluded, using similar methods, that scarlatinal streptococci fell into a serologically distinct group. F. A. Stevens and A. R. Dochez, as late as 1926, in an elaborate study ("Antigenic relationship between strains of streptococci from scarlet fever and erysipelas," J. Exper. Med., 43:379, 1926) still maintained that scarlatinal and erysipelas streptococci fell into essentially different immunological groups. This position was, however, already being questioned by the Dicks (Ref. 18), by A. W. Williams, H. D. Hussey, and E. J. Banzhof ("Culture filtrates of hemolytic streptococci from scarlet fever: intracutaneous reactions in test animals," Proc. Soc. Exper. Biol. & Med., 21:291, 1924), and by British workers (J. Smith, "The serological classification of haemolytic streptococci obtained from cases of scarlet fever," J. Hyg., 25:165, 1926; Fred Griffith, "Types of haemolytic streptococci in relation to scarlet fever," J. Hyg., 25:385, 1926; and G. R. James, "The relationship of streptococci to scarlet fever," J. Hyg., 25:415, 1926).

The unraveling of this problem was confused by the fact that in a certain locality most cases of scarlet fever may for a season be caused by one predominant type. It was when scarlatinal strains from various countries were compared that lack of identity was readily made out by Griffith typing (Ref. 29).

17. MAIR, W. An immunity reaction in scarlet fever, Lancet, 2:1390, 1923.

In this extremely important paper Mair discusses the immunological problems posed by the Schultz-Charlton test (Ref. 14). He points out that the facts can be explained only on the basis of neutralization by antitoxin of a toxin which produces the rash. Negative reactions with sera drawn early in the disease are due to the fact that antitoxin has not yet developed; the presence of antitoxin in "normals" is due to a previous attack, perhaps subclinical, of scarlet fever. Variations in degree of blanching are due to differences in amount of toxin in the skin and of antitoxin in the test serum. Mair, by examining serum drawn early in the disease, as well as convalescent serum from the same person, demonstrated the development of antitoxin as the infection progressed. The work of the Dicks (Ref. 20) was predicted in Mair's concluding statement: "It seems highly probable that the causal micro-organism will be capable of producing a toxin and, by immunization of animals, an antitoxin, of which the latter should give the Schultz-Charlton reaction in man."

18. DICK, George F., and DICK, Gladys Henry. The etiology of scarlet fever, J.A.M.A., **82**:301, 1924.

The Dicks swabbed the tonsils of two volunteers with a 48-hour culture of hemolytic streptococcus isolated from the throat of a scarlet fever patient. One volunteer remained well; the other developed typical scarlet fever with sore throat, fever, leukocytosis, rash, desquamation, etc. The authors concluded: "Since the streptococci used in these experiments have fulfilled the requirements of Koch's laws, it may be concluded that they cause scarlet fever."

While the Dicks deserve credit for the final proof that streptococcus is the cause of scarlet fever, we believe that the logical, progressive, and systematic approach to the problem by Dochez and his associates was equally important (Ref. 19). In their paper of 1921 entitled "Experimental inoculations in scarlet fever" (J.A.M.A., **77**:782), the Dicks concluded: "The thirty streptococcus throat inoculation experiments constitute a series large enough to discourage further experiments of the same kind with hemolytic streptococci." Seven of their volunteers developed sore throat *but no rash;* the Dicks did not seem to sense at the time that these people were simply immune to the rash toxin. The Dicks also did inoculations with "a pleomorphic organism similar to those previously found in cultures of throat, blood and urine in early uncomplicated scarlet fever," and, although they did not produce frank disease, they definitely rated it as a possible causal agent: "If the pleomorphic organism . . . bears an etiological relation to scarlet fever it should be possible by inoculation of a larger series of volunteers to produce a rash on the skin as well as the palate." This pleomorphic organism is heard of no more in the writings of the Dicks, but in another paper ("Experimental scarlet fever," J.A.M.A., **81**:1166, 1923) they described the inoculation of five volunteers whose tonsils were swabbed with a culture of hemolytic streptococcus obtained from the "sore finger" of a woman with scarlet fever. Three of these volunteers remained well, one developed tonsillitis but no skin rash, and one had scarlet fever with a typical rash, etc. Somewhat similar results were obtained in a second series of inoculations. However, the situation was still not clear to the Dicks, who concluded: "The two cases of experimental scarlet fever reported were probably caused by the hemolytic streptococcus or by some unrecognized organism closely associated with it in cultures. These experiments do not justify the conclusion that all cases of scarlet fever are caused by the hemolytic streptococcus described." Their final experiment was done at a time when all thoughtful students of the subject were already convinced that the hemolytic streptococcus was the primary cause of scarlatina.

19. DOCHEZ, A. R., and SHERMAN, Lillian. The significance of Streptococcus hemolyticus in scarlet fever, J.A.M.A., **82**:542, 1924.

Although his paper appeared three weeks after that of the Dicks (Ref. 18), Dochez seems to deserve equal credit for establishing the streptococcus as the cause of scarlet fever. He concluded: "From the results detailed, it would seem that a specific streptococcus is the cause of scarlet fever, that the disease in its principal characteristics resembles diphtheria, and that both immunity in human beings and the experimental immunity developed by inoculation of animals are antitoxic in nature."[3] Dochez's views were based on the consistent isolation of hemolytic streptococcus from the throat during the first days of the disease, the fact that the organisms seemed to fall into a single immunological group, the production in guinea pigs with this streptococcus of a disease resembling scarlet fever, and the development of an immune serum[4] in the horse which "possesses the capacity to blanch the rash locally in scarlet fever and which when used therapeutically, causes a marked abatement of all the symptoms."

20. DICK, George F., and DICK, Gladys Henry. A skin test for susceptibility to scarlet fever, J.A.M.A., **82**:265, 1924.

The observations of the Dicks on soluble toxins in scarlet fever were of fundamental importance in leading to the final understanding of the disease. Simultaneously with their work, Dochez expressed the view (Ref. 19) that the "principal localization of the infection is in the throat in most instances and that there the streptococcus in question elaborates a toxin which is absorbed and produces the rash and general symptoms." It was the Dicks, however, who first prepared a usable "toxin" from filtrates of cultures of streptococci obtained from scarlet fever patients; they showed that an intracutaneous injection of this filtrate practically never produced a skin reaction in people convalescent from scarlet fever or with a history of a previous attack, whereas 41.6 per cent of persons who had no history of scarlet fever showed a red area up to 5 cm. in diameter in 24–36 hours. These positive tests could be inhibited by convalescent scarlet fever serum, and positive skin tests were reversed after an attack of scarlet fever. This was the basis of the Dick test.

The Dicks raised the question of whether all the symptoms of scarlet fever could be due to this "toxin." They injected "toxin" into healthy people who had never had scarlet fever ("Scarlet fever toxin in preventive immunization," J.A.M.A., **82**:544, 1924) and produced severe local reactions, fever, nausea, and, in some cases, a rash,[5] and found that the previously positive skin test had been reversed. They thought they had produced an active immunization but did not realize at the time that the immunity was primarily to the skin toxin and did not prevent subsequent "scarlet fever without rash."

The Dicks' next communications ("A scarlet fever antitoxin," J.A.M.A., **82**:1246, 1924) dealt with the production of an antitoxic serum by immunizing a horse, not with streptococci as in previous work (Refs. 8, 9, 19), but with the

---

[3] All this had been noted by Bergé in 1893 (Ref. 7).

[4] Dochez's serum was produced by instilling "scarlatinal streptococci into a mass of agar previously injected subcutaneously into the horse. It was hoped that toxins absorbed from such a focus would produce antitoxic, as well as antibacterial, effects."

[5] This had all been shown years before by Gabritchewsky (Ref. 7).

toxic filtrate of cultures. More detailed reports on preventive immunization by injections of "toxin" were reported in a further paper ("The prevention of scarlet fever," *ibid.*, **83**:84, 1924), and soon a report appeared ("Therapeutic results with concentrated scarlet fever antitoxin," *ibid.*, **84**:803, 1925), in which the Dicks described the use of their horse serum in clinical cases. They concluded that the antitoxin blanches the rash,[6] lowers temperatures, and improves the general condition of many scarlet fever patients. If given early, the course of the disease was shortened, and the incidence of complications and sequelae was greatly reduced. The careful production of this serum, its concentration, and standardization, so that only small amounts of horse serum needed to be injected, constituted an important advance in therapy. Unfortunately, it was ultimately shown that the antitoxin acted mainly on the rash and perhaps certain toxic symptoms but did not have the antibacterial action necessary to eliminate the streptococcal infection; it did not furnish a complete cure of the disease.

Finally, all the work described above was amplified in two further papers by the Dicks ("Results with the skin test for susceptibility to scarlet fever," J.A.M.A., **84**:1477, 1925, and "Therapeutic results with concentrated scarlet fever antitoxin," *ibid.*, **85**:1693, 1925). Important points were that not all strains of scarlet fever streptococci were equally good "toxin" producers; the Dicks also failed to substantiate the immunological identity of scarlet fever streptococci as observed by Dochez and his associates (Ref. 16). Sheep immunized with two strains of streptococci which had produced experimental scarlet fever yielded sera which agglutinated the homologous organism in high concentration but gave no cross-agglutination. This position was later confirmed (Ref. 29).

The fundamental importance of all this work is not to be underestimated. It brought clearly into focus the question of what part of the disease was due to the soluble toxin and what part was the result of the local streptococcal infection in the throat. Does the soluble toxin do more than cause the rash? Is it also responsible for part or all of the toxic symptoms? Or do its effects vary in different cases? Be this as it may, the applications of the toxin and antitoxin of the Dicks in immunization and in therapy has gradually fallen into some disuse, partly because there may be severe reactions from the material and partly because the effects are thought to be mainly against the erythrogenic toxin—the rash. Furthermore, modern antibiotics are highly effective in extirpating the infection. The antitoxin may still be useful, however, in certain patients, such as very severe, intensely prostrated cases in which the action of toxin may be predominant.

21. KIRKBRIDE, Mary B., and WHEELER, Mary W. Comparison of reaction in individuals to toxins prepared from three strains of scarlet fever streptococci, Proc. Soc. Exper. Biol. & Med., **26**:85, 1924.

Using "toxins" prepared from three scarlatinal strains of streptococcus, the writers found that most people reacted similarly with skin tests to all three. A few people failed to give a response to one or another "toxin." This suggested that not all these "toxins" were identical and that immunity might exist

---

[6] As predicted by Mair (Ref. 17).

to one of them and not to others. Kirkbride and Wheeler later elaborated these studies ("Studies of the toxins of the hemolytic streptococci associated with scarlet fever," J. Immunol., **11**:477, 1926; **13**:19, 1927). W. H. Park and R. G. Spiegel ("Complexity of the scarlet fever toxin and antitoxin," J. Immunol., **10**:829, 1925) also concluded that a variety of rash-producing toxins might be formed by different strains of streptococci, although in most cases toxin production seemed to be similar. J. D. Trask, Jr., and F. G. Blake still later ("Heterologous scarlet fever," J.A.M.A., **101**:753, 1933) offered further evidence of heterogenicity among the toxins found in the blood in scarlet fever as well as among the scarlatinal antitoxins naturally found in man, and they concluded that "polyvalency is desirable in therapeutic scarlatinal antitoxin." These observations may explain the discordant results obtained with the early scarlatinal antisera (Refs. 8, 9).

The important paper of H. Aranow and W. B. Wood, Jr. ("Staphylococcic infection simulating scarlet fever," J.A.M.A., **119**:1491, 1942) should also be noted in this connection. From a case of staphylococcic osteomyelitis with typical scarlatiniform rash no hemolytic streptococci could be grown, but the hemolytic staphylococcus which was isolated from the lesion and from the blood produced an erythrogenic toxin which was neutralized by commercial scarlatinal antitoxin.

22. ZINGHER, Abraham. The Dick test in normal persons and in acute and convalescent cases of scarlet fever, J.A.M.A., **83**:432, 1924.

The widest application of the work of the Dicks (Ref. 20) is the use of "toxin" as a skin test for susceptibility to scarlet fever—the Dick reaction. The contemporary position is comprehensively and authoritatively stated in this paper.

23. BLAKE, Francis G., TRASK, James D., Jr., and LYNCH, John F. Observations on the treatment of scarlet fever with scarlatinal antistreptococcic serum, J.A.M.A., **82**:712, 1924.

Blake and his associates report clinical results with Dochez's antiscarlatinal horse serum (Ref. 19). They laid stress on its value in diagnosis and described its capacity locally to blanch the rash in scarlet fever patients. Also, "the serum would appear to possess very marked curative properties." In some toxic cases there was complete recovery within 24–36 hours. Forty to 60 cc. of serum was usually adequate. Blake was doubtful whether the serum would be effective in septic complications. K. Birkhaug ("Studies in scarlet fever," Bull. Johns Hopkins Hosp., **36**:134, 1925) also reported favorable results with Dochez's serum. Forty cc. administered during the first 3 days caused a prompt disappearance of the toxemia, a critical fall in temperature and pulse rate, and prompt fading of the rash. The incidence of septic complications was low in cases treated prior to the fourth day.

One is not convinced that these results are materially different from those obtained years earlier by Moser (Ref. 9). Although scarlet fever is usually treated nowadays by penicillin (Ref. 32), immune sera containing antibodies against the rash toxin and other possible soluble toxins would still seem indicated in very severe cases with intense initial toxemia.

24. TRASK, James D., Jr., and BLAKE, Francis G. Observations on the presence of a toxic substance in the blood and urine of patients with scarlet fever, J. Exper. Med., **40**:381, 1924.

Although the possibility that a soluble toxin elaborated in the throat is responsible for the rash and perhaps other symptoms was suggested long before (Ref. 7), it was not until the work of the Dicks (Ref. 20) that the evidence became convincing. Trask and Blake went a step further and actually demonstrated the presence of toxin in the blood. They found that sera drawn early in the disease from scarlet fever patients produced large areas of erythema in "susceptibles," whose own serum contained no rash-blanching substance. The toxic substance was neutralized by serum which gave a blanching test but not by negative sera. The toxin was also neutralized by Dochez's immune-horse serum (Ref. 19) but not by normal horse serum.

Trask and Blake still regarded the streptococci of scarlet fever as a specific group, and they believed that all the generalized manifestations of the disease were due to the soluble "toxin." These concepts were later shown to be open to question.

25. STEVENS, Franklin A., and DOCHEZ, A. R. The occurrence of throat infection with Streptococcus scarlatinae without a rash, J.A.M.A., **86**:1110, 1926. The epidemiology of scarlatinal throat infections sine exanthemate, *ibid.*, **87**:2137, 1926.

There were already many clinical observations of contacts with scarlet fever patients who developed sore throat without rash (Refs. 2, 7). It remained for Stevens and Dochez to isolate strains of streptococci from the throats of such patients and to prove by agglutination and absorption tests that they were identical in subjects with and without rash. They also showed that in the type of infection without rash the Dick test was negative, although the strain could be demonstrated to produce toxin, which, in turn, was neutralized by antitoxin. Throat infections without rash were found to occur in people who had previously had scarlet fever, although the organism was a "Streptococcus scarlatinae" and produced toxin.

Stevens and Dochez concluded that scarlatinal antitoxin was an efficient therapeutic agent in scarlatinal throat infections without rash, a position which is not strongly supported with the type of scarlet fever seen today. They were uncertain whether the absence of rash was always due to immunity to rash toxin or to failure of the streptococcus to produce the toxin, and, in general, they raised the question of which components of the disease were the result of the local throat infection and which were caused by soluble poisons, including the rash toxin.

26. TRASK, James D. Studies in scarlet fever. I. The amount of scarlatinal toxin in the blood of patients with scarlet fever, J. Clin. Investigation, **3**:391, 1926.

In an important series of papers from Blake's laboratory, the studies which demonstrated the presence of erythrogenic toxin in the blood (Ref. 24) were extended. Trask worked out a system of measuring the amount of toxin in the blood of patients in terms of Dick skin-test units (Ref. 20). In different patients toxin varied from 0.25 to 300 units, but these values bore no relation to the general severity of the disease. Blake and Trask amplified these observations ("Studies in scarlet fever. II. The relation of the specific toxemia of scarlet fever to the course of the disease," J. Clin. Investigation, **3**:397, 1926) and now showed that the presence of toxin ran parallel to the occurrence of the rash but did not follow all the manifestations of the disease, especially the (late) septic features. "The results suggest that the duration of the specific toxemia is measured by the duration of the rash," which fades as the patient develops his own antitoxin or as therapeutic antitoxin is given. E. E. Nicholls continued these studies ("III. Infections with Streptococcus scarlatinae in persons with scarlatinal antitoxic immunity," J. Clin. Investigation, **3**:411, 1926) and showed that the old observation of scarlet fever without rash was to be explained by the subject's possessing specific antitoxic immunity, even though the streptococci isolated from the throat produced toxin. Nicholls' final conclusion was important: "Immunity to the toxin of Streptococcus scarlatinae as determined by the Dick test does not necessarily provide the immunity to local pyogenic infections with Streptococcus scarlatinae."

27. GUNN, William, and GRIFFITH, Fred. Bacteriological and clinical study of one hundred cases of scarlet fever, J. Hyg., **28**:250, 1929.

The writers isolated and classified, by the Griffith method of typing (Ref. 29), the streptococci present in the throats of cases of scarlet fever. Examinations were repeated at weekly intervals, and in half the cases the same type of streptococcus remained. In the others there was a change of type one or more times; this was considered to be a reinfection. V. D. Allison and W. A. Brown ("Reinfection as a cause of complications in scarlet fever wards," J. Hyg., **37**:153, 1937) confirmed and amplified these studies, and H. L. de Waal ("The serological types of haemolytic streptococci in relation to the epidemiology of scarlet fever and its complications," J. Hyg., **40**:172, 1940) undertook the incredibly difficult task of making repeated cultures during the course of hundreds of cases of scarlet fever. The most important of his interesting observations was that, when a complication occurred, it was associated with a streptococcus of a different type from that which was present on entry in 61.5 per cent of the cases.

All this suggests that the streptococcus which is the primary cause of scarlet fever is at the time not behaving exactly like a non-specific pyogen. An analogy is the behavior of the pneumococcus in acute lobar pneumonia; the pneumococcus produces a specific disease but may on occasion behave as a non-specific pyogen causing suppuration in joints, meninges, or elsewhere. The typhoid bacillus, which primarily causes a specific non-pyogenic disease—typhoid fever —may also alter its activity so as to produce an abscess.

28. LANCEFIELD, Rebecca C. A serological differentiation of human and other groups of hemolytic streptococci, J. Exper. Med., **57**:571, 1933.

Although Dochez and others (Ref. 16) had concluded on the basis of agglutination reactions that the streptococci of scarlet fever fell into a single specific immunological group, considerable evidence against this view soon accumulated. Lancefield, herself one of Dochez's original associates, later criticized the agglutination reaction "on account of (*a*) the troublesome spontaneous agglutination so commonly encountered among streptococci; (*b*) the nonspecific cross-agglutination difficult of interpretation and (*c*) the existence of so many specific types as to make identification of strains impractical by type-specific agglutination." In this extremely important paper she showed that immune sera satisfactory for precipitin tests with extracts of streptococci could be readily prepared. By this method practically all hemolytic streptococci fell into five groups "which bear a definite relationship to the sources of the cultures." Most pathogenic strains from human disease, including scarlet fever, fall into group A, which can be further subdivided by appropriate methods (Ref. 29). This work made possible the final conclusion that the only feature which scarlatinal streptococci necessarily have in common is the ability to produce erythrogenic toxin and that such toxin may be produced by serologically distinct types.

29. GRIFFITH, F. The serological classification of Streptococcus pyogenes, J. Hyg., **34**:542, 1934.

Griffith had already developed his method of rapid slide agglutination ("Types of haemolytic streptococci in relation to scarlet fever," J. Hyg., **25**:385, 1926), but in this paper he showed that the group A strains of Lancefield (Ref. 28) could be subdivided into a large number of serological types. Twenty-seven types are described. Many of these were isolated from cases of scarlet fever, so that this work finally put an end to the idea of a specific race of scarlatinal streptococci.

L. A. Rantz ("The serological typing of hemolytic streptococci of the Lancefield Group A," J. Clin. Investigation, **21**:217, 1942) gives a definitive summary of the Griffith types of hemolytic streptococci reported in various outbreaks of scarlet fever in different localities. It is pointed out that in any one season the types responsible are relatively few but that the same types do not predominate every season.

30. STOCK, Aaron A. Studies on the hemolytic streptococcus. I. Isolation and concentration of erythrogenic toxin of the N.Y. 5 strain of hemolytic streptococcus, J. Immunol., **36**:489, 1939.

Attempts to concentrate and purify the rash toxin were obviously desirable. In this work Stock prepared material of which 0.0001 μg. was equivalent to one skin-test dose (Dick). Later Stock ("IV. Further purification and concentration of scarlet fever toxin," J. Biol. Chem., **142**:777, 1942) prepared material which contained 200,000,000 skin-test doses per milligram, and he also found (L. E. Krejci, A. H. Stock, E. B. Sanigar, and E. O. Kraemer, "V. The electrophoretic isolation of the erythrogenic toxin of scarlet fever and the determination of its chemical and physical properties," J. Biol. Chem., **142**:785, 1942), by electrophoretic analysis, that the material contained five distinct constituents and was a protein.

31. BLOOMFIELD, Arthur L., and RANTZ, Lowell A. An outbreak of streptococcic septic sore throat in an army camp, J.A.M.A., **121**:315, 1943.

An important question is whether the soluble toxins of scarlatinal streptococci produce any clinical effects besides the rash. The writers studied a mass infection of young men in an army camp, presumably resulting from contaminated milk or food. Several hundred men were taken sick almost simultaneously with an acute streptococcic sore throat. It was shown that one strain—Type 15—was responsible. Approximately one-fourth of the patients had a typical scarlatinal rash; in most cases no rash was seen. As far as one could tell by clinical observation, there was no over-all difference in the severity, course, or complications in the two groups. This would suggest that, in this outbreak at least, the effect of the "toxin" was confined to production of the rash. It is hard to escape the conviction, however, that the hyperacute variety of scarlet fever with death from "toxemia" in the first few days must be due to other or more potent soluble toxins. This view is supported by the undoubted beneficial effects of antitoxic sera observed in such cases in the past (Refs. 9, 22).

The whole question of the interpretation of "scarlet fever without rash" is analyzed in this paper.

32. HIRSH, Harold L., ROTMAN-KAVKA, Georgine, DOWLING, Harry F., and SWEET, Lewis K. Penicillin therapy of scarlet fever—comparison with antitoxic and symptomatic therapy, J.A.M.A., **133**:657, 1947.

The discovery of penicillin revolutionized the treatment of scarlet fever. The writers clearly define the different effects of penicillin and of scarlatinal antitoxin in a large series of cases. Penicillin resulted in fall in temperature, lessening of sore throat, lessened "toxicity," and marked lowering of incidence of pyogenic complications; its effect was essentially antibacterial and reduced the number of carriers. Antitoxin caused more rapid decline of temperature than did penicillin.

An important point previously emphasized by W. W. Spink and his associates ("Sulfadiazine and penicillin for hemolytic streptococcus infection of the upper respiratory tract," Arch. Int. Med., **77**:260, 1946) is that, unless one continues penicillin in adequate dosage for a fairly long period—7 to 10 days—relapse is likely to occur, and the carrier state is likely to persist. M. Meads and his associates had also found ("Penicillin treatment of scarlet fever," J.A.M.A., **129**:785, 1945), in a small but carefully studied series, that with even as little as 10,000 units of penicillin every 3 hours hemolytic streptococci disappeared from the throat cultures within 48 hours, and if treatment was continued for 7 days, the original types did not reappear. Finally, L. Weinstein and L. F. Potsubay ("A comparison of 'symptomatic treatment,' gamma globulin and penicillin in the treatment of scarlet fever," J. Pediat., **37**:291, 1950) reviewed the growing literature on modern therapy and reported the results of treatment in 255 patients with "proved" scarlet fever. Gamma globulin (presumably antitoxic) blanched the rash but had no effect on the streptococci in the pharynx; did not seem to prevent carrier state; and had little, if any, effect in preventing complications. Penicillin, on the other hand, caused rapid disappearance of streptococci from the local focus, terminated the carrier state, and decreased the incidence of suppurative complications.

From all this, one may conclude that penicillin is adequate in the general run of scarlet fever patients and is the method of choice, but in hyperacute "toxic" cases antitoxin should be given in addition.

However, penicillin has completely altered the outlook on scarlet fever, which is no longer to be dreaded as it was fifty years ago.

ERYSIPELAS

Clinical	Refs. 1, 2, 5
Epidemiology	Ref. 1
General	Refs. 1, 2, 5
Pathogenesis	Refs. 3, 6
Penicillin in	Ref. 9
Serological reactions in	Ref. 7
Serum therapy	Ref. 4
Streptococcus in	Refs. 3, 6
Sulfonamides in	Ref. 8
Therapy	Refs. 2, 8, 9

THE early literature on erysipelas is confused and difficult, first, because many of the papers are inaccessible and, second, because erysipelas so often occurred in association with other clinical forms of streptococcal infection such as sore throat, pyogenic abscess, and puerperal fever. The best general treatise still remains that of Lenhartz (Ref. 5), although the long article by A. Vautrin, P. Spillman, and L. Ganzinotti ("Érysipèle," in *Dictionnaire ency-clopédique des sciences médicales*, 1st Ser., **35** [Paris: G. Masson (1887?)], 461) contains much interesting material.

The bibliography of erysipelas should be considered in connection with that of scarlet fever (see pp. 108 ff.).

1. M'DOWEL, Ephraim. Observations on erysipelas, Dublin J.M. Sc., **6**:161, 1835.

In reading the early literature on erysipelas, one is struck by the powerful epidemic tendency which was so often in evidence. M'Dowel's observations are a good illustration: "As far back as November, more than the usual number of cases of erysipelas were observed . . . but within the last three months it appeared to have assumed an epidemic character . . . every kind of injury almost was followed by it; it occurred after bleeding and leeching, after burns, simple as well as compound fractures, venereal ulcers on the genitals, and in the throat, after the application of blisters, sinapisms, irritating ointments or liniments; it occurred so constantly after operations, that unless when absolutely necessary, they were postponed frequently as long as was compatible with the safety of the patient." In addition to the epidemic character, one is struck by the great number of cases in which a violent sore throat with swelling of regional lymph nodes preceded or followed facial erysipelas. In all forms, abscesses or suppurative complications were frequent. One cannot help wondering whether there were active at the time strains of streptococci which had a special tendency to produce erysipelas. At any rate, the violent epidemic character and the association with outbreaks of puerperal fever are noted again and again. A. Hirsch (*Handbuch der historisch-geographischen Pathologie* [2d ed.; Stuttgart: Ferdinand Enke, 1883], **2**:270) gives a comprehensive review of such epidemics up to 1880. The subject is also discussed by Lenhartz (Ref. 5, p. 3).

2. TROUSSEAU, A. Clinique médicale de l'Hôtel-Dieu de Paris, On erysipelas, and especially erysipelas of the face, **1**:296. Paris: J.-B. Baillière et fils, 1861.

In this article Trousseau did not give a systematic description of erysipelas, but he raised innumerable important questions. In spite of the fact that he could not, of course, understand the dual role of the streptococcus which at one moment produces the characteristic superficial lymphangitis of facial erysipelas and in the next acts as an ordinary pus-producer, he sensed the answers to many vexing questions.

He wondered what made erysipelas at times violent and epidemic, following the least surgical interference, whereas, at other times in the same surgical ward, years might elapse without a case. He noted the association of epidemics of puerperal fever and of erysipelas. He considered erysipelas definitely contagious, although there were exciting causes. He distinguished surgical erysipelas and medical erysipelas. The latter, although apparently idiopathic, he believed could originally be traced to a small lesion on the lip, in the nose, etc., thus bringing the two varieties in a sense together. He noted the frequent appearance of fever and malaise for a day or two before the erysipelatous eruption appeared. He stressed the benign course and low mortality of "medical" facial erysipelas in contrast to erysipelas arising in the course of another acute disease such as smallpox or in a patient reduced by tuberculosis. He described "érysipèle ambulant," the variety which slowly wended its way over the whole body or jumped here and there. He described in graphic style epidemics of erysipelas or instances in which a number of people in a household successively contracted the disease; such outbreaks are much less often seen today and give credence to the activity of special strains of erysipelas streptococci.

Trousseau's treatment was far ahead of the times. "Expectancy is then my treatment of facial erysipelas. But, gentlemen, I feed them, I feed them even if there is fever or delirium. Thus, instead of depleting the patients by loss of blood or the application of leeches behind the ears, in place of giving emetics or repeated purgatives, in place of keeping them on a restricted diet, I remain a spectator of the struggle in which I know nature will emerge victorious, if I do not disturb her operations. . . . To know how to wait is a great science in our art, prudent waiting often explains successes; it explains, above all, those obtained sometimes by those of the Hahnemann sect."

3. FEHLEISEN, [F.]. Ueber Erysipel, Deutsche Ztschr. f. Chir., **16**:391, 1882.

According to Fehleisen, the first claim that erysipelas was due to a living organism was made by Hueter ("Verhandlungen ärztlicher Gesellschaften," Berl. klin. Wchnschr., **6**:358, 1869), but an inspection of the article yields nothing worthy of mention. Wladimir Lukomsky ("Untersuchungen über Erysipel," Virchows Arch. f. path. Anat., **60**:418, 1874) described in fatal cases of erysipelas, among other findings, "lymph vessels filled with micrococci." Th. Billroth and F. Ehrlich ("Untersuchungen über Coccobacteria septica," Arch. f. klin. Chir., **20**:403, 1877) observed cocci in a mélange of septic infections, some of which were associated with erysipelas. The important fact, however, was that the idea of infection as a cause of erysipelas was in the air, and the way was paved for the work of Fehleisen. He first reported one fatal case ("Untersuchungen über Erysipel," Sitzungsb. d. phys.-med. Gesellsch. Würzburg, 1881, p. 126) in which he clearly saw micrococci in the superficial lymphatics, but in the present definitive paper he described the process more in detail. He saw and pictured beautifully the lymph channels of the epidermal and subepidermal layers of the skin choked with masses of cocci. He concluded: "Erysipelas is to be distinguished from the various forms of acute phlegmon . . . not only by the clinical picture but by the peculiar micrococcus which differs from all hitherto described pathogenic bacteria . . . and seems to be a special species." Thus Fehleisen anticipated later claims (Ref. 6) of a special erysipelas streptococcus, which in the end turned out to be incorrect (Ref. 6). Soon thereafter Fehleisen summarized his work on erysipelas in a little book (*Die Aetiologie des Erysipel* [Berlin: Theodor Fischer, 1883]). In almost all of a series of rabbits and to a lesser extent in humans, in whom cultures of "erysipelas cocci" were injected, erysipelas was produced. He also described the regression of superficial malignant tumors following the artificial production of erysipelas in their vicinity. He felt that erysipelas was definitely contagious and was spread from person to person by direct contact or by the mediation of instruments, etc.

Fehleisen isolated streptococci from erysipelas in pure culture; as we said above, he felt that this organism was specific for erysipelas and differed from the ordinary *Streptococcus pyogenes* both morphologically and biologically.

Fehleisen's work on streptococci in the lymphatics in erysipelas was promptly confirmed by R. Koch ("Zur Untersuchung von pathogenen Organismen," Mitt. a. d. k. Gsndhtsamte, **1**:38, 1881), using a similar method of biopsy. Koch does not allude to Fehleisen by name and perhaps worked independently of him. It is a question who really deserves priority.

4. CHANTEMESSE. Die Serumtherapie des Erysipels, München. med. Wchnschr., **43**:43, 1896.[1]

Shortly after A. Marmorek ("Le Streptocoque et le sérum antistreptococcique," Ann. Inst. Pasteur, **9**:593, 1895) produced his antistreptococcal serum, Chantemesse reported the effects of it in erysipelas. He thought the results better than with other methods of therapy. Of 501 treated cases, the mortality was only 2.59 per cent. The general condition was said to be improved, but the spread of the eruption was not stopped in its tracks. The treatment had a vogue for many years, always with conflicting and questionable results. Aside from the early work, W. S. McCann ("The serum therapy of erysipelas," J.A.M.A., **91**:78, 1928) in a critical study questioned the value of serum therapy, although D. Symmers and K. M. Lewis ("The antitoxin treatment of erysipelas," J.A.M.A., **99**:1082, 1932) felt that treatment with "antitoxin" often shortened the disease and reduced the mortality. However, serum therapy has become a dead letter in the treatment of erysipelas since the advent of penicillin.

5. LENHARTZ, Hermann. Erysipelas (Rose, Rothlauf) und Erysipeloid. Vienna: Alfred Hölder, 1899.

Lenhartz' monograph, definitive to date, with bibliography, takes up every phase of the subject, bacteriological, clinical, epidemiological.

6. FRANCIS, Thomas, Jr. Studies on pathogenesis and recovery in erysipelas, J. Clin. Investigation, **6**:221, 1928.

Following Fehleisen's pioneer work, there was a great debate as to whether there was a specific erysipelas streptococcus or whether any pyogenic streptococcus could on occasion produce erysipelas. The early observations dealing with this question, pro and con, are summarized in Lenhartz (Ref. 5, p. 17). J. Petruschky ("Entscheidungversuche zur Frage der Specificität des Erysipel-Streptococcus," Ztschr. f. Hyg. u. Infectionskr., **23**:142, 1896) pointed out that

---

[1] We have been unable to trace the original French paper.

the alleged cultural and morphological differences between erysipelas and other streptococci described by Fehleisen did not hold. He also emphasized the common clinical experience of one form of streptococcal infection passing over into another, such as an infant who developed erysipelas by nursing a mother with a streptococcal mastitis. Petruschky inoculated women who had cancer with strains of streptococci from non-erysipelatous sources and with these produced erysipelas. He pointed out that the sort of disease to be caused by a given streptococcus depended rather on site of infection, virulence of organism, resistance of the infected person, and the influence of already existing diseases. "Certain it is that one cannot determine the specificity of a streptococcus from the disease picture. The designations 'Streptococcus erysipelatis' and 'Streptococcus pyogenes' cannot be maintained as originally claimed." R. Koch and J. Petruschky ("Beobachtungen über Erysipel-Impfungen am Menschen," Ztschr. f. Hyg. u. Infektionskr., **23**:477, 1896) soon confirmed and amplified these observations, and Petruschky ("Untersuchungen über Infection mit pyogenen Kokken," Ztschr. f. Hyg. u. Infektionskr., **18**:413, 1894) had already furnished impressive clinical examples of the non-specificity of pyogenic cocci. He summarized: "There are pure streptococcol infections in which erysipelas develops in direct connection with a primary suppurative process . . . contrariwise, there are suppurative processes which begin in connection with a primary erysipelas and are caused by the same streptococcus." Marmorek, too—the pioneer in streptococcal serum therapy—concluded that strains from human disease were all of one sort. A. L. Bloomfield ("The association of susceptibility to scarlet fever and acute tonsillitis," California & West. Med., **28**:477, 1928) reported the case of a young woman who had, in immediate succession, streptococcal otitis media, acute tonsillitis, infection of right maxillary antrum, scarlet fever, erysipelas, and thrombophlebitis, all presumably caused by the same strain of streptococcus.

In spite of these facts, K. E. Birkhaug ("Studies on the biology of the Streptococcus erysipelatis. I. Agglutination and agglutinin absorption with the Streptococcus erysipelatis," Bull. Johns Hopkins Hosp., **36**:248, 1925) concluded that erysipelas was produced by a group of immunologically specific strains of streptococcus. "These experiments indicate that it is possible to differentiate by immunological methods a group of hemolytic streptococci causing erysipelas from the group of hemolytic stretococci responsible for scarlet fever on the one hand, and on the other, from the large series of miscellaneous hemolytic streptococci producing a variety of pyogenic infections." F. A. Stevens and A. R. Dochez ("Antigenic relationship between strains of streptococci from scarlet fever and erysipelas," J. Exper. Med., **43**:379, 1926) sustained the same thesis, although it was soon questioned and finally disposed of by F. Griffith ("The serological classification of Streptococcus pyogenes," J. Hyg., **34**:542, 1934).

Meanwhile, Francis discussed the whole question of the pathogenesis and recovery in erysipelas and demolished the claims of Birkhaug ("IV. Toxin production of the Streptococcus erysipelatis," Proc. Soc. Exper. Biol. & Med., **23**:201, 1925; "Erysipelas. V. Observations on the etiology and treatment of erysipelas with antistreptococcus serum," J.A.M.A., **86**:1411, 1926) that recovery from erysipelas was associated with the neutralization of a soluble circulating toxin analogous to the rash toxin of scarlet fever.

7. SPINK, W. W., and KEEFER, C. S. Studies of hemolytic streptococcal infection. II. The serological reactions of the blood during erysipelas, J. Clin. Investigation, **15**:21, 1936.

Spink and Keefer analyzed the mechanism of recovery from erysipelas in the light of the development of antibodies. They found that the antistreptolysin of the blood serum increased during the disease and that the streptococcidal power of the blood might also increase. Some patients nonetheless developed erysipelas in the face of titers of these substances as high as in controls. The writers bring out clearly the complexity of the situation.

8. SNODGRASS, W. R., and ANDERSON, T. Sulphanilamide in the treatment of erysipelas, Brit. M.J., **2**:1056, 1937.

Snodgrass and Anderson had reported favorable results in the treatment of erysipelas with prontosil ("Prontosil in the treatment of erysipelas," Brit. M.J., **2**:101, 1937). They now reported similar success with sulfanilamide, and a little later Snodgrass, Anderson, and Rennie ("Sulphamido-chrysoidine, sulphanilamide, and benzyl-sulphanilamide in the treatment of erysipelas," Brit. M.J., **2**:399, 1938) reported a mortality of only 2.06 per cent in 242 cases treated with sulphanilamide and related drugs.

9. MORTENSEN, Ole. The efficacy of penicillin and 2-sulfanilamido-5-methyl-1,3,4-thiodiazole ("Lucosil") in the treatment of erysipelas, Acta med. scandinav., **139**:465, 1951.

Although there are earlier reports of treatment with penicillin of single cases of erysipelas such as that of A. L. Bloomfield, W. M. M. Kirby, and C. D. Armstrong ("A study of penicillin failures," J.A.M.A., **126**:685, 1944), we have been unable to find an account of a large series until the present paper. Ninety-eight patients were treated with penicillin and fifty-two with "Lucosil." Although the difference in results with the sulfonamides and penicillin were slight, penicillin seemed to produce a more rapid fall of temperature and subsidence of cutaneous symptoms. It is now (1956) regarded as the treatment of choice.

RHEUMATIC FEVER

(*Continued on following page*)

Section 9

RHEUMATIC FEVER

SO MUCH has been written on every phase of rheumatic fever that the bibliographer is confronted with an almost hopeless task. We call the reader's attention again to the fact that the present list is compiled not for specialists but for general doctors and medical students; although it is certainly incomplete, we have tried to mention every reference which deals with a really fundamental advance in knowledge of the subject.

Excellent older accounts of acute rheumatic fever are those of Senator ("Polyarthritis rheumatica acuta," in H. von Ziemssen, *Handbuch der speciellen Pathologie und Therapie* [Leipzig: F. C. W. Vogel, 1875], **13**:12) and of A. Pribram (*Der acute Gelenkrheumatismus*. [Vienna: Alfred Hölder, 1901]). The latter monograph, of some five hundred pages, is especially comprehensive; it leaves no phase of the disease to date untouched, and it concludes with a bibliography of nearly two thousand titles. Among the numerous briefer English books should be mentioned especially that of Cheadle (Ref. 14). The monographs on the relation of streptococci to rheumatic fever (Ann. Pickett-Thomson Res. Lab. [London: Baillière, Tindall & Cox, 1928], Vol. 4, Part 1) contain useful bibliographies. The books by Coburn (Ref. 22) and by Wilson (Ref. 11) deal with certain special phases of the subject but are of general interest and have good bibliographies. Finally, there is assembled in a symposium on *Rheumatic Fever*, edited by L. Thomas (Minneapolis: University of Minnesota Press, 1952), a series of recent articles which really cover the whole subject. An excellent brief summary of the disease is given by L. A. Rantz (Ref. 24).

Invaluable critical bibliographies of recent literature on rheumatic fever are included in the "rheumatism reviews," which have appeared under the leadership of P. S. Hench in Ann. Int. Med., **9**:883, 1936; **10**:754, 1936; **11**:1089, 1938; **12**:1005, 1939; **13**:1655, 1940; **14**:1383, 1941; **15**:1002, 1941; **28**:66, 1948; **39**:498, 1953. To these should be added the article by C. B. Perry ("Review of the literature on acute rheumatism during the years 1939–1945," Ann. Rheumat. Dis., **6**:162, 1947).

1. BAILLIE, M. The morbid anatomy of some of the most important parts of the human body, p. 46. 2d ed. London: J. Johnson, 1797.

Baillie gives a good description of mitral disease: "The valvular apparatus between the auricles and ventricles is also occasionally thickened, having lost all its transparency, and having an opaque white color. The chordae tendineae likewise become thicker than natural . . ." (p. 32). And as to symptoms, he says: "When the heart is much enlarged, it is attended with palpitations . . . but more commonly the pulse is feeble and irregular. . . . The causes which produce a marked growth of the heart are but little known; one of them would seem to be *rheumatism attacking this organ* [italics ours]." In a footnote, he adds: "Dr Pitcairn has observed this in several cases."

Here, then, is one of the first hints of a relation between rheumatic fever and valvular heart disease. For the most part, however, no one at the time suspected such a relation. John Abernethy ("On a diminution [in consequence of disease]

135

of the area of the aperture by which the left auricle of the heart communicates with the ventricle of the same side," Med.-Chir. Tr., 1:27, 1815), for example, describes accurately the clinical features and autopsy findings in two cases of mitral stenosis, with no hint of "rheumatism" preceding the heart disease.

2. HAYGARTH, J. A clinical history of diseases. Part first. Being 1. A clinical history of the acute rheumatism. London: Cadell & Davies, 1805.

In this little monograph, Haygarth gives an excellent clinical description of acute rheumatic fever: "The symptom peculiar to this disease is an inflammation of the joints which often increases to great violence, with swelling, soreness to touch, and sometimes redness of the skin. It attacks most, if not all the joints of the body in different patients, often two, three or more joints at a time, leaving some and going to others in succession, frequently returning again to each of them several times during the disease [p. 16]. . . . Exposure to cold or moisture is the chief cause of the acute rheumatism [p. 17]. . . . This very formidable and extremely painful disease continues for many weeks; more or less. . . . The remedies usually employed in the acute Rheumatism are bleeding by the lancet or leeches, blisters, antimony, sudorifics, saline medicines, and the warm Bath. The principal purpose of this publication is to recommend the Peruvian Bark in preference to all other remedies [p. 18]." For whatever it means, we quote the following: "Hence we learn that persons who have been previously affected with the acute or chronical Rheumatism, the gout or *sore throat* [italics ours], especially the first are most liable to suffer attacks of this disease" (p. 30).

But throughout the book, including numerous case reports, there is not a word to indicate that the writer had any idea of an association with heart disease.

3. DUNDAS, D. An account of a peculiar disease of the heart, Med.-Chir. Tr., 1:37, 1809.

"There is a disease of the heart, which I apprehend is not very uncommon, no less than nine cases of it having, in the course of thirty-six years, fallen under my care. I have heard of several other cases, and yet I do not believe any account of it is to be found in any medical author." Dundas then gives a good description of what is clearly mitral disease with auricular fibrillation. But significant is the following paragraph: "In all of the cases which I have seen, this disease has succeeded one or more attacks of rheumatic fever . . . the inflammation, pain and swelling of the extremities, after having shifted from one joint to another for many weeks, subsided; but the affection of the heart continued . . . producing in the progress of the disease, and towards its close, a considerable disposition to dropsy, under which the patient lingered for ten months. . . . All those I have seen were young persons. . . . One . . . I think can not recover; and one is apparently well, having survived the attack four years. He has had no rheumatic affection for two years and a half, but the action of the heart is still very violent, and easily increased by exercise. His recovery is attributed to a very strict adherence for a long time to a vegetable and milk diet, and great attention to avoid any considerable exertion." At autopsy, cardiac enlargement was always present, and in one case "upon opening the left ventricle was found an irregular excrescence of the nature of polypus, attached to and nearly occupying the whole of one of the valvulae mitrales." Could this be an instance of bacterial endocarditis? Others were also aware of the relationship, since Mr. Pemberton described a patient who "had been in his youth and indeed even to the time he was taken ill (aged 36) subject to acute rheumatism." Then comes an exquisite description of what was probably the onset of auricular fibrillation: "He was seized with a considerable pain at the heart, and a difficulty of respiration, great palpitation and great anxiety. He conceived that the smallest motion of the body would have instantly destroyed him, and this dread seemed to have totally bereft him of the power of utterance." So, too, Dr. Marcet gave an account of "two cases of translation of rheumatism from the extremities to the chest. . . ."

Dundas concludes: "The knowledge that this disease is always the consequence of, or is connected with, rheumatic affection, points out the necessity of attending to the translation of rheumatism to the chest; and shews the importance of employing very vigorous measures to remove it as soon as possible; but wherever it has made any considerable progress, I fear it will baffle every effort," words still as good today as 150 years ago. At any rate, it is clear that the relation of rheumatic fever to mitral disease was becoming common knowledge in the early nineteenth century.

4. WELLS, W. C. On rheumatism of the heart, Tr. Soc. Improvement M. & Chir. Knowledge, 3:373, 1812.

Wells tried to set the record straight to date. He emphasized the unpublished observations of Dr. David Pitcairn, who "about the year 1788, began to remark, that persons subject to rheumatism were attacked more frequently than others, with symptoms of an organic disease of the heart." He then alluded to Baillie's observations, which are certainly brief and inadequate (Ref. 1). He mentioned the work of Dr. Odier[1] of Geneva and of Dr. Dundas (Ref. 3) and then reported cases of his own which were undoubtedly rheumatic valvular disease but not nearly so well described as those of Dundas. Wells clearly described subcutaneous fibroid nodules in his Case II: "Many of the tendons of the superficial muscles in this patient were studded with numerous small hard tumours, an appearance I have observed only in one other person . . ." (see also Ref. 9).

5. BOUILLAUD, J. New researches on acute articular rheumatism in general. Translated by James Kitchen. Philadelphia: Haswell, Barrington & Haswell, 1837.[2]

Bouillaud's ideas of rheumatic fever were as follows: "Pain, heat, redness, tumefaction, with or without fluctuation of the affected joints—such are the local symptoms of acute articular rheumatism. . . . The pain is increased by touching

[1] Odier's book, *Manuel de médicine practique etc. par Louis Odier* (Geneva: J. J. Paschaud Librairie, 1803), is reviewed in detail in the Edinburgh M. & Surg. J., 2:446, 1806. The reviewer states: "Among the various symptoms which are apt to supervene on acute rheumatism, and to degenerate afterwards into a chronic complaint, Dr. Odier mentions an affection of the heart. . . . Its characteristic symptoms are frequency and irregularity of the pulse, oppression and cough. It is frequently accompanied with anasarcous swellings. . . ."

[2] The original French edition, *Nouvelles recherches sur le rhumatisme articulaire* (Paris, 1836), was unfortunately not available to us.

and by the slightest motion. . . . Fluctuation, a sign of articular effusion, can only be well discovered in the large joints and especially in the knees. . . . Violent fever . . . accompanies above local symptoms. . . . Articular rheumatism, considered by itself and apart from various complications, shows itself with great variety both in extent and intensity. Thus as to extent, it sometimes is so slight as to be dissipated in twenty four hours; then, again, so severe as to resist whole months, unless the most energetic measures are used. . . . Whilst the acute rheumatism easily leaves one or more joints, it generally does so to invade others, whatever may be the mechanism which presides over this displacement. . . . By the acknowledgment of every observer . . . the duration of this disease is very long; the medium term being from 40 to fifty days [pp. 31–34]. The termination of acute articular rheumatism, although often of some duration, is rarely fatal. But yet endocarditis, pericarditis, pleuritis, with which it coincides, sometimes produces death [p. 35]."

It is clear, then, that Bouillaud had a much less complete view of rheumatic fever than we have today. He thought that the disease consisted simply of acute inflammation of joints, which often spread to the heart. He believed that acute rheumatism was in the group of phlegmasias or acute inflammations. "Can any one indeed refuse the title of phlegmasia to a disease which at its height is characterized, in reference to its local symptoms, by pain, heat, swelling, and redness; and with respect to its general state by a most violent fever [p. 43]. As to the determining causes, they may be reduced, on final analysis, to one alone: viz., the impression of cold, especially when humid [p. 40]." Bouillaud also thought that fatigue was a contributory cause. The fact, however, that he and his contemporaries at times found frank pus in the joints of patients with "acute articular rheumatism" shows that they confused the disease with pyogenic arthritis, possibly gonococcal, which may well mimic rheumatic fever.

Bouillaud was a curious mixture of the new clinicopathological school and of old Galenic ideas. He recommended, following Sydenham, bleeding as an almost specific cure for rheumatic fever. In Case III, for example, the procedure consisted of the following: "First day of treatment—bleeding to six bowls in the morning and four in the evening. In the interval scarified cups over the precordial region to the extent of three bowls (in all 52 oz.). Second day four bowls; forty leeches. Third day—four bowls. Fourth day—three bowls. Fifth day —most of the joints are free from swelling; the pain and the fever have disappeared. Convalescent—soup."

Bouillaud was emphatic about the relation of rheumatic fever to heart disease: "It is, I will venture to say, a discovery worthy of some attention; to wit, the almost constant coincidence, either of endocarditis, or of pericarditis, or endo-pericarditis, with violent acute articular rheumatism. This fact . . . is of such vast importance that it constitutes, in some measure, a true revolution in the history of acute articular rheumatism" (Preface, p. iii). It was following Laënnec's introduction of the stethoscope that diagnosis of valve lesions during life became possible, in contrast to the anatomical diagnosis of the earlier observers (Refs. 1, 3, and 4). Bouillaud was a pioneer in physical examination of the heart (see, e.g., his *Traité clinique des maladies du cœur* [Paris: J.-B. Baillière, 1835]): "In auscultating the sounds of the heart, in some individuals still laboring under, or convalescing from, acute articular rheumatism, I was not a little surprised to hear a strong, file, saw or bellows sound [*bruit de râpe, de scie ou de soufflet*], such as I had often met with in chronic or organic induration of the valves, with contraction of the orifices of the heart [p. 9]. Pericarditis exists in about half the patients affected with acute articular rheumatism [p. 12]. Endocarditis, like pericarditis, manifests itself under the same influences as acute articular rheumatism [p. 12]. But in these phlegmasias . . . there exist nice degrees; and I acknowledge that in such cases the diagnosis is both difficult and uncertain [p. 16]." He also clearly described cases of valve lesions persisting or becoming evident long after all signs of articular rheumatism had disappeared.

Bouillaud was apparently unfamiliar with, or at least gave no credit to, the earlier observers (Refs. 1, 3, and 4) on the relation of rheumatism to heart disease.

6. SÉE. De la chorée: rapports du rhumatisme et des maladies du cœur avec les affections, nerveuses et convulsives, Mém. Acad. méd., Paris, **15**:373, 1850.

As early as 1821, the association of chorea with rheumatic fever was clearly recognized. James Copland ("Case of chorea, etc., with an account of post-mortem appearances," London M. Repository, **15**:23, 1821), for example, stated that "Pritchard, the subject of the following case, was attacked, at the age of nine years, with acute rheumatism. Soon after his recovery, chorea St. Viti supervened." Later he had another violent bout of rheumatic fever with cardiac involvement and "he had become again seized by chorea, similar in all its symptoms, with the attack from which he had recovered fourteen months before."

The patient died, and, at autopsy, the cord, which itself appeared normal, was surrounded with coagulable lymph and turbid serum. The interpretation of these findings is difficult. J. Roeser ("Carditis unter der Form von Chorea St. Viti," J. d. pract. Heilk., **67**:54, 1828) reports a child suffering from typical chorea who at death showed pericarditis and inflammation of the heart. Richard Bright ("Cases of spasmodic disease accompanying affections of the pericardium," Med.-Chir. Tr., **22**:1, 1839) describes the case of a young man whose trouble began with "general rheumatic symptoms, pains in the limbs, with puffiness and swelling of the wrists, and some other joints." When all this was subsiding, "I found him labouring under the most fully marked symptoms of severe chorea. His head was constantly thrown from one side of the bed to the other. His lips were closed, and opened with a smacking sound, and when he desired to put out his tongue it was protruded with all the forced grimace and difficulty observed in chorea." There were signs of organic heart disease. He died, and at autopsy there was found acute pericarditis and endocarditis. Dr. Yonge, of Plymouth ("Case of cerebral disturbance, dependent upon disease of the pericardium," Guy's Hosp. Rep., **5**:276, 1840), reports a somewhat similar case: "He states that about a fortnight since he was confined to bed by rheumatic fever, caused by exposure to night-air and damp, from falling asleep in a graveyard, where he was watching a corpse." He then developed chorea and at death was found to have acute endocarditis. H. M. Hughes ("Digest of 100 cases of chorea," Guy's Hosp. Rep., **4**:2d ser., 360, 1846) presents a careful analysis of cases, many of which were clearly associated with rheumatism and/or endocarditis.

But these case reports are insignificant in comparison with the monumental monograph of Sée, which occupies 150 quarto pages. Among the characteristics of chorea, "most constant and most essential are irregular and disordered movements, almost always continuous and unmotivated, which, without absolutely impairing the action of the will on the affected muscles, removes all synergism from their contractions, all precision from their efforts. . . ." Every feature of the disease is taken up in detail too great for us to review, but the section on association with rheumatism is of special importance. In 128 cases of chorea, Sée found that 61 coincided with articular inflammation or pain. In the vast majority, articular rheumatism preceded the chorea, but there were also cases concomitant with, or preceding, the rheumatic fever. The material is well documented by references to the literature. There is a good deal of matter in this long essay which today seems irrelevant and incorrect, but the association of chorea with rheumatic fever is emphatically emphasized. The essential anatomical lesions were "phlegmasias [inflammations], pseudo-membranous or purulent, of the serous membranes, especially of the pericardium or the arachnoid. . . . The anatomical findings in the acute phase are a pseudo-membranous inflammation, a serous congestion, or a simple hyperemia. In the chronic stage one finds the products of plastic lymph organized in the manner of patches, opacities, thickenings, adhesions, fibrous indurations, sometimes fibro-cartilaginous or bony." One doubts whether all these cases were simple chorea. J. Godwin Greenfield and J. M. Wolfsohn ("The pathology of Sydenham's chorea," Lancet, **2**:603, 1922) give an excellent historical review and then report histological studies of a fatal case of chorea. They describe thrombosis of vessels, round-cell infiltration, and changes in nerve cells and conclude that chorea is "a meningo-encephalitis of rheumatic origin."

7. SUTTON, H. G. Cases of rheumatic fever treated for the most part by mint water: collected from the clinical books of Dr. Gull, with some remarks on the natural history of that disease, Guy's Hosp. Rep., **11**:3d ser., 392, 1865.

"In studying the treatment of acute disease it is impossible not to observe how confidently remedies, various and even opposite in their modes of action, have been recommended. . . . It is probably while endeavouring to explain the effects, so little to be expected from such different kinds of treatment, an opinion has been gradually formed that the natural course of the disease had more to do with the result than the remedy." Gull and Sutton therefore proceeded to study the natural course of the disease in patients treated only by rest and safeguarding. They noted that all the symptoms might subside in 5, 6, 7, or 8 days, unaided by treatment. Every type of case is described: brief, long, recurrent, with and without cardiac involvement. "It would appear . . . that those cases in which the symptoms are acute tend to get well much sooner than those in which the symptoms are sub-acute. . . ."

Since mention of antecedent sore throat or respiratory infection, so much stressed today, is conspicuous by its absence in the early descriptions, the following case in Sutton's report is of special interest and importance: "A young lady was suffering from sore throat; she was very subject to enlarged tonsils. Some yellow cheesy-looking substance was noted on the tonsils. She appeared depressed, and was sweating freely, but no acid odour. She was kept in bed for

3 days, then appearing much better, she was allowed to get up. . . . One day, about a month after she had had this throat affection, she complained of pain in the right knee. . . . There was pain, first in one knee, then in the other, also in the ankles, but no swelling; so she continued for eight or ten days." About the end of that time she became worse, and "a harsh grating to-and-fro murmur was heard over the heart."

"In relation to the rheumatic state, is the very important question, when we have lost all the symptoms of rheumatic fever,—has the patient lost the rheumatic condition of the system. The case of Dr. Rees would lead us to think not."

"A perusal of the above cases tends to show that the best treatment for rheumatic fever has still to be determined. . . . The cases show that too much importance has been attached to the use of medicines, especially in those acute cases where the tendency to a natural cure is the greatest."

In a subsequent number ("A second report of cases of acute rheumatism," Guy's Hosp. Rep., **12**:3d ser., 509, 1866), Sutton gives admirable descriptions of more cases of rheumatic fever; both these papers are preliminary to the study of Gull and Sutton (Ref. 8).

8. GULL, W. W., and SUTTON, H. G. Remarks on the natural history of rheumatic fever, Med.-Chir. Tr., **52**:43, 1869.

In the first half of the century, students of rheumatic fever devoted themselves largely to the trial of various remedies. Many papers appeared in which claims were made for the virtue of one or another form of medication. There was much special pleading and many post hoc fallacious conclusions. We have already pointed out Bouillaud's emphasis on bleeding as the only useful remedy (Ref. 5). D. J. Corrigan, on the other hand ("Observations on the treatment of acute rheumatism by opium," Dublin J.M. Sc., **16**:256, 1840), strongly advocated the use of opium. "The most important rule to be remembered . . . is that *full and sufficient* doses shall be exhibited." He prescribed it in increasing amounts until a beneficial effect was obtained. The first indication that the proper dose had been reached is "the statement of the patient, who in reply to an inquiry as to how he has passed the night, probably says that he has not slept, but that he is free from pain and feels comfortable." Kersten ("Beiträge zur Behandlung des hitzigen Gelenk-Rheumatismus," Deutsche Klin., **1**:16, 1849) also described a rigid dosage scheme for opium; he was not so certain as Corrigan, however, that this treatment prevented cardiac complications. J. J. Furnivall ("On the pathology of acute rheumatism, and on the prevention of heart disease," Lancet, **1**:304, 1844), after commenting on the obscurity which enveloped the pathology of acute rheumatism, concluded that alkali was the proper treatment because of the acid predominant in the system and "as a thinner of the fibrine superabounding in the blood." Innumerable other medicines and schemes of treatment had their advocates.

Soon, however, critical papers began to appear. Thomas K. Chambers ("Statistics of the treatment of rheumatic fever," Brit. M.J., **2**:237, 1863) found that patients treated with nitrate of potash remained in hospital for a mean stay of 40 days, those treated with bicarbonate of potash q. 2 h. stayed 34.3 days, those treated with "a less quantity of the same" stayed 40.0 days, and those treated without drugs stayed 30.0 days. When patients were bedded in blankets instead of in sheets, the occurrence of pericarditis and endocarditis was lower. Obviously, these figures do not speak strongly for the virtue of medicines.

But Gull and Sutton approached the problem in a highly unbiased attitude. "In this paper we are desirous of bringing under the notice of the profession the particulars of a few more cases of rheumatic fever which have been treated by mint-water, or, in other words, by absolute rest and regulated diet, unaided by medicine. . . . We are now desirous of pointing out what appears to be the natural course of rheumatic fever with reference to the heart; to show in what proportion of cases the heart has become diseased when the patients were treated by mint-water; and to consider if there be any evidence to prove that the heart is more frequently involved where cases are treated by alkalies, lemon-juice, or by the application of blisters to the joints." They concluded emphatically that none of these methods of therapy influenced the course or duration of the disease or prevented cardiac complications. "The reason why the heart did not become diseased when rheumatic fever was treated by alkalies or blisters to the joints is to be attributed not to the influence of drugs but to the natural course of the disease. . . . At present, therefore, as regards treatment, our cases seem to show that we are limited to a careful regimen of the patients. Rest, mechanical and physiological, rest in the very outset of the disease. We ought not to wait until the rheumatic process has become well developed in the joints, for it appears to us that the heart becomes involved simultaneously with the joints, and by rest we hope to quiet the heart's action, and so prevent it becoming diseased."

Gull and Sutton's study is a model of critical approach and reasoning. It gave a sound orientation to therapy and prepared the way for the introduction of salicylates in treatment of rheumatic fever (Ref. 10).

9. MEYNET, P. Rhumatisme articulaire subaigu avec production de tumeurs multiples dans les tissus fibreux périarticulaires et sur le périoste d'un grand nombre d'os, Lyon méd., **20**:495, 1875.

Wells (Ref. 4) appears to have been the first to mention "fibroid nodules," but his account is brief and inadequate. In his textbook on *Diseases of Children* (Philadelphia: Lindsay & Blakiston, 1868) Thomas Hillier, however, referred to a child with "aggravated chorea" who developed under his scalp "a number of hard round lumps, about the size of peas and horse beans; the skin moves over them, but they are firmly attached to the bone. They are neither red nor tender on pressure." Later there appeared a swelling on the inner condyle of the femur. "Dr. Jenner saw him with me and feared that these growths might be malignant," but in favor of rheumatism "is the circumstance that there is now a loud systolic murmur at the heart's apex." The boy got well, and the lumps disappeared.

But Meynet seems to have been the first to direct special attention to subcutaneous fibroid nodules. He reported the case of a boy who had several rheumatic relapses: "Along the course of each of these tendons one found a rosary of little lumps about the size of a lentil or of a pea, hard to the touch, not painful and intimately adherent to these tendons . . . all around these joints one finds little tumors. . . . Furthermore, a point of importance to note, these nodosities appear and disappear with great speed; we have seen them so to speak spring up under our eyes from day to day, and we have likewise seen them disappear. Which is the native and precise seat of these neoplasms? It is evident to us that they are due to rheumatism. . . . In our young subject it is evident that it is, above all, the fibrous tissues which are involved—joints, periosteum, and tendons." Meynet left little to be described further as regards the clinical features. E. Troisier and L. Brocq ("Les Nodosités sous-cutanées éphémères et le rhumatisme," Rev. méd. Paris, 1:297, 1881) reported another case and gave a thorough discussion of the subject. At about the same time there appeared the report of H. Hirschsprung ("Eine eigenthümliche Localisation des Rheumatismus acutus im Kindesalter," Jahrb. f. Kinderh. 16:324, 1881), in which he gave detailed reports of several cases. He concluded: "The nodules must be considered as new growths of connective tissue of a chronic inflammatory sort with a tendency to necrobiosis. They are probably derived from tendons, the tissues of which they resemble."

To T. Barlow and F. Warner ("On subcutaneous nodules connected with fibroid structures occurring in children the subjects of rheumatism and chorea," Tr. Internat. M. Cong., 14:116, 1881), however, goes the credit for the first detailed and comprehensive account. They gave an analysis of 27 cases and described the natural history of these nodules in great detail. A nodule was removed during life, and microscopic sections were made, which showed "wavy strands of fibrous tissue, with caudate, spindle-shaped, nucleated cells and abundant vessels. It had indeed, many of the characters of organizing granulation tissue." B. F. Massell, J. R. Mote, and T. D. Jones ("The artificial induction of subcutaneous nodules in patients with rheumatic fever," J. Clin. Investigation, 16:125, 1937) found that "the injection of the patient's own blood into the subcutaneous tissues of subjects with rheumatic fever frequently results in the appearance of subcutaneous nodules in the area injected. They are clinically indistinguishable from nodules occurring spontaneously."

Every phase of the subcutaneous fibroid nodule is fully discussed in H. Keil's definitive monograph ("The rheumatic subcutaneous nodules and simulating lesions," Medicine, 17:261, 1938), with over three hundred references.

10. MACLAGAN, T. The treatment of acute rheumatim by salicin, Lancet, 1:342, 1876.

"The idea of treating acute rheumatism by salicin occurred to me in November 1874. I had at that time under my care a well-marked case of the disease (Case 1) which was being treated by alkalies, but was not improving. I determined to give salicin; but before doing so, took myself first five, then ten, and then thirty grains without experiencing the least inconvenience or discomfort. . . . I gave to the patient referred to twelve grains every three hours. The result exceeded my most sanguine expectations. . . . On the following day, after 84 grains of salicin had been taken, the pulse had gone down to 100, the temperature to 99.6° (from 102.8° the previous day), a fall of over 3°, the pain and swelling of joints, but especially the pain, had much abated, the joints could be moved a little, and the patient expressed himself as being much better." Maclagan reported eight cases, with graphic charts showing striking drops in temperature. He concluded that salicin was a valuable remedy in acute rheumatic fever; that, the more acute the fever, the more marked the benefit, usually within 24–48 hours; and that there was great relief of pain. "I shall be greatly obliged if those who try the remedy, and do not care to publish their observations, would kindly forward to me the results of their experience, be it favourable or otherwise."

At about the same time, Stricker ("Über die Resultäte der Behandlung der Polyarthritis rheumatica mit Salicylsäure," Berl. klin. Wchnschr., **13**:1, 15, 1876), no doubt independently, treated patients with acute rheumatic fever in Traube's clinic with salicylic acid. All the patients were freed of fever and local manifestations within 24–48 hours. He emphasized that this effect was something apart from the general antipyretic action of the drug. L. Reiss ("Nachtrag zur innerlichen Anwendung der Salicylsäure, inbesondere bei dem acuten Gelenkrheumatismus," Berl. klin. Wchnschr., **13**:86, 1876) soon amplified Stricker's report. Meanwhile, Broadbent ("Treatment of rheumatic fever by salicylic acid," Lancet, **1**:530, 1876), who was unaware of Maclagan's report but who knew of Stricker's work, reported similar excellent results. "Few diseases have had brought against them a heavier armament of drugs than has acute rheumatism. It has been stormed by alkalies and salines, attacked by acids, assaulted by perchloride of iron and by quinine, surprised by propylamine and ethylchlorüre, drained by venesection and purgatives, flooded alternately with hot and cold water, alarmed with blisters, blasted with hot air, lulled by opium and appeased by chloralhydrate. In addition to these, it has been constantly harassed by the raids of lesser foes, such as lemon juice, citric acid, belladonna and iodide of potassium. . . . Salicylic acid has been shown by Stricker to be able to prevail against some cases of acute rheumatism and Dr. Broadbent's experience seems to confirm this character." In a letter to the Lancet (**1**:585, 1876) Maclagan complained that Broadbent did not grant him due priority, to which Broadbent replied with a gracious explanation (*ibid.*, p. 619).

The use of salicylic acid or salicylate was promptly accepted as of real value. J. L. Miller ("The specific action of salicylates in acute articular rheumatism," J.A.M.A., **63**:1107, 1914) studied the length of time that patients with acute rheumatic fever treated with and without salicylates remained in the hospital; 1,907 patients with salicylates averaged a 32.28 days' stay; 1,600 without salicylates, 33.6 days. Miller concluded, therefore, that "statistics show that patients receiving salicylate are free from pain much earlier than those not treated. As the treated patients much more frequently relapse . . . the period of stay in the hospital . . . is the same." P. J. Hanzlik ("Actions and uses of the salicylates and cinchopen in medicine," Medicine, **5**:197, 1926) presented a monumental review of the whole subject, superseded only by Martin Gross and Leon Greenberg's monograph, *The Salicylates: A Critical Bibliographical Review* (New Haven: Hellhouse, 1948) with bibliography of some four thousand titles.

In 1943, A. F. Coburn ("Salicylate therapy in rheumatic fever: a rational technique," Bull. Johns Hopkins Hosp., **73**:345, 1943) proposed the treatment of acute rheumatic fever by large doses of salicylates intravenously with control of blood levels. He thought that this method was more effective in preventing cardiac involvement than standard oral administration. The method was extensively taken up, but G. E. Murphy (Bull. Johns Hopkins Hosp., **77**:1, 1945), in a careful study, showed that in several patients given intravenous salicylates in large doses "characteristic rheumatic lesions developed in a variety of sites during the course of salicylate therapy." B. V. Jager and R. Alway ("The treatment of acute rheumatic fever with large doses of sodium salicylate," Am. J.M.

Sc., **211**:273, 1946) were also unenthusiastic about Coburn's method, and now (1956) it seems to have dropped into disuse.

11. GOODHART, J. F. On the rheumatic diathesis in childhood, Guy's Hosp. Rep., **25**:3d ser., 103, 1880.

The large number of reports in the modern literature on the occurrence of rheumatic fever in families makes one forget that this fact was recognized over seventy-five years ago. P. H. Pye-Smith ("Analysis of the cases of rheumatism and other diseases of the joints," Guy's Hosp. Rep., **19**:3d ser., 311, 1874) is quite emphatic: "There can be no doubt that a tendency to rheumatic fever is inherited." He gives an analysis of 68 cases in which the patient asserted that one or more of his blood relatives had been attacked by rheumatic fever. Goodhart goes into the matter much more thoroughly: "Acute rheumatism in children is in the majority of cases inherited." His paper concludes with a table of cases indicating the occurrence of rheumatic manifestations in the family. For example, of children with acute rheumatic fever, we have statements such as the following: Girl, aged 9. Father has had rheumatic fever. Boy, aged 9. Mother has had rheumatic fever. Girl, aged 4. Father died with rheumatic fever and heart disease, etc. A. E. Garrod and E. H. Cooke ("An attempt to determine the frequency of rheumatic family histories amongst non-rheumatic patients," Lancet **2**:110, 1888) state: "It is universally admitted that rheumatism is an extremely hereditary disease." Nonetheless, the writers attempted to find out how often the relatives of non-rheumatic patients gave a history of rheumatic disease. The figure was about 20 per cent, as against 30–35 per cent in the relatives of rheumatic patients.

But Cheadle's discussion (Ref. 14, "Occasional lectures on the practice of medicine," p. 227) is most impressive. "The second personal factor, viz., hereditary predisposition, is one of the most potent. . . . The tendency to rheumatism is transmitted as strongly as the tendency to gout. . . . In thirty-two consecutive cases out of my private notebooks . . . in twenty-three, that is 70 per cent, there was a definite history of rheumatic fever in near blood relations. If chorea and erythema be taken as sufficient evidence of rheumatism, the proportion is raised to . . . 93 per cent. . . . A case is recorded . . . which shows remarkable family proclivity to the disease. A rheumatic mother had twelve children, and eleven of them had rheumatism before the age of twenty . . . as might be inferred, when the proclivity is inherited from both parents the tendency is greatly intensified; not only is the liability to the disease increased . . . but its severity and persistence are increased also. . . . Now it occurred to me that this extraordinary tendency of rheumatism to develop in certain families might be due to some special faults of locality or circumstances, but careful inquiry into a number of cases showed me that they arose in various localities, in members of the family when in different places and under different conditions."

During subsequent years many papers which added little were published on the same question. The recent studies of M. G. Wilson and M. D. Schweitzer ("Rheumatic fever as a familial disease, environment, communicability and heredity in their relation to the observed familial incidence of the disease," J. Clin. Investigation, **16**:555, 1937) seem, however, to carry the subject further. In a careful study of families under controlled conditions, they found, as had Cheadle, that "there did not appear to be a direct relation between the environments studied and the incidence of rheumatic fever. There was no direct relation between the type and source of exposure and the resulting activity. . . . Intimate contact ('familial exposure') and casual contact ('extrafamilial exposure') were equally effective. . . . The hereditary mechanism involved was a single autosomal recessive gene." Their general conclusion is that "susceptible" persons acquire rheumatic fever much more readily than others, but they do not determine from these studies the exact role of environment and contagion in the acquisition of the disease. J. R. Paul and R. Salinger ("The spread of rheumatic fever through families," J. Clin. Investigation, **10**:33, 1931) had come to similar conclusions and thought that the spread of rheumatic fever through families strongly suggested infection, with the role of environment and hereditary predisposition as yet undetermined. It was of interest that rheumatic activity was often accompanied by evidence of respiratory tract infection. An intensive analysis of the whole problem, with full bibliography, is given by Wilson in her book, *Rheumatic Fever* (New York: Commonwealth Fund, 1940), p. 21. Wilson has also recently summarized her views ("Heredity and rheumatic disease," Am. J. Med., **2**:190, 1947).

12. FOWLER, J. K. On the association of affections of the throat with acute rheumatism, Lancet, **2**:933, 1880.

The relation of hemolytic streptococcus sore throat to rheumatic fever is a relatively modern concept. Indeed, in the older literature one scans series after series of cases (Refs. 3, 4, and 5) without finding any allusion to sore throat at all. Senator ("Die Krankheiten des Bewegungsapparatus," in Von Ziemssen, *Handbuch der speciellen Pathologie und Therapie* [Leipzig: F. C. W. Vogel, 1875], **13**:12), for example, in his comprehensive article makes no mention of sore throat. Sutton's case (Ref. 7) is an exception to the general rule. When attention began to be centered on the throat and tonsils, confusion arose, since sore throats are mentioned with all sorts of bacteriological findings, and in many cases rheumatic fever, on the basis of the old theory of focal infection (F. Billings, "Focal infection: its broader application in the etiology of general disease," J.A.M.A., **63**:899, 1914), was attributed to "septic tonsils," that is to say, tonsils which were simply large and which contained bacteria of all sorts. We should make it clear that the current view of the relation of sore throat to rheumatic fever refers to a specific acute group A tonsillitis or pharyngitis, even if mild. Much of the older literature is therefore worthless; it is comprehensively reviewed by David and Robert Thomson ("An historical survey of researches on the role of the streptococci in acute articular rheumatism or rheumatic fever. G. The association of tonsillitis with rheumatic fever and its manifestations," Ann. Pickett-Thomson Res. Lab., 4 [Pt. 1]: 56, 1928).

Fowler is, however, quite clear on the subject: "I have for some time past made it a rule in all cases of acute rheumatism . . . to inquire carefully for any history of tonsillitis or catarrh of the pharynx having preceded the attack. I was led to do this by a remark from Dr. Garrod, F.R.S., when he was attending me for a severe attack of rheumatic fever in the winter of 1874. A month before my illness I had a sharp attack of acute tonsillitis, and Dr. Garrod told me he noticed that the two affections were not uncommonly associated. . . . Without at present being able to give an exact percentage of cases presenting this premonitory symptom, I think I should not exaggerate if I were to put it at 80 per cent." Fowler proceeds to describe the details of 20 patients in whom a bad sore throat preceded evidence of articular rheumatism by intervals of 7–21 days. This paper is a masterpiece of precise reporting and leaves no doubt as to the association of tonsillitis and rheumatic fever. This association is discussed in detail in the elaborate "Reports of the Collective Investigative Committee of the British Medical Association" (Ref. 13). Among 655 cases of articular rheumatism, 158 were "the subjects of tonsillitis." One patient, a woman aged thirty, had had three attacks of tonsillitis "each followed by acute rheumatism." A. Mantle ("The etiology of rheumatism from a bacterial point of view," Brit. M.J., 1:1381, 1887) later noted that "rheumatism and scarlatina were not infrequently observed in the same house, scarlatina attacking the younger members of the family, rheumatic fever the older, scarlatina usually entering the house first. . . . Acute tonsillitis had frequently been observed under the same conditions." E. Roos ("Über rheumatische Angina," Berl. klin. Wchnschr., 31:575, 1894) comments on the lack of recognition of this association in Germany and reports a case of typical tonsillitis followed in 12 days by acute arthritis. He gives an excellent comprehensive review of the early literature on the subject, as does E. Bloch ("Zur Aetiologie des Rheumatismus," München. med. Wchnschr., 45:445, 1898).

One of the most important points of all this work was the recognition of a latent period between the sore throat and the symptoms of rheumatic fever. Later, B. Schick ("Über die Nachkrankheiten des Scharlach," Jahrb f. Kinderh., 1907, Ergänzungsband, p. 132) formulated the latent period between scarlet fever and its sequels as an allergic manifestation, and, while he mentioned postscarlatinal "rheumatism" as one of the sequels, the evidence is that he did not identify such rheumatism with acute rheumatic fever but regarded it as a specific consequence of scarlatina. This view was challenged on good evidence by J. R. Paul, R. Salinger, and B. Zuger ("The relation of rheumatic fever to post-scarlatinal arthritis and post-scarlatinal heart disease: a familial study," J. Clin. Investigation, 13:503, 1934). Recently, E. E. Fischel ("The role of allergy in the pathogenesis of rheumatic fever," Am. J. Med., 7:772, 1949) has given a definitive review of this phase of the subject, with a bibliography of nearly three hundred titles. J. K. Aikawa ("Hypersensitivity and rheumatic fever," Ann. Int. Med., 41:576, 1954) also discusses the subject in interesting fashion.

Turning now to more modern material, J. A. Glover ("Incidence of rheumatic disease," Lancet, 1:199, 1930) tells of an interesting outbreak in a training school where two thousand boys lived in crowded quarters. "There was a sharp epidemic of tonsillitis, followed by an outbreak of acute rheumatism. Again we see the peak of the tonsillitis epidemic precedes the crest of the rheumatic wave by some two or three weeks." The situation was now getting "warm" as to incriminating in some way the hemolytic streptococcus. A. F. Coburn and R. H. Pauli ("Studies on the relationship of Streptococcus hemolyticus to the rheumatic process. I. Observations on the ecology of hemolytic streptococcus in relation to the epidemiology of rheumatic fever," J. Exper. Med., 56:609, 1932) were among the first to go further and insist on infection with hemolytic streptococcus. "The majority of rheumatic patients who contract hemolytic streptococcus pharyngitis experience shortly afterward a definite recrudescence of their disease. In conclusion there is a close relationship between respiratory infection with hemolytic streptococcus and activity of the rheumatic process in susceptible individuals." In another paper, Coburn and Pauli ("Studies on the relationship of Streptococcus hemolyticus to the rheumatic process. II. Observations on the biological character of Streptococcus hemolyticus associated with rheumatic disease," J. Exper. Med., **56**:633, 1932) showed that the streptococci isolated from the throats of rheumatic persons were not of a single Lancefield type but fell into six antigenic groups.

W. R. F. Collis ("Acute rheumatism and haemolytic streptococci," Lancet, **1**:1341, 1931) quotes Dr. F. Griffith, who investigated an outbreak of tonsillitis at a public school which was followed in several instances by primary acute rheumatism. "Griffith found that a haemolytic streptococcus of a well-defined serological type was responsible for the cases and suggested (private communication) that there might be direct aetiological connexion between this streptococcal infection and rheumatic attacks." It is of interest in this connection that recent work has shown that post-streptococcal nephritis almost always is preceded by Type 12 hemolytic streptococcal throat infection (C. N. Stetson, C. H. Rammelkamp, Jr., R. M. Krause, R. J. Kohen, and W. D. Perry, "Epidemic acute nephritis: studies on etiology, natural history, and prevention," Medicine, **34**:431, 1955). Collis himself showed, in an epidemic of acute tonsillitis, that "rheumatic relapses occurred in 9 out of 11 children who developed acute streptococcal infection, while similar febrile disorders not associated with the hemolytic streptococcus caused no relapse." J. A. Glover and F. Griffith ("Acute tonsillitis and some of its sequels: epidemiological and bacteriological observations," Brit. M.J., **2**:521, 1931) conclude that "infection of the throat with hemolytic streptococci produces varying clinical pictures in different persons. These include first, a symptomless infection . . . secondly, tonsillitis; thirdly, febricula, feverish catarrh or pharyngitis, without noticeable sore throat. Any of the latter three conditions may be followed by otitis media or by acute rheumatism." Glover, in contrast to the American experience, found most cases of scarlet fever to be caused by Types 1, 2, 3, and 4. W. H. Bradley ("Epidemic acute rheumatism in a public school," Quart. J. Med., **1**:79, 1932) reports on an interesting outbreak in a boys' school. "Two epidemics of rheumatism are recorded and their relation to parallel waves of hemolytic streptococcal sore throat are demonstrated: the causal streptococci being of two distinct strains." L. A. Rantz, working in the army camps on outbreaks of acute rheumatic fever during World War II, confirmed and amplified the early observations (L. A. Rantz, P. J. Boisvert, and W. W. Spink, "Etiology and pathogenesis of rheumatic fever," Arch. Int. Med., **76**:131, 1945; and "Hemolytic streptococcic sore throat: the post-streptococcic state," *ibid.*, **79**:401, 1947). Rantz and his associates found that the alleged latent period between throat infection and outburst of rheumatic fever was really featured by various abnormalities. They worked out details of the streptococcal infection with reference to definition of strains, and they designated all the non-suppurative late events as the "post-streptococcic state"; there were many other interesting findings.

While attacks of acute rheumatism are, then, so often preceded by hemolytic streptococcus throat infections, not all outbreaks of streptococcal tonsillitis are followed by rheumatic fever. A. L. Bloomfield and A. R. Felty ("Bacteriological observations on acute tonsillitis with reference to epidemiology and susceptibility," Arch. Int. Med., **32**:483, 1923), for example, studied with the greatest care the clinical and bacteriological features of acute follicular tonsil-litis in a closed group. During one season there were 39 cases, all caused by hemolytic streptococcus; in not a single instance was there any evidence of rheumatic fever. So, too, A. L. Bloomfield and L. A. Rantz ("An outbreak of streptococcic septic sore throat in an army camp," J.A.M.A., **121**:315, 1943) studied an outbreak of acute streptococcus sore throat affecting several hundred soldiers due to Type 15 hemolytic streptococcus. Within three weeks there was no evidence of rheumatic fever in a single man. Possibly the organisms involved were not "rheumatogenic."

13. WHIPHAM, T. Reports of the Collective Investigating Committee of the British Medical Association: Report on Inquiry No. III: Acute rheu-matism, Brit. M.J., **1**:387, 1888.

The committee invited doctors to send in reports of cases of acute rheumatism; observations on 655 patients were received. These reports are analyzed from every conceivable standpoint and furnish a mine of information. Some of the points discussed are sex, age, occupation, class in society, habits, food, locality, atmosphere, antecedent tonsillitis, antecedent scarlet fever, chorea, influence of treatment, relapsing cases, etc.

14. CHEADLE, W. B. Harveian lectures on the various manifestations of the rheumatic state as exemplified in childhood and early life, Lancet **1**:821, 871, 921, 1889.

We have already pointed out how the concept of rheumatic fever widened in scope from simple acute arthritis during the first three quarters of the century. It remained for someone to organize and codify all this information, and this Cheadle did in these lectures, which are a landmark in the clinical study of the subject. The material was published as a book, *The Various Manifestations of the Rheumatic State as Exemplified in Childhood and Early Life* (London: Smith, Elder & Co., 1889), and later on in revised form in Cheadle's mono-graph, *Occasional Lectures on the Practice of Medicine* (London: Smith, Elder & Co., 1900).

Cheadle enumerates the various manifestations of the rheumatic state. Endo-carditis and pericarditis, pleurisy, and tonsillitis are seen in both adults and children. Subcutaneous tendinous nodules, chorea, and exudative erythema are commoner in children. "For my present purpose I shall assume the connexion and speak of these seven phases, together with arthritis, as the rheumatic series." Each of these manifestations is systematically discussed, with illustrative case reports. "The account of the various phases of rheumatism would be in-complete without some reference to the scarlatinal affection. Articular inflamma-tion appears now and again in the course of scarlet fever, which can in no way be distinguished from that of acute rheumatism. It is often accompanied by endocarditis or pericarditis, and sometimes by chorea." In this point of view Cheadle was far ahead of his time.

T. Duckett Jones ("The diagnosis of rheumatic fever," J.A.M.A., **126**:481, 1944) later classified the various manifestations of rheumatic fever from the standpoint of value in diagnosis. He divided the criteria into major (carditis, polyarthritis, chorea, subcutaneous nodules, and erythema marginatum) and minor (fever, arthralgia, prolonged P-R in the electrocardiogram, preceding hemolytic streptococcal infection, previous rheumatic fever, or inactive rheumatic heart disease). These criteria have been modified by the American Heart Association (*Modern Concepts of Cardiovascular Disease: Jones Criteria* [Modified] *for Guidance in the Diagnosis of Rheumatic Fever* [1955], Vol. **24**, No. 9).

15. NEWSHOLME, A. The natural history and affinities of rheumatic fever: a study in epidemiology, Lancet, **1**:589, 657, 1895.

"The thesis which will be advanced and supported . . . is that rheumatic fever is a specific febrile disease, caused by . . . a pathogenic micro-organism. . . . Such a view of the causation of rheumatic fever does not cover the entire ground. Assuming that rheumatic fever only occurs when a special pathogenic micro-organism is introduced . . . its causation is by no means exhausted. It occurs chiefly or only in predisposed persons, in certain states of health, and under the influence of certain excitants—as fatigue, injury and chill, the exact value of which in its causation will be hereafter discussed. Further, it occurs by preference at certain seasons of the year, in certain localities, or perhaps on certain soils. . . . We have to consider, on the one hand, the influences determining an individual attack of rheumatic fever; and on the other hand, the wider influences determining the extent of its varying prevalence in different countries in successive years."

A more precise statement of the problem could not be made today (1957). The following factors Newsholme regards as essential: the active infective agent, conditions of environment, and personal factors. He reviewed some earlier reports on "epidemic" outbreaks but concluded: "There has, however, so far as I am aware been no wide and thorough investigation of the epidemiology of rheumatic fever." First, Newsholme traced the incidence of rheumatic fever in various hospitals through the years and concluded that there was at times a definite epidemic prevalence; then the influences of the various ancillary factors enumerated above are analyzed. Newsholme felt that the influence of heredity had been exaggerated but that injury and fatigue were definite predisposing factors and that dust perhaps had some influence. He also found a close relationship between rainfall, level of ground water, and the amount of rheumatic fever: "There is abundant evidence of seasonal incidence of rheumatic fever."

Meanwhile, A. Hirsch (*Handbuch der historisch-geographischen Pathologie* [2d ed.; Stuttgart: Ferdinand Enke, 1886], **3**:530) gave a list of outbreaks, from which he concluded that "polyarthritis is a specific infectious disease." The subject may be pursued further in the paper of D. Seegal and B. C. Seegal ("Studies in the epidemiology of rheumatic fever," J.A.M.A., **89**:11, 1927) and in that of R. M. Atwater ("Studies in the epidemiology of acute rheumatic fever and related diseases in the United States based on mortality statistics," Am. J. Hyg., **7**:343, 1927), who concludes that "acute rheumatic fever appears to be related to the family of streptococcal infections, because of bacteriological indications, clinical resemblances and epidemiological kinship." The subject is dealt with fully and systematically by J. R. Paul (*The Epidemiology of Rheumatic Fever* [New York: Metropolitan Life Insurance Co., 1930]; *The Epidemiology of Rheumatic Fever and Some of Its Public Health Aspects* [New York: Metropolitan Life Insurance Co., 1943]). Finally, F. F. Schwentker

("The epidemiology of rheumatic fever," in *Rheumatic Fever*, ed. L. Thomas [Minneapolis: University of Minnesota Press, 1952], p. 17) gives a precise recent review.

16. ASCHOFF, L. Zur Myocarditisfrage, Verhandl. d. deutsch. path. Gesellsch., **8**:46, 1904.

William Stokes (*The Diseases of the Heart and Aorta* [Dublin: Hodges & Smith, 1854]) clearly recognized disease of the heart muscle as of importance apart from valve lesions (pp. 109 and 113). There are also a number of hints in the early literature as to the presence of anatomical myocardial changes in cases of rheumatic fever. S. West ("Analysis of 40 cases of rheumatic fever," St. Bart's Hosp. Rep., **14**:221, 1878), for example, stated in regard to dilatation of the heart: "This may depend upon organic changes in the muscular tissue and in one case was proved to do so by microscopical examination," which showed that "in these white patches the muscular tissue had undergone acute granular (fatty) degeneration, its fibers being converted into granular cylinders." In James F. Goodhart's case of rapid enlargement of the heart (Tr. Path. Soc., London, **30**:279, 1879) myocardial changes were found also: "I examined sections of the muscular wall microscopically and there was a considerable quantity of interstitial cell-growth around the vessels and between muscular fasciculi." But these observations were highly rudimentary, and it was L. Krehl ("Beitrag zur Pathologie der Herzklappenfehler," Deutsches Arch. f. klin. Med., **46**:454, 1890) and E. Romberg ("Über die Bedeutung des Herzmuskels für die Symptome und den Verlauf der acuten Endocarditis und der chronischen Klappenfehler," Deutsches Arch. f. klin. Med., **53**:141, 1894) who were pioneers in emphasizing the importance of the anatomical and functional state of the myocardium apart from valve lesions. While they did not describe the specific lesion of rheumatic fever, they did stress changes in the myocardium as a result of rheumatic fever and other infections.

It was Aschoff, however, who first described the specific rheumatic lesion in the myocardium—the Aschoff body. "We succeeded in defining more closely the histological makeup of the products of inflammation and, indeed, in finding peculiar nodules which seem to be specific for rheumatic myocarditis. To be sure, full-blown nodules were found in only two cases of recurring endocarditis, but they correspond in their situation with the cellular proliferation found in the other cases. They are regularly situated in the vicinity of small or medium blood vessels and often show an intimate relation to the adventitia. Or there may be a lesion of all the vessel coats such as is described in arteritis nodosa. The actual nodules are very small, submiliary, and consist of the approximation of strikingly large cells with one or more abnormally large, slightly indented or polymorphous nuclei." He goes on in much more detail: "While in one case the nodule makes the impression of a fresh cell proliferation, in another a partial or total fibrous change can be demonstrated." Aschoff strongly supported the Leipzig school—Krehl and Romberg—in their contention that cardiac failure was due more to weakness resulting from changes in the myocardium than from valve lesions.

P. Geipel soon confirmed Aschoff's findings ("Untersuchungen über rheumatische Myokarditis," Deutsches Arch. f. klin. Med., **85**:75, 1905), as did C. Coombs ("The myocardial lesions of the rheumatic infection," Brit. M.J.,

8:1513, 1907), in England. Meanwhile, Aschoff ("A discussion of some aspects of heart block," Brit. M.J., **2**:1103, 1906) described the nodules in English. E. Bracht and Wächter ("Beitrag zur Aetiologie und pathologische Anatomie der Myocarditis rheumatica," Deutsches Arch. f. klin. Med., **96**:493, 1909) found the nodules in three cases of definite acute rheumatism but in no patient dying of other infectious diseases. Finally, W. Thalhimer and M. A. Rothschild ("On the significance of the submiliary, myocardial nodules of Aschoff in rheumatic fever," J. Exper. Med., **19**:417, 1914) reviewed the literature and reported their own studies. They regarded the nodules as characteristic of rheumatic infection and, even in the absence of a rheumatic history, believed that the presence of Aschoff bodies signified a previous attack of rheumatism. The nodules were found in three cases of chorea, proving the close relation of this condition to rheumatism. Thalhimer and Rothschild found the nodules most often in the walls of the left ventricle; where infection antedated death by a long period, fresh Aschoff bodies were not always in evidence, but the healed remains represented by sclerotic patches were present. C. McEwen ("Cytological studies on rheumatic fever. I. The characteristic cell of the rheumatic granuloma," J. Exper. Med., **55**:745, 1932) later studied, by supravital stains, material aspirated from subcutaneous fibroid nodules. He concluded that the characteristic large cells "probably arise from the undifferentiated mesenchymal elements of loose connective tissue, although it is possible that endothelial cells take part in their formation in some instances. Since there is little doubt that the subcutaneous rheumatic nodules are pathologically identical with rheumatic granulomata elsewhere in the body, these conclusions are considered applicable also to the Aschoff body cells of the myocardial submiliary nodules." But the subject has continued in dispute, and recently G. E. Murphy ("Evidence that Aschoff bodies of rheumatic myocarditis develop from injured myofibers," J. Exper. Med. **95**:319, 1952) sustained the thesis that the essential lesion appeared to be "damaged muscle fibers, their fragments, and syncitial cell masses of probable muscular origin that proliferate from beneath the sarcolemma."

Other important general articles on the Aschoff body are those of W. C. von Glahn ("Auricular endocarditis of rheumatic origin," Am. J. Path., **2**:1, 1926) and of B. J. Clawson ("The Aschoff nodule," Arch. Path., **8**:664, 1929). The latter has an extensive review of the literature.

This may also be the appropriate spot to refer to the somewhat disputed subject of rheumatic arterial lesions (O. Klotz, "Arterial lesions associated with rheumatic fever," J. Path. & Bact., **18**:259, 1913; A. M. Pappenheimer and W. C. von Glahn, "Lesions of the aorta associated with acute rheumatic fever and with chronic cardiac disease of rheumatic origin," J.M. Res., **44**:489, 1924).

> 17. FABER, H. K. Experimental arthritis in the rabbit: a contribution to the pathogeny of arthritis in rheumatic fever, J. Exper. Med., **22**:615, 1915.

This time, as we have pointed out (Ref. 23), was the era of isolation of nonhemolytic streptococci from cases of rheumatic fever and the production of lesions in rabbits with them. Faber noted that in the literature, especially when strains of low virulence were used, there was a latent period between the injection of organisms and the occurrence of arthritis, or it might even be necessary to give more than one injection to produce disease. He therefore thought that perhaps the joint needed to be prepared, or "sensitized," by a preliminary contact with the antigen before an arthritic reaction could take place. He showed experimentally that streptococci of "low virulence were frequently not able to produce arthritis at the first attack but at this time prepare the way for such an effect in a later attack." It was found that the exciting injection must be the same as that used for the sensitizing injection and, furthermore, that the preparation might be made by the introduction directly into the joint of organisms living or dead. By intravenous inoculation, without previous sensitization, it was possible to cause arthritis in rabbits only after three or more injections. An analogy between these experiments and the relapses of human rheumatic fever was suggested, as well as a further analogy with the primary lesion in human rheumatic fever.

H. F. Swift and R. H. Boots ("The question of sensitization of joints with non-hemolytic streptococci," J. Exper. Med., **38**:573, 1923) did not, however, confirm Faber's work. They concluded that joints of rabbits first treated with streptococci "were no more liable to involvement than were other untreated joints of the same animals."

18. COHN, A. E., and SWIFT, H. F. Electrocardiographic evidence of myocardial involvement in rheumatic fever, J. Exper. Med., **39**:1, 1924.

Disturbance of cardiac mechanism, especially prolongation of conduction time, occurs so frequently in rheumatic fever that Jones (Ref. 14) sets it down as one of the minor diagnostic criteria. J. Parkinson, A. H. Gosse, and E. B. Gunson ("The heart and its rhythm in acute rheumatism," Quart. J. Med., **13**:363, 1919) reviewed the literature on disturbances of cardiac mechanism in rheumatic fever and reported observations on 50 cases of their own which were studied clinically and with polygraphic tracings. They described various disorders. But Cohn and Swift first dealt with the subject comprehensively with electrocardiographic studies. They found that "in one way or other the heart was affected in 35 of 37 cases of rheumatic fever." A-V block occurred in eight cases and was the most frequent disturbance next to premature auricular contractions. Such observations have now become standard practice in the study of acute rheumatic fever (L. A. Rantz, P. J. Boisvert, and W. W. Spink, "Hemolytic streptococcic sore throat: the poststreptococcic state," Arch. Int. Med., **79**:401, 1947).

19. SWIFT, H. F. The pathogenesis of rheumatic fever, J. Exper. Med., **39**:497, 1924.

Physicians had gradually recognized the association of a variety of apparently unrelated disturbances (Ref. 14) with classical acute articular rheumatism: endocarditis, pericarditis, myocarditis, chorea, subcutaneous fibroid nodules, and other lesions. Swift, in this important paper, brought out and pictured an identity of the underlying pathological changes in all these various manifestations. "The perivascular proliferative type of lesion, resembling an infectious granuloma, explains the subacute and chronic character of the clinical symptoms in many patients with this disease. Marked exudation of serum into the periarticular tissues and of serum and cells into the joint cavities are concomitants of the acute arthritis." A short while later there appeared the authoritative review of W. G. MacCallum ("Rheumatism," J.A.M.A., **84**:1545, 1925), with a brilliant description of the lesions, including the diffuse rheumatic changes in the left auricle to which he first drew attention ("Rheumatic lesions of the left auricle of the heart," Bull. Johns Hopkins Hosp., **35**:329, 1924). In 1940, Swift ("Rheumatic heart disease: pathogenesis and etiology in their relation to therapy and prophylaxis," Medicine, **19**:417, 1940) developed the whole subject further. Other comprehensive reviews of the pathological changes are those of B. Sacks ("Pathology of rheumatic fever: a critical review," Am. Heart J., **1**:750, 1926), of W. C. von Glahn ("The pathology of rheumatism," Am. J. Med., **2**:76, 1947), and of G. E. Murphy ("The histopathology of rheumatic fever: a critical review," in *Rheumatic Fever*, ed. L. Thomas [Minneapolis: University of Minnesota Press, 1952], p. 28). These articles have extensive bibliographies.

> 20. SWIFT, H. F. Rheumatic fever, J.A.M.A., **92**:2071, 1929.

In this masterly lecture Swift brings every phase of acute rheumatic fever—clinical variations, pathology, etiology—up to date. He touches on his own hypothesis of hypersensitivity to non-hemolytic streptococci.

> 21. PAUL, J. R. Pleural and pulmonary lesions in rheumatic fever, Medicine, **7**:383, 1928.

Paul reviews critically this whole somewhat confused and indefinite subject, and, more recently, E. E. Muirhead and A. E. Haley ("Rheumatic pneumonitis," Arch. Int. Med., **80**:328, 1947) again go over the question and report anatomical studies of their own.

> 22. COBURN, A. F. The factor of infection in the rheumatic state. Baltimore: Williams & Wilkins Co., 1931.

Modern views on rheumatic fever, at least in America, were much influenced by Coburn's book. Instead of a narrow concept of acute rheumatic fever, he looked on the disease from a wider aspect as "the rheumatic state." Thus under this head he included a great variety of manifestations, the significance of some of which was not generally recognized. While Coburn's spectrum is perhaps too broad, he deserves credit for expanding the older narrow limits of the disease. All sorts of material—environmental, bacteriological—are discussed in detail. Coburn also deserves credit for being one of the first to point the finger at the hemolytic streptococcus as a specific causal agent (see also Ref. 12).

But, as one goes back in the literature, one usually finds that things have been said before, and it must be stated that Coburn's views on the natural history of the disease were anticipated by Cheadle (Ref. 14), who actually used the term "the rheumatic state."

> 23. LICHTMAN, S. S. and GROSS, L. Streptococci in the blood in rheumatic fever, rheumatoid arthritis and other diseases: based on a study of 5,233 consecutive blood cultures, Arch. Int. Med., **49**:1078, 1932.

It was inevitable that, with the advent of the bacteriological era, a disease like rheumatic fever should be regarded as due to a living agent. The long series of reports of cultivation of various organisms from patients with rheumatic fever or at autopsy is thoroughly summarized by David and Robert Thomson ("An historical survey of researches on the role of the streptococci in acute articular rheumatism or rheumatic fever," Ann. Pickett-Thomson Res. Lab., 4:1, 1928), and only a few can be listed in this bibliography. Throughout the history of the subject, however, three errors constantly recur. First, undoubtedly there was often confusion between acute rheumatic fever and subacute bacterial endocarditis; streptococci isolated from cases of the latter condition were often assigned as the cause of rheumatic fever. Second, there was at the time no realization that non-hemolytic streptococci are basic members of the normal flora of the throat and bowel and that they may on occasion be isolated from the blood of healthy people. Third, it was not realized that any streptococcus injected intravenously into rabbits in adequate dosage may produce multiple lesions of joints and of endocardium. Observations of this sort were used as arguments that organisms isolated from patients were the cause of rheumatic fever. R. I. Cole ("Experimental streptococcus arthritis in relation to the etiology of acute articular rheumatism," J. Infect. Dis., 1:714, 1904) early pointed out the latter error. First, he reported his own work to the effect that, over a three-year period, cultures from blood and joint effusions in every case of rheumatic fever seen in the Johns Hopkins Hospital were sterile. He then injected into rabbits strains of streptococci from sources definitely not rheumatic and concluded: "Arthritis and endocarditis may be produced by the intravenous inoculation of rabbits with streptococci from various sources, and the results obtained are quite similar to those described as resulting from the inoculation of the so-called 'Micrococcus' or 'Diplococcus rheumaticus.' Therefore the description of a distinct variety or species of streptococci based on this property of causing endocarditis and arthritis [in rabbits], is unwarranted."

A few of the early bacteriological claims must, however, be listed because of their importance in the history of the subject. F. J. Poynton and A. Paine ("The etiology of rheumatic fever," Lancet, 2:861, 932, 1900) cultivated from blood and joints in eight cases of rheumatic fever a Gram-positive coccus with which they produced lesions in rabbits. This work drew wide attention and served for some years as a focal point for discussion of the etiology of rheumatic fever. Poynton and Paine finally embodied all their work in a volume entitled Researches on Rheumatism (London: J. & A. Churchill, Ltd., 1913). It is of interest that years later Poynton gave ground from his strong position, doubted that a streptococcus was the sole cause of rheumatic fever, and suggested looking elsewhere—for example, for a filter passer ("The prevention of acute rheumatism," Lancet, 2:1000, 1924). H. F. Swift and R. A. Kinsella ("Bacteriological studies in acute rheumatic fever," Arch. Int. Med., 19:381, 1917) were able to cultivate non-hemolytic streptococci from somewhat less than 10 per cent of typical cases of acute rheumatic fever. They concluded with the rather vague statement that "it seems evident that no type of streptococcus has been constantly associated with acute rheumatic fever." B. J. Clawson ("Studies on the etiology of acute rheumatic fever," J. Infect. Dis., 36:44, 1925), using large amounts of blood (50 cc.) for culture, isolated non-hemolytic streptococci from a considerable percentage of cases of acute rheumatic fever and produced lesions in rabbits. He erroneously thought that "rheumatic endocarditis and subacute bacterial endocarditis may be produced by the same agent and are but different degrees of the same process." Similarly, J. C. Small ("The bacterium causing rheumatic fever and a preliminary account of the therapeutic action of its specific antiserum," Am. J.M. Sc. **173**:101, 1927) described the isolation of "a serologically specific nonhemolytic streptococcus with distinctive biological characteristics" from blood and throats of patients with rheumatic fever; with this organism he produced the usual rabbit lesions. "We, therefore, have named this microorganism Streptococcus cardioarthritidis, and offer it upon the basis of these observations as the cause of rheumatic fever." Finally, R. L. Cecil, E. E. Nicholls, and W. J. Stainsby ("Bacteriology of the blood and joints in rheumatic fever," J. Exper. Med., **50**:617, 1929) were able to cultivate streptococci from the blood in the amazingly high figure of 83.9 per cent of cases. "These findings corroborate those of previous investigators and make it difficult to escape the conclusion that rheumatic fever is a streptococcal infection usually of the alpha or viridans type."

Interestingly enough, R. N. Nye and E. Waxelbaum ("Streptococci in infectious [atrophic] arthritis and rheumatic fever," J. Exper. Med., **52**:885, 1930), following Cecil, Nicholls, and Stainsby's technique with meticulous care, were unable to confirm their results.

On the other side of the argument, R. N. Nye and D. Seegal ("Non-hemolytic streptococci and acute rheumatic fever," J. Exper. Med., **49**:539, 1929) found that blood cultures from 25 cases of acute rheumatic fever were negative for non-hemolytic streptococci. They emphasized quite properly that non-hemolytic streptococci are invariably present in immeasurable numbers in the throats of all human beings and that their cultivation from the throats of rheumatic fever patients is meaningless. "The foregoing facts seem to invalidate the assumption that any of these non-hemolytic streptococci play a specific role in the etiology of acute rheumatic fever." Another blow was struck by L. Gross, L. Loewe, and B. Eliasoph ("Attempts to reproduce rheumatic fever in animals," J. Exper. Med., **50**:41, 1929), who claimed that streptococci isolated from rheumatic fever did not produce true lesions of the disease (Aschoff bodies) in rabbits. "Judged by these criteria, we have failed to reproduce the disease. This conclusion, we believer, holds true for all the work thus far reported in the literature." It remained for Lichtman and Gross, with a truly devastating attack, to demolish the theory that rheumatic fever was a direct infection with non-hemolytic streptococci. They began by listing 11 major fallacies in the previous work and concluded that "study of 5,233 consecutive blood cultures shows [that] . . . an incidence of non-hemolytic streptococcemia between 4 and 15.5 per cent occurs in at least 9 diseases," some of which, such as aplastic anemia, anemia, leukemia, and colitis, obviously had nothing to do with rheumatic fever. "On the basis of the incidence of the 'transient' streptococcemia alone, these organisms cannot justifiably be considered causative agents of these diseases."

Thus, at long last, the ghost of this controversy which had been waged for forty years was finally laid.

24. MYERS, W. K., and KEEFER, C. S. Antistreptolysin content of the blood serum in rheumatic fever and rheumatoid arthritis, J. Clin. Investigation, **13**:155, 1934.

Since hemolytic streptococcal throat infections were often found to precede bouts of acute rheumatic fever, it was natural to look for antibodies against streptococci or their products in the blood serum of patients. B. Schlesinger and

A. G. Signy ("Precipitin reactions in the blood of rheumatic patients following acute throat infections," Quart. J. Med., **2**:255, 1933), for example, studied precipitin reactions; and C. S. Keefer, W. K. Myers, and T. W. Oppel ("Streptococcal agglutinins in patients with rheumatoid [atrophic] arthritis and acute rheumatic fever," J. Clin. Investigation, **12**:267, 1933) measured agglutinins. The determination of antistreptolysin titer has remained the popular method, however, of investigating antibodies against hemolytic streptococcus. E. W. Todd ("Antihaemolysin titres in haemolytic streptococcal infections and their significance in rheumatic fever," Brit. J. Exper. Path., **13**:248, 1932) made early studies, as did A. F. Coburn and R. Pauli ("Studies on the relationship of Streptococcus hemolyticus to the rheumatic process. III. Observations on the immunological responses of rheumatic subjects to hemolytic streptococcus, J. Exper. Med., **56**:651, 1932). Both these groups of workers found increased titers of antistreptolysin during acute attacks of rheumatic fever. The observations of Myers and Keefer are, however, of special interest because of the large number of controls. Thus they found that the antistreptolysin serum levels of patients with rheumatic fever fell in the same range as those with overt hemolytic streptococcal infections, such as scarlet fever and erysipelas, and that these levels were often higher than ever attained in normal persons. However, many patients with rheumatic fever had titers not above those reached in normals. J. J. Bunim and C. McEwen ("The antistreptolysin titer in rheumatic fever, arthritis and other diseases," J. Clin. Investigation, **19**:75, 1940) found that the "incidence of elevated titers bore no relation to the various clinical manifestations of rheumatic infection," but those whose illness was preceded by a memorable upper respiratory infection showed a response more commonly than those without such a history.

Through the years stress has been placed on abnormally high titers as an indication of hemolytic streptococcal infection or of rheumatic fever in doubtful cases where there is no overt sore throat or positive culture for a hemolytic streptococcus. L. A. Rantz (*Rheumatic Fever* [Chicago: Year Book Publishers, Inc., 1954]) finds antistreptolysin measurements most useful for the exclusion of rheumatic fever: "It is evident that titers of 50 units or less are virtually incompatible with the early stages of rheumatic fever." Rantz and his group have reported other important studies on antistreptolysin (L. A. Rantz, M. Maroney, and J. M. Di Caprio, "Antistreptolysin 'O' response following hemolytic streptococcus infection in early childhood," Arch. Int. Med., **87**:360, 1951; L. A. Rantz, E. Randall, and H. H. Rantz, "Antistreptolysin 'O': a study of this antibody in health and in hemolytic streptococcus respiratory disease in man," Am. J. Med., **5**:3, 1948). Numerous other antistreptococcal antibodies have been studied to the same general effect, but their use has not yet become feasible in routine clinical work (L. A. Rantz, *The Prevention of Rheumatic Fever* [Springfield, Ill.: Charles C Thomas, 1952], pp. 16 ff.). The earlier work is also reviewed by Wilson (*Rheumatic Fever* [New York: Commonwealth Fund, 1940], pp. 96 ff.). Other serological tests, not including streptococcal antibodies, have been suggested. Their use is reviewed by M. McCarty ("Present status of diagnostic tests for rheumatic fever," Ann. Int. Med., **37**:1027, 1952). A penetrating analysis of this phase of the subject is also given by H. F. Swift ("The etiology of rheumatic fever," Ann. Int. Med., **31**:715, 1949), by R. A. Good ("Acute-phase reactions in rheumatic fever," in *Rheumatic Fever*, ed. L.

Thomas [Minneapolis: University of Minnesota Press, 1952], p. 115), and by M. McCarty ("The immune response in rheumatic fever [*ibid.*, p. 136]).

Recently, stress has been placed on tests which may reveal the "activity" of the rheumatic process. Such a test is the measurement of C-reactive protein in the blood. G. H. Stollerman, S. Glick, D. J. Patel, I. Hirschfeld, and J. H. Rusoff ("Determination of C-reactive protein in serum as a guide to the treatment and management of rheumatic fever," Am. J. Med., **15**:645, 1953) and R. J. Roantree and L. A. Rantz ("Clinical experience with the C-reactive protein test," Arch. Int. Med., **96**:674, 1955) attempt to evaluate this test, upon which the last word is not yet said. The subject is summarized editorially by J. J. Bunim ("Laboratory tests for rheumatic activity" [editorial], J. Chronic Dis., **3**:230, 1956).

25. COBURN, A. F., and MOORE, L. V. The prophylactic use of sulfanilamide in streptococcal respiratory infections, with special reference to rheumatic fever, J. Clin. Investigation, **18**:147, 1939.

Having found that sulfanilamide used prophylactically prevented the development of induced hemolytic streptococcal infections in guinea pigs, even though it did not cure them when established, it occurred to Coburn and Moore to see whether the drug had any prophylactic effect against rheumatic fever in children. Seventy-nine of eighty rheumatic children escaped "hemolytic streptococcal infection and signs of rheumatic activity" while under treatment. C. B. Thomas and R. France ("A preliminary report of the prophylactic use of sulfanilamide in patients susceptible to rheumatic fever," Bull. Johns Hopkins Hosp., **64**:67, 1939) and C. B. Thomas, R. France, and F. Reichsman ("The prophylactic use of sulfanilamide in patients susceptible to rheumatic fever," J.A.M.A., **116**:551, 1941) reported similar favorable results. No major rheumatic episodes occurred during the 79 person-seasons in the treated group, whereas there were 10 per cent recurrences in the controls. A. G. Kuttner and G. Reyersbach ("The prevention of streptococcal upper respirotory infections and rheumatic recurrences in rheumatic children by the prophylactic use of sulfanilamide," J. Clin. Investigation, **22**:77, 1943) strongly supported the above findings, as did R. H. Feldt ("Sulfanilamide as a prophylactic measure in recurrent rheumatic infection: a controlled study involving 131 'patient-seasons,'" Am. J.M. Sc., **207**:483, 1944). C. R. Messeloff and M. H. Robbins ("Prophylactic use of sulfonamides in children with rheumatic fever," J. Lab. & Clin. Med., **28**:1323, 1943), on the other hand, failed to find a significant difference between the test group and the controls. A. J. Morris, R. Chamovitz, F. J. Catanzaro, and C. H. Rammelkamp, Jr. ("Prevention of rheumatic fever by treatment of previous streptococcic infections: effect of sulfadiazine," J.A.M.A., **160**:114, 1956) found that the treatment of the acute sore throat with sulfadiazine neither eradicated the streptococcus nor prevented subsequent rheumatic fever. However, they regarded sulfonamides as of value in prophylaxis.

All this work has now become rather a dead issue because sulfonamides have been almost universally replaced by penicillin (Ref. 27), but it served to bring out a principle in the prophylaxis of rheumatic fever which is generally recognized as sound—the prevention of hemolytic streptococcus throat infections protects against the evidences of rheumatic fever, which so often follow such infection.

26. RICH, A. R., and GREGORY, J. E. Experimental evidence that lesions with the basic characteristics of rheumatic carditis can result from anaphylactic hypersensitivity, Bull. Johns Hopkins Hosp., **73**:239, 1943.

We have already referred to the concept of hypersensitivity in rheumatic fever (Ref. 12). The observations of Rich and Gregory seem, however, particularly striking: "The experimental procedure in this study has consisted in the sensitization of rabbits to sterile horse serum, under conditions that produce serum sickness." They picture beautiful lesions that "in their basic characteristics, resemble closely those of rheumatic carditis." In a further paper, Rich and Gregory ("Further experimental cardiac lesions of the rheumatic type produced by anaphylactic hypersensitivity," Bull. Johns Hopkins Hosp., **75**:115, 1944) show, side by side, experimental lesions and the lesions of human rheumatic carditis; they appear practically identical. S. D. Kobernick ("Experimental rheumatic carditis, periarteritis nodosa and glomerulonephritis," Am. J.M. Sc., **224**:329, 1952) gives a comprehensive review of the entire subject, with full bibliography.

27. MASSELL, B. F., DOW, J. W., and JONES, T. D. Orally administered penicillin in patients with rheumatic fever, J.A.M.A., **138**:1030, 1948.

The authors report pioneer observations of the effect of penicillin on hemolytic streptococcus carriage in the throat. Orally administered penicillin in doses of 300,000–1,000,000 units per day for 10 days suppressed hemolytic streptococci in the throats of all but 2.1 per cent of patients with rheumatic fever. Many papers soon followed, describing all sorts of permutations and combinations of methods of administration, dosage, and type of preparation of penicillin. Some of the important reports are the following: F. W. Denny, L. W. Wannamaker, W. R. Brink, C. H. Rammelkamp, Jr., and E. A. Custer, "Prevention of rheumatic fever," J.A.M.A., **143**:151, 1950; L. W. Wannamaker, C. H. Rammelkamp, Jr., F. W. Denny, W. R. Brink, H. B. Houser, E. O. Hahn, and J. H. Dingle, "Prophylaxis of acute rheumatic fever, by treatment of the preceding streptococcal infection with various amounts of depot penicillin," Am. J. Med., **10**:673, 1951; B. F. Massell, G. P. Sturgis, J. D. Knobloch, R. B. Streeper, T. N. Hall, and P. Norcross, "Prevention of rheumatic fever by prompt penicillin therapy of hemolytic streptococcic respiratory infections," J.A.M.A., **146**:1469, 1951; B. B. Breese, chairman, "Prevention of rheumatic fever," in *Modern Concepts of Cardiovascular Disease* (1953), Vol. **22**: No. 1; R. L. Chancey, A. J. Morris, R. H. Conner, F. J. Catanzaro, R. Chamovitz, and C. H. Rammelkamp, Jr., "Studies of streptococcal prophylaxis: comparison of oral penicillin and benzanthine penicillin," Am. J.M. Sc., **229**:165, 1955; and, finally, G. H. Stollerman, J. H. Rusoff, and I. Hirschfeld, "Prophylaxis against group A streptococci in rheumatic fever," New England J. Med., **252**:787, 1955. Stollerman observed no recurrences among 145 patients with rheumatic fever who received monthly injections of benzanthine penicillin during a 2-year period. As a result of all this work, the various heart associations are now urging that children who have had evidence of rheumatic fever receive penicillin prophylaxis over long periods. The final details of this procedure are not yet defined.

The whole subject of prevention of rheumatic fever is critically discussed in L. A. Rantz, *The Prevention of Rheumatic Fever* (Springfield, Ill.: Charles C Thomas, 1952).

28. MURPHY, G. E., and SWIFT, H. F. Induction of cardiac lesions, closely resembling those of rheumatic fever, in rabbits following repeated skin infections with group A streptococci, J. Exper. Med., **89**:687, 1949.

Although Faber's views (Ref. 17) demand some modification in the light of recent work, he deserves credit for opposing the idea that rheumatic fever was a simple direct infection with streptococci and for promoting the concept of altered reactivity (allergy) in the mechanism of production of the clinical phenomena of the disease.

We must now turn to the work of Swift, since it dominated the stage in America for many years. Swift, too, regarded hypersensitivity as implicit in the reaction of rheumatic fever and, with his associates, developed a hypothesis which they formulated as follows: "The theory is advanced that the pathogenesis of rheumatic fever can be explained by the existence in certain individuals of a condition of hypersensitiveness (allergy or hyperergy) to streptococci resulting from repeated low-grade infections or from the persistence of foci of infection in the body. When under suitable circumstances streptococci or products of streptococci are disseminated to the tissues these tissues over-react and the characteristic picture of the disease results" (H. F. Swift, C. L. Derick, and C. H. Hitchcock, "Rheumatic fever as a manifestation of hypersensitiveness [allergy or hyperergy] to streptococci," Tr. A. Am. Physicians, **43**:192, 1928). In another paper ("Bacterial allergy [hyperergy] to nonhemolytic streptococci, in its relation to rheumatic fever," J.A.M.A., **90**:906, 1928), these writers further set forth their hypothesis and express the feeling that reactions which have been ascribed to hemolytic streptococci were not obtained in their experiments.

It would serve no purpose to give in detail the analogies with syphilis and tuberculosis upon which Swift's hypothesis was based or to recite the experimental evidence with which Swift and his associates sought to support their views during the next decade. A list of the principal papers is as follows: C. L. Derick and H. F. Swift, "Reaction of rabbits to non-hemolytic streptococci. I. General tuberculin-like hypersensitiveness, allergy or hyperergy following the secondary reaction," J. Exper. Med., **49**:615, 1929; C. H. Hitchcock and H. F. Swift, "Studies on indifferent streptococci. III. The allergizing capacity of different strains," J. Exper. Med., **49**:637, 1929; H. F. Swift and C. L. Derick, "Reactions of rabbits to non-hemolytic streptococci. II. Skin reactions in intravenously immunized animals," J. Exper. Med., **49**:883, 1929; H. F. Swift, C. H. Hitchcock, C. L. Derick, and Currer McEwen, "Intravenous vaccination with streptococci in rheumatic fever," Am. J.M. Sc., **181**:1, 1931; C. L. Derick and M. N. Fulton, "Skin reactions of patients and normal individuals to protein extracts of streptococci," J. Clin. Investigation, **10**:121, 1931; M. P. Schultz and H. F. Swift, "Reactions of rabbits to streptococci: comparative sensitizing effect of intracutaneous and intravenous inocula in minute doses," J. Exper. Med., **55**:591, 1932.

The obvious error in interpretation of this work is that, while Swift and his associates clearly produced evidence of allergic reactions to non-hemolytic streptococci and their products, they did not produce rheumatic fever.

But, by 1940, Swift seemed to have modified his views on the relation of non-hemolytic streptococci to rheumatic fever ("Rheumatic heart disease: pathogenesis and etiology in their relation to therapy and prophylaxis," Medicine, **19**:417, 1940). He now inclined to the hemolytic streptococcus as the causal agent: "At present the hemolytic streptococcus seems to bear a more intimate relationship to the disease than any other known pathogenic agent." He referred to outbreaks of tonsillitis followed by rheumatic fever (Ref. 12). Later, Swift ("The relationship of streptococcal infections to rheumatic fever," Am. J. Med., **2**:168, 1947) spoke out even more strongly for hemolytic streptococcus on the basis of patients with scarlet fever who later developed evidence of rheumatic fever. The investigations of Swift culminated in his important work with Murphy. They found that rabbits, after sustaining two to ten infections with hemolytic streptococci of different serological types within 3–20 months, sickened and developed various symptoms. "In the hearts of the . . . infected rabbits . . . there have been found on microscopic examination focal alterations in the connective tissue framework in blood vessel adventitia, valves, mural endocardium, epicardium and in the myocardial interstitium." These and other lesions "closely resembling those found in rheumatic fever, have developed in rabbits that sickened following multiple successive skin infections with several serological types of Group A streptococci." The lesions are beautifully pictured. Finally, a most interesting report is that of R. J. Glaser, W. A. Thomas, S. J. Morse, and J. E. Darnell, Jr., "The incidence and pathogenesis of myocarditis in rabbits after group A streptococcal pharyngeal infections," J. Exper. Med., **103**:173, 1956. These workers devised a method of producing acute streptococcal pharyngeal infections in rabbits, which in many cases were followed by myocardial lesions thought to be typical of rheumatic fever. When intradermal infections with the same organism were produced, the lesions appeared in a much smaller number of animals.

29. HENCH, P. S., SLOCUMB, C. H., BARNES, A. R., SMITH, H. L., POLLEY, H. F., and KENDALL, E. C. The effects of the adrenal cortical hormone 17-hydroxy-11-dehydrocorticosterone (compound E) on acute phase of rheumatic fever: preliminary report, Proc. Staff. Meet. Mayo Clin., **24**:277, 1949.

Hench and his associates first observed that cortisone had favorable effects on rheumatic fever. This brief report was promptly followed by extensive use both of cortisone and of corticotropin (ACTH) in other cases of the disease. Within a year it was possible for B. F. Massell, J. E. Warren, G. P. Sturgis, B. Hall, and E. Craige ("The clinical response of rheumatic fever and acute carditis to ACTH," New England J. Med., **242**:641, 1950) to make an extensive report on the subject. In general, the results were favorable, although on long usage the untoward effects of adrenal steroids manifested themselves. Reports now came in rapidly; some of the important ones were the following: M. G. Wilson and H. N. Helper, "Effect of pituitary adrenocorticotropic hormone [ACTH] in acute rheumatic carditis," J.A.M.A., **145**:133, 1951; T. N. Harris, W. B. Abrams, T. F. P. Leo, and J. P. Hubbard, "Cortisone therapy in acute rheumatic carditis: preliminary observations," Circulation, **3**:215, 1951; A. G. Kuttner, J. S. Baldwin, C. McEwen, J. J. Bunim, M. Ziff, and D. K. Ford, "Effect of ACTH and cortisone on rheumatic carditis," J.A.M.A., **148**:628, 1952; and A. R. Barnes, "The effects of cortisone and ACTH on the acute phase of rheumatic fever," Circulation, **3**:770, 1951. A. Golden and J. W. Hurst ("Alterations of the lesions of acute rheumatic myocarditis during cortisone therapy," Circulation, **7**:218, 1953) reported the changes in the cardiac lesions of a patient dying with acute rheumatic heart disease treated with cortisone. An inhibition of the inflammatory reaction was found without demonstrable alteration of the collagen injury. So, too, L. M. Taran, G. A. Gulotta, N. Szilagyi, J. M. Jablon, and W. K. Lane ("Effect of cortisone and ACTH on the protracted phase of rheumatic carditis in children," Am. J. Med., **14**:275, 1953) found that the exudative manifestations responded readily so long as therapy was maintained but that there was no convincing indication of definite arrest of active carditis. B. F. Massell ("Medical progress: ACTH and cortisone therapy of rheumatic fever and rheumatic carditis," New England J. Med., **251**:183, 221, 263, 1954) carefully reviews the entire literature to date. He points out that the original hope of a total rapid cure of rheumatic fever by steroid therapy is not to be realized, whereas a suppression of various inflammatory components of the disease may be achieved—especially fever and polyarthritis. Finally, a report by the United Kingdom and United States co-operative group ("The treatment of acute rheumatic fever in children: a cooperative clinical trial of ACTH, cortisone, and aspirin," Circulation, **11**:343, 1955) concludes: "There was no evidence that any of the three agents resulted in uniform termination of the disease and on all treatments some patients developed fresh manifestations during treatment. . . . At the end of one year there was no significant difference between the three treatment groups in the status of the heart." The use of steroids is therefore (January, 1957) still *sub judice.*

30. PINNIGER, J. L. The left auricular appendage in mitral stenosis: a study of 15 cases submitted to valvulotomy, St. Thomas's Hosp. Rep., **7**: ser. 2, 54, 1951.

It had come to be generally accepted not only that the Aschoff body was evidence of the "rheumatic state" but that "fresh"-looking nodules indicated an "active" stage of the disease. With the development of mitral valvulotomy for mitral stenosis, there came into vogue the excision of the tip of the auricular appendage, partly for purposes of biopsy. Pinniger was the first to report examinations of auricular appendages removed at operation: "Aschoff node formation was present . . . in no fewer than 10 (65 per cent) of these cases. These findings give strong support to the view that activity of the rheumatic process persists in a high proportion of patients with clinically quiescent rheumatic valvular disease." A little later M. Kuschner, M. I. Ferrer, R. M. Harvey, and R. H. Wylie ("Rheumatic carditis in surgically removed auricular appendages," Am. Heart J., **43**:286, 1952), found Aschoff bodies in 4 of appendages excised in 11 patients who were clinically regarded as definitely inactive. D. Sabiston and R. H. Follis, Jr. ("Lesions in auricular appendages removed at operations for mitral stenosis of presumed rheumatic origin," Bull. Johns Hopkins Hosp., **91**:178, 1952) made similar studies of the material from Blalock's clinic and also found the histological changes of rheumatic fever in a number of cases. "Of particular significance would appear to be the discovery of such changes in patients who did not give a history of ever having had symptoms of a rheumatic episode." Similarly, J. P. Decker, C. Van Z. Hawn, and S. L. Robbins found Aschoff bodies in 83 of 183 excised auricular appendages ("Rheumatic 'activity' as judged by the presence of Aschoff bodies in auricular appendages of patients with mitral stenosis. I. Anatomic aspects," Circulation, **8**:161, 1953). Review of the clinical records of these patients by W. F. McNeely, L. B. Ellis, and D. E. Harken ("Rheumatic 'activity' as judged by the presence of Aschoff bodies in auricular appendages of patients with mitral stenosis. II. Clinical aspects," Circulation, **8**:337, 1953) showed no correlation between the presence of Aschoff bodies and the usual clinical or laboratory criteria of rheumatic activity. Finally, J. R. Gil, H. Rodriguez, and J. J. Ibarra ("Incidence of asymptomatic active rheumatic cardiac lesions in patients submitted to mitral commissurotomy and the effect of cortisone on these lesions," Am. Heart J., **50**:912, 1955) concluded from similar findings that "a large group (60 per cent) of patients submitted to commissurotomy show active but asymptomatic cardiac lesions."

But is there not another possible interpretation of all these findings? If Aschoff bodies are frequently found in patients with no evidence of rheumatic activity, are the nodules absolutely reliable evidence of such activity? This thought would seem to be supported by the observations of W. A. Thomas, J. H. Averill, B. Castleman, and E. F. Bland ("The significance of Aschoff bodies in the left atrial appendage," New England J. Med., **249**:761, 1953), who found that "the Aschoff lesions, and other histological changes in the atrial appendage of patients with fatal rheumatic fever are identical with those found in the surgical specimens from patients with mitral stenosis who show no recognizable clinical or laboratory signs of recent rheumatic activity," even though the authors themselves draw the opposite conclusion.

31. SOLOFF, L. A., ZATUCHNI, J., JANTON, O. H., O'NEILL, T. J. E., and GLOVER, R. P. Reactivation of rheumatic fever following mitral commissurotomy, Circulation, **8**:481, 1953.

The writers give a systematic description of the "postcommissurotomy" syndrome. The syndrome occurred in 24 per cent of 179 consecutive persons subjected to the operation. It is characterized by precordial pain and by fever, is frequently associated with the precipitation or intensification of heart failure, and is at times accompanied by migratory joint pains, arrhythmias, hemoptysis, or psychosis and sometimes terminates in death. The writers give arguments in favor of this syndrome being rheumatic activation and speculate as to the exact mechanism of action.

MENINGOCOCCAL INFECTION

Antibiotic therapy	Refs. 31, 32
Bacteriology	Refs. 9, 11, 12, 19
Carriers of meningococci	Refs. 15, 16, 19, 26
Chemotherapy	Refs. 29, 30
Clinical	Refs. 1, 2, 3, 4, 5, 13
Epidemics	Refs. 8, 19
General	Refs. 23, 25, 27
Kernig's sign	Ref. 7
Meningococcus bacteremia	Refs. 14, 20
Meningococcus types	Refs. 22, 24
Nasopharyngitis	Ref. 6
Pathology	Refs. 1, 2, 3, 4, 5
Serum therapy	Refs. 17, 18, 21, 28

MENINGOCOCCAL INFECTION

THE situation as regards meningococcal infection is confused by the great variety of syndromes caused by the meningococcus—epidemic meningitis, sporadic meningitis, chronic meningococcus sepsis without meningitis, acute meningococcal bacteremia without meningitis—the unity of which was not suspected until isolation and identification of the organism were possible. We have found no comprehensive modern bibliography of the subject. The early literature is largely concerned with the descriptions of epidemics; it is thoroughly reviewed and documented by Hirsch (Ref. 8). Good general bibliographies are to be found in Foster and Gaskell's book (Ref. 25) and in the treatise of C. Worster-Drought and Alexander Mills Kennedy, *Cerebro-spinal Fever* (London: A. & C. Black, Ltd., 1919).

1. VIEUSSEUX. Mémoire sur la maladie qui régné à Genève au printemps de 1805, J. méd. chir. et pharm., Paris, **11**:163, 1806.

The outbreak at Geneva in 1805 described by Vieusseux is generally taken as the starting point of the modern study of epidemic meningitis. As here described, one was dealing with a new and violent disease of high mortality, featured by sudden prostration or collapse, intense headache, vomiting, at times convulsions, rapid feeble pulse, and often death in a few hours. Most of those who survived several days recovered. There is no clear description of petechial spots during life or of stiff neck or opisthotonos. At autopsy one saw only a congestion and reddening of the meninges. Vieusseux regarded this disease as definite and distinct from other fevers and named it "malignant non-contagious cerebral fever." In one family four children were rapidly stricken, and all died. Tartar emetic was thought to be the best remedy.

One would not be absolutely certain of the nature of this disease, however, were it not for the autopsy reports of Matthey (A. Matthey, "Recherches sur une maladie particulière qui a régné à Genève en 1805," J. méd. chir. et pharm., Paris, **11**:243, 1806). "The vessels of the meninges were greatly injected. A gelatinous 'humor,' colored by blood was spread over the entire surface of the brain. Over the posterior part of the lobes of the brain and in the interior one saw a yellowish, puriform matter without manifest alteration of the cerebral tissue" (p. 246). "The nervous system seems strongly and directly attacked, for all the symptoms proclaim a brain lesion. One sees the bloody engorgement, the lymphatic and puriform effusions which explain the inefficiency of the methods which are tried to prevent or dissipate them" (p. 249).

2. NORTH, E. A treatise on a malignant epidemic commonly called spotted fever. New York: T. & F. Swords, 1811.

"It is between four and five years since a new and singular disease, which has obtained the name of Spotted Fever first appeared in Medfield, in Massachusetts," says North in his Preface (p. vii). "Since this time it has prevailed as an epidemic and has proved a most tremendous plague in a considerable number of towns in this state, in Massachusetts, in Rhode-Island, in the state of

New-York, in Vermont, and elsewhere sweeping off great numbers of inhabitants. No regular treatise, calculated to give the public an entire view of this disease, has hitherto been published" (p. vii).

"Whether the spotted fever may be considered as only a variety of cynanche maligna or scarlatina, and be arranged under the order *phlegmasia* or *exanthemata;* or whether it ought to be regarded as only a variety of the malignant petechial fever of authors; or whether it is a new species of disease, to be added to the list of human calamities, is yet to be determined" (p. 6).

The disease frequently occurred in a very violent form; the descriptions resemble those of the bacteremic cases seen in World War I (Ref. 14). North mentions in his description "a great surprising sudden loss of strength," "violent pain of the head and many times of the limbs," "syncope," "coma," "mania," "delirium," and "petechiae" (pp. 10–12). "So frequent indeed was this species of hemorrhage during the first season in which the disease prevailed, that it was considered as one of its most striking characteristics, and gave rise to the name *petechial* or *spotted fever,* which has been very generally, though very improperly, applied to the disease. In size they [the spots] were various, commonly the head of a pin and a six cent bit would mark the two extremes" (p. 13). Under Section III (p. 15), "On the More Unusual Symptoms of the Fever," it is stated: "These are a dilatation, and, in some, a contraction of the pupils of the eyes, redness and suffusion of the eyes; blindness in some, in others double or treble vision; a drawing back of the head, with a kind of clonic spasm of the muscles of the neck." It seems clear that these cases which correspond more with the present-day sporadic type were relatively less common than the hyperacute (bacteremic?) form. As to the cause, North is straight eighteenth century: "The spotted fever is asthenic in its nature. Hence the remote and predisponent causes must be such as debilitate the system" (p. 25). There is no suggestion of contagion. The long section on treatment is hardly worthy of review; North leans heavily on Sydenham and on Huxham.

Indeed, it would be difficult to be sure of the nature of this disease, were there not appended autopsy notes of two cases by Drs. L. Danielson and E. Mann: "The second examination was made twelve hours after death, on the body of a girl of five years old, of the same family. Between the dura and the pia mater was effused a fluid resembling pus" (p. 95).

The last half of the book is of special interest; it consists of letters from physicians, copies of reports of cases, and other material dealing with the epidemic.

A great problem in the bibliography of cerebrospinal meningitis is the fact that for nearly a century the only recognized form was the epidemic. Most of the outbreaks occurred in small towns, in garrisons, or in other odd places and were described by local doctors with inadequate documentation and usually in obscure or inaccessible medical journals. Two examples are *An Inquiry into the Nature and Treatment of the Prevailing Epidemic Called Spotted Fever,* by Job Wilson, M.D. (Boston: Bradford & Read, 1815), and *A History and Description of an Epidemic Fever Commonly Called Spotted Fever,* by E. Hale, Jr., M.D. (Boston: Wells & Lilly, 1818). Little was added, therefore, to the knowledge of the disease until the discovery of the causal organism (Ref. 9). As to sporadic cases, one searches in vain through the older treatises for anything definite. Without bacteriological study and without lumbar puncture, everything was in confusion, and whether the case was one of tuberculous meningitis, of pyogenic meningitis, or of meningococcus meningitis cannot be told. In Andral's great collection, for example (G. Andral, *Clinique médicale ou choix d'observations recueillies à l'Hôpital de la Charité* [Paris: Fortier, Masson et Cie, 1840] one finds (**5**:65, 17th observation) a report of a case of "intense headache at start, with vomiting. Tendency to sleepiness and immobility. Gradual development of coma, more and more profound." At autopsy, "purulent infiltration of the pia mater at the base of the brain and cerebellum." Whether this was meningococcus meningitis one cannot, of course, say. The various epidemics are, however, listed in Hirsch (Ref. 8).

3. BROUSSAIS, C. Histoire des méningites cérébro-spinales. Paris: Moquet & Hanquelon, 1845.

During the years preceding this book there had been numerous and severe outbreaks of epidemic meningitis in troops in garrisons all over France. The explanation of this distribution of the disease, now well understood (Ref. 26), was a cause of great perplexity to contemporary observers. At any rate, the army doctors rendered reports of various local outbreaks, and Broussais abstracted and condensed them in his book, the special virtue of which is the numerous careful case reports with autopsy studies. Broussais clearly defined the disease. Aside from the excellent descriptions, however, there is little of value. Broussais missed his chance of making a fundamental epidemiological observation. "Do the migrations of the various regiments from one part of France to another account for the propagation of the epidemic?" he says (p. 14) and then adds, "We shall see that it is impossible to accept this explanation."

4. NIEMEYER, F. Die epidemische Cerebro-spinal-Meningitis. Berlin: August Hirschwald, 1865.

Niemeyer's monograph was based mostly on personal observations of epidemics in Freiburg, Karlsruhe, and Rastat. Epidemic meningitis had long been thought, especially by the French, to be a variant of typhus, typhoid, or some sort of "spotted" fever. Niemeyer took issue with this point of view. He insisted that the important symptoms all pertained to intracranial disease and that, when convalescence was delayed, "it depends in unmistakable fashion wholly on the residuals of the meningitis" (p. 9). This is all confirmed at autopsy, where the only significant change is "a widespread inflammation of the coverings of the brain and spinal cord" (p. 10). Furthermore, "the changes in the brain coverings in epidemic meningitis are exactly the same as those found in the sporadic form" (p. 10). There are no significant changes in the lymph glands or spleen. Niemeyer was, however, not sure that the disease was an infection, and he was willing to admit that atmospheric or telluric causes might be at fault, although he declined to rule out the probability of infection, mainly on epidemiological grounds. He evidently saw no fulminating hyperacute cases such as those described by the Americans (Ref. 5).

The introductory chapter is followed by a detailed description of the pathological anatomy based on fifteen cases. Under symptoms are listed severe headache, pains in the neck and back, stiffness of neck, pains in the extremities, hyperesthesia, tetanic cramps in the neck and back muscles, convulsions, cranial nerve and other palsies, psychic disturbances, deafness, ptosis, diplopia, pupillary disturbances, inflammatory exudate in joints, fever, etc. He concludes this section with the following dicta: "All symptoms observed in the course of epidemic cerebrospinal meningitis are clearly accounted for by the purulent inflammation of the pia of the brain and cord" (p. 67). Of those affected, 69.9 per cent died; some of the survivors were deaf or had visual disturbances. "The treatment consisted mainly in the energetic use of cold in the form of ice packs to the head, leeches behind the ears and calomel internally" (p. 71).

The monograph of Mannkopff (*Ueber Meningitis cerebrospinalis epidemica* [Braunschweig: Friedrich Viewig & Sohn, 1866]) is noteworthy because of its excellent historical introduction; brilliant and detailed clinical account, including that of opisthotonus; and complete pathological description. There is a long philosophical discussion of the etiology and nature of the disease which leads to nothing definite.

5. STILLÉ, A. On the proper designation of the present epidemic (cerebrospinal meningitis), Am. J.M. Sc., **49**:121, 1865.

The extensive recrudescence of epidemic meningitis during the preceding ten years had stimulated an immense amount of discussion as to the nature of the disease and how to classify it. The American journals are full of brief articles reporting a few cases, usually without autopsy. Stillé gives a critical discussion of the whole subject which throws important light on contemporary views. He points out that, although the disease was first named "spotted fever," even in the early descriptions skin hemorrhages were by no means constantly present; he makes a plea for the designation "cerebrospinal meningitis." He then points out the confusion which has arisen with typhus. This was evidently due to the occurrence of very acute cases (probably with bacteremia) in which, at autopsy, when the skull was opened, bloody serum gushed out but no actual pus. In patients who lived longer, however, with a less fulminating disease, when the pia was opened frank pus was found. Stillé did useful work in tracing this spectrum. J. A. Lidell ("On epidemic cerebro-spinal meningitis or spotted fever, with cases," Am. J.M. Sc., **49**:17, 1865) reports patients who died in a day or two after onset. "While sawing off the calvarium and subsequently removing the brain, a *large quantity of serum* coloured with blood flowed away." W. H. Draper ("Cerebro-spinal meningitis, or spotted fever," Am. M. Times, **9**:99, 111, 1864) described cases he had seen "with terrible fatality at Carbondale, in the coal regions of Pennsylvania." "Many cases terminated within 12 hours." "In cases which are rapidly fatal, the lesion consists simply in an intense engorgement of the sinuses, veins, and minute vessels of the pia mater, with varying amounts of serous subarachnoid and ventricular effusion. In more protracted cases . . . the arachnoid is lifted, and the surface of the brain obscured by a layer of consistent greenish pus. . . . These inflammatory exudations are sometimes confined to the surface of the convolutions, sometimes to the base of the brain, and in many instances are found in both localities." The very high mortality—in some outbreaks nearly 100 per cent—was stressed and the futility of known therapy emphasized. In the discussion on etiology Draper stated: "The question of contagion in this malady is one of great interest and importance. Most authorities agree that it is non-contagious. This, I believe, is the conclusion, without exception of all observers of the disease in this country." Stillé also embodied his ideas in a book, *Epidemic Meningitis, or Cerebrospinal Meningitis* (Philadelphia: Lindsay & Blakiston, 1867).

6. STRÜMPELL, A. Zur Pathologie und pathologischen Anatomie der epidemischen Cerebrospinal-Meningitis, Deutsches Arch. f. klin. Med., **30**:500, 1882.

Important clinical and pathological observations on epidemic meningitis. Strümpell quotes a finding of Professor Weigert of "an intensive purulent inflammation of the superior nasopharynx. This stimulated the thought that the inflammation in the nasopharynx could furnish a starting point for the investigation of the manner in which the infectious material of epidemic meningitis enters the body, especially the areas apparently so shut off as the brain and spinal cord." To this observation many later German writers trace the doctrine of the nasopharynx as portal of entry for the meningococcus.

7. KERNIG, W. Ueber ein wenig bemerktes Meningitis Symptom, Berl. klin. Wchnschr., **21**:829, 1884 (original: Vrach, St. Petersburg, **5**:427, 446, 1884).

Kernig describes his well-known sign, emphasizing its occurrence in epidemic meningitis. With the leg flexed at the hip, it is mechanically impossible to extend the knee (*Beugestarre*).

8. HIRSCH, A. Handbuch der historisch-geographischen Pathologie, **3**:379. 2d ed. Stuttgart: Ferdinand Enke, 1886. (English translation by Charles Creighton [London: New Sydenham Society, 1886], **3**:547.)

A detailed, extremely well-documented account of the innumerable epidemics of "meningitis cerebro-spinalis epidemica," which, first described in Geneva in 1805 (Ref. 1), occurred with increasing frequency throughout Europe and the United States. Even as late as 1886 the disease was thought of as essentially epidemic, and Hirsch made no particular mention of sporadic cases. He noted that some epidemics were largely confined to children; he also pointed out the frequency of epidemics in soldiers in barracks, the explanation of which is now, of course, clear (Ref. 26); writing at the beginning of the bacteriological era, Hirsch questioned the claims of various bacteriologists (Ref. 9) and concluded that the virus was unknown and the disease "not contagious but transportable."

9. WEICHSELBAUM, A. Ueber die Ätiologie der akuten Meningitis cerebro-spinalis, Fortschr. d. Med., **5**:573, 1887.

The paper is a model of precise work. It was based on post-mortem examination of six instances of cerebrospinal meningitis in which Weichselbaum found "an entirely different kind of bacteria" than the pneumococci and miscellaneous organisms which were recovered from most sporadic cases of meningitis. In the first case there were found in the meningitis exudate and in the ventricular fluid in cover-slip preparations a moderate number of cocci, usually arranged in pairs, with the side toward each other flattened so that each coccus represented a half-sphere. "They lie either free between the pus cells or inside them where they are present in considerable numbers and remind one of gonococci." Similar organisms were seen in all the other five cases. Weichselbaum was able to cultivate them on agar; the growth was fairly delicate, and transfer through many generations was difficult. They appeared in smears of cultures in pairs, tetrads, or small clumps. Some diplococci were larger than other cells. They were stained well with methylene blue and were decolorized by Gram's method. They were abundant in sections through the meninges. "Because of its characteristic form, I will designate this variety of coccus as Diplococcus intracellularis meningitidis." Weichselbaum did not isolate the organism during life; this was first done by Heubner (Ref. 12). Injections of culture in rather large quantities killed mice, guinea pigs, rabbits, and dogs with various lesions and organisms in the blood stream. Weichselbaum suggested the paranasal sinuses or the middle ear as the portal of entry in human cases. Interestingly enough, Weichselbaum discussed his organisms simply as a cause of one group of meningitis cases; he said nothing about having discovered the cause of epidemic meningitis.

10. JAEGER, H. Die Transportmittel gewisser Infectionsstoffe und Vorschläge zur Vernichtung derselben am Krankenbette, im Haushalt im Verkehr, Deutsche med. Wchnschr., **20**:409, 1894.

The German ministry of health as early as 1888 ("Erlass des kgl. Ministers der 2 Cl. Medizinal-Angelegenheiten, die epidemische Genickstarre [Meningitis cerebrospinalis] betreffend," Veröffentl. d. k. Gsndhtsamte, **12**:751, 1888) laid down rules for the isolation and handling of cases of meningitis based on the conviction that the disease was "communicable and contagious." The disease was made reportable; the patients were to be isolated; the room and its contents, especially handkerchiefs, were to be cleaned and disinfected.

Jaeger reached the conclusion that the portal of entry for epidemic meningitis was from the nose through the lamina cribrosa to the meninges. He therefore examined nasal secretions and in four of five cases found "unequivocal" meningococci, and from contaminated handkerchiefs he grew the organism in pure culture. No meningococci were recovered from the secretions of eight healthy people.

This appears to be the first study of meningococcus carriers, assuming, which seems to us very doubtful, that the organisms were meningococci and not *Micrococcus catarrhalis*.

11. JAEGER, H. Zur Ätiologie der Meningitis cerebrospinalis epidemica, Ztschr. f. Hyg. u. Infectionskr., **19**:351, 1895.

Weichselbaum described his cocci in sporadic cases of meningitis which were difficult to distinguish from those due to various other organisms, especially pneumococcus. He was not too emphatic in his claims, especially as he was unable to produce the typical disease in animals. Otto Leichtenstern ("Ueber Meningitis cerebro-spinalis epidemica," Deutsche med. Wchnschr., **11**:391, 537, 1885) had already found organisms, which seemed partly to meet Weichselbaum's description, in several cases of meningitis; and F. Goldschmidt ("Zur Aetiologie der Meningitis cerebrospinalis," Centralbl. f. Bakt., **2**:649, 1887) reported similar confirmatory findings. Nonetheless, the matter remained in dispute, and little more work was done for a number of years. Jaeger studied an outbreak of definite epidemic meningitis and uniformly isolated from the meninges of fatal cases an organism which he regarded as that of Weichselbaum. He also found it in sections of tissues and grew it in culture. As to animal inoculation, he found, as did Weichselbaum, that subcutaneous injection was totally ineffective. He concluded that the meningococcus was a different organism from the pneumococcus, of which not everyone had as yet been convinced, and he definitely insisted that the organism of Weichselbaum was the significant finding in epidemic meningitis.

However, there were several odd points in the findings of Jaeger. His organisms did not always decolorize with the Gram stain; they sometimes occurred in chains; and they could be isolated from dried nasal secretions. What was Jaeger actually dealing with? At any rate, it remained for H. Albrecht and A. Ghon ("Ueber die Aetiologie und pathologische Anatomie der Meningitis cerebrospinalis epidemica," Wien. klin. Wchnschr., **14**: 984, 1901) to give a complete and critical analysis of the literature to date, as well as observations of their own, and to settle definitely that the cause of epidemic meningitis was the organism of Weichselbaum, to explain that it was always Gram-negative, always fragile and difficult to cultivate, and essentially non-pathogenic for small animals. The findings reported by others of Gram-positive forms, or organisms resembling pneumococci, of readily cultivable organisms were clearly either contaminations or mixed infections. This paper is definitive and settled for all time a much-vexed question. Albrecht and Ghon were also among the first definitely to isolate true meningococci from the nasopharynx.

12. HEUBNER, O. Beobachtungen und Versuche über den Meningokoccus intracellularis (Weichselbaum-Jaeger), Jahrb. f. Kinderh., **43**:1, 1896.

Heubner was the first, by means of lumbar puncture, to recover Meningococcus from the spinal fluid during life. He found typical "biscuit-shaped" diplococci in pus cells; they are also described as like a pair of coffee beans side by side. He injected pus containing meningococci intraspinally into goats and produced definite meningitis. He grew the organism in pure culture. He emphasized the value of spinal puncture in clinical practice in differentiating various forms of meningitis, although others, such as Lichtheim ("Zur Diagnose der Meningitis," Berl. klin. Wchnschr., **32**:269, 1895), had already dealt with the general subject following Quincke's introduction of lumbar puncture and detailed description of the technique (H. Quincke, "Ueber Hydrocephalus," *Verhandl. d. Kong. f. inn. Med.* [Wiesbaden: J. F. Bergman, 1891], **10**:321).

13. COUNCILMAN, W. T., MALLORY, F. B., and WRIGHT, J. H. Epidemic cerebro-spinal meningitis and its relation to other forms of meningitis: a report of the State Board of Health of Massachusetts. Boston: Wright & Potter, 1898.

A comprehensive summary of all phases of the disease, supplemented by the authors' own early observations, in which they confirmed the work of Weichselbaum (Ref. 9). There is an excellent historical section.

14. OSLER, W. The arthritis of cerebro-spinal fever, Boston M. & S.J., **139**:641, 1898.

In the course of a report of a case of epidemic meningitis with inflammation of the joints and other evidence of sepsis, Osler stated that meningococcus was isolated from the blood during life. N. B. Gwyn ("A case of general infection by the Diplococcus intracellularis of Weichselbaum," Bull. Johns Hopkins Hosp., **10**:112, 1899) reported on the bacteriology of the patient. Two blood cultures were positive for meningococcus. "This is believed to be the first instance recorded in which general infection, or septicemia has been demonstrated in this disease." H. Cochez and Lemaire ("Relation de l'épidémie de méningite cérébrospinale à Alger et dans les environs," Arch. gén. de méd., **189**:574, 1902) were able to grow meningococci from the blood of two patients with meningitis who recovered.

H. Salomon ("Ueber Meningococcenseptikämie," Berl. klin. Wchnschr., **39**:1045, 1902) describes a patient who obviously had a septic fever with purpura (spotted fever) from whose blood meningococcus was recovered. Irregular septic fever continued, however, for several months, with repeated isolation of meningococcus from the blood. Eventually, the patient developed signs of meningitis, but recovered. "For two months the meningococcus circulated in the blood while we waited from day to day for meningitis to appear. But finally it found its accustomed localization in the intracranial space." This, of course, is a classical case of chronic meningococcus sepsis. However, meningococci were soon isolated from the blood in regular cases of meningitis, as, for example, that of A. Marcovich ("Meningococcen im kreisenden Blute," Wien, klin. Wchnschr., **19**:1312, 1906), who reviewed the early literature.

Meanwhile, F. W. Andrewes ("A case of acute meningococcal septicemia," Lancet, **1**:1172, 1906) described a patient in collapse, covered with purpura, from whose blood meningococci were grown and in whose blood meningococci were seen *intra vitam* within the leukocytes. At autopsy there were hemorrhages everywhere and "both suprarenals were in an intensely hemorrhagic condition, dark purple in color, swollen, and contrasting strongly with the kidneys which were but slightly congested"; the case was obviously one of the Waterhouse-Friederichsen syndrome.[1]

Elser and Huntoon ("Studies on meningitis," J.M. Research, **20**:377, 1909) isolated meningococci from the blood in eleven of forty-one cases of meningitis. They thought that the organism first gained access to the blood and secondarily localized in the meninges. The idea of a preliminary bacteremic stage in epidemic meningitis was strongly emphasized by W. W. Herrick ("The intravenous serum treatment of epidemic cerebrospinal meningitis," Arch. Int. Med., **21**:541, 1918). He recognized, in an epidemic in an army camp, "primary meningococcus sepsis in almost half of the cases before the characteristic selective action on the meninges has been exerted," and he advocated brisk use of serum intravenously as well as intraspinally.

[1] Thus Andrewes antedated Waterhouse' case by five years (R. Waterhouse, "A case of suprarenal apoplexy," Lancet, **1**:577, 1911). It is of interest that in the report of the pathologist in the Middlesex Hospital Reports for 1894, there is a pathological report (p. 279) of a case with profuse purpura and bilateral hemorrhages into the suprarenal capsules. The modern literature is reviewed by L. D. Weinstein and T. H. McGavack, "The Waterhouse-Friederichsen syndrome," New England J. Med., **232**:95, 1945.

Thus all types of meningococcus infection are illustrated, and with any there may be a bacteremia.

15. GOODWIN, M. E., and VON SHOLLY, A. L. The frequent occurrence of meningococci in the nasal cavities of meningitis patients and of those in direct contact with them, J. Infect. Dis., Suppl. 2, p. 21, 1906.

The writers review the earlier papers in which meningococci were claimed to have been isolated from the nasal sinuses or nasopharynx. They conclude that the cultures of only fourteen cases in the literature were studied with sufficient care to warrant their acceptance as true meningococci, and they point out that meningococci are easily confused with other Gram-negative organisms of the catarrhalis group. A. Ghon and H. Pfeiffer ("Der Micrococcus catarrhalis [R. Pfeiffer] als Krankheitserreger," Ztschr. f. klin. Med., 44:262, 1902) give a detailed discussion of this group, point out their frequent occurrence in the upper air passages, and discuss the differentiation of them from gonococci and meningococci. They emphasize the coarse opaque colonies with ragged edges and the spontaneous agglutinability. Although they were not clear that catarrhalis was a member of the normal basic flora of the upper air passages, they assigned it a very subordinate role in disease. H. Jaeger ("Die specifische Agglutination der Meningococcen als Hilfsmittel in ihrer Artbestimmung und zur bacteriologischen Diagnose der epidemischen Genickstarre," Ztschr. f. Hyg. u. Infectionskr., 44:223, 1903) prepared immune sera in rabbits with meningococci and with these was able to recognize specifically other strains and, in general, emphasized the value of the procedure. *Micrococcus catarrhalis* uniformly failed to agglutinate in these sera. Goodwin and von Sholly made nasal cultures with the greatest care. Meningococci were isolated from seventeen of thirty-seven patients with meningitis when culture was made during the first 2 weeks of the disease, whereas meningococci were also isolated in five of forty-five healthy persons living in close contact with meningitis patients. The organisms were identified by careful morphological and cultural criteria and by agglutination tests. Goodwin and von Sholly concluded: "Meningococci were isolated from nasal mucus of 50 per cent of meningitis patients and from about 10 per cent of the people in closest contact with them. They were frequently present in enormous numbers. The finding of meningococci in great numbers in the nasal mucus of such a large proportion of the patients and of those caring for them, and the absence of meningococci from the nasal mucus of a large number of normal persons examined would strongly indicate the necessity of isolating cases of cerebro-spinal meningitis," a conclusion reached by the Germans as early as 1888 (Ref. 10).

16. KUTSCHER, K. Ueber Untersuchungen der Nasenrachenhöhle gesunder Menschen auf Meningococcen, Deutsche med. Wchnschr., 32:1071, 1906.

It was already common knowledge that meningococci are frequently found in the nasopharynx of patients with meningitis and of contacts. Kutscher made cultures from healthy people who had no known contact with meningitis patients at a time when no clinical cases existed. In fifty-six people he isolated meningococci four times; all were agglutinated by specific sera in a titer of

1:500 to 1:1,000. The source of these organisms and the epidemiological implications are discussed. Similar findings have since been obtained innumerable times by others.

17. JOCHMANN, G. Versuche zur Serodiagnostik und Serotherapie der epidemischen Genickstarre, Deutsche med. Wchnschr., **32**:788, 1906. It occurred to Jochmann to try to prepare a potent antimeningococcus serum as a therapeutic agent and also for diagnostic purposes, especially to separate true meningococci from other Gram-negative cocci. He immunized a horse first with dead and then with living culture; the serum attained a titer of 1:1,500. The serum specifically agglutinated true meningococci, as Jaeger found (Ref. 11); Jochmann soon discovered that a considerable number of healthy people in the vicinity of an epidemic harbored meningococci in the nasopharynx, as Goodwin and von Sholly had found (Ref. 15). *Micrococcus catarrhalis* was not agglutinated. Jochmann laid the ghost of widespread claims that there were Gram-positive varieties of meningococci by showing that specifically agglutinable strains were always Gram-negative. He also stressed the fact that his serum was polyvalent. The serum protected mice and guinea pigs against intraperitoneal injection of meningococci. Jochmann then treated some forty human cases, first with subcutaneous injection and later with intraspinal serum. Some of the patients seemed to be helped, but Jochmann concluded with the greatest conservatism that the serum at least did no harm. These observations opened the long era of serotherapy of epidemic meningitis, which did not end until about 1940. Kolle and Wassermann ("Versuche zur Gewinnung und Wertbestimmung eines Meningococcenserum," Deutsche med. Wchnschr., **32**:609, 1906) also did important early work on preparing an immune serum.

18. FLEXNER, S. Concerning a serum therapy for experimental infection with *Diplococcus intracellularis*, J. Exper. Med., **9**:168, 1907.

Flexner's interest in meningitis began in connection with the New York epidemic of 1904–5. His first paper (S. Flexner, "Contributions to the biology of *Diplococcus intracellularis*," J. Exper. Med., **9**:105, 1907) dealt with the cultural and other biological characteristics of meningococcus. Although Annibal Bettencourt and Carlos França ("Ueber die Meningitis cerebrospinalis epidemica und ihren specifischen Erreger," Ztschr. f. Hyg. u. Infectionskr., **46**:463, 1904) had failed to produce experimental meningitis in various animals, including monkeys, Flexner ("Experimental meningitis in monkeys," J. Exper. Med., **9**:142, 1907) attempted again to produce the disease by lumbar puncture. He used huge quantities of bacteria. The animals usually died in a few hours or recovered promptly. In the fatal cases "meningitis" was found, but the organisms tended to die out quickly, and it is doubtful whether Flexner produced a condition really analogous to the human disease. From this point he went on to treat the experimental disease with immune serum. "In summarizing these experiments, it may be said that by employment of an homologous antidiplococcus serum several monkeys were saved from death due to experimental infection with Diplococcus intracellularis. The monkeys could, by simultaneous injection of serum and culture be prevented from developing severe symptoms." However, Flexner found "a certain definite protective value" in normal monkey serum also. Flexner suggested the possibility of developing "more active antisera" for use in human meningitis.

A preliminary report of all the above work appeared in August, 1906 (S. Flexner, "Experimental cerebrospinal meningitis and its serum treatment," J.A.M.A., 47:560, 1906).

19. FLÜGGE, [C.]. Die Verbreitungsweise und Bekämpfung der epidemische Genickstarre, München. med. Wchnschr., 54:1059, 1907.

Flügge summarized concisely the situation as regards distribution of meningococci in relation to the spread of the disease. He stated that all patients with epidemic meningitis harbored meningococci in the nasopharynx for the first 5 days, after which the organisms usually disappeared rapidly. Among contacts, about 70 per cent were found to be carriers for 3 weeks or so. Since the meningococcus is a delicate organism, which does not survive well outside the body, the disease must be spread by carriers. Flügge had already become interested in meningitis during the German epidemic of 1905 ("Die im Hygienischen Institut der Königl. Universität Breslau während der Genickstarre-Epidemie im Jahre 1905 ausgefürten Untersuchungen," Klin. Jahrb., 15:353, 1906). This volume also contains many articles by German authorities such as Kolle and Wassermann, von Lingelsheim, and others which are a mine of information on the details of the disease; they are all based on the material studied in this great epidemic.

20. LIEBERMEISTER, G. Ueber Meningococcensepsis, München. med. Wchnschr., 55:1978, 1908.

Liebermeister seems to have been the first to recognize chronic meningococcus spesis as a definite clinical entity apart from epidemic meningitis. He reports a classical case with arthralgia, prolonged irregular fever, positive blood cultures, but normal spinal fluid, with recovery. The voluminous literature on this syndrome is comprehensively reviewed by Dopter (Ref. 27, pp. 136 ff.). Poorly documented cases are, however, found in earlier reports, such as those of E. Sacquépée and E. Peltier ("Méningites cérébrospinales grippales," Arch. gén. de méd., 187:537, 1901) and of A. Cochez and Lemaire (Ref. 14). W. Dock in 1924 ("Intermittent fever of 7 months' duration due to meningococcemia," J.A.M.A., 83:31, 1924) was able to collect sixty-eight cases from the literature.

21. FLEXNER, S., and JOBLING, J. W. Serum treatment of epidemic cerebro-spinal meningitis, J. Exper. Med., 10:141, 1908.

The writers immunized a horse with a mixture of meningococcus strains, first given subcutaneously and later intravenously. The titer of the serum is not stated. Forty-seven cases of epidemic meningitis were treated by one to three intraspinal injections of the serum. Of the patients, 72.3 per cent recovered, whereas of untreated cases in the same epidemic about 70 per cent died. Flexner and Jobling were conservative but hopeful in their conclusions. A little later they reported ("An analysis of 400 cases of epidemic meningitis treated with the anti-meningitis serum," J. Exper. Med., 10:690, 1908) a large number of cases with a detailed tabulation of results. Of these cases, only 11–50 per cent died, depending upon age, as against an over-all mortality of at least 75 per cent in untreated cases. They concluded: "The antimeningitis serum when used by the subdural method of injection, in suitable doses and at proper intervals, is capable of reducing the period of illness; of preventing, in large measure, the chronic lesions and types of the infection; of bringing about complete restoration to health in all but a very small number of the recovered, thus lessening the serious deformity and permanent consequences of meningitis; and of greatly diminishing fatalities due to the disease." Meanwhile, Harvey Cushing and Frank J. Sladen ("Obstructive hydrocephalus following cerebrospinal meningitis, intraventricular injection of antimeningitis serum [Flexner]," J. Exper. Med., **10**:548, 1908) called attention to the possible introduction of serum directly into the ventricles in cases with hydrocephalus and block.

But the Germans had not been idle. A. Wassermann ("Ueber die bisherigen Erfahrungen mit dem Meningococcen-Heilserum bei Genickstarrekranken," Deutsche med. Wchnschr., **33**:1585, 1907) reported several cases treated by subcutaneous and intraspinal injections of Jochmann's serum with promising results; and C. Schöne ("Ueberblick über die Behandlung von 30 Genickstarrekranken mit Jochmann'schen Meningococcenserum," Therap. d. Gegenwart, **48**:52, 1907) reported on thirty treated cases. They achieved results comparable with those of Flexner after intraspinal injection.

Flexner later ("The results of the serum treatment in 1,300 cases of epidemic meningitis," J. Exper. Med., **17**:553, 1913) gave a comprehensive summary of the results of treatment with his serum of cases all over the world. The mortality of all treated patients was 30.9 per cent; of those treated on the first to third day, only 18.1 per cent died. At the same time, the mortality of untreated cases varied from 70 per cent to 90 per cent. Flexner discussed at length the difficulties and complications of serum therapy.

With World War I there developed numerous intense epidemics of meningitis, especially in the armed forces. These epidemics stimulated the studies not only on classification (Ref. 24) but on standardization of therapeutic sera, taking into account the different strains of meningococcus. H. L. Amoss and M. Wollstein ("A method for the rapid preparation of anti-meningitis serum," J. Exper. Med., **23**:403, 1916) led the way in the preparation of potent polyvalent sera with a further report (H. L. Amoss and P. Marsh, "Standardization of antimeningitis serum," J. Exper. Med., **28**:779, 1918), dealing largely with criteria for standardization. Serum therapy subsequently had a checkered career. In the late 1920's and 1930's there were severe outbreaks of meningitis which appeared refractory to available sera and had a mortality rate of 70–80 per cent. The complexities of this situation in relation to classification of strains is reviewed by Branham (Ref. 24). It is interesting to note the way in which things have come full circle, so that in 1940 there were again emphasized only two groups of meningococci—Group I, responsible for most of the recent epidemics, and Group II, responsible for most endemic cases and carriers.

22. DOPTER, C. Étude de quelques germes isolés du rhinopharynx voisins du méningocoque (paraméningococcus), Compt. rend. Soc. de biol., **67**:74, 1909.

It did not occur to the early writers that there were different types of meningococci, distinguishable serologically. Dopter isolated organisms from the nasopharynx which were morphologically and culturally indistinguishable from meningococci and which gave the same reactions in sugars but which differed in certain serological respects. These organisms were to be differentiated from the pseudomeningococci of von Lingelsheim, which gave different reactions in sugars from true meningococci. Dopter felt that his parameningococci had, however, the same clinical significance as true meningococci. Dopter and Pauron ("Différenciation des paraméningocoques entre eux par le saturation des agglutinins," Compt. rend. Soc. de biol., **77**:231, 1914) later extended these studies and differentiated various types of parameningococci. Up to this time, however, little or no attention had been paid to differences in strains in clinical work, and the sera of Flexner and of Jochmann were prepared from various meningococci, selected in empirical and haphazard fashion. Dopter led the way in purposeful and intelligent classification of meningococcus strains.

23. NETTER, A., and DEBRÉ, R. La méningite cérébrospinale. Paris, Masson et Cie, 1911.

This classical monograph fully summarizes knowledge of every phase of meningococcus meningitis to date. The clinical descriptions are comprehensive and admirable and include such complications as paralysis and visual and auditory troubles. The chapter on the nasopharynx as the habitat of the meningococcus is an especially valuable summary. The authors offer an explanation for the widely varying number of carriers found by different observers, and they conclude that the intensity of the outbreak of meningitis and the carrier rate correspond. This was well shown later by Glover (Ref. 26).

24. GORDON, M. H., and MURRAY, E. G. Identification of the meningococcus, J. Roy. Army M. Corps, **24**:411, 1915.

It was thought at first that all meningococci were identical. From about 1905 on, however, numerous workers began to distinguish various races or strains. The differentiation was made partly by morphological study, partly by fermentation of sugars, and partly by serological tests. Some of the early papers of importance are those of J. A. Arkwright ("On variations of the meningococcus and its differentiation from other cocci occurring in the cerebro-spinal fluid," J. Hyg., **7**:193, 1907; "Varieties of the meningococcus with special reference to a comparison of strains from epidemic and sporadic sources," *ibid.*, **9**:104, 1909); K. Kutscher ("Ueber Untersuchungen der Nasenrachenhöhle gesunder Menschen auf Meningococcen," Deutsche med. Wchnschr., **32**:1071, 1906); William J. Elser and Frank M. Huntoon ("Studies on meningitis," J.M. Research, **20**:377, 1909), and Dopter (Ref. 22). None of these students, however, arrived at any definitive or uniform classification of meningococci. Arthur W. M. Ellis ("A classification of meningococci based on group agglutination obtained with monovalent immune rabbit serums," Brit. M.J., **2**:881, 1915) was able to divide meningococci into two groups by agglutination tests, and J. A. Arkwright ("Grouping of strains of meningococcus isolated during the epidemic of cerebrospinal meningitis in 1915," Brit. M.J., **2**:885, 1915) came to the same conclusion. His two main groups corresponded to Dopter's meningococci and parameningococci (Ref. 22).

Gordon and Murray, using improved methods for agglutination and absorption tests, were able to distinguish four definite serological types of meningococci among patients in the army. Further reports by Gordon appeared ("Identification of meningococcus," J. Hyg., **17**:290, 1918; *Cerebrospinal Fever* (M. Res. Council, Spec. Rep. Ser., No. 50 [London: His Majesty's Stationery Office, 1920]). This work had important implications in serum therapy and in epidemiological studies. Meanwhile, similar studies were being made in France by M. Nicolle, E. Debains, and C. Jouan ("Études sur les méningocoques et les sérums antiméningococciques," Ann. Inst. Pasteur, **32**:150, 1918). While strains of meningococci have been found which do not fit Gordon's types, he brought order into the whole subject, and his results have been of practical use. For recent comprehensive discussion of the meningococcus see Sara E. Branham ("The meningococcus [*Neisseria intracellularis*]," Bact. Rev., **4**:59, 1940; "The significance of serological types among meningococci," J.A.M.A., **108**:692, 1937).

25. FOSTER, M., and GASKELL, J. F. Cerebro-spinal fever. London: Cambridge University Press, 1916.

An excellent survey to date of meningitis, based largely on recent military experience. The historical section is especially valuable.

26. GLOVER, J. A. Observations of the meningococcus carrier rates, and their application to the prevention of cerebrospinal fever, *in* Cerebrospinal fever, p. 133. (M. Res. Council, Spec. Rep. Ser., No. 50.) London: His Majesty's Stationery Office, 1920.

Glover carefully followed the carrier rate in a military installation where there was great crowding. Under these conditions, with beds only 6 inches apart, the carrier rate was found to rise from the normal of 2–4 per cent to the amazing figure of over 70 per cent, following which clinical meningitis broke out. When the beds were spaced 3 feet apart, the outbreak promptly subsided, and the carrier rate fell to a low level. This phenomenon was repeated several times during periods of crowding. Here was final proof that carriers were the source of meningitis and that danger of clinical infection varied with the density of the healthy carrier population. A review of this subject is that of K. F. Maxey ("The relationship of meningococcus carriers to the incidence of cerbrospinal fever," Am. J.M. Sc., **193**:438, 1937). Of special interest are the studies of Geoffrey Rake ("Studies on meningococcus infection. VI. The carrier problem," J. Exper. Med., **59**:553, 1934). Rake carefully followed a small group of carriers and found that they fell into three categories, namely, chronic, intermittent, and transient.

27. DOPTER, C. L'Infection méningococcique. Paris: J.-B. Baillière et fils, 1921.

This comprehensive work deals, like that of Netter and Debré (Ref. 23), with every phase of the subject and leaves little to be added today.

28. BLACKFAN, K. D. The treatment of meningococcus meningitis, Medicine, **1**:139, 1922.

Blackfan reviews the whole history of treatment of meningococcus meningitis, including serum therapy.

29. BANKS, H. S. Chemotherapy of meningococcal meningitis, Lancet, **2**:921, 1939.

The advent of the sulfonamides sounded the death knell of serum therapy for epidemic meningitis. Banks reported 31 cases treated with sulfanilamide without a death and 36 cases treated with M&B 693 with 1 death. On the whole, patients improved more rapidly with chemotherapy than with serum, and the doing-away with intraspinal therapy was a great advantage. "No evidence in favour of auxiliary treatment with serum was obtained." By 1943, Paul B. Beeson and Ethel Westerman ("Cerebrospinal fever," Brit. M.J., **1**:497, 1943) were able to discuss sulfonamide therapy in 3,575 cases, with an over-all fatality rate of 15.94 per cent. Serum was also used in some cases; among 2,591 cases in whom sulfonamides were used alone, the fatality rate was 14.3 per cent. Among patients from fifteen to twenty-five years old, only 5–8 per cent died. Similarly, A. A. Jubb ("Chemotherapy and serotherapy in cerebrospinal [meningococcal] meningitis," Brit. M.J., **1**:501, 1943) found a death rate of 9.2 per cent in 2,357 cases treated by chemotherapy alone.

An earlier note is that of F. F. Schwentker, S. Gilman, and P. H. Long ("The treatment of meningococcic meningitis with sulfanilamide," J.A.M.A., **108**:1407, 1937), who treated 11 patients with sulfanilamide subcutaneously and intraspinally, with a mortality of 9 per cent.

30. MEEHAN, J. F., and MERRILEES, C. R. An outbreak of cerebrospinal meningitis in a foundling hospital: the treatment of carriers with "M. and B. 693," M.J. Australia, **2**:84, 1940.

It was known that outbreaks of meningitis ran parallel to the carrier rate, but no simple secure method of extirpating meningococci from the nasopharynx had been discovered. The writers treated carrier children after an outbreak of meningitis in a foundling hospital with "B. and M. 693" (a sulfonamide) and immediately reduced the carriers from 75 to 3. Similarly, R. W. Fairbrother "Cerebrospinal meningitis: the use of sulphonamide derivatives in prophylaxis," Brit. M.J., **2**:859, 1940), in a very careful study, found that "adequate dosage with sulphapyridine is a satisfactory method of clearing meningococci from the nasopharyngeal mucosa." Finally, F. S. Cheever, B. B. Breese, and H. C. Upham ("The treatment of meningococcus carriers with sulfadiazine," Ann. Int. Med., **19**:602, 1943) found that "sulfadiazine is effective, since all of 161 meningococcus carriers receiving 8 grams of the drug over a period of 72 hours yielded negative cultures on the fourth day."

31. MILLER, C. P., and FOSTER, A. Z. Studies on the action of penicillin. II. Therapeutic action of penicillin on experimental meningococcal infection in mice, Proc. Soc. Exper. Biol. & Med., **56**:166, 1944.

The writers studied the effect of penicillin on experimental meningococcus peritonitis in mice. There was a definite curative effect. Similarly ("III. Bactericidal action of penicillin on meningococcus in vitro," *ibid.*, p. 205), they found that "meningococci are readily killed by penicillin in nutrient broth at 37°."

32. ROSENBERG, D. H., and ARLING, P. A. Penicillin in the treatment of meningitis, J.A.M.A., **125**:1011, 1944.

The writers reported the first sizable series of meningitis cases treated with penicillin. They gave an intrathecal injection of 10,000 units every day as well as small doses intramuscularly. Sixty-four of sixty-five patients recovered. Finland and his associates also in an early report (M. Meads, W. H. Hams, B. A. Samper, and M. Finland, "Treatment of meningococcal meningitis with penicillin," New England J. Med., **231**:509, 1944) concluded that penicillin was less satisfactory than sulfonamides and acted more slowly. However, they had available only small doses of penicillin. Recently, Lepper and his associates (H. H. Lepper, H. F. Dowling, P. F. Wehrle, N. H. Blatt, H. W. Spies, and M. Brown, "Meningococcic meningitis: treatment with large doses of penicillin compared to treatment with Gantrisin," J. Lab. & Clin. Med., **40**:891, 1952) treated meningococcus meningitis with injections of 1,000,000 units of penicillin intramuscularly or intravenously every 2 hours without intrathecal injections. Of forty patients, only one died. These writers conclude that penicillin is just as effective as sulfonamides when large doses are used. The earlier studies (E. D. Dernoff-Stanley, H. F. Dowling, and L. K. Sweet, "The absorption into and distribution of penicillin in the cerebrospinal fluid," J. Clin. Investigation, **25**:87, 1946), which showed little, if any, penicillin in the spinal fluid after parenteral injections, were done, as it turned out, with too small doses of the antibiotic. On the other hand, Schwenlen and his associates (G. T. Schwenlen, R. L. Barton, T. J. Bauer, L. Loewe, H. N. Bundeson, and R. M. Craig, "Penicillin in spinal fluid after intravenous administration," J.A.M.A., **130**:340, 1946) found, working with syphilitics, that significant amounts of penicillin were demonstrated in the spinal fluid after intravenous drip of 10,000,000–25,000,000 units of penicillin in 24 hours.

GONORRHEA AND GONOCOCCAL INFECTION

Clinical	Refs. 1, 2, 10
Differentiation from syphilis	Refs. 1, 2
General	Refs. 1, 2, 10
Gonococcal arthritis	Ref. 13
Gonococcal endocarditis	Ref. 15
Gonococcal infection in females	Refs. 9, 10, 11
Gonococcal lesions of the skin	Ref. 14
Gonococcal ophthalmia	Ref. 5
Gonococcus	Refs. 3, 4, 6, 7, 8, 10, 12
Treatment with antibiotics	Ref. 16

Section 11

GONORRHEA AND GONOCOCCAL INFECTION

THE early literature on gonorrhea is concerned largely with the differentiation of the disease from syphilis, and the reader is referred to the section on syphilis of this bibliography for pertinent references. Innumerable books are available on the subject of gonorrhea, of which that by Ernst Finger (*Die Blenorrhöe der Sexualorgane und ihre Complicationen* [Leipzig and Vienna: Frantz Deuticke, 1888]) is the classical text which ran through many editions and translations. Gonorrhea is usually discussed in the general textbooks on venereal and genitourinary diseases, and many important articles lie buried in journals on the eye and other special branches. Much, of course, is to be found in the gynecological literature from the time of Bumm (Ref. 10) on. Among modern texts one should mention the large, well-documented treatise by Charles C. Norris (*Gonorrhea in Women* [Philadelphia and London: W. B. Saunders Co., 1913]) and the standard text by P. S. Pelouze (*Gonorrhea in the Male and Female* [3d ed.; Philadelphia and London: W. B. Saunders Co., 1939]), which ran through many editions.

We have not attempted to follow the bibliography through all the ramifications of the special domains in which the gonococcus may cause disease; we have had in mind that this bibliography is primarily for medical students and physicians with general interests.

1. BELL, Benjamin. A treatise on gonorrhea virulenta and lues venerea. 2 vols. Edinburgh: James Watson & Co., 1793.

Bell was the first clearly to differentiate gonorrhea from syphilis and to insist that it was an independent disease. After a general introduction he devotes a full volume to the discussion of the "gonorrhea virulenta." "Every discharge of matter from the urethra, excited by impure coition, is termed Gonorrhoea Virulenta." There follow chapters on clinical features of the disease, going into minutest details of symptoms and course. "The duration of gonorrhoea has always been a matter of much uncertainty." He points out that, with simple urethritis, "the disease will not commonly endure a fortnight . . . but, wherever the lower parts of the urethra are affected, particularly when the prostate gland and other parts about the neck of the bladder are diseased, the running, in almost every instance proves obstinate" (p. 67). Bell, along with others, questioned the value of the medicines in vogue: "A low diet, mercury, and evacuants of different kinds, did much harm, as we have already observed, by inducing such a degree of debility and relaxation as materially affected the constitution" (p. 74). The pros and cons of local injections and the use of sounds are discussed. The first part of the book ends with an excellent recapitulation: "It appears that Gonorrhoea is a local disease, proceeding from a specific contagion, and not necessarily connected with any other . . . that the discharge of matter which takes place is not the effect of ulceration, but proceeds from an inflamed state of the urethra and contiguous parts . . . that the disease is always formidable in proportion to the depth of parts that are affected . . . that in the cure of Gonorrhoea no advantage is derived from mercury, or any remedy acting altogether upon the constitution [in contrast to syphilis] . . . that where the membrane of the urethra is alone affected, no remedy proves so successful as astringent injections . . . but that they are never employed but with much risk of doing harm where the inflammation has reached Cowper's glands, to the prostate gland or to the bladder . . . that when the bladder is affected, opium or hyoscyamus are in like manner to be used to relieve pain" (pp. 168 ff.). Bell described all sorts of local complications of gonorrhea but was entirely unaware of distant metastases, such as arthritis, ophthalmia, etc. The book is nonetheless a masterpiece, based as it is on accurate observation of clinical cases.

2. RICORD, Ph. Traité pratique des maladies vénériennes. Paris: De Just Rouvier & E. le Bouvier, 1838.

The book by Ricord, the great French expert on venereal disease, deals with both syphilis and gonorrhea, although he believed them to be different diseases and proved his point by a great many intradermal inoculations of gonorrheal pus into volunteers without result, whereas, if the material were syphilitic, chancres would be expected to appear. Ricord went further than Bell in recognizing some distant complications, such as gonococcal ophthalmia. "Its development must be attributed to the direct application of the gonorrheal matter to the conjunctiva . . . the first thing to be urged is speed and energy. . . . Hesitation and uncertainty are often followed by loss of the eyes . . . one must always insist on applications of silver nitrate" (p. 761). The method of application is described in detail. Ricord does not, however, mention the common occurrence of gonococcal arthritis.

3. NEISSER, Albert. Ueber eine der Gonorrhoe eigentümliche Micrococcusform, Centralbl. f. d. med. Wissensch., **17**:497, 1879.

The idea of a bacterial cause of gonorrhea was in the air. Thus Lebert (in H. von Ziemssen, *Handbuch der speciellen Pathologie und Therapie* [Leipzig: F. C. W. Vogel, 1875], **9**, Part II, 295) four years before Neisser's discovery said: "It is therefore highly probable that gonorrheal pus contains a contagious principle which frankly the microscope and chemical analysis have so far not found. . . . One can suppose that germs develop in the depths of the urethral mucosa." Various workers were searching for such a cause at the time. In this modest and conservative report Neisser announced the discovery of the gonococcus. The organisms were seen in pus from gonococcal urethritis spread thin on slides and stained with methyl violet. The intracellular predominance, the biscuit-shaped pairs of recently divided cocci, are well described. These bacteria were found in thirty-five cases of gonorrhea varying in duration—3 days to 13 weeks—but not in a chronic case of 1½ years. The gonococcus seemed to be the only organism present. Neisser isolated it from nine purulent urethritides in women and from two patients with gonorrheal conjunctivitis. Neisser reserved final judgment as to the significance of the organisms, pending cultural and inoculation experiments.

Neisser's work was soon confirmed in other countries, as, for example, by P. Weiss (Thèse de Nancy, Iʳᵉ sér., No. 119 [1880]), an abstract of whose work is reported in Ann. de dermat. et syph. ("Le microbe du pus blennorhagique"), **2**:189, 1881. Weiss found Neisser's coccus in the gonorrheal discharges of both men and women and apparently was the first to advise the use of potassium permanganate irrigations, 0.25 per 1,000, later much employed. O. Haab ("Kleinere ophthalmologische Mittheilungen. II. Parasitäre Augenkrankheiten," Cor.-Bl. f. schweiz. Aerzte, **11**:79, 1881) early confirmed the finding of typical cocci in the discharge of conjunctivitis of the newborn and in gonorrheal ophthalmia. He was unable, however, to grow the organisms in culture.

4. LEISTIKOW. Ueber Bacterien bei den venerischen Krankheiten, Charité-Ann., **7**:750, 1880.

Leistikow reports confirmation of Neisser's work. He also undertook culture studies with Löffler, and, after many failures, the "cultures finally throve in a blood serum gelatin at body temperature." They tried many inoculation experiments in rabbits, dogs, rats, mice, guinea pigs, and horses, with failure in all to produce disease. The results in a monkey were uncertain. Leistikow was probably the first to report successful cultivation of the gonococcus. Chemotherapy was already under way, and he discussed the relative merits of injections of bichloride, zinc solutions, tannic acid, lead acetate, silver nitrate, and carbolic acid. The results were hard to evaluate, since gonorrheal discharges ceased of themselves with time.

5. CREDÉ, [C.]. Die Verhütung der Augenentzündung der Neugeborenen, Arch. f. Gynaecol., **17**:50, 1881.

Starting from the assumption that conjunctivitis of the newborn was acquired from gonococcal infection of the mother during the baby's passage through the birth canal, Credé began prophylactic treatment of all newborn babies in the Leipzig clinic. He first used various solutions but "from 1 June 1880 all eyes without exception were disinfected directly after birth . . . with a single drop of nitrate of silver (1:50)." At the same time, douching of the mother was discontinued: "All the children so treated have escaped eye inflammation of even slight grade." Mild hyperemia and increased secretion might be present in the first 24 hours, but no harm was ever done to the eyes. "The main point is in the experience that not disinfection of the vagina but only of the eye achieves the goal." The incidence of conjunctivitis fell in the clinic from 13.6 in 1874 to 0.5 in 1880. In a further communication (*ibid.*, **18**:367, 1881) Credé reported 400 new cases in addition to 200 previously recorded. The babies' eyes were wiped with a cloth dipped in plain water and then "one drop of 2 per cent solution of silver nitrate was instilled. No child so treated developed ophthalmia neonatorum in the first 7 days of life." Credé's method was soon generally in use the world over and was relied upon for many years. His work was summarized in a book (*Die Verhütung der Augenentzündung der Neugeborenen* [Berlin: A. Hirschwald, 1884]).

Penicillin has recently been tried in place of silver nitrate as a prophylactic against gonococcal conjunctivitis. The relative merits of the two are analyzed by H. C. Franklin ("Prophylaxis against ophthalmia neonatorum, clinical comparison of penicillin and silver nitrate; preliminary report," J.A.M.A., **134**:1230, 1947). He leans, on the whole, toward penicillin, although the diminished frequency of maternal gonorrhea makes the problem much less urgent than in Credé's day.

6. KRAUSE, Fedor. II. Die Micrococcen der Blennorrhoea neonatorum, Centralbl. f. prakt. Augenh., **6**:134, 1882.

Krause succeeded in growing gonococci from blenorrhea neonatorum, using coagulated blood serum as a culture medium. He obtained diplococci in pure culture from 12 children. Inoculation of the conjunctivae of various small animals was unsuccessful. This work was done in Hirschberg's clinic, and Hirschberg himself is reported ("Gesellschaft der Charité-Aerzte in Berlin, 16 Feb., 1882," Berl. klin. Wchnschr., **19**:500, 1882) to have made inoculations with gonorrheal pus into the human eye and invariably to have produced disease, although animal inoculation failed. At the same meeting early attempts at treatment of gonorrheal urethritis are reported. Lewin used bichloride of mercury injections (1:20,000), Güterbock reported that irrigations with water were just as effective, and Leistikow found that patients recovered equaly well without any irrigations.

7. NEISSER, Albert. IV. Die Micrococcen der Gonorrhoe, Deutsche med. Wchnschr., **8**:279, 1882.

Neisser gives a definitive review of the subject to date. He first makes it clear that the gonococcus is a specific organism and again describes its morphological features: biscuit-shaped diplococci, "adherent" to pus cells. "Gonococci are absolutely constant in every case of gonorrhea . . . and are not found in any other disease. . . . Furthermore, the gonococci are the only organisms which are found in gonococcal pus." He now reports success in cultivation of gonococci on meat-extract–peptone gelatin. "As far as one can ever tell anything by microscopic examination, all the doctors who looked at the preparations say that the cultures are pure growths of gonococci (H. A. Cohnheim, Koch, Ehrlich)." Inoculation of humans with cultures failed, however, as well as animal inoculations. Neisser was unable to find gonococci in pus from gonococcal arthritis and epididymitis, but he stressed the occurrence of the germs in ophthalmia.

However, not everyone accepted the gonococcus as the specific cause of the disease, and various conflicting reports in the literature on the specificity and pathogenicity of "gonococci" are reviewed by Bumm (Ref. 10).

8. BOCKHART, Max. Beitrag zur Aetiologie und Pathologie des Harnröhrentrippers, Vrtljschr. f. Dermat. u. Syph., **15**:3, 1883.

Bockhart undertook to inoculate a normal male urethra with a pure culture of gonococci which he received from Dr. Fehleisen. The subject was a man with advanced dementia paralytica. Four days later, there was a full-blown urethritis with countless gonococci in the secretion. A few days later the patient died, and at autopsy the sections of the urethra showed gonococci. Here, then, seemed to be undoubted proof that the gonococcus was the pathogenic agent in urethritis. Bockhart built up a theory of the pathogenesis of gonorrhea on the basis of lymphatic invasion. The distant complications—endocarditis, arthritis—he felt come from extension of infection into the blood stream.

9. ARNING, E. Ueber das Vorkommen von Gonococcen bei Bartolinitis, Vrtljschr. f. Dermat. u. Syph., **15**:371, 1883.

Arning found gonococci regularly in acute and chronic inflammation of Bartho-in's glands in women. At about the same time, E. Bumm ("Beitrag zur Kentniss

der Gonorrhoe der weiblichen Genitalien," Arch. f. Gynaecol., **23**:328, 1884),
the gynecologist, made a systemic study of gonococcal infection in women and
pointed out the "most frequent site of gonorrhea is the mucosa of the cervix
uteri." But, to confuse matters, Bumm found organisms resembling gonococci in
the genitals of women "where the possibility of gonorrhea was absolutely excluded." These cocci were biscuit-shaped diplo-forms and were readily cultivable on artificial media, where they grew out as milk-white plaques, which produced no lesion when inoculated on mucous membranes. One suspects that
these bacteria were members of the *N. catarrhalis* group. They were also found
in ulcerative processes in the mouth and in sputum.

10. BUMM, Ernst. Der Micro-Organismus der gonorrhoischen Schleimhaut-
Erkrankungen, "Gonococcus-Neisser." Wiesbaden: J. F. Bergmann, 1885.

This little book, which is a definite landmark in the subject, opens with a critical
review to date of the literature on the gonococcus. There follows a description
of the morphology and staining and a discussion of numerous biscuit-shaped
diplococci other than gonococci—a lemon-yellow diplococcus, not pathogenic; a
milk-white diplococcus, not pathogenic; a yellow-white diplococcus, pathogenic; a pink diplococcus, not pathogenic. All these need to be differentiated
from the gonococcus. Bumm lists the "pathological secretions" in which the
gonococci occur: male and female urethritis, bladder and kidney, periurethral
abscesses, knee joint, conjunctiva, rectum, body and cervix of the uterus, Bar-
tholin's glands. Bumm summarizes the position of the gonococcus in diagnosis:
"The presence of Neisser's gonococcus in the secretions proves the infectious
origin of the disease of the mucous membrane, and, conversely, gonococcus-free
secretion has no virulent characteristics." Bumm gradually assembled a considerable amount of pathological tissue from which he was able to build up the
histological appearance of gonococcal infection day by day until the thirty-third
day—a fundamental piece of work. He next summarizes the literature on attempts to cultivate the gonococcus on artificial media and describes his own
successful work, pointing out the difficulties and the ease with which confusion
could arise with other diplococci which were readily cultivable. He feels that
Neisser did not grow genuine gonococci, whereas Fehleisen probably and Leistikow definitely did. Bumm inoculated the urethra of a healthy woman and produced gonococcal urethritis, once more proving the pathogenic specificity of the
organism.

Bumm's summary brings out very well the difficulties of the subject at the
time, principally the confusion of gonococci with other diplococci in smear and
in culture. He also speculated about distant lesions, as to whether they were due
to spread of gonococci through the body or whether they were "sympathetic" or
due to an absorbed toxin—questions which vexed everyone at the time. However, his monograph was definitive to date and left relatively little of importance
untouched.

11. FRAENKEL, Eugen. Bericht über eine bei Kindern beobachtete En-
demie infectiöser Colpitis, Virchows Arch. f. path. Anat., **99**:251, 1885

The syndrome of vulvovaginitis in little girls was recognized in the early part of
the nineteenth century, as pointed out in the excellent reviews of the literature
of Cahen-Broch ("Die Urogenital-Blenorrhoe der kleinen Mädchen," Jahrb. f

Kinderh., **34**:369, 1892) and of A. Epstein ("Ueber Vulvovaginitis gonorrhoica bei kleinen Mädchen," Arch. f. Dermat. u. Syph., **23**:3, 1891). The occurrence in little girls, the relative immunity of boys and of girls after menstruation started, the usual non-venereal nature of the spread of the disease, the association of the child with a mother who had gonorrhea, the occurrence in institutions where many children were in close contact and where a common bathtub and towels were used, were all stressed. R. Pott ("Die specifische Vulvo-Vaginitis im Kindesalter und ihre Behandlung," Jahrb. f. Kinderh., **19**:71, 1883) was among the first to insist that this disease was "the expression of a specific communicable disease of the mucous membrane" and to point out how widespread it was in the general population. The above writers give detailed descriptions of the findings and clinical course of the condition, and the chronic character and great resistance to disinfectants and astringents were noted by everyone. Fraenkel, however, was the first to establish definitively the gonococcus as cause of the disease. He studied the discharges and "the finding was very striking, since there was success in demonstrating in every preparation the presence of a micro-organism which differed in no respect from the gonococcus of Neisser."

The large modern literature on the subject is reviewed by R. A. Benson and A. Steer ("Vaginitis of children," Am. J. Dis. Child., **53**:806, 1937). Recently, A. Cohn, A. Steer, and E. L. Adler ("Gonococcal vaginitis," Ven. Dis. Inform., **21**:208, 1940) could only prove that 23.3 per cent of cases of juvenile vaginitis were definitely gonococcal, and they placed more emphasis than most observers on actual sexual contact. However, both sulfanilamide and sulfapyridine produced rapid cures. Like all other manifestations of the gonococcus, vaginitis responds promptly to penicillin (B. G. Clarke and H. H. Eisenberg, "Gonococcic vaginitis in children treated with single injection of penicillin in beeswax and peanut oil; report of twenty cases," Am. J. Dis. Child., **74**:707, 1947).

12. WERTHEIM, Ernst. Reinzüchtung des Gonococcus Neisser mittels des Plattenverfahrens, Deutsche med. Wchnschr., **17**:1351, 1891.

Wertheim modified previous cultural procedures so that he readily grew gonococci in plates of serum-peptone agar. He inoculated the urethras of five men with general paresis and in every case produced typical gonorrhea, from which the gonococci were again recovered. Wertheim considered that his experiments gave final and indisputable proof that the coccus of Neisser was actually the cause of gonorrhea. The observation has often been repeated by various observers.

Modern work on the complexity of suitable media for growth of the gonococcus is summarized in the article by J. F. Mahoney and J. D. Thayer *in* R. J. Dubos, *Bacterial and Mycotic Infections of Man* (2d ed.; Philadelphia: J. B. Lippincott Co., 1952), page 565. As methods have been improved, cultures have been found to have as valuable a place in diagnosis as direct smears (see C. M. Carpenter *et al.*, "Evaluation of twelve media for the isolation of the gonococcus," Am. J. Syph., **33**:164, 1949; and J. D. Thayer, J. H. Schubert, and M. A. Bucca, "The evaluation of culture mediums for the routine isolation of the gonococcus," J. Ven. Dis. Inform., **28**:37, 1947).

13. HÖCK, Heinrich. Ein Beitrag zur Arthritis blennorrhoica, Wien. klin. Wchnschr., **6**:736, 1893.

The concept of gonococcal arthritis seems to have grown slowly, so that Brandes of Copenhagen ("Du rhumatisme blenorrhagique," Arch. gén. de méd., 4:257, 1854) could open his paper with the question "Does blenorrhagic rheumatism really exist?" Apparently some of the alleged cases were only instances of vague aches and pains, or they may have been some other variety of arthritis. Brandes reports several cases of gonorrhea associated with arthritis, but, as there was no bacteriological confirmation, they are difficult to interpret. He points out that this form of arthritis is much more common in men than in women and that it often accompanies ophthalmia. "The complication of cardiac lesions is rare, very rare, but it is not impossible." The knee is the joint most often affected, although the trouble migrates from joint to joint. Ankyloses of large joints rarely occur. G. Bücker (*Ueber Polyarthritis gonorrhoica* [Inaug. diss., Berlin, 1880]) reviews the whole subject and reports two cases in which pus was withdrawn from joints, but apparently no search was made for Neisser's coccus.

A step forward was made by L. M. Petrone ("Sulla natura parasitaria dell'artrite blenorrhagica," Riv. clin. di Bologna, 3:94, 1883, which is abstracted in Centralbl. f. Chir., 10:586, 1883), who found, in smears from the joint exudate of two cases of urethritis and arthritis, bacteria which corresponded in every respect with Neisser's organisms. One does not know what to make of the statement that the cocci were seen also in the blood, presumably in smears. In the following year F. Kammerer ("Ueber gonorrhoische Gelenkentzündung," Centralbl. f. Chir., 11:49, 1884) also saw typical gonococci in the exudate of an inflamed knee joint, but neither of these observers brought the final proof of the existence of gonococcal infection of joints by cultivating the organism.

Höck seems to have been the first to isolate gonococci from a joint which was the seat of acute arthritis. Interestingly enough, his patient was a baby with gonococcal ophthalmia; he reviews a number of other instances of arthritis following gonococcal ophthalmitis in which organisms were seen in smears but were not cultured. Neisser ("Ueber die Züchtung der Gonococcen bei einen Fall von Arthritis gonorrhoica," Deutsche med. Wchnschr., 20:160, 1894) shortly after reported culture from the knee and finger of an adult with gonococcal arthritis; and, finally, Bordoni-Uffreduzzi ("Ueber die Localization des Gonococcus im inneren des Organismus [durch den Gonococcus herforgerufene Pleuritis und Arthritis]," Deutsche med. Wchnschr., 20:484, 1894) produced urethritis in a volunteer with a culture of gonococcus obtained from a case of arthritis. That the gonococcus could spread in the body and produce distant lesions now seemed understandable.

C. S. Keefer and W. W. Spink ("Gonococcic arthritis: pathogenesis, mechanism of recovery and treatment," J.A.M.A., 109:1448, 1937) give a definitive modern discussion of the subject up to the antibiotic era. They point out certain associated lesions, such as metastatic catarrhal conjunctivitis, iridocyclitis, and keratodermia blenorrhagicum, and the occasional occurrence of bacteremia even without endocardial involvement. In another paper ("Latent gonorrhoea as a cause of acute polyarticular arthritis," J.A.M.A., 109:325, 1937) they emphasize the fact that gonococcal arthritis may occur when the primary urethral infection gave no overt manifestations.

The modern therapy of gonococcal arthritis begins with the use of artificial fever, the results of which are summarized by R. M. Stecher and W. M. Solomon ("The treatment of gonorrhoeal arthritis with artificial fever," Am. J.M. Sc., **192**:497, 1936). Of a series of fifty cases, twenty-six were relieved of all joint symptoms, eleven received benefit, while thirteen were not helped. Because of the strenuous and complicated character of fever therapy, it was soon replaced by chemotherapy when the sulfonamides were found effective. C. S. Keefer and L. A. Rantz ("Sulphanilamide in the treatment of gonococcal arthritis," Am. J.M. Sc., **197**:168, 1939) were the first to report a careful study. They found that in adequate dosage the drug diffused into the synovial fluid, which was sterilized in several days. The "results are encouraging and all patients with gonococcal arthritis should be treated intensively with the drug." J. H. Linner ("Suppurative myositis and purulent arthritis complicating acute gonorrhoea," J.A.M.A., **123**:757, 1943) was the first to report a case treated with penicillin. N. Spitzer and O. Steinbrocker ("The treatment of gonococcal arthritis with penicillin," Am. J.M. Sc., **218**:138, 1949) later reviewed the subject and found that, among twenty-eight cases, "23 were regarded as cured or greatly improved, 5 as failures."

14. VIDAL, Émile. Éruption généralisée et symétrique de croûtes cornées avec chute des ongles, d'origine blenorrhagique, coincidante avec une polyarthrite de même nature. Recédive à la suite d'une nouvelle blenor-rhagie, deux ans après la guérison de la première maladie, Ann. de dermat. et syph., **4**:3, 1893.

Vidal appears to have been the first to describe thoroughly the skin lesions of gonorrhea and to note their association with arthritis. "The recurrence of these lesions, the pathogenesis of which was in doubt in 1890, shows that they are a direct manifestation of the gonorrheal infection, just as arthritis is." J. G. Downing ("Keratoderma blenorrhagicum," J.A.M.A., **102**:829, 1934) reviews the literature with a case report of his own, as do W. W. Spink and C. S. Keefer ("The renal and dermatologic complications of gonococcal infection," New England. J. Med., **217**:241, 1937). The first American case was that of F. E. Simpson ("Keratodermie blenorrhagique," J.A.M.A., **59**:607, 1912), whose paper is especially useful because it contains abstracts of the previously reported cases. A. W. Frerich, S. Schwartz, and O. Steinbrocker ("Penicillin in the treatment of keratosis blenorrhagica with polyarthritis," Arch. Int. Med., **79**:239, 1947) treated three cases with penicillin, with brilliant cures in two of them.

15. THAYER, William Sidney, and BLUMER, George. Ulcerative endo-carditis due to the gonococcus; gonorrhoeal septicemia, Bull. Johns Hopkins Hosp., **7**:57, 1896.

J. Marty ("De l'endocardite blenorrhagique," Arch. gén. de méd., **28**:660, 1876) gives brief excerpts of several cases from the literature and reports two of his own in which an attack of gonorrhea was followed by arthritis and signs of endocarditis. He gives an excellent discussion of the whole subject, but, as his own patients did not die and as there was no bacteriological confirmation, it remains uncertain whether these were really cases of gonococcal endocarditis. Previously, Lacassagne ("Des complications cardiaques de la blenorrhagie,"

Arch. gén. de méd., **19**:15, 1872) reviewed the subject of serous membrane involvement with gonorrhea, and he reports a number of cases of pericarditis, including one of his own which he regards as of gonococcal origin. Thayer and Blumer review the reports of several recent cases of endocarditis in which gonococci were presumably seen in smears from the heart valves at autopsy, but the final proof of cultures was not obtained. Their own patient ran the typical course of ulcerative endocarditis. At autopsy there were vegetations of the mitral valve containing what were morphologically typical gonococci. The organisms were recovered in blood culture during life and were grown from the valve after death. Here, then, was the first proved case of gonococcal sepsis with ulcerative endocarditis. Modern statistics on this lesion may be found in Thayer's monograph, "Studies on bacterial (infective) endocarditis," Johns Hopkins Hosp. Rep., Vol. **22**, Fasc. I, 1926. W. S. Thayer and J. W. Lazear ("A second case of gonococcal septicemia and ulcerative endocarditis with observations upon the cardiac complications of gonorrhoea," J. Exper. Med., **4**:81, 1899) soon reported a second case of gonococcal bacteremia with extensive vegetations on the tricuspid valve and multiple purulent lesions. They review the literature and point out that there are five cases (including their own two) in which the gonococcal nature of the infection is definitely proved. But they go further and emphasize that the gonococcus may on occasion act exactly like the pyogenic cocci and produce a general sepsis with multiple purulent lesions and bacteremia. "Grave myocardial changes, necrosis, purulent infiltration, embolic abscesses are common in severe gonococcal septicaemias . . . the diagnosis may in some cases be made during life by cultures taken from the circulating blood." The article is a classic. Thayer later ("On the cardiac complications of gonorrhoea," Bull. Johns Hopkins Hosp., **33**:361, 1922) again wrote on the subject.

One wonders what effect modern drugs and antibiotics would have on this serious disease. E. S. Orgain and M. A. Poston ("Gonococcal endocarditis, with recovery after sulfapyridine," New England J. Med., **221**:167, 1939) report a case with recovery after treatment with sulfapyridine; and P. H. Futcher and V. C. Scott ("Four cases of gonococcal endocarditis treated with sulfanilamide, with recovery of one," Bull. Johns Hopkins Hosp., **65**:377, 1939), using strict criteria, had one recovery after transfusion and sulfanilamide, whereas three other patients treated with sulfanilamide died. Further to complicate the interpretation, spontaneous recovery or recovery following transfusion alone has been reported fairly often. Futcher and Scott review the literature on "spontaneous" recovery from gonococcal endocarditis and bacteremia.

16. HERRELL, W. E., COOK, E. N., and THOMPSON, L. Use of penicillin in sulfonamide resistant gonorrheal infections, J.A.M.A., **122**:289, 1943.

E. P. Abraham *et al.* ("Further observations on penicillin," Lancet, **2**:177, 1941) had shown that the gonococcus was highly sensitive to penicillin in the test tube; Herrell and his associates confirmed this observation and seem to have been the first to use the material in clinical gonorrhea. Because of very limited amounts of penicillin available, they treated only sulfonamide-resistant cases. "The complete absence of toxicity following the intravenous administration of pyrogen free penicillin, the lack of any discomfort to the patient and the rather rapid disappearance of clinical symptoms have been observed in three cases of sulfonamide resistant gonorrheal infection. . . . In all the cases reported, in addition to the clinical response noted, negative bacterial cultures were obtained some time between seventeen and forty-eight hours after the institution of penicillin therapy." A little later, J. F. Mahoney, C. Ferguson, M. Bucholtz, and C. J. Van Slyke ("The use of penicillin sodium in the treatment of sulfonamide-resistant gonorrhea in men," Am. J. Syph., **27**:525, 1943) reported cure of seventy-two of seventy-five cases of gonorrhea with a total of only 160,000 units of penicillin over a treatment period of 45 hours. Since then, the supremacy of penicillin in treatment of gonorrhea has been universally confirmed, as, for example, by T. H. Sternberg and T. B. Turner ("The treatment of sulfonamide resistant gonorrhea with penicillin sodium," J.A.M.A., **126**:157, 1944). C. P. Miller, W. W. Scott, and V. Moeller ("Studies on the action of penicillin. I. The rapidity of its therapeutic effect on gonococcic urethritis," J.A.M.A., **125**:607, 1944) found that intramuscular doses of 50,000–100,000 units of penicillin were followed by rapid disappearance of gonococci from cases of urethritis.

TUBERCULOSIS

Allergy	Refs. 51, 59, 60
Bacteriology	Refs. 28, 29, 32, 37, 65, 66
Bovine	Refs. 23, 31, 45, 52
Childhood type	Refs. 25, 53, 56
Clinical features	Refs. 1, 2, 4, 5, 8, 10, 17, 19
Etiology	Refs. 13, 15, 16, 18, 20, 23, 28, 31, 32, 37, 44, 52, 56, 58, 61
Immunity and resistance	Refs. 36, 38, 39, 40, 41, 43, 49, 51, 56, 57, 58, 59, 60, 61, 67, 70
Mass surveys	Ref. 61
Pathology	Refs. 1, 2, 4, 5, 13, 17, 19, 21, 34, 47
Prevention	Refs. 9, 37, 38, 39, 40, 41, 44, 57, 61
Reinfection	Refs. 56, 58, 61
Skin test	Ref. 49

(*Continued on following page*)

Section 12

TUBERCULOSIS

It HAS been our purpose in this bibliography, beginning with the nineteenth century, to list all the fundamental contributions to a subject; so far, this has not seemed an insuperable task. With tuberculosis, however, we confess that our courage has been daunted. The vast size of the subject, the limitless literature, and the innumerable facets have, we fear, made it impossible to include every major contribution, especially those of recent years. Perhaps this list should be called "high spots" of tuberculosis rather than a "bibliography." On the other hand, we have been heartened by the fact that no such effort seems to have been made previously, by the conviction that anyone perusing this chapter will gain a good general conception of the history of tuberculosis and the significance of the disease, and, finally, by the knowledge that the references which we have listed give ready access to further pursuit of the literature.

It is difficult for the modern student to realize how vague and rudimentary the knowledge of tuberculosis was at the beginning of the nineteenth century. Medicine was just emerging from the Galenic doctrine of humors; little was known about morbid anatomy; and cellular pathology was still in the future. Jaundice, dropsy, and fever were thought of as diseases in themselves rather than as symptoms, and so, too, those people who wasted away with cough, blood-spitting, and "hectic" fever were loosely spoken of as "consumptives." As more and more autopsies were done, especially by the early-nineteenth-century French clinician-pathologists, certain distinct appearances were noted in the lungs of many of those who died. It was the clearer definition of the clinical features of consumption by physical examination, along with formulation of the various anatomical changes found at autopsy, that dispelled some of the obscurity, which was not lifted until the transmission experiments of Villemin (Refs. 18, 22) and the discovery of the bacillus by Koch (Ref. 28).

The modern student must also realize that a hundred and fifty years ago what we now think of as early tuberculosis was completely unrecognized. Doctors dealt largely with advanced disease, and such disease was highly prevalent. As the young Brontës dropped off one by one of consumption, this was accepted more or less as a matter of course; Anne consented to see a physician only on the day of her death. Laënnec himself was consumptive, and Keats, hardly more than a boy, died in the arms of his friend Joseph Severn, a wraith racked by cough and hemorrhage.

As in the case of so many diseases, it is almost impossible to decide who among all those who wrote on consumption and on tubercle first really sensed their true relationship. Matthew Baillie and G. L. Bayle certainly deserve mention before one goes on to Laënnec, who towers above all contemporaries in the field.

We know of no really complete bibliography of tuberculosis. The little *Historical Chronology of Tuberculosis* is of great value but unfortunately contains few actual references. The modern literature on infection and immunity is well covered in the Bibliography of Rich's monumental work (Ref. 67). The

197

masterful "Essays on Tuberculosis," by Allen Krause, which lie buried in the *Journal of Outdoor Life* for the years 1918–23, should be reprinted. Flick's large volume is full of generous quotations but again gives no systematic bibliography. Pinner's book is especially useful because the numerous references are each followed by a critical abstract. Finally, Dubos' readable volume lists a number of the most comprehensive reviews, as well as many books ancillary to the main subject but of great interest.

Burke, Richard M. *A Historical Chronology of Tuberculosis.* Springfield: Charles C Thomas, 1938.

Flick, Lawrence F. *Development of Our Knowledge of Tuberculosis.* Philadelphia, 1925.

Pinner, Max. *Pulmonary Tuberculosis in the Adult.* Springfield: Charles C Thomas, 1925.

Dubos, René, and Dubos, Jean. *The White Plague.* Boston: Little, Brown & Co., 1952.

1. BAILLIE, Matthew. The morbid anatomy of some of the most important parts of the human body. 3d ed. London: J. Johnson, 1807.

This must be regarded as one of the great medical books of the nineteenth century; in a day when writing about disease was usually fanciful and speculative, we find here clear and precise descriptions based on objective observation. Not only was Baillie a great physician in his day, but he was not "dated."

"The object of this work is to explain more minutely than has hitherto been done the changes in structure arising from morbid action in . . . the human body." "The human mind is prone to form opinions upon every subject which is presented to it, but from a natural indolence is frequently averse to inquire into the circumstances which can alone form a sufficient ground for them. This is the most general cause of false opinions, which have not only pervaded medicine, but almost every other branch of knowledge. When, however, the mind shall be obliged to observe facts which can not be reconciled with such opinions, it will be evident that the opinions are ill-founded, and they will be laid aside. We grant, it does not always happen that men are induced to give up their opinions, or even to think them wrong, upon observing facts which do not agree with them, but surely it is the best means of producing this effect; and whatever change may be wrought on the individuals themselves, the world will be convinced, who have fewer prejudices to combat." These remarks from the Preface strike the keynote to the descriptions which follow.

As regards tuberculosis, what Baillie had to say seems sound as far as it goes. But both the anatomical description and the clinical remarks are brief and obviously inadequate. Under the heading of "Tubercles" we read: "There is no morbid appearance so common in the lungs as that of tubercles. These consist of rounded firm white bodies interspersed through their substance." "They are at first very small, being not larger than the heads of very small pins, and in this case are frequently accumulated in small clusters. The smaller tubercles of a cluster probably grow together, and form one large tubercle." "When cut into they are found to consist of a white smooth substance, having a firm texture, and often contain in part a thick curdy pus." "When several tubercles of considerable size are grown together so as to form a pretty large tuberculated mass, pus is very generally found upon cutting into it." "When tubercles are converted into abscesses, phthisis pulmonalis is produced, one of the most destructive diseases in this island." "In cutting into the lungs, a considerable portion of their structure sometimes appears to be changed into a whitish soft matter, somewhat intermediate between a solid and a fluid, like a scrofulous gland just beginning to suppurate."

The clinical side is described as follows: "When tubercles are forming in the lungs but have not advanced to suppuration, they are attended with a slight cough, with occasional difficulty of breathing, and a pulse somewhat accelerated. These are symptoms which commonly usher in phthisis pulmonalis and are frequently overlooked. . . ." "When the tubercles have begun to suppurate and abscesses to be formed, then there is an expectoration of a thick pus which is occasionally tinged with blood, emaciation, debility and . . . hectic fever."

Baillie is sternly objective. There is no hint as to his views (perhaps he had none) on cause, contagion, etc.

2. BAYLE, G. L. Recherches sur la phthisie pulmonaire. Paris: Gabon, 1810.

By this time, the concept of tubercle as a small "tumor" was well established. Now there began an era of lively discussion: Are all tubercles the same? What is the significance of the lesions often seen with tubercle, such as diffuse infiltrations, caseation, and abscess? Are tubercles in other organs the same process as in the lung? What clinical symptoms go with various lesions? How does tubercle arise? Is it contagious? These and many other questions were soon under violent debate, often with special pleading. Bayle was prominent in these discussions and often reported on the subject to the society of the Paris school of medicine. Laënnec frequently refers to his work. However, Bayle's treatise of 428 closely printed pages is rather disappointing, beginning with his definition of the *essential character* of phthisis: "Pulmonary phthisis should include *every lesion of the lung which, left to itself, produces a progressive disorganization of this viscus, in the train of which ulceration supervenes and finally death*" (p. 5). This is a bad start, since this definition obviously includes abscess, tumor, mycoses, etc. Nor is one encouraged by reading (p. 18) that there are six forms of phthisis—tuberculous, granular, melanotic, ulcerous, calculous, and cancerous.

However, under the heading of "Tuberculous Phthisis" there are descriptions of what was doubtless tuberculosis, although there is no clear recognition of evolution from tubercle to cavity. On the whole, Bayle's discussions seem confused, even though there are bits of good description. They are usually impaired, furthermore, by extraneous and inconsequential material. One wonders whether Bayle's reputation as a phthisiologist is not largely due to his recognition by Laënnec, although, actually, Laënnec usually refers to him only to disagree. Certainly Bayle's book is not so satisfying as Baillie's brief discourse on tubercle.

3. CARSON, James. Essays, physiological and practical, pp. 61–65. Liverpool: Printed by F. B. Wright, 1822.

One would hardly mention Carson's recommendation of artificial pneumothorax in pulmonary tuberculosis if it were only a casual suggestion. But in these essays he reports careful physiological experiments in which he recognized the problems of lung elasticity and intrathoracic pressure relations, and he studied artificial pneumothorax in animals. "It is my recollection to have read of cases of consumption having been cured by the chest being deeply wounded in battle. . . . I am now disposed to place in those histories a degree of credit which I confess I did not formerly yield to them. The cure . . . depended upon the reduction of the diseased and wounded lung to a state of collapse. The operation which I have ventured to suggest should be purposely performed, was in these cases, roughly indeed, made by accident." He recognized that sudden total collapse might be risky: "To obviate these dangers, the plain and simple means are to reduce the lung . . . to a state of collapse by degrees only. This might be accomplished, by admitting a small quantity of air into the cavity of the chest at one time, and allowing an interval to exist between the successive admissions." "It has long been my opinion that if ever this disease (consumption) is to be cured, and it is an event of which I am by no means disposed to despair, it must be accomplished by mechanical means, or in other words by a surgical operation."

Carson thought in terms of open pneumothorax, and it was not until years later that closed pneumothorax was developed by Forlanini and others. The history of the whole subject is set forth in Otto Mistal, *Die Vorläufer von Forlanini in der Pneumothorax-Therapie* (Zurich and Leipzig: O. Füssli, 1929), and by L. R. Davidson, M. Furhman, and V. J. Rella, "The precursors of Forlanini and Murphy," Am. Rev. Tuberc., **40**:292, 1939.

4. LAËNNEC, R. T. H. Traité de l'auscultation médiate et des maladies des poumons et du cœur. Seconde édition entièrement refondue. Paris: J. S. Chaudé, 1826.

The second and most complete edition of Laënnec's classic appeared in 1826, the year of his death from consumption. The section on tuberculosis occupies pages 532–728 in Volume 1. It is impossible in a bibliography of this sort to do adequate justice to Laënnec's epoch-making work by brief quotations, so packed with new views are these pages. A brief summary, however, would include the following: using the new methods of physical diagnosis, especially the stethoscope, Laënnec recognized and classified the pulmonary lesions of consumptives during life. He clearly showed the relation of anatomical tubercle to the clinical disease and defined the various types of lesion. As Krause has admirably summarized it ("Essays on tuberculosis," J. Outdoor Life, **15**:6, 1918): "He recognized that the yellow tubercles were a later stage of the small round gray tubercles, that as the small tubercles grew and developed their boundaries joined to form more extensive areas or diffuse changes, that these latter in turn could undergo degeneration, disintegration and liquefaction so that in time cavities might result. In other words, all these varied and apparently dissimilar changes were different phases of the same process—tubercle. There was only one disease —consumption, though its symptomatic manifestations might be as kaleidoscopic as the entire range of medicine itself. Consumption was a unity and tubercle was a unity, and consumption and tubercle were indissolubly linked. And as he gazed at such lungs Laënnec saw even more. The cavity at the top, he taught, must be the oldest process; the yellow, diffuse, cheesy patches lower down must have started later; the numerous minute grayish and yellowish points towards the bottom must be the youngest of all the tubercles. There must have been successive *crops* of tubercles or eruptions as he styled them. He recognized, too, that the changes that were often to be found in the bowels, the kidneys, the bones, the glands and other organs of consumptives were tuberculous."

Laënnec did not believe that tuberculosis was infectious or communicable, but he insisted that the disease was curable, especially in the early stages, contrary to general opinion at the time, but, like most, he felt that there was no doubt about hereditary predisposition.

No student of tuberculosis can afford not to read the original text, the masterly exposition of a genius, or at least a good translation.

5. LOUIS, P. Ch. A. Recherches anatomico-pathologiques sur la phthisie. Paris: Gabon et Cie, 1825.

Louis was one of the greatest of the French clinician-pathologists of the early nineteenth century. He had a remarkable capacity for precise unbiased observation and for clear and beautifully written descriptions. Louis opens his Preface by exclaiming that one may be surprised to "see appear new researches on phthisis following the recent work of Bayle and M. Laënnec" (p. vi). Louis did add, however, a great deal. He paid special attention to tubercle in other organs than the lungs. "These researches," says the report to the Royal Academy of Medicine which precedes the actual text (p. 5), "made with minute care, have led M. Louis to a very important conclusion. None of the 358 subjects which he has autopsied has shown tubercles in any other organ unless they were also present in the lung."

Louis confined his observations to tuberculosis, and it seems to us that he gave a clear over-all picture of the disease hardly surpassed by Laënnec. As a matter of fact, Louis's book appeared in the year preceding Laënnec's second (and best) edition.

The book is in two parts: "Pathologic Anatomy" and "'Symptoms and Treatment." The first part deals systematically with the lesions, illustrated by careful autopsy reports, many of which might well have come from a modern department of pathology. In the second part the clinical features are admirably detailed. The various stages of the disease—early, late, etc.—are discussed, as well as the symptoms of involvement of organs other than the lung.

Louis, like everyone in his day, had only vague ideas of etiology and seems to have taken no definite position about the spread of the disease; at any rate, there is no suggestion that he thought tuberculosis communicable.

The section on treatment is brief. When the symptoms were mild, he ordered "an infusion of lichen, a gummy potion and often a small dose of syrup of diacode to calm the cough and procure a little sleep." Leeches, bleeding, blisters, and all sorts of medicines were tried in more severe cases and for hemoptysis.

As with Laënnec, any serious student of tuberculosis must carefully study Louis's book; one cannot do justice to it in a few words. The report of the committee of the academy (p. 16) concludes: "We think that the Academy, specially charged to give a good direction to medical studies, should encourage the number, always very small, of those who, instead of following the crowd with speculative discussions, devote their lives to gathering observations at the bedside; to seeking after death to trace the disorders which have preceded and led to them; and to deduce from the combination of these facts inescapable conclusions."

It should be emphasized that in this entire era the pathogenesis of anatomical tubercle was completely obscure. Many writers regarded it as the result of "inflammation," although this process itself was only vaguely defined, or as an outgrowth of bronchitis or "peripneumonia." All this was very indefinite. Others regarded tubercle as a local secretion.

6. DELPECH, J. L'Orthomorphie,[1] 1:240. Paris: Gabon, 1828.

Delpech seems to have been the first clearly to distinguish tuberculosis from other diseases of the spine. He points out that tubercles of vertebrae are the cause of the "mal vertébral de Pott." "The state of science is such on this point that it is appropriate today to call this disease tuberculosis of the vertebrae; this will be the first time it has received a characteristic name." There follows an excellent and comprehensive description of the clinical features and pathology, amplified by an atlas of fine illustrations. Every orthopedist should be familiar with Delpech's book.

7. [PAPAVOINE, Louis-Nicolas]. Observations d'arachnitis tuberculeuse; par M. Papavoine, interne des hôpitaux. J. hebd. de méd., 6:113, 1830.

An excellent and comprehensive clinical and pathological description of two cases of tuberculous meningitis, which may be contrasted a century later with the recent report of Lorber on 549 cases (John Lorber, "The results of treatment of 549 cases of tuberculous meningitis," Am. Rev. Tuberc., 69:13, 1954).

8. MORTON, Samuel George. Illustrations of pulmonary consumption, its anatomical characters, causes, symptoms and treatment. Philadelphia: Key & Biddle, 1834.

After the pioneer work of Laënnec and of Louis there was little fundamental advance in the subject until Villemin, thirty years later. Most of the contemporary accounts leaned heavily on the great French authorities. At best, there were amplifications, but no one questioned their basic anatomical findings. As to etiology, contagion, and treatment, on the other hand, there were bitter disputes and strong arguments about trivial points. Therapy had advanced but little beyond medieval empiricism; much of it was supported by the fallacious anecdotal method. Clinical descriptions dealt almost entirely with the advanced disease, with wasting, cavitation, and "hectic" fever.

Morton's treatise should be noted because it is the first book printed in the United States on tuberculosis and because it illustrates very well the above points. "My attention was particularly directed to diseases of the lungs, by an attendance on the clinical lectures of the celebrated Laënnec; who with astonishing acuteness of mind and personal urbanity combined the faculty of imparting a portion of his enthusiasm to all who heard him" (p. viii). There is a systematic discussion of lesions and of symptoms illustrated by autopsies and by

---

[1] Full title: *L'Orthomorphie, par rapport à l'espèce humaine: ou recherches anatomico-pathologiques sur les causes, les moyens de prévenir, ceux de guérir les principales difformités et sur les véritables fondemens de l'art appelé: orthopédique.*

colored plates, in which the author took great pride but which seem crude to the modern eye.

Under "Treatment" there are advised, for various indications, bleeding, spirits of turpentine, elixir of vitriol, common salt, opium, sugar of lead, cupping, blisters, issues, rest, gum water, farinaceous food, infusion of sage, prussic acid, digitalis, iodine, uva ursi, sarsaparilla, fumigation from boiling tar and potash ("in truth I have seen it act like a charm," p. 135). There are prescriptions about diet, clothing, exercise, and climate ("a mixture of sea and land air is unfavorable to delicate lungs," p. 145). "Nothing seems to exert a more decidedly favorable influence on the lungs than unmixed sea-air" (p. 150). "Although consumption makes its chief havoc among the poor and the miserable, we often see it invade, without distinction, the abodes of temperance, of refinement and of luxury, and number among its victims the young, the accomplished and the beautiful! The reason is obvious. The midnight application of the student, the imprudence of dress so common among fashionable females, and the various excesses which too often form a part of the recreation of the wealthy, produce those same liabilities to consumption, which, though from different causes, are entailed upon the indigent and the miserable" (p. 164).

9. CLARK, James. A treatise on pulmonary consumption. London, 1835. (American edition, from which we quote [Philadelphia: Carey, Lea & Blanchard, 1835].)

The comments made on Morton's treatise apply equally to Clark's. The latter's claim to distinction was his great emphasis on prevention. He was a pioneer in public health. In the Dedication of his book to Leopold I, king of the Belgians, he says: "It is only by convincing the public of the comparative futility of all attempts to cure consumption and of the signal efficacy of proper measures directed to prevent it that physicians can ever hope to produce those beneficial results in improving public health and in preserving and prolonging human life, which it is the distinguishing privilege of their profession to am at" (p. iii). And from the Preface (p. vii): "My great aim has been to point out the nature and causes of the constitutional affection in which tuberculous diseases have their origins, and on those to found rules for prevention and treatment." But, since Clark had no idea that the disease was infectious or communicable but thought that it "has its origin in a morbid state of the constitution," his praiseworthy ideas could not be put into very successful practice, although some of them happen to coincide with more rational procedures. Clark made useful statistical studies in trying to get at the cause of tuberculosis. He pointed out the pulmonary changes which occurred in workers in dusty trades such as miners and stonemasons, and he undoubtedly described silicosis and silicotuberculosis. But shoemakers, tailors, and weavers were thought prone to tuberculosis because of their sedentary employment and strained posture, whereas seamen, butchers, and tanners were considered more or less exempt because of the "free and regular exercise in the open air which they enjoy." There is an interesting chapter on tuberculous disease in animals. As to cause, almost every conceivable circumstance is mentioned except contagion. "The view which I take of tuberculous cachexia, without which, in my opinion, tuberculous disease of the lungs can not occur, leads me entirely to disbelieve that consumption can be communicated by contagion" (p. 182). Obviously, then, Clark's rules for prevention had no rational basis. He urged that members of families "predisposed to tuberculosis" should not marry because their tuberculous constitution was thought hereditary. "By placing the predisposed child in the most favorable circumstances as regards those agents which exert a constant influence on the health such as food, air, exercise, etc. . . . we may improve the constitution so as to overcome the hereditary predisposition" (p. 207). As to actual therapy, Clark was no better than Morton: the use of emetics in tuberculosis, for example, fills nine pages (pp. 255–64).

10. TROUSSEAU, A., and BELLOC, H. Traité pratique de la phthisie laryngée, etc. Paris: J.-B. Baillière, 1837.

Although this book has been referred to as if it dealt entirely with tuberculosis of the larynx, the authors used phthisis in the general sense, common at that time, of a wasting disease. Actually, only a few pages are devoted to laryngeal tuberculosis, mainly in the form of case reports. These are done, however, in masterly fashion, and there can be no doubt that the authors were dealing with advanced laryngeal lesions in association with pulmonary tuberculosis. These are well illustrated by plates and are clearly distinguished from cancerous, syphilitic, and other forms of laryngeal phthisis. This monograph of nearly five hundred pages is done in Trousseau's best style and was "crowned" by the academy. It brought order where confusion had existed, although Louis and others had had something to say on the subject.

11. BODINGTON, George. An essay on the treatment and cure of pulmonary consumption, on principles natural, rational and successful. London: Longman, Orme, Brown, Greene & Longmans, 1840; also reprinted by the New Sydenham Society *in* Selected essays and monographs (1891).

This essay is a landmark in the history of the treatment of pulmonary consumption. The writer was the first to discredit completely the irrational and useless current methods of treatment: bleeding, tartar emetic, digitalis, demulcents, blisters, leeches, and plasters. Although Bodington's basis for therapy was actually meaningless as we see it today ("the main ground of the treatment has been to preserve or restore to a normal condition the functions of the nervous filaments interwoven with the substance of the lungs, and exercising influence over the capillary system and other parts of the organization"), what he proposed agreed essentially with the best modern management up to the time of surgery and antibiotics. His plan consisted of quiet residence in the country with plenty of fresh air, easing of stress, moderate exercise, an abundant simple diet, and sedatives. There are case reports of patients with advanced disease who recovered under this program, which antedated Brehmer, Dettweiler, and Trudeau by a good many years.

12. RAYER, P. Traité des maladies des reins, etc., **3**:618. Paris: J.-B. Baillière, 1841.

Rayer seems to have been the first to present a comprehensive description of the various forms of tuberculosis of the kidney, ureter, and bladder. In fifty-seven pages the literature is reviewed, the pathology is described, and there are excellent case reports and illustrations.

13. VIRCHOW, Rud. Ueber die Verschiedenheit von Phthise und Tuberculose, Verhandl. d. phys.-med. Gesellsch. Würzburg, **3**:98, 1852.
Virchow criticized Laënnec's views on tuberculosis and insisted on the non-
identity of phthisis and tuberculosis. To the modern student this seven-page
discussion seems almost absurd, since it is based on anatomical criteria which
are meaningless now. Virchow did perhaps rightly claim that Laënnec centered
too much attention on the lungs when tuberculosis was actually a widespread
disease, but, on the whole, he confused and held back the subject until Villemin's transmission experiments. But when one realizes that even today the
various gross appearances of tuberculosis, cancer, and pyogenic and mycotic infections may be confused and that cavitation may take place in tumor, as well
as in tuberculosis or pyogenic infection, Virchow's position does not seem too
illogical. It was perhaps because Virchow knew so much that he became confused.
Virchow's doctrine may be briefly summarized somewhat as follows: The
diffuse, caseating pulmonary lesions described by Laënnec may develop out of
all sorts of lung disease, such as ordinary pneumonia or bronchitis. When these
diffuse lesions occur, the patient has the clinical features of consumption. Discrete small tubercles are something else and have nothing to do with consumption, although they are harmful, and the combination of tubercle and consumption is considered especially serious. Or as Niemeyer said, "The worst thing
that can happen to a consumptive is that he become tuberculous."

14. JAEGER, Eduard. Ueber Choroidealtuberkel, Oesterreich. Ztschr. f.
prakt. Heilk., **1**:9, 1855.
This seems to be the first description of choroidal tubercles. Although brief,
everything worthwhile is said. The tubercles are described as seen with the
ophthalmoscope and at autopsy. It is pointed out that they cause no eye symptoms unless in the macular region. The author raises the question of whether
tuberculosis cannot be diagnosed earlier by recognition of choroidal tubercles
than by other methods.
Choroidal tubercles must have been much more common in the days of extensive disseminated tuberculosis than at present.

15. BREHMER, Herrmann. Die chronische Lungenschwindsucht. Berlin:
Th. Chr. Fr. Enslin, 1857.
The key to Brehmer's character is found on the title page of this book, where
he says of it, "For unprejudiced doctors and critically thinking laymen," and
below: "Motto: In the natural sciences the authority of thousands cannot con-
tradict the simple reasoning of a single man."
Was Brehmer a quack or only an enthusiast? In this his first book—a mass of
pseudo-physiology and superficial rationalism—he may well scoff at the ridiculous ideas of others, but this is hardly a defense of his own. "The abnormally
small heart, the weakness of its walls are the one and only cause of acquired
tuberculosis and consumption" (p. 69). On an elaboration of this thesis he built
up his cosmos of therapy—life in the mountains with a special course of feeding
and of baths. He developed, one after another the great sanatoria of Görbersdorf
in the Silesian "Riesengebirge." Under his system, at a time when consumption
was thought incurable, many of the tuberculous undoubtedly got well; he em-

phasized starting treatment in early cases, and some of his patients probably did not have tuberculosis at all. Like most of the successful sanatorium men, his follower Dettweiler, Trudeau at Saranac, and in modern times others such as Peers of Colfax and Pottenger of Monrovia, he had a tremendous personality. Morale, faith, and hope no doubt played their part in Brehmer's cures, but we can find no shred of rational basis in what he did other than the elimination of the old harmful nostrums and depleting measures, together with a certain amount of rest, although this was not carried out as a purposeful measure. Brehmer reported some of his cases from time to time ("Zur Therapie der chronische Tuberculose," Deutsche Klin., **17**:126, 1865) and later wrote another book (*Die Therapie der chronischen Lungenschwindsucht* [Wiesbaden: J. F. Bergmann, 1887]) as enthusiastic, as polemical, and with as little sound basis as his earlier essay. Like most men of this sort, he was a fighter with a chip on his shoulder and, despite his uncompromising vigor, somewhat on the defensive. Much has been written about Brehmer, mostly with admiration or even reverence, although he was at first scoffed at. Now his work is often approached as one might a shrine. Certainly many of his patients worshiped him. His influence has dominated all subsequent sanatoria and open-air methods of treatment (see, for example, Hugh M. Kinghorn, "Herrmann Brehmer," Tr. Am. Climat. & Clin. A., **37**:193, 1921; Vincent Y. Bowditch, "Visits to Brehmer's and Dettweiler's sanatoria," J. Outdoor Life, **16**:65, 1919).

16. BUHL, [Ludwig]. Bericht über 280 Leichenöffnungen, Ztschr. f. rat. Med., **8**:1, 1857.

Buhl seems to have been the first to emphasize the fact that miliary tuberculosis resulted, by blood-borne dissemination, from an earlier focus. "Miliary tuberculosis appears, therefore, to be a specific infectious disease and has the same relation to its portals of entry as pyemia with its multiple abscesses has to a primary focus of suppuration or acute miliary carcinosis has to its primary growth" (p. 50). In a later paper ("Psoasabscess mit nachgefolgter Miliartuberculose," Wien. med. Wchnschr., **9**:195, 1859) by Buhl's associates, it is stated that "a special poison, the tuberculous element, enters the blood from a caseous or suppurative focus and sets up at innumerable points" military tubercules. These were advanced views which implied an infectious agent, but the matter was still controversial when Buhl's book was published years later (Ludwig Buhl, *Lungenentzündung, Tuberculose und Schwindsucht* [Munich: Rudolph Oldenbourg, 1872], see pp. 112–14). It was Weigert, however, who first described the ulceration of tuberculous foci into the thoracic duct and vena cava ("Die anatomischen Wege des Tuberkelgiftes," Wien. med. Presse, **24**:1373, 1883).

17. VILLEMIN, J. A. Du tubercle au point de vue de son siège, de son évolution et de sa nature. Paris: J.-B. Baillière et fils, 1862.

With the great school of French clinician-pathologists of the early nineteenth century there arose a vast literature on the morbid anatomy of disease. Following Laënnec, innumerable discussions on "tubercle" appeared, most of which are unreadable and meaningless to the modern student. The great Virchow had confused, not clarified, the issue (Ref. 13). Villemin, later to do epoch-making work on transmission (Ref. 18), gives no indication in this little monograph, written only three years earlier, that he considered tubercle communicable. But in this systematic anatomical study he clearly points out that caseation and calcification are later stages of what begins as tubercle. He did not regard the process as a specific disease but thought the sequence might occur in any inflammation. He noted, however, the frequency of tubercle in the lungs and lymph nodes.

We cannot reprint Villemin's thirty-five general conclusions which occupy four pages of his book. A few, however, are as follows: (II) "Later one sees that these tuberculiform processes have a common property: that of transforming themselves after a while into a material of peculiar consistency, which one compares to cheese and to which one applies the epithet *caseous.*" (V) "From this point on, *caseous matter* and *tubercle* become synonymous." (XVI) "The tuberculous process passes thus through fatty, caseous and calcific stages, but this property is not specific (to tuberculosis), it is general to all organic matter." (XXXI) "The intensity of the cause which produces tubercle does not affirm itself by the size of the morbid lesions but by their multiplication and their generalization through the whole economy."

One senses in the record of these dark gropings some confused glimpses of the truth, but no further real progress could be made until communicability of a specific lesion was proved. That was Villemin's great contribution. Up to this point he seems far behind Laënnec.

18. VILLEMIN, J. A. Cause et nature de la tuberculose, Bull. Acad. de méd., Paris, **31**:211, 1865.

From long study of the clinical and pathological features of tuberculosis, Villemin became convinced that "tuberculosis is the result of a specific causal agent, in other words a virus. This agent should be found in the morbid products which it has produced by direct action on the normal elements of the affected tissues. Introduced into a susceptible organism, it should then reproduce itself and, at the same time, the disease of which it is the determining cause." He then presented proof that this was true by a series of precise experiments. This work was so epoch-making that we shall quote in detail from one of the many observations:

"First series of experiments. . . . On March 6 we took two young rabbits about 3 weeks old. . . . In one of these rabbits we made a little wound behind the ear and inserted two small fragments of tubercle and a little purulent liquid taken from a cavity in the lung of a tuberculous man dead 23 hours. . . . On March 30 and April 4 we repeated the inoculations. . . . June 20 we sacrificed the two rabbits. We found in the inoculated one . . . [that] the lungs are filled with large tuberculous masses formed by the agglomeration of several granulations. The control rabbit . . . *showed absolutely no tubercle.*"

Villemin's conclusions from many similar experiments were: "Tuberculosis is a specific affection. Its cause resides in an inoculable agent. Inoculation from man to rabbit works very well. Tuberculosis belongs, then, to the class of virulent diseases and should be placed in the nosological framework side by side with syphilis but even closer to glanders."

In a second paper ("Cause et nature de la tuberculose," Bull. Acad. de méd., Paris, **32**:152, 1866) Villemin continued and elaborated his first experiments. He pointed out, first, that true tuberculosis was pretty much confined to man, monkey, cattle, and rabbit; he believed that so-called tubercles in other animals were due to parasites. He now made systematic studies on inoculation from man to rabbit, cow to rabbit, rabbit to rabbit, man to guinea pig (*cochon d'Inde*). These were all successful, but inoculations from man to dog, cat, sheep, and fowl failed to produce definite tuberculosis.

Villemin's work was so novel and so important, if true, that the academy appointed a commission to appraise it critically. In a long report ("Rapport sur deux communications de M. Villemin ayant pour titre: 'Cause et nature de la tuberculose'—*Commissaires:* MM. Louis, Grisolle, H. Bouley et G. Colin, *rapporteur,*" Bull. Acad. de méd., Paris, **32**:897, 1867), Colin reported that the commission had confirmed and verified Villemin's work and concluded: "Consequently, it [the academy] has the honor to propose:

"1. That the author of the two lectures on tuberculization be thanked;

"2. That he be invited to pursue the studies which he has so well begun;

"3. And, finally, to recommend his work, or at least the unpublished part of it, to your committee for publication."

Thus Villemin was promptly vindicated, and the current textbook legend that he fought for years for recognition by the Paris medical authorities is obviously incorrect.

In the same session of the academy at which Villemin's second report was presented, Lebert ("Quelques expériences sur la transmission par inoculation des tubercles par M. le professeur H. Lebert, à Breslau," p. 119) reported his experiences on the transmission of tubercle, which he clearly reproduced in guinea pigs and rabbits inoculated with human material. Lebert made the valuable observation that, while the lesions varied in the donor, they were quite similar in the recipient animals. Lebert stated that his experiments had been going on for years; no mention was made of Villemin's report of the year before. Nor was there mention of any experimental work in Lebert's large and excellent treatise on tuberculosis (H. Lebert, *Traité pratique des maladies scrofuleuses et tuberculeuses* [Paris: J.-B. Baillière, 1849]).

19. VILLEMIN, J. A. Études sur la tuberculose. Paris: J.-B. Baillière et fils, 1868.

In this monograph of over six hundred pages Villemin elaborated all his work on tuberculosis—clinical, pathological, and experimental. "These experiments prove the great analogy between tuberculosis and the best-understood virulent diseases. The evolution of tubercle depends on the point of inoculation, the time which elapses between the moment of this inoculation and tuberculous eruptions in various organs . . . the initial tubercle developing at the point of insertion of the virulent material becomes the source of the generalization of the disease, just as in syphilis."

One can readily understand the immense importance of Villemin's work.

20. [CHAUVEAU, A.]. Tuberculose expérimentalement produite par l'ingestion de viande tuberculeuse: par M. le professeur Chauveau (résumé d'une lecture faite à l'Académie de Médecine), Gaz. méd. Lyon, **20**:550, 1868.

The transmission experiments of Villemin were not yet generally accepted. Strong support for the communicability of tuberculosis was given by the observations of Chauveau, a veterinarian who fed tuberculous material to young healthy calves. They soon became ill, and when they were sacrificed on the fifty-second day, there were found "the most beautiful lesions of generalized tuberculosis with marked predominance in the intestine and mesentery." The lungs also were studded with tubercles. Chauveau raised the question, then, whether the portal of entry for tuberculosis might not be by way of the digestive tract as well as the lungs, which had previously been regarded as paramount. He immediately saw and emphasized the public health aspects and the dangers "against which it is important to take sanitary police measures." Chauveau's work raised a storm of protest in some quarters, mainly because of the dangerous implications to man.

The early literature on the whole question of contagion of tuberculosis by ingestion as well as by inhalation is vividly analyzed by Krause ("Essays on tuberculosis," J. Outdoor Life, **15**:295, 1918).

21. LANGHANS, Th. Ueber Riesenzellen mit wandständigen Kernen in Tuberkeln und die fibröse Form des Tuberkels, Virchows Arch. f. path. Anat., **42**:382, 1868.

It is difficult to decide from the vast literature who deserves credit for the first adequate histological description of tubercle. Certain it is that the earlier accounts, such as those of G. Gluge (*Atlas der pathologischen Anatomie* [Jena: F. Manke, 1850]), are entirely inadequate. Langhans, at any rate, first clearly emphasized the characteristic giant cell of tubercle, but his pictures are really quite deficient and reflect the primitive histological methods of the day.

22. [VILLEMIN, Jean Antoine]. De la propagation de la phthisie, par le docteur Villemin, professeur au Val-de-Grâce: mémoire lu à l'Académie de Médecine, dans sa séance du 13 avril 1869, Gaz. hebd. de méd., **6**:260, 1869.

Here Villemin reports fundamentally new experiments. He now made subcutaneous injections of fresh sputum into rabbits and also injections of dried powdered sputum. Typical lesions were produced in all the animals. He also showed that, while fresh dried sputum caused lesions, it lost its "inoculability" if the sputum stood for several days before desiccation or if the sputum was dried too long before injection. Infectious material fed or introduced by stomach tube yielded typical lesions, but injections of sweat from tuberculous patients failed to transmit the disease. "Tubercle and expectorated material from the tuberculous behave like virulent substances; they produce tuberculosis by inoculation and by absorption through the natural routes (digestive, respiratory). . . . But what one must never forget in the production of every transmissible disease is that there are two factors: the morbid germ, on the one hand, and the more or less great susceptibility of the organism. It is because one pays no attention to the second that one goes wrong" and blames on anger, fear, fatigue, etc., "nearly every disease such as typhoid, typhus, plague, cholera, as well as scurvy, pellagra, glanders, phthisis, cancer, etc."

23. GERLACH, A. C. Ueber die Impfbarkeit der Tuberculose und der Perlsucht bei Thieren, sowie über die Uebertragbarkeit der letzteren durch Fütterung, Virchows Arch. f. path. Anat., **51**:290, 1870.

The work of Gerlach is a milestone in the understanding of the transmission of tuberculosis and of the significance of bovine tuberculosis. Gerlach first set about to confirm Villemin's experiments, which he did by inoculating into animals material from tuberculous cows. He then turned his attention to milk. Milk from an old tuberculous cow whose disease (*Perlsucht*) was confirmed at autopsy was fed to five animals representing four different species. All developed typical tuberculous lesions. The mesenteric nodes were invariably much enlarged and seemed to represent the oldest lesion, although there were changes in the lungs and elsewhere. Gerlach quite justly concluded that he had produced tubercle and that "Perlsucht," i.e., bovine tuberculosis, was probably the same disease as human tuberculosis. He promptly saw the public health implications—that milk of doubtful origin was no longer safe as a "wet nurse" for children, nor was it safe to eat flesh, even if cooked, of cattle who might be tuberculous. He pointed the way to the extirpation of bovine tuberculosis. The revolutionary character of these observations is clear when one realizes that at the time "Perlsucht" of cattle had been completely exonerated as a source of human tuberculosis.

The correctness of Gerlach's claims was not immediately recognized, nor did everyone accept the tremendous public health implications. A bitter controversy was waged for many years before everyone was convinced by the finding of tubercle bacilli in the udders of cows. The work of T. Smith (Ref. 45) on the different reactions of animals to human and bovine tubercle bacilli helped greatly to clear up some of the misunderstandings. It is of interest that a great deal of this work was done by veterinarians.

The whole subject is skilfully analyzed by A. Krause ("Essays on tuberculosis," J. Outdoor Life, **15**:295, 327, 1918).

24. ARMANINI, Luciano. Sulla specificità e virulenza della sostanze caseose e tuberculose: richerche sperimentali, Movimento med.-chir., **4**:233, 1872.

Although Villemin's great work on transmission of tuberculosis now seems unassailable, it was by no means generally accepted at the time. A huge controversial literature arose, and many able workers thought that they could explain Villemin's findings on other grounds than the transfer of a living virus. To Armanini seems to go the credit for the use of a method later employed by Cohnheim (Ref. 26), which went far to prove transmissibility. Armanini scarified the corneas of guinea pigs with a needle dipped in tuberculous material. At the end of ten days no lesion was apparent. But on the twentieth day small gray nodules which were undoubtedly tubercles appeared, although Armanini himself was conservative in interpreting the findings. This was only a part of Armanini's extensive transmission experiments. The paper is comprehensive and gives full credit to previous workers in other countries. It deserves to be reprinted in English.

25. [PARROT, Joseph Marie Jules]. Abstract of report at the meeting of October 28, 1876, Compt. rend. Soc. de biol., **28**:308, 1876.

The definition of the primary pulmonary lesion of childhood tuberculosis is usually attributed to Ghon (Ref. 53), but he himself disclaimed credit for priority and pointed out that Parrot, as early as 1876, had fully recognized and described the focus in the lung and the associated hilar adenopathy. Parrot's brief communication is very much to the point. He showed that in children (one to seven years old) every tuberculous hilar node is associated with a pulmonary focus, which usually appears the older of the two. Previous students had, in the main, believed that hilar nodes occurred without any lung lesion or that the two might be quite independent. Parrot pointed out the need for meticulous search through the lung if the primary focus was to be found. "At this time of life there is no affection of the lung which is not reflected in the bronchial nodes; they are, as it were, the mirror of the lungs and vice versa. There is no bronchial node adenopathy which does not have a pulmonary origin."

The subject is extensively developed in Georges Küss's book (*De l'hérédité parasitaire de la tuberculose humaine* [Paris, 1898]). Küss reviews the older literature and adds many observations of his own, although the book deals primarily with the question of hereditary tuberculosis.

26. [COHNHEIM, J., and SALOMONSEN]. Reports on experimental tuberculosis, Jahresb. d. Schles. Gesellsch. f. vaterl. Kult., **55**:222, 1877.

Cohnheim was apparently unaware of Armanini's work (Ref. 24) on experimental ocular tuberculosis. The method may, however, have been suggested to him by the work of W. Goldzieher ("Ueber Implantationen in die vordere Augenkammer," Arch. f. exper. Path. u. Pharmakol., **2**:387, 1874), although Goldzieher's experiments dealt with foreign bodies, poisons, etc., and not with infectious material. In this brief report Cohnheim and Salomonsen described the introduction of minute particles of tuberculous material into the anterior chamber of rabbits. As in Armanini's work, the eyes were perfectly clear for a few days, but, after about 2 weeks, there "suddenly appeared in the tissue of the iris one or more tiny light gray nodules." They concluded "(1) that inoculation tuberculosis develops independently of traumatic inflammation and (2) that inoculation tuberculosis has an incubation period in the rabbit of something over 3 weeks."

This work, sponsored by the great German pathologist, went far toward convincing everyone of the transmissibility of tuberculosis. Salomonsen reported the experiments in great detail ("Om Impodning af Tuberculose, särligt; Kaninens iris," Nord. med. ark., **11**:1, 1879), and Cohnheim himself summarized them in his little monograph, *Die Tuberculose vom Standpunkte der Infectionslehre* (Leipzig, 1880). K. Schuchardt finally ("Die Impftuberculose des Auges und ihr Zusammenhang mit der allgemeinen Impftuberculose," Virchows Arch. f. path. Anat., **88**:28, 1882) reviewed the whole subject and analyzed the relation of experimental ocular tuberculosis to generalized experimental lesions.

27. DETTWEILER, P. Die Behandlung der Lungenschwindsucht, in geschlossenen Heilanstalten mit besonderer Beziehung auf Falkenstein i/T. Berlin: G. Reimer, 1880.

Dettweiler, patient and pupil of Brehmer (Ref. 15), is credited with being the first systematically to use complete rest in the treatment of pulmonary tuberculosis. He had no idea, however, that healing of the tuberculous process could be directly promoted by rest but prescribed it for incidental difficulties such as "heart weaknesses" or "severe anemia." If these were marked, he had the patient recline all day in the open air on a comfortable couch. Breathing exercises and mountain climbing are discussed only in relation to their effect on the heart. This treatise of 129 pages, somewhat ponderously written, also stresses plenty of food and goes into innumerable other facets of the cure as practiced at Falkenstein. The influence of Brehmer is clearly evident.

It seems obvious that the rational and purposeful use of rest in pulmonary tuberculosis should be credited to Trudeau (Ref. 55) rather than to Dettweiler. The latter, however, clearly emphasized fresh air and the "outdoor life" and the morale factor in sanitarium life.

Later Dettweiler ("Die Therapie der Phthisis," Verhandl. d. Kong. f. inn. Med., Wiesbaden, **6**:13, 1887) gave a comprehensive lecture on treatment in which he emphasized the same points: liberal upbuilding diet,[2] fresh air, morale, and rest.

Pratt, a modern exponent of the home rest cure, gives a fine summary of the whole subject (J. H. Pratt, "The importance of prolonged bed rest in the treatment of pulmonary tuberculosis," Am. Rev. Tuberc., **1**:637, 1917).

    28. KOCH, Robert. Die Aetiologie der Tuberculose, Berl. klin. Wchnschr., **19**:221, 1882.

Koch's work ranks with that of Laënnec and Villemin as one of the greatest achievements in the study of tuberculosis. Koch had convinced himself, as a result of the work of Villemin, of Cohnheim, and of others, that the dread disease was communicable and was caused by a living "virus." The "bacteriological era" was at its peak, and new organisms were being isolated right and left. Koch was the master technician; he was an expert in staining and in pathological tissue technique. He deliberately set about to demonstrate the organisms of tuberculosis, which he felt must exist. His first stroke of genius, when ordinary stains showed nothing, was to add potash to his methylene blue to intensify its effect, and then there were revealed in tuberculous tissues of all sorts, from man and animal, many typical slender bacilli. Koch noted that these were usually "pure" and that no cocci of the common sort were present to indicate contamination.

Koch then set about growing the bacilli. He used coagulated serum (this was not his own idea), but again his genius was revealed by his patience in waiting several weeks for growth to occur. All known bacteria, at the time, appeared in culture media within a few days; if nothing was visible, the cultures were usually discarded. Just what went on in Koch's mind to make him preserve his cultures of tuberculous material and patiently wait for several weeks he does not say. Perhaps he forgot to discard them, or perhaps he did not know himself; therein lay his genius.

  [2] A dinner at Falkenstein was as follows:

DECEMBER 16

Potato soup
Rabbit ragout with noodles
Filet sauté au madeire. Cauliflower
Stewed duck, salad, compote
Apricot torte. Fruit, etc.

The next step was to inoculate by various routes—subcutaneous, intraperitoneal, intraocular—into animals bacilli which had been subcultured several times. In all these elaborate and conclusive experiments, typical tubercle was produced, just as with inoculation of tuberculous material direct from lesions. And, finally, tubercle bacilli were once more grown from the lesions produced by inoculation with pure cultures. The paper is a masterpiece of exposition and does not leave much more to be said. Indeed, after Koch had read his report at the meeting of the Physiological Society in Berlin on March 24, 1882, when the chairman called for discussion, everyone was silent—even the great Virchow, whose tenacious views about the non-unity of tuberculous lesions were finally shattered.

In his concluding remarks Koch pointed out that tubercle bacilli could be derived only from the animal organism, and he believed that the portal of entry must usually be by inhalation of dust. He found that *dry* sputa retained their virulence for several weeks. Finally, he pointed out the public health aspect and declared that the basic knowledge was now at hand for a logical and successful campaign against tuberculosis.

An excellent and accurate translation of Koch's paper, with a stimulating introduction by Allen Krause, is to be found in the American Review of Tuberculosis (The aetiology of tuberculosis, Dr. Robert Koch, a translation, by Bertha Pinner and Max Pinner," **24**:285, 1932).

29. [EHRLICH, Paul]. Aus dem Verein für innere Medicin zu Berlin. Sitzung vom 1 Mai 1882 (stenographic report of a talk by Ehrlich at the previous meeting), Deutsche med. Wchnschr., **8**:269, 1882.

Ehrlich, later to become renowned in the fields of immunity and chemotherapy, was interested in stains, probably through the influence of his cousin Weigert, the pathologist. Koch had hardly announced his work when Ehrlich set about to improve the difficult staining technique of tubercle bacilli. He found that "analinöl" added to a saturated alcoholic solution of fuchsin or methyl violet made an excellent stain. It shortened the process by many hours, and the specimens were better preserved. He also established the principle of the acid-fastness of tubercle bacilli by decolorizing his preparations with a mixture of one part of nitric acid and two parts of water and finding that the organisms remained brilliantly stained. He pointed out that the capsule seemed impermeable to acid and that therefore alkalis should be effective in destroying the bacilli.

F. Ziehl ("Zur Färbung des Tuberkelbacillus," Deutsche med. Wchnschr., **8**:451, 1882) modified the Ehrlich procedure by using carbolic acid instead of aniline and a weaker acid for decolorization. The contemporary strivings for better straining methods are well summarized by B. Fränkel ("Ueber die Färbung des Koch'schen Bacillus und seine semiotische Bedeutung für die Krankheiten der Respirationsorgane," Berl. klin. Wchschr., **21**:193, 1884).

We cannot go further into the staining and morphology of tubercle bacilli in this bibliography, but the problem is fully discussed in H. G. Wells, L. M. De Witt, and E. R. Long, *The Chemistry of Tuberculosis* (Baltimore: Williams & Wilkins Co., 1923); and in H. S. Willis and M. M. Cummings, *Diagnostic and Experimental Methods in Tuberculosis* (Springfield, Ill.: Charles C Thomas, 1952).

30. FORLANINI, C. A contribuzione della terapia chirurgica della tisi. Ablazione del polmone? Pneumotorace artificiale? Gazz. d. osp., **3**:537, 585, 601, 609, 617, 641, 657, 665, 689, 705, 1882.[3]

Although there had been some previous suggestions (Ref. 3), credit is generally given to Forlanini for popularizing the procedure of induced closed pneumothorax. This, his first paper or, rather, series of papers was, however, long, rambling, and philosophical, with little factual material; artificial pneumothorax by no means immediately came into popular use, and it was only many years later that Forlanini's important monograph defining indications, technique, and results appeared (C. Forlanini, "Die Behandlung der Lungenschwindsucht mit den künstlichen Pneumothorax," Ergebn. inn. Med. u. Kinderh., **9**:621, 1912). The whole subject is reviewed by Eli H. Rubin ("Pneumothorax treatment of pulmonary tuberculosis," Medicine, **16**:351, 1937) with nearly three hundred references. Forlanini's original paper has been translated into English (S. Lojacano, "Forlanini's original communication on artificial pneumothorax," Tubercle, **16**:54, 1934). Extra-pleural pneumonolysis, which falls in the domain of collapse therapy, is comprehensively reviewed by Arthur H. Aufses, "Extrapleural pneumonolysis in the treatment of pulmonary tuberculosis," Medicine, **18**:129, 1939.

It is of interest that pneumothorax, for so many years one of the mainstays of treatment in pulmonary tuberculosis, is now (1954) becoming obsolete. As the lush Mississippi steamboats vanished practically overnight when the railroad was built along the river, so antibiotics and resection are rapidly crowding out pneumothorax, the disadvantages of which are being more and more emphasized. Actually, Forlanini raised the question in 1882 of whether resection would not ultimately be an important method of therapy.

The history of artificial pneumothorax in America is vividly told by James J. Waring (J. Outdoor Life, **30**:305, 1933).

31. BOLLINGER, O. Ueber Tuberkelbacillen im Euter einer tuberculösen Kuh und über die Virulenz des Secretes einer derartig erkrankten Milchdrüse, Ärztl. Intelligenzbl., **30**:163, 1883.

This brief paper was of fundamental importance in the controversy as to whether milk from tuberculous cows was a source of the disease. Bollinger had already shown that a few drops of such milk sufficed on injection to kill a guinea pig in a few weeks. He and his associates in the Munich Pathological Institute now examined a diseased udder from a tuberculous cow, in the tissues and secretions of which they demonstrated innumerable bacteria which had "all the characteristics of tubercle bacilli." Lesions produced in guinea pigs by this material again showed typical tubercle bacilli.

[3] Forlanini's articles on artificial pneumothorax actually appeared in the journal Gazzetta degli ospitali. Curiously enough, Lojacano states in his literal translation in Tubercle that the journal was the Gazetta degli ospadeli e delle cliniche di Milano of the same date. This error has been repeated in the bibliography of Rubin's article. The explanation of this odd mistake is that the Gazzetta degli ospitali in 1895 changed its name to the longer and more pompous title of Gazetta degli ospedali, etc. The error is the same as giving credit to the New England Journal of Medicine for an article which appeared in its predecessor, the Boston Medical and Surgical Journal.

32. KOCH, R. Die Aetiologie der Tuberculose, Mitt. a. d. k. Gsndhtsamte, Berlin, **2**:1, 1884.

In this important article of eighty-six folio pages Koch made his definitive presentation of the discovery and isolation of the tubercle bacillus and the proof of its causal relation to the disease. It is really a masterful elaboration of his preliminary communication. As Krause has well put it (J. Outdoor Life, **15**:109, 1918): "Years have slipped by since then, and in this time a tremendous lot of grist has gone through the tuberculosis mill. But today Koch's great work . . . remains what it was when it first saw the light: as regards the character and life history of the tubercle bacillus, complete and unassailable in every detail, without a flaw, without a leak to be plugged." Koch also discussed the clinical and anatomical features of various forms of spontaneous tuberculosis in man and in animals. This treatise is undoubtedly one of the great pieces of medical writing of all time. It should be read and the beautiful plates examined by every doctor.

33. STRASSMANN, Fritz. Ueber Tuberculose der Tonsillen, Virchows Arch. f. path. Anat., **96**:319, 1884.

In any discussion of the portal of entry of the tubercle bacillus the question of tonsillar involvement is paramount. Strassmann found a high incidence of small tubercles in the tonsils from cadavers which showed extensive lesions of various organs, usually with cavitation of the lungs. In only one case was caseation of glands of the neck noted. In tonsils excised during life, S. J. Crowe, S. S. Watkins, and A. S. Rothholz ("Relation of tonsillar and nasopharyngeal infections to general systemic disorders," Bull. Johns Hopkins Hosp., **28**:1, 1917) found that 4–8 per cent showed tuberculosis, in some cases extensive and with caseation. In over half the patients with tuberculous tonsils, there was clinical evidence of tuberculous glands of the neck. These observations emphasized the tonsil as perhaps an important portal of entry for the tubercle bacillus.

34. BAUMGARTEN, I. Die Histogenese des tuberculösen Processes, Centralbl. f. klin. Med., **5**:233, 1884.

By studying material derived from the anterior chamber of the eyes of rabbits which had been inoculated with tubercle bacilli, Baumgarten gave the first comprehensive and correct interpretation of the histology of tubercle. He showed that epithelial and giant cells arise from fixed tissue cells and not from the colorless blood corpuscles, as had been previously claimed.

Study of this subject has continued through the years (see, for example, Arthur J. Vorwald, "The early cellular reactions in the lungs of rabbits injected intravenously with human tubercle bacilli," Am. Rev. Tuberc., **25**:74, 1932; Florence R. Sabin, "Cellular studies in tuberculosis," Am. Rev. Tuberc., **25**:153; Esmond R. Long, "The inflammatory reaction in tuberculosis," Am. J.M. Sc., **185**:749, 1933).

35. DE CÉRENVILLE, [Édouard]. De l'intervention opératoire dans les maladies du poumon, Rev. méd. de la Suisse rom., **5**:441, 1885.

It is difficult to trace priority in connection with thoracoplasty for tuberculosis, since the procedure was really an outgrowth of the general concept of collapse therapy. Collapse operations, also, were not originally designed exclusively for tuberculosis but were tried in all sorts of pulmonary suppurations. De Cérenville, however, clearly grasped the concept that rib resection might be practiced not only as an approach to drainage of a cavity but for its value as a collapse measure. "Ablation of the ribs achieved an important mechanical effect. This mechanical factor is the *retraction of the thorax* indispensable in certain instances for complete success." "In another case of tuberculous cavity with resection of two ribs, the cavity was not opened. Operation July 18, by July 28 the gap between the ends of the resected ribs had manifestly retracted." In another case after rib resection: "The thorax showed a marked retraction in the zone corresponding to the cavity. At the same time the cavity contracted." It must be remembered that this sort of "eosurgery" was really ancillary to the primary objective of opening and draining cavities. Nonetheless, it was inevitable that De Cérenville's work should be followed by further development of thoracoplasty. Everyone interested in the subject should study this paper. H. Quincke ("Zur operativen Behandlung der Lungenabscesse," Berl. klin. Wchnschr., **25**:349, 1888) also recognized the importance of collapse, although he was primarily interested in non-tuberculous abscesses. By 1890 Carl Spengler ("Zur Behandlung starrwandiger Höhlen bei Lungenphthise," Verhandl. d. Gesellsch. Deutscher Naturforsch. u. Ärzte, **63**:236, 1890–91) clearly enunciated the principles of more modern therapy. In cases of rigid cavities it was advisable to treat by "mobilization of the stiff walls, in our case by rib-resection and mobilization of the thoracic wall, that is by a thoracoplasty without opening the pleural cavity." Spengler seems to have been the first to use the term "thoracoplasty." The next landmark in the subject was Brauer's comprehensive article (L. Brauer, "Erfahrungen und Ueberlegungen zur Lungenkollapstherapie," Beitr. z. klin. Tuberk., **12**:49, 1906), and to these should be added the authoritative review, with their own contributions, of F. Sauerbruch and H. Elving, "Die extrapleurale Thorakoplastik," Ergebn. inn. Med. u. Kinderh., **10**:869, 1913. The whole subject is well summarized in John Alexander, *The Surgery of Pulmonary Tuberculosis* (Philadelphia: Lea & Febiger, 1925), and in Alexander's more recent comprehensive treatise, *The Collapse Therapy of Pulmonary Tuberculosis* (Springfield, Ill.: Charles C Thomas, 1937).

We cannot attempt to refer to the colossal current literature, which requires a special bibliography of its own.

36. MARFAN, A. De l'immunité conférée par la guérison d'une tuberculose locale pour la phthisie pulmonaire, Arch. gén. de méd., **157**:423, 1886.

No sooner had the bacillus been discovered than many workers began to occupy themselves with the question of prevention and immunization of tuberculosis. Marfan in a paper which is definitely a landmark pointed out that "local tuberculosis," such as glands of the neck (scrofula), was really only a local manifestation of a "general" infection and that one must not expect a complete cure by local excision. He also noted that pulmonary tuberculosis was mild or absent in those having lupus or scrofula. He raised the question, "Will it be possible one day to vaccinate against tuberculosis? One day perhaps experiment will answer this question; until now tuberculosis, even attenuated, is a disease too serious, with evolution too insidious and uncertain, for one to attempt preventive inoculation." This was years before vaccination with BCG was tried (Ref. 57).

37. CORNET, Georg. Die Verbreitung der Tuberkelbacillen ausserhalb des Körpers, Ztschr. f. Hyg. u. Infectionskr., **5**:191, 1888.

The discovery of the tubercle bacillus by Koch was greeted with high enthusiasm on all sides. Soon, however, troubled thoughts arose. It was believed at first that consumptives exhaled tubercle bacilli at every breath and that they might be projected into the air by wind currents blowing over sputum. If this was so, the inspired air and the environment in general must be full of bacilli all the time, and how could anyone escape infection when one of every seven people already had consumption? In the near-hysteria aroused by these views, it was even proposed to ship all consumptives to an island isolated in mid-ocean.

These speculations, however, had the merit of arousing on all sides an acute awareness of the public health aspects of the problem, and they stimulated a vast amount of experimental work. Cornet's paper, or rather monograph, since it occupies 141 pages, explores the subject in great detail. Cornet was a pupil of Koch, and this work was done under the master's sponsorship. First, others as well as Cornet showed that tubercle bacilli were not expelled on ordinary breathing and that moist sputum did not readily lead to clouds of bacilli in the air. Cornet's main work, remarkable in extent and detail, consisted of collecting dust from walls and floors in the vicinity of coughing consumptives. With this dust he was able by inoculation to produce tuberculosis in laboratory animals. He also showed that dust from areas where there were no consumptives did not produce tuberculosis.

Cornet enunciated the theory that tuberculosis of the lungs was acquired by the inhalation of bacilli swept up in dust containing dried sputum (Cornet's dust theory). While this view, which was widely accepted, turns out, of course, to be true only in part, if at all, it gave an immense impetus to study of the problem; emphasized the danger of careless expectoration of sputum on floors, into handkerchiefs, etc.; and started the movements for sputum control and sterilization so important in tuberculosis. The paper is especially outstanding because of the careful and thorough methods and the astute and detailed reasoning.

38. GRANCHER, J., and MARTIN, H. Tuberculose expérimentale. Sur une mode de traitement et de vaccination, Compt. rend. Acad. d. sc., **111**:333, 1890.

After the discovery of the bacillus, many workers tried every conceivable method of "immunization" with preparations of tubercle bacilli of all sorts. Grancher and Martin, although their experiments were primitive, seemed to show that rabbits prepared by injections of attenuated bacilli (method of attenuation not clearly stated but suggested by Pasteur's rabies immunization) developed increased resistance to subsequent injections of virulent bacilli. The validity of these observations cannot be tested now, but they clearly anticipated later attempts at human immunization (Ref. 57).

39. KOCH, R. I. Weitere Mittheilungen über ein Heilmittel gegen Tuberculose, Deutsche med. Wchnschr., **16**:1029, 1890.

This was the famous report which shook the medical world, since Koch here claimed that the new preparation, tuberculin,[4] was a curative agent in tuberculosis. Koch first discussed the subject at the International Medical Congress (Berlin, August 4, 1890). He stated in this paper that he did not intend to publish until his observations were complete but that irresponsible publicity had forced his hand. Actually, he said nothing about the preparation or composition of tuberculin; he stated only that it was derived from cultures of the bacillus.

Although Koch discussed the diagnostic value of his material and pointed out that recovery might be indicated by a waning reaction, he considered the substance to be primarily a therapeutic agent. He emphasized that it was ineffective when given by mouth. No reaction occurred in healthy guinea pigs, but Koch regarded this as a species difference between guinea pig and man. He did not realize that a non-tuberculous man would also not react, and his healthy (*gesunde*) people who gave mild reactions of course had latent tuberculosis. The classical symptoms of a tuberculin reaction following subcutaneous injection are graphically described, and the specificity is emphasized.

The conviction that tuberculin was a curative agent in tuberculosis was based primarily on observation of visible lesions, such as lupus vulgaris. "With these lesions, changes occur which allow one to recognize a really surprising specific antituberculosis action." Koch then gave a graphic description of the sequence of events—exacerbation followed by crusting, desquammation, and healing by healthy scar. Curative action was less dramatic with lymph node and bone lesions, and the results with advanced consumption were dubious enough to make him admit that one could do better with the very early stages of pulmonary disease. Koch also insisted that tuberculin did not kill the bacilli but only the living tuberculous tissue. Dead tuberculous masses must either slough off or be removed surgically. Throughout the paper one should remember that Koch had no idea of the concepts of hypersensitivity and allergy which were to be developed a few years later (Ref. 48).

Koch closed on a conservative note. He had to depend largely on the reports given to him by his clinical associates. One reads between the lines that this sound and critical observer was not yet absolutely sure of his ground. One may wonder whether he later regretted being forced into hasty publication of material not yet large enough for statistical analysis.

40. TRUDEAU, E. L. An experimental study of preventive inoculations in tuberculosis, M. Rec., **38**:565, 1890.

Only a few weeks after Koch had announced his great discovery (Ref. 39) of cure and prevention of tuberculosis by "tuberculin," Trudeau, working obscurely in Saranac Lake and using essentially the same material as Koch, published this important study in which he was unable to show any preventive effect of

---

[4] The term "tuberculin" was not used by Koch, who spoke only of his curative material (*Heilmittel*). It was introduced later, perhaps by Doutrelpoint (Deutsche med. Wchnschr., **17**:348, 1891), or perhaps by O. Bujwid ("Doswiadzema na zwierzetach z. tuberkulina," Gaz. lek. Warszawa, 2d ser., **11**:582, 1891).

culture filtrates against experimental tuberculosis. Trudeau was right, and Koch was wrong: no animal has ever been protected against tuberculosis by pretreatment with tuberculin. This paper is also of interest because Trudeau describes the origin of the famous attenuated R_1 strain used for so many years in experimental tuberculosis.

A little later (E. L. Trudeau, "The treatment of experimental tuberculosis by Koch's tuberculin, etc.," M. News, **61**:253, 1892) he concluded that "Koch's tuberculin does not cure experimental tuberculosis in the guinea pig," but he thought that experimental tuberculosis in the rabbit's eye could be healed by injections of the culture filtrates. Trudeau did not, of course, understand at the time that success with tuberculin as a therapeutic measure depends on the character of the lesion and the setting-up of just the right amount of reaction, criteria which for the most part have rendered tuberculin impractical. At about the same time, as Trudeau points out, W. Donitz ("Ueber die Wirkung des Tuberculins auf die experimentelle Augentuberculose des Kaninchens," Deutsche med. Wchnschr., **17**:1289, 1891) reported on the cure by tuberculin of experimental tuberculosis of the anterior chamber of the eye in the rabbit. "To get healing, it is necessary to give increasing doses of tuberculin and for a long time to maintain a not too slight reaction."

41. KOCH, R. Fortsetzung der Mittheilungen über ein Heilmittel gegen Tuberculose, Deutsche med. Wchnschr., **17**:101, 1891.

It is difficult now to appreciate the sensation made by Koch's announcement of a curative agent for tuberculosis (Ref. 39). In this brief supplementary paper, he again describes the classical experiment which led him to believe in its healing powers: if a guinea pig with a tuberculous nodule of the skin from a first injection is reinjected with a suspension of tubercle bacilli, the original nodule becomes acutely inflamed and necrotic but then leaves a clean ulcer, which heals completely. Since the injection of bacilli led at times to local abscesses, Koch thought an extract of the organisms might suffice, and in this paper he now divulges the nature of the curative agent. "This substance . . . is a glycerin extract of pure cultures of tubercle bacilli."

Meanwhile, intensive clinical trials were being made by doctors to whom Koch furnished the material, and in this volume of the Deutsche medizinische Wochenschrift (1891) there are no fewer than seventy-four reports of its use under various circumstances on the patients who flocked from all sides. Everyone agreed on its great and specific value in diagnosis, but there were many reservations and doubts about its therapeutic effects, and some even declared that it was dangerous and furthered the tuberculous process.

In still another paper Koch ("Weitere Mittheilung über das Tuberculin, *ibid.,* p. 1189) provides details of the preparation of tuberculin and of attempts to purify it. Injections were given to a number of healthy doctors, who all "reacted." In trying to explain this, Koch was again at a disadvantage in working before the elementary concepts of allergy had been defined.

An excellent early summary of the whole status of tuberculin is given in the monograph of L. Hamman and E. Wolman, *Tuberculin in Diagnosis and Treatment* (New York: D. Appleton & Co., 1912).

42. TUFFIER, [Théodore]. De la résection du sommet du poumon, Semaine méd., 2:201, 1891.

Aside from some primitive and unsuccessful attempts, Tuffier seems to have been the first successfully to extirpate part of a lung for tuberculosis. The case is reported in detail, and the patient was presented as cured. In his comprehensive lecture before the Twelfth International Congress of Medicine in Moscow in 1897 ("Chirurgie du poumon, en particulier dans les cavernes tuberculeuses et la gangrène pulmonaire," Compte-rend. du XIIe Cong. Internat. de Méd. Moscou, 1897, p. 5, pub. S. P. Yokovlev, Moscou, 1899), Tuffier develops the whole subject of pneumonectomy, which he amplified into his book, *Chirurgie du poumon* (Paris: Masson et Cie, 1897). It is of interest that the surgery of pulmonary tuberculosis, in view of its present vogue, was not pursued further for many years. As recently as 1935 a report of lobectomy (S. O. Freedlander "Lobectomy in pulmonary tuberculosis," J. Thoracic Surg., 5:132, 1935) was hailed as an original achievement by those surgeons who discussed the paper. The rapid development, especially in very recent years (1950—), of lobectomy and segmental resection goes hand in hand with the availability of effective antibiotics (Ref. 63).

There is now a large and rapidly growing literature which cannot be reviewed in detail and which is indeed still controversial (see, for example, Edward J. O'Brien et al., "The present chaos regarding resection of residual and caseous lesions in pulmonary tuberculosis," J. Thoracic Surg., 26:441, 1953; J. Maxwell Chamberlain, Clifford F. Storey, Robert Klopstock, and Charles F. Daniels, "Segmental resection for pulmonary tuberculosis," J. Thoracic Surg., 26:471, 1953, 300 cases; Lyman A. Brewer III, Harlow W. Harrison, Rodney P. Smith, and Angel F. Bai, "Indications for segmental resection in pulmonary tuberculosis," Am. Rev. Tuberc., 69:554, 1954).

43. TRUDEAU, E. L. Eye tuberculosis and anti-tubercular inoculation in the rabbit, Tr. A. Am. Physicians, 8:108, 1893.

Although Grancher and Martin (Ref. 38) thought that they had produced resistance to tuberculosis by injection of "attenuated" strains of bacilli, Trudeau's experiments were much more convincing. After injecting avian bacilli into rabbits, subsequent inoculations into the eye were made with strains derived from "tuberculous lesions of the rabbit." In the previously vaccinated animals, injections of mammalian bacilli into the eye were followed by a sharp reaction, often with subsequent recovery, in distinction to progressive tuberculosis of the eye in the untreated controls. Trudeau recognized that the immunity or resistance conferred was only partial. "I do not lay claim, therefore, to have produced a complete or permanent immunity by a safe method," concluded this sound and careful investigator. In a follow-up study of these rabbits ("A report of the ultimate results obtained in experimental eye tuberculosis by tuberculin treatment and anti-tubercular inoculation," Tr. A. Am. Physicians, 9:168, 1894) Trudeau noted that the eye lesions recurred and progressed in many of the animals. "The extent to which the tubercular process can be influenced favorably seems to depend rather upon the degree and character of the irritation induced about the tubercle . . . than upon any direct germicidal effect or upon the production of a lasting immunity."

Trudeau sensed the fact that significant immunity could be stimulated only by the production of tubercle in the body (preferably with living bacilli) and that soluble culture products were ineffective.

44. FLÜGGE, C. Ueber Luftinfection, Ztschr. f. Hyg. u. Infectionskr., **25**:179, 1897.

Flügge and his associates convinced themselves that the transmission of tubercle bacilli dried in dust, as promoted by Cornet (Ref. 37), was not of practical importance in human pathology. They thought it more likely that direct transmission took place from person to person. They were also aware, as had been shown by others, that the quietly exhaled breath was sterile and that actual particles of sputum or saliva must be expelled in order for bacteria to leave the respiratory passages. This led to the development of Flügge's "droplet theory." Even though it was shown that prolonged and close contact in direct line with the patient's cough was necessary in order to inhale any large number of bacilli, Flügge concluded that pulmonary tuberculosis was most likely transmitted by the inhalation of bacillus-containing droplets.

It is in this paper that Flügge laid the experimental groundwork for the droplet theory. During the next few years, a large number of papers appeared in the same journal by Flügge ("Die Verbreitung der Phthise durch staubformiges Sputum und durch beim Husten verspritzte Tröpfchen," Ztschr. f. Hyg. u. Infectionskr., **30**:107, 1899) and by his associates, probing every conceivable phase of transmission of bacterial infection. One particularly important paper was that of Bruno Heyman ("Ueber die Ausstreuung infectioser Tröpfchen beim Husten der Phthisiker," Ztschr. f. Hyg. u. Infectionskr., **30**:139, 1899), who demonstrated the great difficulty of infecting guinea pigs by having consumptives cough directly at them. In spite of this, the droplet theory was widely accepted at the time. An authoritative and critical analysis of this whole problem is to be found in Allen Krause's "Essays on tuberculosis. VII. Infection by inhalation: Flügge's theory of droplet infection," J. Outdoor Life, **15**:225, 1918.

45. SMITH, Theobald. A comparative study of bovine tubercle bacilli and of human bacilli from sputum, J. Exper. Med., **3**:451, 1898.

Koch believed that all tubercle bacilli from mammalian sources were the same "species," and this view was generally held until the work of Smith. In a report before the Association of American Physicians ("Two varieties of the tubercle bacillus from mammals," Tr. A. Am. Physicians, **11**:75, 1896) he studied a strain of the bacillus from a tuberculous raccoon, presumably infected from a human source, and a strain from a tuberculous bull. Striking differences were shown, which were extended by the elaborate studies reported in the present paper. Smith clearly defined the cultural and pathogenic differences (in guinea pigs, in rabbits, and in cattle) which are standard knowledge today. He opened the way for clarification of human infection with bovine strains. "Now that we have established some . . . differences between bovine and sputum bacilli . . . the time has come . . . to study with care the tubercle bacilli from cases of supposed animal origin, so that . . . some basis may be found upon which to found statistics. . . . It will take much time. . . . In the meantime the relation of bovine to human tuberculosis must be somehow defined before a fairly helpless and frightened public." Smith's work explained many previously perplexing problems, such as the difficulty of producing tuberculosis in cattle with material from human sources.

46. FRÄNKEL, Albert. Das Tuberculinum Kochii als Diagnosticum, Ztschr. f. Tuberk., **1**:291, 1900.

The significance of the tuberculin reaction was greatly confused by the occurrence of many positive reactions in apparently healthy men. E. Peiper, for example ("Ueber die Wirkung des Koch'schen Mittels auf gesunde oder nichtuberculose Individuen," Deutsche med. Wchnschr., **17**:160, 1891), with this point in mind found that eighteen of twenty-two patients with absolutely no evidence of tuberculosis gave positive reactions. The obvious solution of this paradox was autopsy material, which would give a more accurate idea of the presence of tubercle than would clinical examination. The first comprehensive studies were made in cattle. Fränkel collected the results of eight thousand autopsies. In only an occasional case (2–3 per cent) was there a discrepancy between the tuberculin test and the anatomical findings. This suggested that the (apparently) healthy people who reacted to tuberculin were nonetheless infected and harbored anatomical tuberculosis. Fränkel's results were promptly confirmed by others.

47. NÄGELI, Otto. Ueber Häufigkeit, Localization und Ausheilung der Tuberculose, Virchows Arch. f. path Anat., **160**:426, 1900.

Although the frequency of tuberculous foci in miscellaneous autopsy material was being recognized, Schlenker (Virchows Arch. of path. Anat., **134**:145, 1893) made the first purposeful study; in 100 autopsies he found tuberculous foci in 66. It was the classical studies of Nägeli, however, which really settled the matter in man, as Fränkel (Ref. 46) had in cattle. Nägeli reported 508 careful autopsies; in 406 there was evidence of tuberculous infection. Among 420 adults, 93 per cent had tubercle. Later, A. Burkhardt ("Ueber Häufigkeit und Uhrsache menschlicher Tuberculose auf Grund von *ca.* 1400 Sectionen," Ztschr. f. Hyg. u. Infectionskr., **53**:139, 1906) published more extensive statistics and pointed out the almost universal finding of tuberculous foci in adults, the infrequency of such lesions in small children, but the very high death rate from tuberculosis in early adult life. The findings in children were extended by the careful studies of F. Hamburger (Wien klin. Wchnschr., **20**:1069, 1907).

All this work explained the apparent paradox of the tuberculin test; "healthy" people who reacted were actually infected and harbored tuberculous foci.

48. LOWENSTEIN, E., and RAPPAPORT, E. Ueber den Mechanismus der Tuberculinimmunität, Ztschr. f. Tuberk., **5**:485, 1904.

It is hardly worthwhile going into the early (and erroneous) views as to the nature of the tuberculin reaction. They are well reviewed by Hamman and Wolman (Ref. 41). It was not until the pioneer work on anaphylaxis and hypersensitivity of Richet and Portier ("De l'action anaphylactique de certains venins," Compt. rend. Soc. de biol., **54**:170, 1902) or Arthus ("Infections répétées de sérum de cheval chez le lapin," Compt. rend. Soc. de biol., **55**:817,

1903), and of Von Pirquet and Schick ("Zur Theorie der Inkubationszeit," Wien klin. Wchnschr., **16**:1244, 1903) that the groundwork was laid for an understanding of the tuberculin reaction. The vast contemporary literature on anaphylaxis cannot be further enumerated here. While Von Pirquet and Schick, Von Behring, and others were evidently aware of the resemblance of the tuberculin reaction to hypersensitivity, Lowenstein and Rappaport seem to have been the first to discuss clearly the mechanism in immunological terms and to define it as a hypersensitive reaction rather than a cumulative effect. Here again the early work was followed by an immense and, at points, controversial literature.

49. VON PIRQUET, C. Der diagnostische Wert der kutanen Tuberculinreaktion bei der Tuberculose des Kindesalters auf Grund von 100 Sektionen, Wien klin. Wchnschr., **20**:1123, 1907.

No procedure has been more important in the study of immunity and epidemiology of tuberculosis than the tuberculin skin test. In this definitive paper Von Pirquet compared the results of his test with autopsies in 100 children. Detailed results and case reports are given. Von Pirquet recognized the significance of variations in the strength of tuberculin: that a high dilution might give no skin reaction when more concentrated material gave a positive test. He found that most of the negative tests were in very young children and, in general, showed that skin tests ran parallel with the results of general tuberculin reactions. The specificity of the procedure was clearly proved. As far as we can find out, Von Pirquet's first published note on the skin test was a report before the Berlin Medical Society, May 8, 1907 ("Tuberculindiagnose durch cutane Impfung," Berl. klin. Wchnschr., **44**:644, 1907). He said that the test was suggested by the immediate reaction to smallpox revaccination, and he described the technique of applying the tuberculin.

In 1908 G. Mantoux ("Intradermo-réaction de la tuberculine. Note de M. Ch. Mantoux présentée par M. E. Roux," Compt. rend. Acad. d. sc., **147**:355, 1908) described the intradermal tuberculin test, which subsequently became standard practice in place of Von Pirquet's method.

50. HAMBURGER, Franz. Ueber die Wirkung des Alttuberculins auf den tuberculosefreien Menschen, München. med. Wchnschr., **55**:1220, 1908.

It took a long while before there was general acceptance of the principle that a positive tuberculin reaction depended on the presence of specific tubercle in the body. Newborn babies who did not react were thought to have a peculiar resistance to tuberculin, and it was not fully understood that absence of reaction in them was due to absence of tubercle. Hamburger's studies were definitive. He gave to children who had negative cutaneous tests as much as 500 mg. of O.T. with no reaction of any sort. These studies, along with anatomical examinations, made it obvious that resistance to tuberculin reaction was due to the absence of infection.

51. RÖMER, Paul H. Spezifische Ueberempfindlichkeit und Tuberculoseimmunität, Beitr. z. klin. Tuberk., **9**:79, 1908.

Work on hypersensitivity and on the tuberculin reaction led almost imperceptibly to the problem of immunity in tuberculosis. The extensive original studies on hypersensitivity are reviewed in this classical paper by Römer, and the applications to tuberculosis are discussed. The early observations dealt largely with resistance to reinfection. The problem was further studied by Römer and Joseph in a series of beautifully controlled experiments ("Die Tuberculose Reinfection," Beitr. z. klin. Tuberk., **17**:287, 1910). Whether the mechanism of immunity was associated with the allergic reaction of reinfection, as Römer believed, was for years vigorously debated and was strongly supported in America by A. Krause (Ref. 59) until Rich (Ref. 60) emphasized that the two phenomena—allergic reaction and immunity—could be dissociated.

Römer and Joseph concluded that immunity in tuberculosis was a specific allergic phenomenon conditioned by the character of the original infection and by the size and circumstances of the reinfecting dose.

There were, however, even in the early days of the subject, conservative individuals who felt that allergy and immunity were not necessarily the same (see, e.g., the important paper of F. Hamburger, "Ueber Tuberculoseimmunität," Beitr., z. klin. Tuberk., **12**:259, 1909).

52. PARK, William H., and KRUMWIEDE, Charles, Jr. The relative importance of the bovine and human type of tubercle bacilli in the different forms of tuberculosis, J.M. Research, **27**:109, 1912.

Beginning with Koch (Ref. 28), a huge controversial literature grew up as to whether bovine tuberculosis was caused by a different race of bacilli from the human disease and whether man could acquire tuberculosis from animals. Although many contradictions were answered by T. Smith's studies (Ref. 45), the definitive report of Park and Krumwiede demonstrated beyond question that the bovine bacillus was at fault in a high percentage of cases of tuberculosis in children who had ingested cow's milk, in intestinal tuberculosis, and in tuberculosis of the glands of the neck. Elaborate tables are given which cannot be reproduced here, but sample figures of infection with bovine bacilli in children under five years of age are as follows: pulmonary, 2.8 per cent; cervical adenitis, 61 per cent; abdominal tuberculosis, 58 per cent. All this seemed finally to show that tuberculosis could result from either inhalation or ingestion and that it might be caused by either human or bovine bacilli. With the elimination of infected milk, tuberculosis of the "glands of the neck" and abdominal tuberculosis have largely disappeared. A later careful study along similar lines is that of R. M. Price, "Summary of a study of the types of tubercle bacilli isolated from human lesions," Am. Rev. Tuberc., **25**:383, 1932.

53. GHON, Anton. Der primäre Lungenherd bei der Tuberculose der Kinder. Berlin and Vienna: Urban & Schwartzenberg, 1912.

This book, profusely illustrated and documented by innumerable autopsy reports, is a classic in the field of the primary tuberculous lung lesion of childhood. Ghon emphasized the need of very careful search for the primary lesion, which might be in any part of the lung, and the associated hilar adenopathy. So fundamental were these studies that such a lesion is still often spoken of as a "Ghon focus" or a "Ghon tubercle." But see Parrot (Ref. 25).

54. SAUERBRUCH, F. Beeinflussung von Lungenerkrankungen durch künstliche Lähmung des Zwerchfells (Phrenicotomie), München. med. Wchnschr., **60**:625, 1913.

Although Stuertz ("Künstliche Zwerchfellähmung bei schweren chronischen einseitigen Lungenerkrankungen," Deutsche med. Wchnschr., **37**:2224, 1911) appears to have suggested artificial paralysis of the diaphragm for chronic unilateral lung disease, Sauerbruch seems to have been the first to report phrenic nerve section in tuberculosis. It was not until some years later that Goetze advocated more effective paralysis by phrenic exairesis. The attention which was paid to this method of therapy will be appreciated if one reads A. H. Aufses' monograph, "Phrenic nerve operations in the treatment of pulmonary tuberculosis," Medicine, **16**:139, 1937, which includes 593 references.

55. TRUDEAU, Edward Livingston. An autobiography. Philadelphia and New York: Lea & Febiger, 1916.

This book is a really great piece of biographical writing; it ranks, in our opinion, with Lockhart's *Scott,* Southey's *Nelson,* and Trevelyan's *Macaulay* for its charm and vividness. No chronicle, furthermore, could be of more interest to the student of tuberculosis, recapitulating as it does that exciting era of the 1880's when the bacillus was discovered and real knowledge of the disease began to advance.

Trudeau was the founder of the sanitarium movement in this country; although influenced by Brehmer and Dettweiler (Refs. 15, 27), he learned the value of rest from his own case, when over and over, as he so vividly tells, effort was followed by fever and prostration. A pioneer in the cultivation of the bacillus and in the study of experimental tuberculosis, it is interesting to hear how long it took after Koch's discovery—eight or nine years—before doctors in general accepted the little red rods as the cause of consumption. Trudeau's scientific work, perhaps not sufficiently recognized, was of the highest caliber and was a real contribution to the understanding of tuberculosis; the Saranac Laboratory with E. Baldwin, A. Krause, and others soon was recognized for its fundamental work.[5] But even today, with chemotherapy and lobectomy, the principles of rest and hygiene developed at the Adirondack Cottage Sanitarium are still paramount in the management of tuberculosis.

56. OPIE, Eugene L. The relation of apical tuberculosis of adults to the focal tuberculosis of children, J. Exper. Med., **26**:263, 1917.

Following the early work on resistance (Ref. 51), it was generally believed that adult tuberculosis occurred not by reinfection from the outside (because the patient had immunity from his childhood infection) but by autoinfection from a focus already present. Attention came to be devoted not so much to external sources of contagion as to mechanisms of alleged lowering of resistance which allowed extension from the subject's already existing, though perhaps latent, focus. This point of view for a long time inhibited proper epidemiological studies and effective public health measures.

[5] Much of this work is reviewed in Edward R. Baldwin, S. A. Petroff, and Le Roy S. Gardner, *Tuberculosis: Bacteriology, Pathology, and Laboratory Diagnosis* (Philadelphia: Lea & Febiger, 1927).

Opie, following Ghon (Ref. 53) (see also "The focal pulmonary tuberculosis of children and adults," J. Exper. Med., **25**:855, 1917), reinvestigated the incidence and character of childhood lesions and of adult tuberculosis by meticulous anatomical studies, as well as by X-rays of lungs removed at autopsy. These studies led Opie to the conclusion that "apical tuberculosis of adults is not the result of infantile tuberculosis but is caused by subsequent infection." A complete investigation of ideas of reinfection followed, and Opie's views were supported (Ref. 61) by meticulous epidemiological studies.

Some other workers held views similar to Opie's, however, and J. Orth, for example, summarized his position (*Ueber einige Tuberculosefragen* [Jena: Gustav Fischer, 1918]) by saying: "It is wrong that the idea of exogenous infection should be held in discredit by some, since its existence is unfortunately only too certain, as the frequent tuberculous illnesses of nurses and attendants bear witness."

57. CALMETTE, A., GUERIN, K., NÈGRE, L., and BOQUET, A. Prémunition des nouveau-nés contre la tuberculose par le vaccin BCG (1921 à 1926), Ann. Inst. Pasteur, **40**:89, 1926.

In this article Calmette and his associates set forth the philosophy and the technique of protective vaccination with a living attenuated bovine bacillus (BCG). Although trials are being continued today (1957), there is still no entire agreement as to its practical value. The difficulty with all procedures of this sort is that, if the "immunizing" dose is too small, inadequate protection is conferred; if it is too large, there is danger of producing progressive tuberculosis. The difficulties in standardizing the vaccine and of interpretation of results are also great—hence the conflicting claims and results. Calmette elaborated this report in another article ("Sur la vaccination préventive des enfants nouveau-nés contre la tuberculose par le BCG," Am. Inst. Pasteur, **41**:201, 1927), and shortly after gave an English summary (A. Calmette and Harry Plotz, "Protective inoculation against tuberculosis with BCG," Am. Rev. Tuberc., **19**:567, 1929).

For a review of the whole subject see K. N. Irvine, *B.C.G. Vaccination in Theory and Practice* (Oxford: Humphrey Milford, 1949). R. Dubos has authoritatively summarized the immunological aspects of BCG vaccination (Am. Rev. Tuberc., **60**:670, 1949). Recent elaborate studies with attempts at careful control are reported by Aronson and his associates (Samuel C. Stein and Joseph D. Aronson, "The occurrence of pulmonary lesions in BCG-vaccinated and unvaccinated persons," Am. Rev. Tuberc., **68**:695, 1953; Joseph D. Aronson and Charlotte Ferguson Aronson, "The correlation of the tuberculin reaction with roentgenographically demonstrable pulmonary lesions in BCG-vaccinated and control persons," Am. Rev. Tuberc., **68**:713).

58. OPIE, Eugene L., and McPHEDRAN, F. Maurice. The contagion of tuberculosis, Am. Rev. Tuberc., **14**:347, 1926.

Following the work of Opie (Ref. 56), Opie and McPhedran, using tuberculin tests, X-rays, and meticulous follow-up procedures, studied the contagion of tuberculosis in families. They showed that when latent tuberculosis, especially as revealed by X-ray, is taken into consideration, "tuberculosis exhibits the characteristics of a contagious disease." While latent lesions could, by extension, lead to spread even to other organs, adult infection seemed to be usually acquired from external sources and not by spread of the subject's "childhood" lesion. Opie's many important studies are summarized in his papers, "Pathology of the tuberculosis of childhood and its bearing on clinical work," Brit. M.J., 2:1130, 1927, and "The pathogenesis of and transmission of tuberculosis," Am. J.M. Sc., 179:104, 1930. He emphasized especially the importance of the latent lesion—without symptoms or physical signs—revealed by tuberculin tests and X-rays in the pathogenesis of overt clinical tuberculosis. In this connection, E. M. Brieger's book, *The Papworth Families* (London: W. Heinemann, Ltd., 1944), is of interest.

59. KRAUSE, Allen K. The dissemination of tubercle bacilli in the immune guinea pig, with a discussion of the probable factors involved in tuberculo-immunity, Am. Rev. Tuberc., 14:211, 1926.

During the early decades of the century an immense amount of work was done on the problem of immunity to tuberculosis. Krause, working first at the Saranac Laboratory and later at the Kenneth Dows Laboratory in Baltimore, dominated this field in America because of his ingenious and elaborate experiments. Krause, following the classical observations of Römer (Ref. 51), sustained the thesis that the allergic reaction associated with reinfection fixed bacilli at their portal of entry and largely prevented invasion and spread. This he considered the essence of immunity, and in his conclusions to this paper he said: "It is believed more probable that, upon being re-infected, the tissues of the immune guinea pig react promptly with some process that serves to impede the further passage of bacilli." "It is submitted that this process is the allergic exudative or inflammatory reaction which invariably sets in upon re-infection of the tuberculous immune guinea pig which is otherwise normal." Innumerable papers by Krause and his associates dealing with this subject are to be found in the American Review of Tuberculosis from 1918 to 1928. Of special importance are the following: H. S. Willis, "The early dissemination of tubercle bacilli after intracutaneous inoculation of guinea pigs of first infection," 11:173, 1925; "The early dissemination of tubercle bacilli after intracutaneous inoculation of immune guinea pigs of reinfection," p. 185; A. K. Krause and H. S. Willis, "The influence of frequently repeated reinfection on allergy and immunity in tuberculosis," 14:316, 1926. Even though they thought it paramount, they did not believe, of course, that the allergic reaction of reinfection was the only influence involved in resistance, and they did much work on dose of bacilli, environment, and other factors. Krause's associate, H. S. Willis ("The waning of cutaneous hypersensitiveness of tuberculin and the relation of tuberculo-immunity to tuberculo-allergy," Am. Rev. Tuberc., 17:240, 1928) even showed in guinea pigs that cutaneous allergy might wane and that "notwithstanding this greatly reduced and practically absent allergy, such guinea pigs, at thirty months after infection, were found to possess a high specific immunity to reinfection with virulent tubercle bacilli," a finding hard to reconcile with Krause's thesis.

Krause held sway over tuberculosis research in America for a good many years, and his views were widely accepted. In addition to being a great scientist, he was a man of brilliant and convincing personality. The objective quality of his experiments leaves them unimpaired, although his main thesis, first systematically questioned by Rich (Ref. 60), has now been weakened.

60. RICH, Arnold Rice, and McCORDOCK, Howard A. An enquiry concerning the role of allergy, immunity and other factors of importance in the pathogenesis of human tuberculosis, Bull. Johns Hopkins Hosp., **44**:273, 1929.

In this extensive critical analysis the prevailing view (Ref. 59), that immunity in tuberculosis was effected by the allergic reaction of reinfection, was challenged by Rich, who adduced an impressive collection of evidence to the contrary. This article was subsequently elaborated into Rich's monumental monograph on *The Pathogenesis of Tuberculosis* (Ref. 67). Rich's views were further exposed in another article ("The role of allergy in tuberculosis," Arch. Int. Med., **43**:691, 1929). In subsequent papers (Arnold R. Rich, Frederick B. Jennings, Jr., and Lillian M. Downing, "The persistence of immunity after the abolition of allergy by desensitization," Bull. Johns Hopkins Hosp., **53**:172, 1933; Herbert Rothschild, Jonas S. Friedenwald, and Clarence Bernstein, "The relation of allergy to immunity in tuberculosis," Bull. Johns Hopkins Hosp., **54**:232, 1934) experimental evidence was produced to show that immunity was unimpaired in animals desensitized so that no recognizable allergic reaction any longer occurred. From this time on, little was heard of the view that the allergic reaction of reinfection was the mechanism of immunity.

61. HETHERINGTON, H. W., McPHEDRAN, F. Maurice, LANDIS, H. R. M., and OPIE, Eugene L. Tuberculosis in medical and college students, Arch. Int. Med., **48**:734, 1931.

The work of Opie and his associates, in which the acquisition of tuberculosis of adults by reinfection from the outside rather than by endogenous flareup of an old lesion was stressed (Ref. 56), was followed by the development of intensive methods of case finding among various groups using tuberculin skin tests, X-rays of the chest, and, to a lesser extent, physical examination and search for bacilli. We cannot review here the vast literature on mass surveys. The subject is covered in Herbert R. Edwards' monograph, *Tuberculosis case-finding: studies in mass surveys* (Suppl. to Am. Rev. Tuberc., Vol. **41**, 1940).

The question of whether medical students and nurses are particularly liable to contract tuberculosis is, however, of immediate practical importance to the student of the epidemiology of the disease. Hetherington and his associates seem to have been the first systematically to investigate this subject. They found a rapidly increasing incidence of apical lesions in medical students and concluded that "they were peculiarly subject to advanced tuberculous infection."

Here again a vast amount of similar work has been and is being done, the general implication of which is that medical students and nurses acquire tuberculosis by contagion with greater frequency than does the population in general. The studies of J. A. Myers and his associates carried the subject forward ("Tuberculosis among students and graduates of medicine," Ann. Int. Med., **14**:1575, 1941; "Tuberculosis among students and graduates in nursing," *ibid.*,

p. 873, 1940), but the immense literature cannot be further reviewed here. A recent study with a plea for standardized comparable methods in case finding is that of R. Bates and W. Davey ("Tuberculosis in medical and nursing students," Am. Rev. Tuberc., **63**:332, 1951). The subject has also been thoroughly reviewed by Eleanor C. Connolly in *Tuberculosis among Hospital Personnel* (New York: National Tuberculosis Association, 1950).

62. FELDMAN, W. H., and HINSHAW, H. C. Effects of streptomycin on experimental tuberculosis in guinea pigs: a preliminary report, Proc. Staff Meet. Mayo Clin., **19**:593, 1944.

The subject of the chemotherapy of tuberculosis really requires a bibliography of its own. Numerous trials have been made in the past with all sorts of agents, including gold salts, derivatives of the sulfonamide group, and many others. Indeed, no sooner had the bacillus been discovered than the dream of the physician was to find some substance which would destroy the bacillus in the human body. Trudeau (Ref. 55, p. 204) tells graphically of his early attempts to cure tuberculous rabbits and guinea pigs by injections of creosote, carbolic acid, and other germicides. But always "the tubercle bacillus bore cheerfully a degree of medication which proved fatal to its host!"

The era of modern effective chemotherapy begins with the work of Feldman and Hinshaw. Following the finding of S. Waksman and others that streptomycin had bactericidal effects on a strain of *Mycobacterium tuberculosis* in the test tube, they tried this agent in guinea-pig tuberculosis. Only enough streptomycin was at first available to treat four animals, but there was a striking result. The material (75 mg. daily per guinea pig) did not seem toxic, and the lesions were absent or insignificant in the treated compared with the untreated controls. A second experiment confirmed the first. The writers are to be commended for their conservative conclusions: "Streptomycin is an antibiotic substance well tolerated by guinea pigs which is capable under the conditions imposed of creating a striking suppressive effect on the pathogenic proclivities in guinea pigs of the human variety of Mycobacterium tuberculosis."

63. HINSHAW, H. C., and FELDMAN, W. H. Streptomycin in treatment of clinical tuberculosis: a preliminary report, Proc. Staff Meet. Mayo Clin., **20**:313, 1945.

Although the first observations in man were made with small amounts of the early material, the writers believed that it produced "a limited suppressive effect." Again they are justified in their caution; they did not wish to disappoint countless hopeful patients by too enthusiastic statements.

By 1953 standardized schemes of antibiotic therapy of tuberculosis had been worked out, as may be read, for example, in the *Transactions of the 12th Conference on the Chemotherapy of Tuberculosis* sponsored by the Veterans Administration, the Army, and the Navy (1953). But the last word has not yet been said on the ultimate potentialities of these forms of therapy (see "Chemotherapy of tuberculosis in man. Present status. Report to the Council on Pharmacy and Chemistry," prepared by Nicholas D'Esopo, J.A.M.A., **154**:52, 1954).

64. LEHMANN, Jörgen. Para-aminosalicylic acid in the treatment of tuberculosis, Lancet, **1**:15, 1946.

In previous work on the intermediate metabolism of tubercle bacilli (*ibid.*, p. 14) Lehmann concluded that derivatives of salicylic acid might be effective in inhibiting growth. In investigating many synthetic substances, he found that *p*-aminosalicylic acid produced definite inhibition. The material was found to have little toxicity for rat, guinea pig, or man, and early trials suggested that it might have a therapeutic effect in clinical tuberculosis. After 10–14 gm. a day by mouth, temperature fell, and this effect was not thought due to a non-specific antipyretic action. Later work has, of course, confirmed the value of *p*-aminosalicylic acid as a useful agent in the therapy of tuberculosis, especially in association with other antibiotics, such as streptomycin. An excellent review is that of E. Bogen, R. N. Loomis, and W. W. Drake, "Para-aminosalicylic acid treatment of tuberculosis," Am. Rev. Tuberc., **61**:226, 1950.

65. DUBOS, René J. Rapid and submerged growth of mycobacteria in liquid media, Proc. Soc. Exper. Biol. & Med., **58**:361, 1945.

Although many attempts had been made to devise a satisfactory medium for the growth of tubercle bacilli, the difficulties were such that inoculation of guinea pigs with suspected material remained the standard method of isolation. Dubos made the important discovery that addition to Long's synthetic medium of various lipids, natural and synthetic, allowed very rapid and diffuse growth of tubercle bacilli. In numerous subsequent papers by Dubos and his associates this brief note is amplified (for references see Dubos, "The tubercle bacillus and tuberculosis," Am. Scientist, **37**:353, 1949).

Dubos' methods have made practicable the routine use of cultures for the isolation of tubercle bacilli.

66. MIDDLEBROOK, Gardner, DUBOS, René J., and PIERCE, Cynthia. Virulence and morphological characteristics of mammalian tubercle bacilli, J. Exper. Med., **86**:175, 1947.

Although previous attempts had been made to correlate growth characteristics and virulence, Dubos and his associates gave the first clear demonstration. In a synthetic medium containing a wetting agent, "Tween 80," virulent cultures tended to form "microscopically demonstrable serpentine cords of varying thickness and length consisting of highly acid-fast bacilli oriented along the long axis of the cord. . . . Avirulent bacilli grow in a more or less nonoriented fashion. They have never been observed to form cords." In this connection one should refer to the monograph by William F. Drea and Anatole Andrejew, *The Metabolism of the Tubercle Bacillus* (Springfield, Ill.: Charles C Thomas, 1953).

67. RICH, Arnold R. The pathogenesis of tuberculosis. Springfield, Ill.: Charles C Thomas, 1944; 2d ed., 1951.

This monumental book is an important milestone in the literature on tuberculosis. It represents a critical analysis of resistance, infection, immunity, and hypersensitivity from every possible standpoint, documented with fifteen hundred references. While reviewers have differed with Rich on small points, all agree on the great skill with which a vast amount of material has been synthesized. Every serious student of tuberculosis must carefully study this outstanding monograph.

68. BERNSTEIN, Jack, LOTT, William A., STEINBERG, Bernard A., and YALE, Harry L. Chemotherapy of experimental tuberculosis. V. Isonicotinic acid hydrazide (Nydrazid) and related compounds, Am. Rev. Tuberc., **65**:357, 1952.

"A class of compounds showing high antituberculous activity is reported for the first time. Of these the most active is isonicotinic acid hydrazide (Nydrazid). In a standardized infection of mice with the Ravenal strain of M. tuberculosis, the minimal effective dose of this compound is 1/700 that of *p*-aminosalicylic acid." This experimental work in mice was soon followed by a flood of clinical reports (Ref. 69). The situation is somewhat confused, since two pharmaceutical houses seem to have developed the same compound practically simultaneously. A number of other articles on the pharmacology of these compounds and on their effects in experimental tuberculosis are to be found in this same number of the review (April, 1952).

69. ELMENDORF, DuMont F., Jr., CAWTHORN, William V., MUSCHEN-HEIM, Carl, and McDERMOTT, Walsh. The absorption, distribution, excretion and short-term toxicity of isonicotinic acid hydrazide (Nydrazid) in man, Am. Rev. Tuberc., **65**:429, 1952.

These workers made a thorough study of the above points in tuberculous patients over periods of from 4 to 16 weeks. They found the drug well tolerated but thought that it was not possible from their observations to "make any positive statement concerning the therapeutic value of this compound in the treatment of tuberculosis." Meanwhile, E. Robitzek and I. Selikoff ("Hydrazine derivatives of isonicotinic acid [Rumifon, Marsilid] in the treatment of active progressive caseous-pneumonic tuberculosis," Am. Rev. Tuberc., **65**:402), publishing at the same time, found that these compounds "exert an impressive therapeutic effect." Slightly antedating these were several reports in the Sea View Hosp. Quart. Bull., **13**:3, 12, 17, 27, and 52, 1952.

Current appraisal of izoniazid is well presented in "Present concepts of antimicrobial therapy in pulmonary tuberculosis" (Am. Rev. Tuberc., **68**:819, 1953), a panel discussion in which differences of opinion are freely expressed, and in E. A. Riley's excellent review, "Chemotherapy of tuberculosis" (Am. J.M. Sc., **226**:552, 1953). However, the whole subject is still in the investigative stage, and the definitive bibliography must await the work of future years.

70. LURIE, Max B., ABRAMSON, Samuel, and HEPPLESTON, A. G. On the response of genetically resistant and susceptible rabbits to the quantitative inhalation of human type tubercle bacilli and the nature of resistance to tuberculosis, J. Exper. Med., **95**:119, 1952.

We have given some of the early references on the development of ideas about immunity (Refs. 51, 59). In recent years the subject has been gone into more from the standpoint of the new views on antibodies which deal with them as concrete definable and measurable substances rather than the hypothetical lock-and-key pictographs of the Ehrlich side-chain theory. The present paper is given simply as an example of this sort of modern study; it is of interest to note the reappraisal of allergy in relation to immunity.

Section 13

LEPROSY

Bacteriology	Refs. 4, 5, 6
Clinical	Refs. 1, 8, 10, 11, 12
General	Refs. 1, 8, 10, 11, 12
Lepromin test	Ref. 17
Pathology	Refs. 3, 7
Therapy, chaulmoogra	Ref. 2
Therapy, general	Ref. 10
Therapy, streptomycin	Ref. 16
Therapy, sulfones	Refs. 14, 15
Transmission	Refs. 1, 6, 7, 9, 10, 13

Section 13

LEPROSY

W HY the bibliography of leprosy presents an almost insuperable problem is not far to seek; very few facts of the disease are settled and agreed upon by all workers—indeed, almost every point is still in dispute. Thus there is yet doubt whether the bacillus of leprosy has been artificially cultivated and whether the disease has actually been transmitted to animals. The question of communicability in man and the modes of adequate exposure are still unsettled. Therapy, even with the modern drugs, remains in a state of trial, and the results are extremely difficult to appraise. As one goes through the literature, then, one can find no definitive papers on any of these points, no one man who clearly proved anything. Hence one must depend on critical discussions, such as are found in the books to which we refer below, of various topics by experts (who often disagree).

Few diseases have a more romantic past in legend and folklore than leprosy. Most of the books enumerated here contain excellent historical sections, especially that of Jeanselme (Ref. 12). In addition, there are to be mentioned the interesting article by Sir James Y. Simpson ("Antiquarian notes of leprosy and leper hospitals in Scotland and England," Edinburgh M. & S.J., **56**:301, 1841; **57**:121, 394, 1842) and the tremendous compilation by R. Virchow ("Zur Geschichte des Aussatzes, besonders in Deutschland, nebst einer Aufforderung an Aerzte und Geschichtsforscher," Virchows Arch. f. path. Anat., **18**:138, 273; **19**:43, 1860; **20**:166, 459, 1861), both of which contain much source material. A good brief historical discussion is that of Kaposi in F. Hebra and M. Kaposi's book, *On Diseases of the Skin* (London: New Sydenham Society, 1875), p. 118, translated by Warren Tay. J. Lowe's paper, "Comments on the history of leprosy," Indian M. Gaz., **77**:680, 1942, is also of interest. The article on leprosy in August Hirsch, *Handbuch der historisch-geographischen Pathologie* (2d ed.; Stuttgart: Ferdinand Enke, 1883), **2**:1, contains much material of historical and epidemiological importance.

As to bibliographies, Danielssen and Boeck (Ref. 1) give an interesting list of older titles, whereas Babes (Ref. 11) has a comprehensive bibliography to date. In Jadassohn's monograph, *Lepra* (Jena: Gustav Fischer, 1928), is an extensive reference list to titles after 1916, and McKinley's article (Ref. 4) is documented by some five hundred references. Bibliographies, more or less extensive, are also found in the books listed below. However, the monumental book by V. Klingmüller (*Die Lepra* [Berlin: Julius Springer, 1930]) is what amounts to an annotated bibliography of the whole subject, with sixty closely printed pages of references which the author has tried to make complete to 1930. The last chapter, on "Lepra in literature and art" by K. Grön, is of special interest. Finally, there should be mentioned the tremendous bibliography of leprosy (Luiza Keffer, *Índice biblográfico de lepra, 1500–1943* [3 vols.; São Paulo, Brazil, 1944, 1946, 1948]), which requires three large volumes to cover all the references.

There are a great many books and monographs dealing with the whole subject of leprosy. Worthy of mention are, of course, Danielssen and Boeck's classic (Ref. 1) and the treatises of G. A. Hansen and C. Looft (Ref. 10), J. Jadassohn (*loc. cit.*), E. Jeanselme (Ref. 12), R. G. Cochrane (*A Practical Textbook of Leprosy* [Oxford, 1947]), and R. Chaussinand (*La Lèpre* [2d ed.; Paris: Expansion Scientifique Française, 1955]). The standard work today is, however, that of L. Rogers and E. Muir (*Leprosy* [Baltimore: Williams & Wilkins Co., 3d ed.; 1946]). The precise brochure by H. L. Arnold (*Modern Concepts of Leprosy* [Springfield, Ill.: Charles C Thomas, 1953]) forms an excellent introduction to the subject. The important topics of prophylaxis, isolation, and leprosaria are dealt with at length in Jeanselme (Ref. 12, p. 566) and in Cochrane (*op. cit.*, p. 191).

A great many journals are devoted solely to the subject of leprosy. Of these, some of the most important are the International Journal of Leprosy, Manila, sponsored by the International Leprosy Association; the Leprosy Review, London, the British Empire Leprosy Relief Association; Leprosy in India, Calcutta, Indian Leprosy Association; and the Lepra Bibliotheca Internationalis, Leipzig. There are journals devoted to leprosy published in foreign languages, such as the Leper Quarterly, Shanghai, sponsored by the Chinese Mission to Lepers, and several South American journals.

Finally there are transactions and reports of innumerable conferences and congresses on leprosy which have been held around the world from time to time.

1. DANIELSSEN, D.-C., and BOECK, Wilhelm. Traité de la spédalskhed, ou éléphantiasis des Grecs, traduit du Norvégien, sous les yeux de M. D. Danielssen, par L.-A. Cosson (de Nogaret). Paris: J.-B. Baillière, 1848. (Original edition: *Om spedalskheden* [Christiania, 1847].)

This monograph of some five hundred pages is generally accepted as the beginning of the modern study of leprosy. Stimulated by and under the auspices of the Norwegian government, Danielssen undertook to study leprosy in St. George's Hospital in Bergen, and, like all studies based on careful observation of facts, his turned out to be a valuable contribution. Danielssen and Boeck divided cases of leprosy into the tuberculous form and the anesthetic form, the former implicating especially the skin and the latter the nerves. This classification, with its sharp differentiation of two groups of cases, has not quite stood the test of time, but as a beginning it was useful. "In the tuberculous form, which has chosen the skin for the theater of its ravages, we have the morbid changes exposed daily before our eyes. In the anesthetic form, which, on the contrary, affects by choice the centers of the nervous system, we have found a series of very interesting nervous phenomena" (Preface, p. xi).

Every aspect of the disease is discussed and documented by case reports. "Under the heading of treatment of leprosy we have little to report." Arsenicals, iodides, and potassium salts are mentioned without much enthusiasm. Bleeding was tried in some cases. As to etiology, the authors incline to accept heredity and to reject contagion. "There are few facts which are more commonly agreed on by authors ancient and modern than the transmission of the disease from parents to children [p. 81]. . . . If we run through modern authors we find them almost unanimous on the non-existence of any contagion" (p. 91). The views of Danielssen and Boeck had great influence on contemporary thought and led for years to almost general acceptance of the theory that the disease was hereditary (see also Ref. 13).

This interesting book, which must be read to grasp its scope, stands on the threshold of past and present. Heavily documented, the ancient and old authors are constantly referred to, while the carefully reported cases give a distinctly modern tone.

2. MOUAT, F. J. Notes on native remedies. No. 1. The chaulmoogra. Indian Ann. M. Sc., **1**:646, 1854.

The treatment of leprosy is very difficult to evaluate because of the long and variable course of the disease and the tendency to spontaneous remission. Thus *post hoc* inferences have been common, and chance, faith, and unknown variables have had an opportunity to influence judgment. To conclude that a drug is effective, therefore, there should either be immediate improvement, or, if slow, improvement should be marked. Slight improvement coming over a long time means nothing. As to the effects of the innumerable drugs and procedures which have been tried in leprosy, they are discussed in the sections on treatment in the various books listed in the introduction. Sir Leonard Rogers ("Recent advances in the treatment and prophylaxis of leprosy," Edinburgh M.J., **37**:1, 1930), writing fairly recently, states that "the advances made in the treatment of leprosy in the last decade or so have opened up a new era of hope for the unfortunate leper, and for the first time in three thousand years the disease has been known there are good grounds for believing that this dreaded disease will become greatly reduced."

However, until the introduction of the sulfones (Ref. 14), chaulmoogra oil or related substances were the backbone of drug therapy, even though the results were variously judged by different observers. Mouat turned his attention to native remedies in India and introduced the chaulmoogra into European practice. "The seeds[1] yield by expression a bland fixed oil with a peculiar and slightly unpleasant smell and taste, with the faintest possible after flavour of the bitter almond. . . . It appears to have been long known to, and prized by the Natives in the treatment of leprosy. . . . I was first informed of its value by Mr. Jones, the Headmaster of the Hindoo College . . . at whose recommendation it was tried in the Leper Asylum, with a favorable result." Mouat then reports three cases in which he thought that brilliant effects were obtained. "With regard to the exhibition of the remedy, it may be taken in the form of a pill, or the seed itself. . . . Six grains in the former case, or three seeds in the latter, may be given daily. . . . In large quantity, however, it is apt to disagree, causing nausea and irritability of the stomach. A more elegant way of administering it would be in the form of the oil."

The development of the use of chaulmoogra oil and its esters is fully discussed by L. Rogers in the article referred to above.

3. VIRCHOW, Rudolph. Die krankhaften Geschwülste, **2**:494 (article on leprosy). Berlin: August Hischwald, 1864.

In this interesting and scholarly article on leprosy, Virchow's histological description of the lesions is of special interest. Virchow discusses his "leprosy

[1] For beautiful photographs of the plant and its seeds, see Jeanselme (Ref. 12, pp. 626 ff.).

cells." "With reference to these cells I note that at the height of their development they consist of round, pale, faintly granular, fragile elements with a moderately large and also granulated nucleus. In the fresh I was specially struck by their tendency to form a sort of vacuole, probably through taking up water. . . . Their size is variable. Many are not much larger than a red blood cell . . . many reach the appearance of the largest mucous corpuscle [*Schleimkörper*]."

4. HANSEN, [Gerhard Henrik Armauer]. Indberetning til det Norske mediciniske Selskab i Christiania om en med understøttelse af selskabet foretagen reise for at anstille undersøgelser angående spedalskhedens årseger tildels udførte sammen med forstander Hartwig, Norsk mag. laegevidensk., 3d ser., **4**:1, 1874. (English translation: I. On the etiology of leprosy by G. Armauer Hansen, Brit. & Foreign M.-Chir. Rev., **55**:459, 1875.)

Hansen had been working on the bacteriology of leprosy for several years before he presented his paper at the medical society of Christiania. Actually, this long communication deals mainly with the question of whether or not leprosy is a hereditary disease. It is not until the last page that an organism is mentioned: "There are to be found in every leprous tubercle extirpated from a living individual . . . small staff-like bodies, much resembling bacteria, lying within the cells. . . . Though unable to discover any difference between these bodies and true bacteria, I will not venture to declare them to be actually identical. Further, while it seems evident that these low forms of organic life engender some of the most acute infectious diseases, the attributing of the origin of such a chronic disease as leprosy to the apparently same matter must, of course, be attended with still greater doubts. It is worthy of notice, however, that the large brown elements found in all leprous proliferations in advanced stages, of which I have in 1869 already given engravings . . . bear a striking likeness to bacteria in certain states of development, as these are represented by Klebs . . . and further, that in almost every preparation from a leprous tubercle, made with the utmost care to avoid contamination and kept for a number of days in the damp chamber, are developed conglobate masses of spherical bacteria or zoogloea."

What, then, was Hansen dealing with? Actually, he seems himself in doubt— "unpregnant of his cause," and certainly Klebs, who was nearly always wrong, was an enthusiastic but unsound leader to follow.

In his next communication Hansen ("Bacillus leprae," Virchows Arch. f. path. Anat., **79**:32, 1880)[2] opens by complaining that Dr. Eklund, to whom he had shown his preparations and declared his views on the parasitic nature of leprosy, had taken credit in a brochure "Om sptelska," recently published, for the discovery of a micrococcus in the tissues and that Dr. Neisser from Breslau had visited in Bergen to study leprosy and had taken home material and published (Ref. 5) to the effect that the preparations were everywhere loaded with bacteria which he, as well as Ferd. Cohn and Koch, considered a new species and the cause of leprosy. Thus Hansen felt that his hand had been forced and that he was obliged to publish his results more at length. Hansen for the most

[2] This paper also appeared in English (G. Armaner [*sic*] Hansen, "The bacillus of leprosy," Quart. J. Micr. Sc., **20**:92, 1880) and in Norwegian ("Bacillus leprae," Nord. med. ark., **12**:1, 1880).

part examined scrapings of leprous material suspended in water and saw all sorts of granules and "bacteria." Only one preparation, after immersion in osmic acid and staining with methyl violet, showed masses which seemed to consist of little rods. "From the various notes of my investigations in 1873 every one will be easily able to see that I had good reason for supposing that bacteria appear in leprous products, but also that I, supported alone by these investigations, could not propound a theory on this subject, and still more decide whether these bacteria really were the virus, which, introduced into the system, produced the disease." The paper is dated October, 1871, and there is a brief addendum: "I have succeeded after the suggestion of Dr. Koch in seeing the bacilli beautifully in sections hardened in absolute alcohol and intensively stained. They are present sometimes singly but usually in clumps, which fits in with their occurrence *in* the cells." The drawings in Plate I are rather unsatisfactory and show nothing which could be identified as lepra bacilli. It appears, then, that Hansen, like Jenner, was inspired with an idea which turned out to be correct, but he does not really present adequate evidence to support it.

Earle B. McKinley's monograph ("The etiology of leprosy," Medicine, **13**:377, 1934) is a vast storehouse of information on the bacteriology, cultivation, and pathogenicity of the lepra bacillus, documented by 525 references, which supersedes any compilations previously published.[3] McKinley summarized the vexed question of whether the bacillus had been successfully cultivated by saying: "There does not exist today any absolute proof that any investigator has actually succeeded in the artificial cultivation of the leprosy bacillus." Furthermore, Chaussinand quite recently (*op. cit.*, p. 33), in going over the subject, comes to similar conclusions: "We have been able to show that Dubos' medium, which allows the cultivation of the tubercle bacillus in a few days, in no way favors growth of the bacillus of Hansen."

5. NEISSER, [A.]. Ueber die Aetiologie des Aussatses, Jahresb. d. Schles. Gesellsch. f. vaterl. Cultur, **57**:65, 1879.

Neisser tells the story of his trip to Norway to study leprosy. He points out that most doctors, following Danielssen, believed that hereditary influences caused leprosy, whereas the view of Hansen that the disease was contagious had practically no adherents. Hansen had found conglomerate masses of bodies in leprosy tissue, inoculation and culture experiments with which yielded no results, "so that he was unable to conclude that he had before him the presumed virus of leprosy." Neisser took home much leprosy tissue, in which, with modern staining methods, he saw innumerable "rods." There follows a detailed description of the organisms and of their relation to the tissue cells. But "in anesthetic macroscopically undiseased skin, I could see neither bacilli nor any other pathological change. . . . I think that these bacilli are related to the pathological changes in Lepra, in other words that Lepra is a bacterial disease. . . . The constancy of the finding of such a tremendous occurrence of this one form of bacillus in the most different organs speaks for my hypothesis."

In a second major paper Neisser ("Weitere Beiträge zur Aetiologie der Lepra," Virchows Arch. f. path. Anat., **84**:514, 1881) straightens out the ques-

---

[3] One is perplexed by the fact that in dealing with the discovery of the bacillus the work of Neisser is not even mentioned (see Ref. 5).

tion of priority. "When I was in Bergen in July and August, 1879, Hansen had the idea that rodlike structures played a role in the cause of leprosy. But even his colleagues in Bergen did not regard his findings as of any importance, although they had been familiar with them for years. Indeed, some were antagonistic to the idea of contagion. . . . At the time there was no question of an actual bacillus and even less of staining and culture technique. . . . I take credit, therefore, for establishing these bodies in their place as pathogenic bacteria, since I was the first who applied in exact fashion the new staining methods of Weigert and Robert Koch and brought evidence that a specific variety of bacteria is concerned in leprosy which can be brought into causal relationship with all the pathological phenomena of the disease." There seems little doubt that Neisser deserves credit for going beyond the vague hypothetical stage and bringing real evidence. Who should have priority for discovering the bacillus we leave to our readers to decide.

Neisser found the bacilli in the skin lesions; in the mucous membranes of the mouth, gums, and larynx; in the interstitium of peripheral nerves; in the cornea, cartilages, testes, lymph glands, spleen, and liver. The bacilli were seen inside the large "lepra cells" described by Virchow (Ref. 3). Neisser describes the histology of the lesions. Some cells are stuffed with bacilli, as shown with aniline stains. Later the cells and bacteria disintegrate, leaving the well-known "vacuole formation" evident. Very few bacilli occur outside cells in the connective tissue. The bacilli are difficult to see unstained. Tinctorial characteristics are described. When properly stained, the organisms appear as "fine slender rods of the length of one-half to three-quarters of a human red cell." They are straight or slightly bent. Some of the bacilli have round swellings at the ends or in the middle. These Neisser regarded as spores. His main argument that the bacilli were the cause of leprosy was their constant presence in all lesions, as well as the histological appearance. He thought the evidence favored lymphatic spread rather than hematogenous distribution. "Leprosy is probably an infectious disease, and its specific production is contagious." Contagion may be direct or indirect. "Leprosy, according to my view, is not transmissible by heredity." Neisser thought that he had succeeded in culturing the bacilli, although he was a little uncertain on this point. The paper contains so much material that the original must be read to get the full implications; at any rate, this is the first really adequate account of leprosy bacilli, Neisser being wrong on only two points—the cultivability of the organisms and the idea that they formed spores.

At about the same time, confirmatory notes began to appear, such as that of V. Cornil and Suchard ("Note sur le siège des parasites de la lèpre," Bull. et mém. Soc. méd. d. hôp., **18:**151, 1881), who describe the same intracellular appearance as had Neisser; and of V. Cornil ("Second note sur le siège des bactéries de la lèpre et sur les lésions des organes dans cette malade," *ibid.*, p. 155), who discusses the histological appearance of the lesions but adds little, if anything, to Neisser's description. He found, as had Neisser, that "in most fibrous tissue, the bacteria throw out long filaments in the interstices of the fibers, the fixed cells of the fibrous tissue being little altered or normal, but there results often a sclerosis, a thickening of these fibrous tissues."

From this point on, the confirmatory studies on the presence of the bacilli in leprosy are too numerous to quote. They are referred to in detail in McKinley's review (Ref. 4).

6. HANSEN, G. Armauer. Studien über Bacillus leprae, Virchows Arch. f. path. Anat., **90**:542, 1882.

From the very discovery of the bacillus, several questions were under debate: (1) whether the organism was cultivatable, (2) whether it could be found in the blood, and (3) whether the disease could be transmitted by it to animals. Neisser (Ref. 5) thought that perhaps he had transmitted the disease to dogs, although he stated later (Ref. 7): "The result of all experiments to date is: Leprosy has thus far not been produced in animals." He also thought that he had cultivated the bacillus. H. Köbner ("Uebertragungsversuche von Lepra auf Thiere," Virchows Arch. f. path. Anat., **88**:282, 1882) tried systematically to transmit the disease to monkeys, guinea pigs, mice, rabbits, pigeons, eels, and frogs, always with negative results. Hansen in the above paper also failed to produce lepra in a monkey and could not find bacilli in the blood. Hansen found bacilli readily in the nodular form of leprosy but not in the anesthetic form. He thought, however, that "spore formation obviously takes place in the human body."

In summary, all this brings out how difficult these matters were to settle with early inadequate methods. Evidently most observers *expected* the bacilli to grow and to be found in the blood and to produce lesions in animals.

7. NEISSER, A. Histologische und bacteriologische Leprauntersuchungen, Virchows Arch. f. path. Anat., **103**:355, 1886.

P. G. Unna, the great German dermatologist ("Leprastudien. Zur Histologie der leprösen Haut," Monatshefte f. prakt. Dermatol., 1885, Ergänzungsheft, p. 34, and "Die Leprabacillen in ihrem Verhältnis zur Hautgewebe" in *Dermatologische Studien* [Hamburg and Leipzig: Leopold Voss, 1886], **1**:1) in elaborate studies challenged the view of Hansen and of Neisser that leprosy bacilli occurred intracellularly; he thought that, for the most part, they lay without the cells in the lymph spaces. This work stimulated Neisser to retort in this long paper, in which he sustained his thesis and added other conclusions, such as his inability to transmit lepra to animals and the fact that, while contagion was possible, the probability was slight. He still insisted on spores and believed that multiplication outside the body was improbable. "At any rate, man is to be regarded as the chief carrier of the leprosy virus, and therefore one should not protest so emphatically 'in the name of humanity' against his isolation." Hansen ("Die Lage der Leprabacillen," Virchows Arch. f. path. Anat., **103**:388, 1886) joined shoulders with Neisser to support the intracellular position of the bacilli. After all, he said, one can answer this question only by seeing, and "Neisser and I have pictured cells, fresh and stained, in which we have seen the bacilli"(!) K. Touton ("Zur Topographie der Bacillien in der Leprahaut," Virchows Arch. f. path. Anat., **104**:381, 1886) also took sides with Hansen and Neisser.

8. NEISSER, A. Der Aussatz, Lepra, *in* H. von Ziemssen, Handbuch der speciellen Pathologie und Therapie, Vol. **14**, Part I: Handbuch der Hautkrankheiten, p. 620. Leipzig, 1883.

A systematic article by a great authority on the disease, giving its contemporary status. Neisser, following Danielssen and Boeck (Ref. 1) and Virchow (Ref. 3), still divided the cases sharply into Lepra tuberculosa and Lepra nervorum. It is of interest that in most of the older discussions leprosy was placed in the category of skin diseases.

9. [Editorial]. The inoculation of a condemned criminal, M. Rec., **29**:449, 1886.

An account is given of the inoculation in Hawaii of a condemned criminal. "Finally, by permission of the Privy Council, Dr. Arning was allowed to make an inoculation upon the condemned criminal Keanu, whose sentence was commuted to imprisonment for life . . . an inoculation was made of leprous matter in the convict's arm. Bacilli were found in the sore or the scar until fourteen months later, but no constitutional symptoms were observed. . . . We regret to learn that owing to difficulties with the Health Board, Dr. Arning's work will probably be discontinued." We have been unable to see Arning's own report (referred to by Porritt and Olsen). If correct, this is a most important observation which fits in with the prevailing view that leprosy is transmitted with great difficulty. The case is questioned by Rogers and Muir (*op. cit.*, p. 89), who say that the subject "may have contracted his subsequently developing disease [leprosy] through contact with two infected relatives."

R. J. Porritt and R. E. Olsen ("Two simultaneous cases of leprosy developing in tattoos," Am. J. Path., **23**:805, 1947) reviewed the literature on transmission by human inoculation and felt that the matter was still in doubt until their observation of two United States Marines, who were tattooed successively by the same man on the same day. Both developed maculo-anesthetic leprosy in the tattoos about 2½ years later. "These two cases provide strong evidence for the spread of leprosy by inoculation."

Interesting material on human inoculations is also to be found in the paper by A. A. St. Mouritz, "Human inoculation experiments in Hawaii including notes on those of Arning and of Fitch. Condensed, arranged and annotated by H. W. Wade," Internat. J. Leprosy, **19**:203, 1951.

10. HANSEN, G. Armauer, and LOOFT, Carl. Leprosy: in its clinical and pathological aspects. Translated by Norman Walker, M.D., F.R.C.P. Bristol: John Wright & Co., 1895.

This book is of special interest and importance because in it Hansen summarizes his mature views on leprosy, formulated after many years of study of the disease.

The introductory chapter deals with the important question of classification. The authors make some criticism of Danielssen and Boeck's "nodular" and "anesthetic" forms and suggest that the terms "Lepra tuberosa" (tuberculosa) and "Lepra maculo-anesthetica" be used, because, sooner or later, both nodules, macules, and anesthesia, are present. The matter of classification has perhaps been needlessly overstressed in the literature; it is thoroughly discussed by Arnold (*op. cit.*, pp. 17 ff.) and by Chaussinand (*op. cit.*, p. 185), who presents the problem in the form of an elaborate table.

There next follow thorough descriptions of the clinical features, with discussion of the pathological changes. As to prognosis, Hansen and Looft state that both forms of leprosy may recover, although "patients rarely live more than eight or nine years after the definite outbreak of the disease" (p. 85). The chapter on etiology is especially important. The writers defend the view that the disease is acquired by contagion and not by heredity, as most workers thought at the time. "It is well known that the Belgian Father Damien became a leper in the Sandwich Islands. If the Father was of pure Belgian ancestry, and his disease was caused by latent hereditary bacilli, then these bacilli must have been at least several hundred years old, unless one assumes that one of his nearer ancestors had had connection with a leper, and that in this way the Father had acquired his bacilli. Against this in the explanation that the Father who tended the lepers on Molokai, with self-sacrificing love, was, through some want of care or caution, infected as he went in and out among the lepers. The choice between the two explanations does not appear to us a difficult one" (p. 93) (see also Ref. 13). "That leprosy is really contagious is primarily evident from its nature as a bacillary disease. . . . Unfortunately all attempts to inoculate animals have failed" (p. 95). "How leprosy is 'caught' we do not know, but we think it is probably by inoculation" (p. 102). Under treatment, the usual mélange of medicine—mader, cashew-nut oil, Gurjun oil, chaulmoogra, phosphorus, arsenic, ichthyol, carbolic acid, creasote [*sic*], mercury, iodide, tuberculin, and many others are mentioned. However, the writers were not deluded by false claims: "The results of the treatment . . . are nothing to boast of, but they show . . . that leprosy at its commencement can be cured. In our opinion this is true, but with the reservation that the cure is not due to treatment, but is the natural development of the disease" (p. 123). "As we are then, in our opinion, unable to destroy the bacilli with remedies, either internal or external, it only remains to us to prevent infection, and that can only be attained by isolation of those affected."

11. BABES, Victor. Die Lepra. Vienna: Alfred Hölder, 1901.

This monograph of some three hundred and fifty pages was the standard reference book on leprosy at the turn of the century. Leprosy was no longer classified as a skin disease, and the differentiation between "nodular" and "nerve leprosy" was less sharply drawn. Every feature of the disease is fully discussed and the work is well illustrated. There is a comprehensive bibliography.

12. JEANSELME, Ed. La Lèpre. Paris: G. Doin, 1934.

This handsome folio volume of some seven hundred pages stands out as a landmark in the literature on leprosy. Well printed on fine paper and beautifully illustrated, the book is a tribute to the printer's art as well as to the scientist's efforts. Of special interest is the excellent historical introduction, as well as the section on prophylaxis and leprosaria, with its many illustrations. Every phase of the disease is discussed, documented, and illustrated.

13. AYCOCK, W. L. Familial susceptibility as a factor in the propagation of leprosy in North America, Internat. J. Leprosy, **8**:137, 1940.

Danielssen and Boeck (Ref. 1) strongly emphasized the role of heredity in the etiology of leprosy, and, even after the discovery of the bacillus, heredity and contagion have both had their adherents. Aycock, a careful epidemiologist, brings evidence that heredity may play an important role, by studying the occurrence of leprosy in certain family stocks regardless of contact. He concludes: "Collected studies covering several generations of family lines in which leprosy continues to occur in several localized areas indicate that hereditary susceptibility is a major factor in the propagation of leprosy on the North American continent. Aycock ("Familial susceptibility to leprosy," Am. J.M. Sc., **201**:450, 1941) also gives a comprehensive review of the literature on the subject, which leads him to the same conclusion.

14. FAGET, G. H., POGGE, R. C., JOHANSEN, F. A., DINAN, J. F., PREJEAN, B. M., and ECCLES, C. G. The promin treatment of leprosy: a progress report, Pub. Health Rep., **58**:1729, 1943.

A new era in the treatment of leprosy began with the introduction of the sulfone derivatives in 1941, although their use spread slowly and only an occasional title is found in the *Index medicus* until 1946. Many more papers were written, for example, on the use of diphtheria toxoid in leprosy. W. H. Feldman, H. C. Hinshaw, and H. E. Moses ("The effect of promin [sodium salt of P,P'-diamino-diphenyl-sulfone-N,N'-dextrose sulfonate] on experimental tuberculosis: a preliminary report," Proc. Staff Meet. Mayo Clin., **15**:695, 1940) tried the drug in experimental tuberculosis and concluded: "The results of this experiment support the possible effectiveness of promin in experimental tuberculosis in guinea-pigs." As a result of this observation, the drug was deemed worthy of trial in leprosy. Faget and his associates began their studies at the National Leprosarium at Carrville, Louisiana, in 1941. The drug was given by mouth to a series of ten patients. Toxic reactions led to a change to the intravenous route, by which 5 gm. nearly every day for long periods was well tolerated. A slowly developing anemia is the major toxic reaction. A number of case reports are given of unselected patients who received the drug for at least 12 months. "Promin appears capable of inhibiting the progress of leprosy in a considerable percentage of cases. As yet no case of leprosy has become arrested under its influence. . . . It is not claimed that promin is a specific for leprosy." Later Faget and Pogge ("The therapeutic effect of promin in leprosy," Pub. Health Rep., **60**:1165, 1945) reported further on results of treatment with promin. "The present study shows that the improvements observed in the earlier report continue to occur, and in a larger percentage of cases than previously reported. . . . Its action is slow and improvements usually become manifest only after 6 or more months of treatment." Faget and Pogge point out that, from the nature of the case, apparent improvement may be due to "psychological responses of patients" or to spontaneous variations in the disease. However, the photographs which they give of patients with nodular leprosy, before and after treatment, are really impressive.

15. FAGET, G. H., and POGGE, R. C. Treatment of leprosy with diasone: a preliminary report, New Orleans M. & S.J., **98**:145, 1945.

Diaminodiphenylsulfone has yielded various derivatives which have been tried in leprosy. One of these is diasone, the disodium formaldehyde sylfoxylate. It has the advantage of being usable when given by mouth. Faget and Pogge gave the drug a careful trial in forty-seven cases, of which only three showed any advance of the disease under treatment. The toxic reactions were relatively mild on an average dose of 1 gm. daily.

The study of various sulfone derivatives has progressed rapidly since these early studies but as yet with no final evaluation. Good brief summaries, with references, of the whole subject of the sulfones in leprosy may be found in the addendum to the third printing of Rogers and Muir (*op. cit.*) (1951); in H. L. Arnold's book (*op. cit.*, p. 8); and in Chaussinand (*op. cit.*, pp. 233 ff.), who says (1955): "The published results [of Faget, Ref. 14] have been confirmed by leprologists all over the world, and at present the sulfones are considered the therapy of choice." Chaussinand's photographs of patients before and after treatment with D.D.S. (4,4'-diamino-diphenylsulfone) are very impressive.

16. FAGET, G. H., and ERICKSON, P. T. Use of streptomycin in the treatment of leprosy, Internat. J. Leprosy, **15**:146, 1947.

It was inevitable that any drug useful in tuberculosis should be tried in leprosy. Faget and Erickson found that streptomycin "produced encouraging results"; but, in the large and continuing dosage which was necessary, toxic effects were too severe to allow it to be the treatment of choice in leprosy. However, streptomycin seemed to be useful in the local treatment of chronic leprous ulcerations. Erickson ("The status of streptomycin and dihydrostreptomycin in the treatment of leprosy," Internat. J. Leprosy, **19**:1, 1951) later reported further observations and stated that "clinical improvement has been almost universal and sustained." Again the toxic effects of prolonged therapy were prohibitive, but he enumerated various situations in which only short-term therapy is necessary —as, for example, for aborting attacks of acute leprous iridocyclitis—and in which streptomycin may be useful.

17. WADE, H. W. Origin of the lepromin test, Internat. J. Leprosy, **19**:221, 1951.

The lepromin test, a term coined by P. Bargeher ("Künstliche lepraspecifische Allergie und active Immunisierung gegen Lepra," Ztschr. f. Immunitätsforsch. u. exper. Therap., **49**:346, 1926), a skin test performed with suspensions of lepromatous material has been much discussed in the literature, although, like so many facets of leprosy, there are disputes as to its significance, technique, and, indeed, its discovery. Wade carefully analyzes the literature with reference to priority. "It has been suggested that the record should be put straight as to when the test which is universally known by Mitsuda's name was first introduced, and to whom credit should be given for its inception. An attempt to [*sic*] this is made here." Fumio Hayashi ("Mitsuda's skin reaction in leprosy," Internat. J. Leprosy, **1**:31, 1933) is much quoted as an early student of the test. In this somewhat dogmatic article Hayashi gives the results of years of work: "The intracutaneous injection of leprosy bacilli produces no reaction in patients who have reached the nodular state, with unlimited proliferation of the bacilli. The positive reaction appears only in normal individuals resistant to leprosy and in lepers in the neuro-macular stage in which a certain degree of resistance is to be presumed."

DIPHTHERIA

Section 14

DIPHTHERIA

MODERN discussion of diphtheria begins clearly with Bretonneau; he had the genius to recognize the disease as a specific entity and to
separate it from the confused welter of sore throats which doctors currently described. When we remember, however, that necrotizing anginas were at the
time common complications of scarlet fever and, indeed, of any severe infection
such as smallpox, typhoid, or typhus and that dirt and neglect of mouth care
added further complicating factors, it is small wonder that most contemporary
authors could do no better than speak of the "putrid" sore throat and the
"malignant ulcerous" sore throat, as, for example, John Huxham did in his
famous *Essay on Fevers* (London: S. A. Cumberlege, 1782). Patients with
communicable disorders were crowded together in the filthy wards of fever
hospitals, and mixed infections were undoubtedly the rule; so that when a
child had "croup" and died from blocking of the air passages, it was indeed
hard to make an accurate diagnosis.

The throat infections of the eighteenth and early nineteenth centuries
occurred for the most part in definite epidemics, often severe and with a high
mortality rate; the benign sporadic cases of the late nineteenth century were
little seen. It was the occurrence in epidemics, however, which gave the clue to
contagion to most serious students of diphtheria. Greenhow (Ref. 4, p. 1), for
example, makes the following observation: "Thus the disease . . . has been
repeatedly observed, whilst very prevalent in certain districts, to pass over
others in their immediate vicinity, of precisely the same character with respect
to soil, climate, aspect, and inhabitants. . . . The two districts are divided by
the River Stour, and the disease prevailed in all the hamlets on the western side
of the river, while scarcely any cases occurred on the eastern, although both are
similar in character, and appeared to be exposed to the same influences."

The much quoted treatises of Francis Home (*An Inquiry into the Nature,
Cause and Cure of the Croup* [Edinburgh: A. Kincaid & J. Bell, 1765]) and of
Samuel Bard (*An Enquiry into the Nature, Cause and Cure of the Angina
suffocativa, or Sore Throat Distemper* [New York: S. Inslee & A. Car, 1771])
are too primitive to be included in a modern bibliography. Actually, one cannot
be certain just what these writers were dealing with. Home's cases, for example,
were found at autopsy to have a tough membrane inside the trachea "but easily
separable as there is always matter behind it." No lesion was found in the
throat. "There appears from the preceding facts, two very different situations of
the *Suffocatio stridula;* the former more inflammatory, and less dangerous; the
latter less inflammatory and highly dangerous [p. 46]. . . . I have observed, that
the urine, which, during the inflammatory state, is thin, had always, after the
purulent state came on, a light ouzy purulent sediment, such as people have
from matter collected anywhere, that has no vent outward" (p. 47). Home did
suggest tracheotomy (p. 59): "When the case is desperate, may we not try
bronchotomy? I can see no weighty objection to that operation, as the membrane can be so easily got at, and is very loose." Bard described a small outbreak
of a disease similar to that reported by Home. The tonsils and back parts of the

246

throat were swollen and covered with white sloughs, but the main lesion was in the windpipe. "The trachea, quite down to its division in the lungs, was lined with an inspissated mucus, in form of a membrane, remarkably tough and firm." Bard stated that the disease was evidently infectious (p. 19); but this means little, since "all infection must be owing to something received into the body, this therefore whatever it is, being drawn in by the breath of a healthy child, irritates the glands of the fauces and trachea as it passes by them and brings about a change in their secretions. . . . In truth, the throat, altho' frequently affected, is not the seat of the disease, and many have died where that has been entirely free from complaint" (p. 34). In a word, both Home and Bard were definitely of the eighteenth century; any remark which suggests a modern out-look is promptly modified by a meaningless statement based on Galenic ideas. Both writers strongly influenced current ideas on sore throats; Home, by imply-ing that croup was a special disease, held back understanding of diphtheria for fifty years until Bretonneau's observations.

Good discussions of the history of diphtheria are to be found in the book by Sanné (Ref. 9); in Adolph Baginsky's monograph (*Diphtherie und diphtheri-tischer Croup* [Vienna: Alfred Hölder, 1899]); in F. Loeffler's chapter in *The Bacteriology of Diphtheria*, edited by George H. F. Nuttall and G. S. Graham-Smith (Cambridge: Cambridge University Press, 1907); and in the monu-mental treatise on *Diphtheria, Its Bacteriology, Pathology and Immunology*, by F. W. Andrewes and others (London: His Majesty's Stationery Office, 1923). Behring's little book (*Die Geschichte der Diphtherie* [Leipzig: Georg Thieme, 1893]) deals especially with the history of immunization in diphtheria. August Hirsch in his *Handbuch der historisch-geographischen Pathologie* (2d ed.; Stuttgart: Ferdinand Enke, 1886), **3:**43, under the title of "Angina maligna" gives a comprehensive list of epidemic outbreaks of diphtheria (English trans-lation by Charles Creighton [London: New Sydenham Society, 1886], **3:**66 ff.).

As to bibliographies, the list of some three thousand titles in Andrewes *et al.* (*loc. cit.*) gives everything of importance up to 1923. The account of the *Corynebacterium diphtheriae* and diphtheroid organisms by R. Tanner Hewlett and W. Bullock in *A System of Bacteriology in Relation to Medicine* (London: His Majesty's Stationery Office, 1930), **5:**67, is precise but thorough. The works of Sanné (Ref. 9) and Baginsky (*loc. cit.*) give classical general accounts of diphtheria; among modern briefer but excellent articles are those of J. Howard Mueller ("The diphtheria bacilli and the diphtheroids" in René J. Dubos [ed.], *Bacterial and Mycotic Infections of Man* [Philadelphia: J. B. Lip-pincott Co., 1952], p. 222) and of F. S. Cheever ("Diphtheria," in R. L. Cecil and R. F. Loeb, *A Textbook of Medicine* [Philadelphia: W. B. Saunders & Co., 1955]).

Innumerable books and treatises which cannot be listed here have been written on the subject of diphtheria.

1. BRETONNEAU, P[ierre]. Des inflammations spéciales du tissu muqueux, et en particulier de la diphthérite, ou inflammation pelliculaire, connue sous le nom de croup, d'angine maligne, d'angine gangreneuse, etc. Paris: Crevot, 1826. (English translation: Memoirs on diphtheria, etc., selected and translated by Robert Hunter Semple. London: New Sydenham Soci-ety, 1859.)

Bretonneau's great book is a collection of four "memoirs," some of which had already been read at the Paris Academy. His chief contribution was his insistence on the identity of syndromes which were regarded as different diseases by Home (*loc. cit.*) and others—namely "diphtheria," "malignant angina," and "croup." "The gist of the work tends to prove that many lesions of the mucous membranes have been confused, while the 'nuances' of one affection have often been taken for different diseases [p. 9]. . . . The exudation which accompanies them presents remarkable differences; sometimes it is serous, sometimes it is mucoid; sometimes it is white and of a cheesy consistency; sometimes it is a membranous substance intimately adherent [p. 10]. . . . I undertake to prove by the witness of facts that the scorbutic gangrene of the gums, the croup, and the angina maligna are one and the same sort of inflammation" (p. 10).

But to this reviewer at least, Bretonneau's book is disappointing. Having stated his great and fundamental thesis, the material with which he sustains it is confused and rambling. He leans heavily on opinions and quotations from authors back to the sixteenth century. His case reports are often obscure and not clearly appropriate. There is a long section on mercurial therapy. The fourth memoir includes translations of the work of Ghisi, Samuel Bard, Nola, and others. In the additions to the second memoir, one finds an interesting section on tracheotomy, in which is presented the case of Élisabeth de Puységur, the daughter of his friend. The operation on this child is described in minute detail.

2. TROUSSEAU, A. Mémoire sur un cas de trachéotomie pratiquée dans la période extrême de croup, J. des connaissances méd. chir., 1:5, 41, 1833.

Sanné (Ref. 9, p. 463) gives Trousseau credit for popularizing tracheotomy in diphtheria. However, the procedure has a stormy history. Home (*loc. cit.*) advised incision of the trachea as a last resort when the patient with croup was suffocating, but he did not himself perform the operation. Apparently, one of the first successfully to execute a tracheotomy was John Andrée, a London surgeon, in 1782. Interestingly enough, his account of the procedure is given secondhand by J. R. Farre (Appendix to the paper on cynanche laryngea, M.-Chir. Tr., 3:323, 1812), who states: "The above interesting report seems to be deficient only in the particulars of the operation, and these, through the kindness of Mr. Astley Cooper, I have obtained. They are given in the words of Mr. Andrée." The operation is described. "The respiration was immediately relieved," and the child recovered. Thomas Chevalier ("Account of a case of croup in which the operation of bronchotomy was successfully performed," M.-Chir. Tr., 6:151, 1815) tells of a seven-year-old boy: "No chance of his recovery now seemed to remain, unless it were by opening the trachea, and I was applied to for this purpose. I exposed the trachea . . . and divided two of the cartilaginous rings vertically, cutting afterwards transversely in the interstice between them." Bloody material gushed forth, the child was able to breathe and recovered. But all were not so lucky; there were more failures than successes, and bitter arguments arose as to the advisability of the procedure. Bretonneau (Ref. 1) argued strongly in favor of tracheotomy and, after two failures, had the good fortune in 1825 to save the daughter of his friend, the Count de Puységur. Trousseau, however, gives with all his brilliance a minute description of the case of a six-and-a-half-year-old child. The disease picture of the child threatened with suffocation is painted with terrifying vividness. "The child, almost breathing his last, let himself be placed on a dining-room table. With a burned match I traced on his neck a line so that my bistoury should not go astray." The operation is then described. The child had a stormy time; there was evidently wound infection. Twelve days after operation the cannula was removed, he breathed through the larynx, and three days later the wound in the neck was healed.

Trousseau knew of twenty-one instances in which tracheotomy was practiced; seven patients were saved—a good record, as all were moribund when the operation was performed. "The operation is easy," whereupon he describes the whole procedure in minute detail. Henri Roget ("Premier exemple de croup guéri à l'hôpital par la trachéotomie," Bull. et mém. Soc. méd. d. hôp. de Paris, 4:209, 1858) after many years gave the story of the first case successfully operated on in the Hôpital des Enfants. By 1839 Gendron ("Nouvelles considérations sur l'angine maligne, l'angine couerineuse, terminée en croup, et sur la trachéotomie," Bull. Acad. de méd., Paris, 3:908, 1839) in a report to the academy advised that tracheotomy not be reserved as a last resort but practiced early; the discussion in which ten authorities—including such men as Velpeau, Baudelocque, Blandin, and Roux—joined is full of interest.

3. BOUCHUT, E. D'une nouvelle méthode de traitement du croup par le tubage du larynx, Bull. Acad. de méd., Paris, 23:1160, 1857–58.

Bouchut seems to have first conceived the idea of intubation for croup. "Children with this disease die either of asphyxia, or diphtheritic poisoning or of pneumonia. Doctors have found nothing better to do when asphyxia is imminent than to open the passages to the air by tracheotomy. M. Bouchut thinks (he has already done it twice) that one could replace this difficult and dangerous operation, which gives a mortality of 80–90 per 100, by a new procedure, not bloody, and free of all danger, no sooner thought of than done: it is intubation of the glottis." The instruments and procedure are described, and two cases are reported. The academy appointed a committee consisting of MM. Blache, Nélaton, and Trousseau, with Trousseau as spokesman, to investigate Bouchut's claims ("Du tubage de la glotte, et de la trachéotomie, Bull. Acad. de méd., Paris, 24:99, 137, 214, 1858–59). Trousseau in a long report was so antagonistic to the procedure that it fell into disuse until Joseph O'Dwyer rediscovered it, apparently independently ("Intubation of the larynx," New York M.J., 42:145, 1885). O'Dwyer devised a new instrument for inserting and withdrawing the tube, which is pictured in his article, and he later reported many successful results with the procedure ("Analysis of fifty cases of croup treated by intubation of the larynx," *ibid.*, 47:33, 1888). A series of excellent photographs illustrating the course of the operation is given by Baginsky (*op. cit.*, pp. 340 ff.).

4. GREENHOW, Edward Headlam. On diphtheria. London: John W. Parker & Sons, 1860.

Greenhow's book summarizes very well the position of diphtheria in the mid-nineteenth century. While Greenhow's description (p. 5) clearly includes diphtheria, it is probable that other types of sore throat, especially scarlet fever, are to some extent confused with it. "Diphtheria is sometimes preceded, and usually accompanied, by fever. . . . There is often a stiffness of the neck at the commencement of an attack and usually more or less swelling and tenderness of the glands at the angles of the lower jaw. The tonsils are commonly swollen and, together with the immediately contiguous parts of the mucous surface, more or less inflamed. Sometimes the swelling and inflammation subside without further local mischief; at others, the inflamed surface presents, from an early stage of the disease, whitish specks or patches, on a continuous covering of a membraniform aspect which . . . usually soon becomes opaque, and in some cases assumes the appearance of wet parchment or chamois leather. This membranous concretion varies in colour from being slightly opaque to white, ash-colour, buff, or brownish, and in rarer instances, to a blackish tint. . . . When the false membrane has been artificially removed, it is apt to be renewed. . . . The severity of the disease is commonly in proportion to the continuity and density of the exudation. . . . If the patches are small and remain distinct, the case ordinarily runs a favourable course [are these cases of follicular tonsillitis?]; if they rapidly coalesce, if the membrane becomes thick and especially if it assumes a brownish or blackish colour, danger is imminent. . . . The surface of the mucous membrane around the exudation is red and vascular, and so tender that in severe cases it bleeds on the slightest touch. . . . The throat is in general the primary seat of the disease; but the inflammation is apt to spread along continuous mucous surfaces, and thus to extend upwards into the nares and the conjunctiva; down the pharynx into the oesophagus; through the glottis into the larynx, trachea, and downwards into the bronchial tubes; or forward on to the buccal mucous membrane, the gums and lips. Wounds and excoriations of the skin . . . are during an epidemic liable to undergo the same process of exudation, which, coagulating, forms a false membrane analogous to that on the tonsils and throat. . . . After a time the false membrane is thrown off, either entire, so as to represent a mould of the parts it covered, or, which is more usual, comes away in shreds or flakes intermingled with mucus. . . . Occasionally sloughing takes place beneath the exudation. . . . The power of swallowing is sometimes so impaired that there has been difficulty in sustaining life during convalescence; and liquids are apt, even after a comparatively slight attack to be regurgitated through the nostrils. Extreme anemia, impairment of vision, a peculiar form of paraplegia, weakness of the hands and arms, numbness, tenderness of the limbs, tingling, wandering pains, and, more rarely, nervous sequelae of a hemiplegic character, are, in the order here written, ulterior consequences of diphtheria." Greenhow observed sudden death, perhaps of cardiac origin, as a frequent mode of termination. It would be hard to find a more exact and precise description today.

Greenhow had trouble in accurately diagnosing many sporadic cases of sore throat, but he was sure that scarlet fever and diphtheria were totally distinct diseases and that an attack of one did not protect against the other. He did not, however, believe that diphtheria was contagious, as Bretonneau insisted. "Facts, already related, have, in my opinion, clearly shown that diphtheria is of indigenous origin, and capable of being generated anew" (p. 138).

Greenhow showed an amazing conservatism as to therapy in an era when medicines were wildly used. As to local treatment of the throat he said: "I am sure much mischief has been produced by its indiscriminate use, especially by the frequent tearing away of the exudation by probangs, or similar con-

rivances for the application of nitrate of silver, or of strong caustic solutions.
. . . I very soon discontinued this rough local medication to the tender and
already enfeebled mucous membrane. . . . In the first place, the application
can but rarely extend to the entire diseased surface; and in the next, the
subjacent tissues are so deeply involved in cases of really malignant diphtheria,
that any application to the mucous membrane could apparently exercise no
beneficial influence upon the disease" (p. 263). He advised mild cleansing
methods such as gargles of tepid water. Upbuilding, safeguarding, and avoid-
ance of bleeding are emphasized. He had no experience with tracheotomy,
which had been "in this country almost always unsuccessful" (p. 270), although
he thought that it might be lifesaving in a certain type of case in which the
air passages were plugged with membrane. "Time is the most important agent
towards recovery from the several forms of nervous affection which follow
diphtheria" (p. 273).

5. CHARCOT and VULPIAN. Note sur l'état des muscles et des nerfs du
   voile du palais dans un cas d'angine diphthéritique, Compt. rend. Soc.
   de biol., 4:173, 1863 (1862).

Postdiphtheritic paralyses are described in practically every general discussion
of diphtheria (Refs. 2, 4, 9) from Bard on. The frequency varies; J. O. Rolles-
on ("Diphtheritic paralysis," Arch. Pediat., 30:335, 1913) among twenty-three
hundred personal cases found an incidence of 20.7 per cent. In very severe
cases the incidence was 48.1 per cent as against 0.0 per cent in mild cases.
There is much more interesting statistical material in this article. "The outlook
in diphtheritic paralyses may be said to depend upon the age of the patient,
the date of onset, and the situation of the paralysis. The older the patient, the
better the prognosis. Cardiac, pharyngeal, and diaphragmatic palsies are the
only kind which need cause anxiety."

There has been great discussion as to the nature of the lesion since Charcot
and Vulpian in their famous case described the muscle fibers of the palate as
appearing normal, whereas "the nerves of the soft palate showed remarkable
alterations. Some of the nerve fibers are represented by tubes entirely void
of medullary substance." The writers continue with more details of the nerve
lesions. P. Meyer, later, in his important review of the subject, with bibliography ("Anatomische Untersuchungen über diphtheritische Lähmung," Virchows Archiv. f. path. Anat., 85:181, 1881), says: "It turns out that the
peripheral nerves are the seat of unequivocal and widespread changes." A
detailed description of these lesions follows. F. R. M. Walshe ("On the pathogenesis of diphtheritic paralysis," Quart. J. Med., 11:191, 1918) studied the
subject extensively and concluded that "diphtheritic paralysis, at any rate . . .
in cranial nerve involvement, is an ascending infection of the central nervous
system: the toxin elaborated in the membrane passing up to the medulla in
the perineural lymph channels of the cranial nerves innervating the tonsils
and fauces." This thesis is sustained in further papers (*ibid.*, 12:14, 32, 1919).
The whole subject is reviewed by Andrewes *et al.* (*op. cit.*, pp. 223 ff.).

6. TROUSSEAU, A. Clinique médicale de l'Hôtel-Dieu de Paris. Paris: J.-B.
   Baillière et fils, 1865; 2d ed.: Diphthérie (Mal égyptiaque), 1:334.

Trousseau, the master clinician, covers the subject in eight lectures. We shal
not quote in detail his admirable description of the various forms of the disease
He differed from Greenhow on the value of local treatment, and, with referenc
to a case of malignant diphtheria, he tells how "I immediately instituted th
treatment which alone offered some chance of success. I cauterized the involve
parts vigorously with a 20 per cent solution of silver nitrate and then insufflate
powdered alum. That evening and the next day the cauterizations were re
peated with a saturated solution of copper sulfate. In the intervals one gav
insufflations alternately of alum and tannic acid. In spite of this, I insisted o
their feeding the child with soup, chocolate and coffee; at the same time
ordered a quinine preparation." Four days later the child was no better, an
it finally died in syncope, "although the local appearance was improved, of th
diphtheritic poison which had infected it." This is a good example of standar
therapy of the day.

Then follows a lecture on the various localizations of diphtheria—palpebra
cutaneous, vulvar, vaginal, anal, and preputial. Trousseau points out that the
are all the same disease: "Diphtheria is, then, par excellence, a specific disease
whose different manifestations, local and general, only constitute variation
within the species, which are all to be traced to the action of a unique morbi
principle, a special virus; it is, in a word, a pestilential disease [*une maladi
pestilentielle*]. Like all specific diseases, it is contagious and perhaps inoculabl
. . . although the experiments designed to give a vigorous demonstration c
the latter have been fruitless." He quotes a good deal of anecdotal materi
on inoculability but is quite certain that the disease is contagious, althoug
"sometimes its mode of transfer from one locality to another is not easy t
grasp."

The next lecture deals comprehensively with postdiphtheritic paralyse
which he says have been overlooked by many recent writers, although "the
existence has been categorically demonstrated by three authors of the midd
and end of the last century, Ghisi, Chomel, and Samuel Bard." Troussea
describes paralysis of the palate, of the sense organs, of the limbs, and of th
muscles of respiration and deglutition. He discusses the nature of these para
yses. He did not believe that they depended on an anatomical lesion b
thought that they were analogous "to what we see in certain cachexias" an
were an effect of the intoxication of the body economy by the poison of th
disease. In the lecture on treatment Trousseau reverts to a host of Galeni
remedies, but there is an excellent discussion of the indications for and th
technique of tracheotomy.

> 7. OERTEL, [M.]. Experimentelle Untersuchungen über Diphtheri
> Deutsches Arch. f. klin. Med., **8**:242, 1871.

Although attempts had early been made to transmit diphtheria to animals,
surgeon, Trendelenburg ("Ueber die Contagiosität und localer Natur der Dipl
theritis," Arch. f. klin. Chir., **10**:720, 1869) seems to have been the first t
have any real success. He performed tracheotomy on rabbits and introduce
tiny particles of diphtheritic false membrane. The animals died in a few da
and at autopsy had lesions resembling diphtheria. Oertel went a step furth
and in an elaborate investigation not only produced diphtheria in rabbits b
passed it from animal to animal. These observations were, of course, not co

irmed bacteriologically, but they seem plausible. At any rate, the authors were convinced that the disease was due to a living agent and was communicable. Dertel thought of the disease as at first localized and then spreading throughout he body.

8. KLEBS, E. Beiträge zur Kenntnis der Micrococcen, Arch. f. exper. Path. u. Pharmakol., **1**:31, 1873.

Credit for discovery of the causal organism of diphtheria is usually given to Klebs and to Loeffler (Klebs-Loeffler bacillus). Klebs's first paper, however, in he very early days of bacteriology, deals with the crudest sort of attempts at cultures. A careful reading of the paper with reference to the bits of membrane from the throats of "diphtheritis" patients, as well as a scrutiny of the illustrative plates, does not give the slightest hint that Klebs saw or isolated the bacilli of diphtheria. Klebs was an energetic, imaginative man, always a step ahead of the field and almost always wrong, as, for example, in his claims of isolating the causal organisms of typhoid fever and of pneumonia. Nor do further instalments of these studies (*ibid.*, **3**:305, 1875; **4**:107, 207, 409, 875) give the slightest hint that Klebs dealt with *Corynebacterium diphtheriae*. Indeed, aside from his enthusiasm and energy, all this material may be pretty much written off as of historical interest only in connection with "eobacteriology." Indeed, Klebs, like Virchow (Ref. 11), was badly confused and tried to differentiate cases of "croup" and of "diphtheria." He did not believe that diphtheria was a specific disease.

Finally, in a symposium on diphtheria (Verhandl. des Congr. f. inn. Med., d Congr. [Wiesbaden: J. F. Bergmann, 1883], III. Sitzung, "Ueber Diphtherie," p. 134), Klebs gave his matured views as follows: He now divided cases of diphtheria into two forms, one caused by a micrococcus and another associated with the presence of "threadlike structures." "By the greatest magnification it appears that very short and narrow rods are regularly seen imbedded in the superficial layer of the false membrane. . . . One can convince himself that groups of rods always lie in the cells. . . . As to the form of these rods, they are uniform and hardly reach the size of a tubercle bacillus. A considerable proportion is spore-bearing, and, indeed, there are always two terminal spores in each rod. As the membrane dries, spores increase notably, so that one finds that many rods contain four spores." In summary, then, as to the bacillary forms of diphtheritis, one finds "the constant presence of a particular form of bacillus in the diseased mucous membrane, which first develops in the epithelial cells and elicits fibrinous exudate as a result of a peculiar vascular lesion."

What was it that Klebs was dealing with? We must leave it to the reader to decide; Loeffler himself (Ref. 10) conceded the fact that Klebs probably saw the specific bacteria which he (Loeffler) later isolated. However, at best, Klebs's demonstration of a causal organism was crude and incomplete.

9. SANNÉ, A. Traité de la diphthérie. Paris: G. Masson, 1877.

This volume of 654 pages is the outstanding treatise to date on diphtheria. It opens with a valuable and well-documented chapter on the history of the disease and then goes on to the pathology, which is discussed in minute detail. Next come sections on clinical symptoms pertaining to all forms of diphtheria; the pages on diphtheritic paralyses are especially detailed and well documented.

Sanné points out that these disturbances are essentially postdiphtheritic and occur usually from the eighth to the fifteenth day of convalescence, the palate and upper portion of the larynx being most frequently affected (p. 152). Their nature seems to be a peripheral neuritis. Circulatory collapse is well described (p. 148): "The adult may have a feeling of impending death and bids his friends goodbye. Respiration is rapid, but on auscultation there are no abnormal murmurs. The pulse is small, irregular, and unequal; soon it becomes thready; it is slowed, it rarely exceeds 80–100 beats; more often it falls to 50 or 40 beats; in one case it did not beat over 26." Here, then, is pretty clear evidence of heart block. Sanné recognized croup as simply a clinical form of diphtheria (p. 193). Under diagnosis he clearly differentiated between acute tonsillitis and diphtheria (p. 276). There is an interesting discussion of epidemics and their origin: "The origin of epidemics of diphtheria can then be explained first by the importation of the causal germs into a healthy locality whether the 'importer' is frankly ill with the disease or whether he brings germs which have long remained latent." Sanné believed that most cases arose by direct contact less often by inoculation, but also by the ambient air. "This is the method, par excellence, of epidemic and contagious diseases"—an idea which was so intrenched in medical thinking that it was hard to extirpate it. Writing at the beginning of the bacteriologic era, he could say about the nature of the diphtheria poison only that the "tendency which comes to us from Germany and which consists in giving in pathology a large place to a parasitic element would make of diphtheria a zymotic disease." Under treatment there is given, first an interminable list of caustics and "dissolvements" to do away with the false membrane and an equal array of every conceivable drug for internal use. Sanné concluded, however: "If the disease was purely local, one would find without trouble in this therapeutic arsenal some means of mastering it. . . . But some such as the cauterizing agents, are dangerous and worse than the disease. The others, milder, are not powerful enough." Most of the remainder of the book is devoted to a 200-page treatise on tracheotomy, too long to review but covering every aspect of the subject with comprehensive bibliography.

> 10. LOEFFLER, Friedrich. Untersuchungen über die Bedeutung der Micro organismen für die Entstehung der Diphtherie beim Menschen, bei der Taube und beim Kalbe, Mitt. a. d. k. Gsndhtsamte, 2:421, 1884.

Loeffler's studies, as definitive as those of Klebs (Ref. 8) were vague and incomplete, appeared appropriately in the same volume as Koch's classical paper on the etiology of tuberculosis. Loeffler, along with Bretonneau, Behring, and a few others, stands out as a giant in the history of diphtheria.

Loeffler begins by firmly supporting Bretonneau's claim that diphtheria was a specific infection and a communicable disease, an "ens morbi" like measles and smallpox, and not simply a group of symptom complexes caused by various agents. While he postulated a bacterial cause, he felt that diphtheria differed from the usual infections insofar as the active disease was confined to the surface of the mucous membranes exposed to the air and hence was liable to invasion by all sorts of organisms. The problem to Loeffler was to sort out these agents and to isolate from among them the essential cause of diphtheria. "Investigation of the internal organs can naturally not be neglected, since several symptoms such as albuminuria, sudden collapse, late paralysis, etc., point to a participation of the kidneys, heart, and central nervous system. Nonetheless, the main interest remains centered in the local affection." There follows an interesting critical review of previous work on the nature and cause of diphtheria. Loeffler concluded: "If we survey this material and ask whether the investigator has fulfilled the modern postulates [for a bacterial cause], the answer is 'No.'" Loeffler saw the masses of bacilli, which were stained well with methylene blue, as well as cocci in sections of false membrane; he differentiated the lesions of scarlet fever, with their preponderant flora of cocci, from the lesions in true diphtheria. He pointed out that in throats not the site of an actual diphtheria infection there was no real false membrane but simply exudate, which was readily scraped away, and that these were coccal infections. Similar lesions were found in smallpox, typhoid, and other infections.

But Loeffler's great contribution was the recovery in pure culture of the causal organism. He described the technique of isolating the bacilli on various media, of which coagulated sheep serum (Loeffler's medium) was best. There follows a long series of experiments in which all sorts of small animals were inoculated with cultures. Guinea pigs were found highly susceptible, with death in 2–5 days. There were local hemorrhagic infiltrations, pleural effusions, brownish lesions in lungs, and congestion of kidneys and suprarenals, but no organisms were recovered except from the local site of inoculation. Rabbits were also susceptible but less so than guinea pigs. Finally, Loeffler gives a critical analysis of the arguments for and against the bacilli as the specific cause of diphtheria and concludes with admirable conservatism: "Strict proof that the rods are the cause of diphtheria has, then, not been brought"; he was thinking in terms of complete fulfilment of Koch's postulates. He was disturbed by finding bacilli indistinguishable from the diphtheria rods in the pharynx of a healthy child and opened the question of carriers by saying: "It is however conceivable that, at a time when many cases of diphtheria are occurring, the presumptive cause of the disease could be found in the pharynx of an occasional child without eliciting symptoms of any sort." He also opened the possibility of a soluble toxin: "The possibility that the bacilli secrete the virus of diphtheria is not excluded."

Thus Loeffler "skimmed the cream" of diphtheria study in a masterful fashion, and his report will always remain a classic.

11. OERTEL, M. J. Die Pathogenese der epidemischen Diphtherie, nach ihrer histologischen Begründung, mit Atlas von 16 chromolithographierten Tafeln. Leipzig: F. C. W. Vogel, 1887.

Although there were already many partial descriptions of the pathological changes in human diphtheria, this monograph of Oertel is a landmark of thoroughness. After a comprehensive review of the previous literature, there are elaborate and detailed descriptions of both gross and microscopic lesions, to which is appended an atlas of colored plates. Of no less importance is the monograph by W. T. Councilman, F. B. Mallory, and R. M. Pearce (*A Study of the Bacteriology and Pathology of Two Hundred and Twenty Fatal Cases of Diphtheria* [Boston: Privately printed, 1901]), to which are appended numerous beautiful photomicrographs and a comprehensive bibliography. The changes in every organ are described in meticulous detail. The whole subject is reviewed in Andrewes *et al.* (*op. cit.*, pp. 216 ff.). It is of historical interest that the influential Virchow, who early contested Bretonneau's ideas on purely anatomical grounds and insisted on the essential difference between diphtheria and croup, stuck to his views as late as 1885 (R. Virchow, "Croup und Diphtherie," Berl. klin. Wchnschr., **22**:129, 1885).

12. ROUX, E., and YERSIN, A. Contribution à l'étude de la diphthérie, Ann. Inst. Pasteur, **2**:629, 1888.

Roux and Yersin were among those who early confirmed the work of Loeffler and isolated from the false membranes of diphtheria the typical bacteria, which they grew in pure culture. They also obtained lesions in animals, as had been done by Loeffler. After the mucous membranes were injured, lesions were readily produced. "The affection which one causes in rabbits recalls the croup in man. The difficulty which the animal has in breathing, the noise made by air passing through the obstructed trachea, the appearance of the trachea congested and plugged by false membrane, the edematous swelling of the tissues and glands of the neck render this resemblance absolutely striking." On subcutaneous injection, guinea pigs were specially susceptible and died usually within 36 hours, with typical local lesions. Roux and Yersin were impressed by the fact that the growth of diphtheria bacilli was confined to the region of inoculation; no diphtheria bacilli could be grown from the internal organs. But, in spite of this, the experimental animals often developed paralyses which were regarded as highly specific of diphtheria. It was these facts which led the writers deliberately to search for a soluble "poison" developed at the local site of growth and thence absorbed to promote remote mischief.

Working with limpid bacteria-free filtrates of diphtheria bacillus cultures, they produced in rabbits, for example, dilatation of blood vessels, especially in the suprarenals and kidneys; ecchymoses along blood vessels; and pleural effusions, as well as muscular paralyses, which often became generalized and affected the muscles of respiration. They concluded, therefore, that the bacilli produced a soluble toxin, and they raised the question of whether it might be an alkaloid or a diastase. Its effect was diminished by heating and by exposure to air. "Is it possible to accustom animals to the poison of diphtheria and to produce in them by this means immunity to diphtheria?" Thus they raised the question which eventually led to modern methods of immunization.

In a second note (*ibid.*, **3**: 273, 1889) Roux and Yersin summarized their findings as follows: "Diphtheria is an intoxication caused by a very active poison formed by the microbe in the local region where it develops. We have proved this by showing that in pure cultures of diphtheria bacilli there is a specific chemical substance which, introduced under the skin of animals, gives them the disease in the absence of a single living organism." The bulk of this paper is devoted to describing the characteristics of the toxin, such as its high potency and the fact that it appears harmless when given by mouth. Finally, they found it difficult to habituate animals to the toxin because of its great potency.

In the third memoir of this series (*ibid.*, **4**:385, 1890) Roux and Yersin again describe the diagnosis of diphtheria by microscopic examination of bits of false membrane and by isolating the specific bacilli in culture. Next they determined how long after clinical recovery bacilli persisted in the throat. "Rapid disappearance of diphtheria bacilli is not always the rule; one can still find them with all their virulence in the throats of people who have had the disease but in whom there is no more false membrane and in whom the mucosa is perfectly healthy." Thus Roux and Yersin raised the important question of healthy carriers (*porteurs*). Later they said again: "Active diphtheria virus can persist in the mouth for a long time after the disease is cured; consequently people who have had diphtheria should not be returned to ordinary life while they are still carriers of the bacillus." Roux and Yersin worked out the guinea-pig test for virulence of diphtheria bacilli and pointed out that there was no regular agreement with the severity of the clinical case. They designated, as pseudo-diphtheria bacilli, organisms morphologically and culturally indistinguishable from virulent bacilli but harmless for animals, which they obtained from non-diphtheritic sore throats and from the throats of healthy children. They found that "virulence" ran parallel to toxin formation, and they presented evidence that "attenuated" or "avirulent" strains might regain their virulence.

Thus Roux and Yersin opened many important questions and plunged into some of the most perplexing problems of diphtheria. Their work was promptly confirmed by various workers, such as A. Kolisko and R. Paltauf ("Zum Wesen des Croups und der Diphtherie," Wien. klin. Wchnschr., **2**:147, 1889).

A full discussion of the production of toxin and of its properties is to be found in Andrewes *et al.* (*op. cit.*, pp. 101 ff.).

13. BRIEGER, L., and FRAENKEL, Carl I. Untersuchungen über Bakteriengifte, Berl. klin. Wchnschr., **27**:241, 268, 1890.

The work of Roux and Yersin (Ref. 12) stimulated an immense amount of study on diphtheria toxin. Loeffler himself ("Der gegenwärtige Stand der Frage nach der Entstehung der Diphtherie," Deutsche med. Wchnschr., **16**:81, 108, 1890) took a hand in the problem. He stated that he had become convinced that diphtheria was a local infection by the fact that in guinea pigs he was never able to find the bacilli except at the site of inoculation. He thought that there might be a soluble toxin, and he tried to extract it. He procured some material which gave local pain and edema on injection but did not produce typical paralyses. Brieger and Fraenkel made a systematic investigation of bacterial poisons, in the course of which they studied bacteria-free filtrates of diphtheria bacillus cultures. Alcohol precipitates were highly toxic and gave the reactions of a protein; hence they named it a "toxalbumen." They measured the great toxicity of the material, of which 2–5 mg/kg were sufficient to kill a rabbit. The animals also developed typical diphtheritic paralyses. This paper really opened the intensive study of the subject, and an immense amount of work was subsequently done on the nature of the toxin. Modern aspects of the subject are reviewed by Mueller (*op. cit.*, p. 226).

14. BEHRING, E., and KITASATO, S. Ueber das Zustandekommen der Diphtherie-Immunität und der Tetanus-Immunität bei Thieren, Deutsche med. Wchnschr., **16**:1113, 1890.

C. Fraenkel's ("II. Immunisierungsversuche bei Diphtherie," Berl. klin Wchnschr., **27**:123, 1890) account of attempts to immunize against diphtheria appeared one day before the classical paper of Behring and Kitasato. The story of the question of priority is told in interesting detail in the book by Professor Behring (*Die Geschichte der Diphtherie* [Leipzig: Georg Thieme, 1893]).

Actually, Fraenkel was confused about the whole subject, and his attempts at immunization consisted of injecting both whole cultures treated in various ways and growth products (toxin). His results were indecisive as regards the production of immunity. Fraenkel thought that toxic and immunizing substances existed side by side in culture fluids; he believed that they could be separated by heating, since the toxic material was destroyed at 55°–60° C., but even with the remainder he was unable to obtain complete protection. The report seems to us of little value, and Fraenkel beclouded, rather than clarified, the issue. The paper of Behring and Kitasato actually dealt mainly with tetanus, but the similarity between the mechanisms of protection in the two diseases was clearly recognized. "The immunity of rabbits and mice which have been immunized against tetanus rests on the ability of the cell-free fluids of the blood to render harmless the toxic substances which tetanus bacilli produce." In these brief words Behring and Kitasato first definitely stated the principle underlying antitoxic immunity.[1] They showed, furthermore, that the antitoxic substances existed in extravascular blood and serum, that this property was so stable that it remained effective when serum was injected into another animal, and that protective properties of the blood are absent in animals which are not immune to tetanus. They predicted that such sera would be useful for the treatment of diphtheria and tetanus in man. A week later Behring's paper ("Untersuchungen über das Zustandekommen der Diphtherie-Immunität bei Thieren," Deutsche med. Wchnschr., **16**:1145, 1890) on diphtheria immunization appeared. While he clearly recognized the antitoxic effects of cell-free blood serum, he did not yet challenge antitoxin by injection of bacteria-free toxin except in the case of sterile pleural effusions produced in rabbits by injections of virulent cultures. He actually used five different methods of immunization, "none of which are applicable to man."

The practical application was slow in developing. Von Behring, Boer, and Kossel ("Zur Behandlung diphtheriekranker Menschen mit Diphtherieheilserum," Deutsche med. Wchnschr., **19**:389, 1893) used a serum derived from sheep which they stated was "as harmless for man as a sterilized solution of physiological saline." They made a rough titration on guinea pigs and found that 5 cc. of this serum protected a 500-gm. guinea pig against 0.8 cc. of diphtheria "toxin" if given 15 minutes in advance. Kossel, in the second part of the paper, reported clinical results which looked promising but were not yet definitive. In another paper von Behring, Boer, and Kossel ("III. Die Werthbestimmung des Diphtherieheilserums," *ibid.*, p. 415) tell in detail of the preparation and use of their sheep serum. In a further instalment von Behring ("IV. Ueber sogenannte 'septische' Fälle von Diphtherie," *ibid.*, p. 543) tells of saving very acute "septic" cases of diphtheria with the serum; and, finally (von Behring, "Die Gewinnung der Blutantitoxin und die Classificierung der Heilbestrebungen bei ansteckenden Krankheiten," *ibid.*, p. 1253), discusses antitoxins in a general way. By 1894 (von Behring and Ehrlich, "III. Zur Diphtherieimmunisierungs und Heilungsfrage," *ibid.*, **20**:437, 1894)

---

[1] In a footnote Behring and Kitasato say: "One may designate these actions against bacterial poisons as 'antitoxic' or 'antifermentative' in contrast to 'antiseptic' and 'disinfectant,' both of which refer to antagonistic action against living infectious material."

serum for both prevention and treatment was being made commercially. Numerous further articles appeared in those years by Behring and his group and others, which cannot be enumerated here.

The nature and preparation of antitoxin are discussed in detail in Andrewes *et al.* (*op. cit.*, pp. 126 ff.).

15. ROMBERG, Ernst. Ueber die Erkrankungen des Herzmuskels bei Typhus abdominalis, Scharlach und Diphtherie, Deutsches Arch. f. klin. Med., **48**:369, 1891.

There has long been a clinical impression that the heart may be seriously affected in diphtheria (Ref. 4). Romberg, a prominent student of the subject, critically reviewed the early literature and presented contemporary views. His own observations revealed definite changes in the heart muscle, especially cellular infiltration and focal degenerative areas. Similar findings were described by Baginsky (*op. cit.*, pp. 189 ff.), who also discussed the clinical features. It is very difficult to tell in these older accounts whether the patient was suffering from cardiac failure in the usual sense or from a shocklike state of peripheral origin.

The upshot of the large and controversial modern literature on the subject is well summarized by E. A. Burkhardt, C. Eggleston, and L. W. Smith ("Electrocardiographic changes and peripheral nerve palsies in toxic diphtheria," Am. J.M. Sc., **195**:391, 1938). Clinically there may be evidence of gross congestive failure, or there may be the syndrome of "peripheral vasomotor shock" such as is seen with cardiac infarction. Arrhythmias are of frequent occurrence, including A-V dissociation. T-wave changes and conduction defects are the principal electrocardiographic alterations. The anatomical changes in the heart muscle are, on the whole, not striking, although patchy areas of degenerated muscle fibers and leukocytic infiltration are seen. I. Gore ("Myocardial changes in fatal diphtheria," Am. J.M. Sc., **215**:257, 1948) in a careful anatomical study of 221 cases found evidence of myocarditis in 70 per cent. He regarded the lesion as a primary toxic myocarditis, which culminated in scarring, a sequel of the pharmacological effect of toxin. If the patient survived, however, T. D. Jones and P. D. White ("The heart after severe diphtheria," Am. Heart J., **3**:190, 1927) found no evidence of appreciable chronic effect on the heart, although N. H. Boyer and L. Weinstein ("Diphtheritic myocarditis," New England J. Med., **239**:913, 1948) believe that, when there have been abnormal electrocardiographic patterns, recovery is probably associated with loss of muscle substance and is therefore never "complete."

16. WELCH, William H., and FLEXNER, Simon. The histological changes in experimental diphtheria, Bull. Johns Hopkins Hosp., **2**:107, 1891.

Although von Babes ("Untersuchungen über den Diphtheriebacillus und die experimentelle Diphtherie," Virchows Arch. f. path. Anat., **119**:460, 1890) had described the pathological changes in experimental diphtheria in rabbits, Welch and Flexner's observations were definitive. They discussed, first, the lesions produced by injection into small animals of living cultures of diphtheria bacilli and described the histological changes in great detail; in a second paper ("The histological lesions produced by the tox-albumen of diphtheria," Bull. Johns Hopkins Hosp., **3**:17, 1892) they compared these with the changes following injection of culture filtrates (toxin). "It may be considered as established now that the toxic products and not the bacilli themselves invade the tissues in diphtheria. This fact would at once suggest that the general lesions . . . were the effects of the soluble poison diffused through the body. Hence, it was desirable to demonstrate this assumption experimentally; and it is not unimportant to know that the lesions in the tissues produced by the bacilli and the toxic principle on the one hand and the toxic principle alone on the other, are in perfect correspondence with each other and, moreover, it would seem not to be superfluous to emphasize the occurrence of definite focal lesions in the tissues of the body, produced by a soluble poison circulating in the blood." Details of the lesions in every sort of animal are given in Andrewes et al. (op. cit., pp. 170 ff.).

17. ROUX, E., and MARTIN, L., Contribution à l'étude de la diphtérie (sérum thérapie), Ann. Inst. Pasteur, **8**:609, 1894.

Roux and Martin's precise and lucid style is a relief after the ponderous and turgid writings of von Behring and his associates. First is given a brief and clear description of how to obtain diphtheria toxin by filtering old cultures of virulent strains of bacilli. In order to get larger quantities of antitoxin, Roux and Martin immunized horses. "The horses which we immunized are not valuable animals [animaux de prix] but cab horses [des chevaux de fiacre] six to nine years old." These horses were desirable because very tolerant of toxin; horse No. 1, for example, in 2 months and 20 days received 800 cc. of toxin. After a few days, the serum of these horses was already antitoxic. When such serum was added to diphtheria toxin, it became harmless both in test tube and in vivo. Antitoxin rendered an animal immune immediately, but for a short time only, several days or at the most a few weeks. Roux and Martin emphasized the quantitative relations of toxin and antitoxin under various circumstances; the antitoxin kept well in the dark and cold. Next are reported prophylactic and curative injections in guinea pigs and rabbits; they describe the subsidence of edema and the melting-away of the false membrane. The treatment of children is reserved for another paper (E. Roux, L. Martin, and A. Chaillou, "Trois cent cas de diphtérie traités par le sérum antidiphtérique," Ann. Inst. Pasteur, **8**:640, 1894). The three hundred children treated had a mortality of 26 per cent as against a usual death rate of 50 per cent. The activity of the serum was 1 : 50,000; that is to say, a guinea pig which received 1/50,000 of its weight of serum survived a dose of toxin which invariably killed in 30 hours. Actually, Roux, Martin, and Chaillou injected 20 cc. of serum under the skin of the flank. Considering the severity of diphtheria in Paris at this time, the results were promising; among 120 cases of pharyngeal diphtheria, only 9 patients died, whereas among 24 cases complicated by severe streptococcal infections, 21 died. So, too, among patients with "croup" requiring tracheotomy, the mortality was 67 per cent. "Could one do better? We are convinced that it is possible. But it will be the consequence not of more medicine but of a better organization of services."[2] The subject of serum therapy of diphtheria is reviewed in Andrewes *et al.* (*op. cit.*, pp. 257 ff.).

18. LEDINGHAM, J. C. G., and ARKWRIGHT, J. A. The carrier problem in infectious diseases. New York: Longmans, Green & Co., 1912.

Indications of the existence of healthy carriers of diphtheria bacilli were already forthcoming in some of the early work on the disease (Ref. 10). Since then a huge literature has sprung up, in which convalescent carriers and healthy contact carriers are differentiated. Early observations on carriers are authoritatively summarized in the book by Ledingham and Arkwright. Much of the work also dealt with the question of the duration of the carrier state, especially in convalescence from clinical diphtheria. An important paper is that of G. H. Weaver ("Diphtheria carriers," J.A.M.A., **76**:832, 1921), which contains statistical material derived from a study of five hundred cases of diphtheria. Weinstein (Ref. 24) reviews the modern literature and points out the disagreement between the figures of various workers. He concludes, however, that the elimination of the carrier state in 3–5 days by adequate dosage of penicillin is statistically valid. "A minimum of 240,000 units of penicillin per day for 12 days is suggested for the treatment of the chronic diphtheria carrier state." It is of interest also that H. D. Wright ("The disappearance of C. diphtheriae from diphtheria patients," J. Path. & Bact., **52**:129, 1941) found that the mitis, intermedius, and gravis types persisted for different lengths of time after acute infection. The matter is further complicated by the question of how many carrier strains are virulent. A. B. Wadsworth has studied this problem ("Virulence of diphtheria bacilli from diphtheria patients and from carriers," J.A.M.A., **74**:1633, 1920). He found that "B. diphtheriae from persons who have had diphtheria or from those who through contact become 'carriers' retains its virulence for several months." J. C. Geiger, F. L. Kelly, and W. M. Bathgate ("Diphtheria carriers," J.A.M.A., **66**:645, 1916) first pointed out the importance of nasal cultures in the detection of carriers and then reported Schick tests which showed that all of a group of contact carriers were immune and hence did not require quarantine; none of these individuals developed diphtheria.

19. SCHICK, B. Die Diphtherietoxin-Hautreaction des Menschen als Vorprobe der prophylaktischen Diphtherieheilseruminjektion, München. med. Wchnschr., **60**:2608, 1913.

Schick ("Kutanreaction bei Impfung mit Diphtherietoxin," München. med. Wchnschr., **55**:504, 1908) had already studied the effect of injecting minute amounts of diphtheria toxin into the skin. He found the reaction specific, since mixtures of toxin and antitoxin produced no visible effect. He concluded, therefore, that a positive test indicates absence of antitoxin in the blood—in other words, susceptibility. He also found that, by means of the skin test, one could estimate accurately the quantity of antitoxin necessary for cure of a clinical case of diphtheria.

[2] In a footnote Roux describes the terrible conditions in the diphtheria wards—crowding, no ventilation, all sorts of infections herded together. "It is, above all, in winter when the pavilion is full, when the windows stay closed, that bronchopneumonia becomes terrible," etc.

In the later paper he gave statistics on the frequency of positive tests and pointed out that almost all the newborn gave negative skin reactions because they still had antitoxin derived from the mother. He now developed the test more as an indication of whether prophylactic injections of antitoxin were necessary in groups of children who had been exposed to the disease. In spite of certain difficulties, the Schick test has been found very useful in epidemiological work. Modern summaries of the problem are those of S. Dudley ("Schick's test and its applications," Quart. J. Med., **22**:321, 1929; *The Schick Test, Diphtheria and Scarlet Fever: A Study in Epidemiology* ["Medical Research Council Special Report Series," No. 75 (London: His Majesty's Stationery Office, 1923)]).

20. BEHRING, E. von. Ueber ein neues Diphtherieschutzmittel, Deutsche med. Wchnschr., **39**:873, 1139, 1913.

In spite of the brilliant discovery of diphtheria antitoxin, cure of clinical cases was not always easy or satisfactory. Toxin rapidly became anchored to body cells and was then no longer susceptible to neutralization by antitoxin; it was necessary, therefore, to treat the patient early if good results were to be obtained in severe cases.

The attention of investigators turned more and more, therefore, to methods of prophylaxis. Von Behring, following the suggestion of Theobald Smith ("The degree and duration of passive immunity to diphtheria toxin transmitted by immunized female guinea pigs to their immediate offspring," J.M. Res., **16**:359, 1907; "Active immunity produced by so-called balanced or neutral mixtures of diphtheria toxin and antitoxin," J. Exper. Med., **11**:241, 1909), who laid the experimental groundwork in guinea pigs, introduced the method of immunizing people by injections of toxin and antitoxin mixtures which therefore is the direct precursor of modern immunization with toxoid. "My new medicine is a mixture of very strong toxin and antitoxin in such proportion as to elicit in guinea pigs none or at most a very slight toxin effect." Injection of this material led to the production of antitoxin in human recipients. Von Behring discusses in detail the quantitative relationships, indications, contraindications, and other relevant matters.

But, despite the fact that toxin-antitoxin injections usually had a high immunizing value, they were not always safe; sometimes toxin and antitoxin became dissociated, or there might be serum reactions (see B. White and E. Robinson, "Effect of exposure to low temperatures on diphtheria toxin-antitoxin mixture," J.A.M.A., **82**:1675, 1924). This led to further attempts to make immunization a harmless procedure (see Ref. 22).

21. DEICHER, H., and AGULNIK, F. Ueber gehäuftes Auftreten ungewöhnlich bösartiger Diphtherie, Deutsche med. Wchnschr., **53**:825, 1927.

Diphtheria incidence had fallen greatly following the introduction of methods of active immunization, and mortality in 1925 had dropped to approximately 5 per cent. Deicher and Agulnik in 1926 became aware of a radical alteration in the character of diphtheria. There appeared patients, mostly with the pharyngeal or nasal type, desperately ill, who apparently died of cardiac failure or vasomotor collapse, highly refractory to ordinary antitoxin therapy and with a mortality of over 25 per cent. "Diphtheria appears recently to have again taken on a 'malignant' character." They emphasized the importance of early intensive therapy, preferably in hospital, if the patient was to be saved. Reports of similar severe epidemics soon came from all over Europe; they are listed by J. S. Anderson, F. C. Happold, J. W. McLeod, and J. G. Thomson ("On the existence of two forms of diphtheria bacillus—*B. diphtheriae gravis* and *B. diphtheriae mitis*—and a new medium for their differentiation and for the bacteriological diagnosis of diphtheria," J. Path. & Bact., **34**:667, 1931). These writers felt that the two types were associated with severe and mild cases and that they could be distinguished by growth on a special medium. A thorough review of the subject with a bibliography of nearly three hundred titles is that of J. W. McLeod ("The types mitis, intermedius and gravis of the Corynebacterium diphtheriae," Bact. Rev., **7**:1, 1943). McLeod accepts three well-defined cultural types of diphtheria bacillus. The mitis strains cause mild diphtheria with occasional deaths from obstructive phenomena; the intermedius and gravis forms may produce the malignant type. The relation of various types to toxin production and response to antitoxin are discussed. A. M. Fisher and S. Cobb ("The clinical manifestations of the severe form of diphtheria," Bull. Johns Hopkins Hosp., **83**:297, 1948) have recently discussed the severe form of diphtheria as seen in this country.

The complexity of the whole problem of factors affecting the incidence of diphtheria is brought out by W. T. Russell (*The Epidemiology of Diphtheria during the Last Forty Years* ["Medical Research Council Special Report Series," No. 247 (London: His Majesty's Stationery Office, 1943)]).

22. RAMON, G. Anatoxine diphtérique, ses propriétés—ses applications, Ann. Inst. Pasteur, **42**:959, 1928.

G. Ramon ("Sur le pouvoir floculant et sur les propriétés immunisantes d'une toxin diphtérique rendu anatoxique [anatoxine]," Compt. rend. Acad. d. sc., **177**:1338, 1923) had worked on this subject for years and had shown that "a diphtheria toxin which has completely lost its toxic effect on animals can still be precipitated by antitoxins." He raised the question to what extent such "anatoxine" still provoked the body to produce antitoxin. "Thanks to its innocuousness and the high degree of immunity which it confers, it seems equally indicated for antidiphtheric vaccination of the child." This work led to Ramon's monumental paper, in which he discussed the preparation of anatoxin by the combined action of addition of formaldehyde to the toxic filtrate and subsequent heating for several weeks at low temperatures (38°–40° C.) until toxicity had disappeared. Guinea pigs injected with this material showed no signs of poisoning and, when challenged with potent toxin after 3 or 4 weeks, were found to be immune. The sera of horses receiving several injections of this anatoxin became highly antitoxic. Ramon quotes references to the literature on early experiences in human immunization by anatoxin. He insisted on a definite technique as follows: "Make a first subcutaneous injection of 0.5 cc., then after an interval of 3 weeks a second injection of 1 cc. and 15 days later an injection of 1½ cc. . . . Such is diphtheria anatoxin. A simple antigen, easy to prepare and handle . . . diphtheria anatoxin gives us a safe and inoffensive means of immunizing animals . . . it gives us a practical and safe method of conferring on man a specific antitoxic immunity, solid and durable and thereby permits us to do battle with diphtheria, an epidemic disease." There follows a long article by L. Martin, G. Loiseau, and A. Laffaille ("L'Immunization antidiphtérique par l'anatoxine chez l'homme. Applications à la prophylaxie de la diphtérie," Ann. Inst. Pasteur, **42**:1010, 1928), which goes into immunization in great statistical detail as checked by Schick tests. Still other articles on the subject follow in the same number of the Annals.

A. T. Glenny, C. G. Pope, H. Waddington, and V. Wallace ("XXIII. The antigenic value of toxoid precipitated by potassium alum," J. Path. & Bact., **29**:38, 1926) first showed that precipitation of toxoid by alum increased its antigenicity. Glenny and Barr ("The precipitation of diphtheria toxoid by potash alum," J. Path. & Bact., **34**:131, 1931) continued this work, and later Barr, Pope, Glenny, and Linggood ("Preparation of alum-precipitated toxoid for use as an immunizing agent," Lancet, **2**:301, 1941) described in detail the practical preparation of the material.

The whole subject of prevention of diphtheria is reviewed by Andrewes *et al.* (*op. cit.*, pp. 349 ff.), and recent discussions are those of J. Jepson ("Immunization of adults against diphtheria and tetanus," New England J. Med., **251**:459, 1954) and of G. Edsall ("Active immunization," New England J. Med., **241**:18, 1949).

23. MUELLER, J. Howard. Nutrition of the diphtheria bacillus, Bact. Rev., **4**:97, 1940.

An authoritative review of the modern problems of bacterial nutrition with reference to diphtheria.

24. WEINSTEIN, Louis. The treatment of acute diphtheria and the chronic carrier state with penicillin, Am. J.M. Sc., **213**:308, 1947.

As long ago as 1929, Alexander Fleming ("On antibacterial action of cultures of a *Penicillium* with special reference to their use in the isolation of *B. influenzae*," Brit. J. Exper. Path., **10**:226, 1929) showed that penicillin had a definitely inhibitory effect on *C. diphtheriae* in the test tube. Weinstein reviews attempts to treat clinical diphtheria with this antibiotic and points out that no definite curative effects have been obtained. His own observations led him to a similar conclusion: "Penicillin has no effect on the clinical course of diphtheria and its use in this disease does not eliminate the necessity of administering adequate amounts of antitoxin." However, penicillin in adequate dosage definitely shortened the duration of the carrier state (see Ref. 18).

TETANUS

CURLING's book on tetanus (Ref. 4) contains a summary of everything of importance known about the disease to date (1836). It also has a thorough bibliography beginning with the year 1668. The monumental volume by Edmund Rose (*Der Starrkrampf beim Menschen* [Stuttgart: Ferdinand Enke, 1897]) deals in its six hundred pages with every phase of the subject. The best general modern account of tetanus, with bibliography, is to be found in G. S. Wilson and A. A. Miles (Topley and Wilson's *Principles of Bacteriology and Immunity* [4th ed.; Baltimore: Williams & Wilkins Co., 1955], 2: 1955).

1. HOWSHIP, John.[1] On lock jaw with tetanus, M. & Phys. J., London, **21**:180, 1808.

This is the first of a series of notes on tetanus by Howship which appeared in this journal over a period of three years, as follows: "Observations on lock jaw, and tetanus, with cases," *ibid.*, p. 407; "Observations upon the phenomena and treatment of tetanus with cases," *ibid.*, p. 446; "Cases of lock jaw and tetanus," *ibid.*, **22**:120, 1809; "Case of tetanus," *ibid.*, p. 185; "Lock jaw and tetanus," *ibid.*, p. 324; "Cases of tetanus," *ibid.*, p. 396; "Cases of tetanus," *ibid.*, p. 479; "Observations upon tetanus," *ibid.*, **23**:15, 1810. These reports give a good idea of the status of the subject a hundred and fifty years ago. "The very limited knowledge we at present possess in the successful treatment of Lock Jaw and Tetanus, must impress the mind of every anxious student in pathology, with the conviction that very much remains to be acquired in this department of medical information. . . . To those who have read of, but have never seen these complaints, the histories already written, and the plans of treatment proposed and described by writers of intelligence, may be satisfactory; but to such as have been in the habit of watching the various changes in this disease at the bedside of the unfortunate sufferer, it does, and must appear, that we are not yet acquainted with any one medicine or application, upon which, from uniform experience we can rely; nor are we possessed of any remedy that can be exhibited in any confidence of its power to afford relief." A number of vivid case reports are presented, with critical evaluation of various methods of therapy, such as mercurial inunctions—a popular method of treatment at the time but useless in Howship's hands. Indeed, William Charles Wells ("A case of tetanus with observations on that disease," Tr. Soc. Improvement M. & Chir. Knowledge, **3**:241, 1812) reported a case occurring "during a salivation from the use of mercury." So intrenched was the use of mercury in tetanus, however, that Wells goes on to say: "It will, perhaps, appear to many, as an obvious conclusion from the preceding case, that mercury ought no longer to be regarded as a remedy for tetanus. But so unstable are the grounds, upon which we frequently build our reasonings in medicine, etc." Sir James Macgregor (Ref. 2) referred to a similar case. He discussed the relation of lockjaw to tetanus and concluded

[1] This was the Howship of Howship's lacunae. His interesting paper on "Microscopic observations on the structure of bone" is to be found in M.-Chir. Tr., **7**:387, 1816.

that they are the same disease. Howship speculated on the nature of tetanus: "It seems to creep as it were, from the wound upwards to the origin of the nerve; from thence, extending its influence to the whole nervous fabric of the sensorium, emanating as from a centre, in the various course of the particular nerves distributed throughout the body and extremities." Here one sees a vague groping toward the theory of neural transmission, although Howship had, of course, no idea of any specific or concrete agent. The question of whether amputation would prevent the progress of tetanus was a live one at the time. Howship reports cases in which amputation was followed by recovery and also those in which it failed. In another case, pressure was tried "to effectually prevent the passing up of the irritating impression from the wound," but the patient was not saved. He reports "a rare case of complete Tetanus from which the Patient recovered" without benefit of special therapy (the wound was in the foot, and the incubation period was 10 days); and also a case in which "Opium certainly checked the Progress of the Disease, and probably saved the life of the patient." Finally, there is a keen essay on the differentiation of the spasms of tetanus from epileptic seizures.

2. LARREY, D. J. Mémoires de chirurgie militaire, et campagnes. Vol. 1: Mémoire sur le tétanos traumatique, p. 235. Paris: J. Smith, 1812.

Although tetanus had been described for centuries and the terms "tetanus," "locked jaw," "opisthotonus," and "trismus," etc., were in common use at the turn of the eighteenth century, most of the current articles were slight and dealt with some special therapeutic agent or method or with a report of a single case. Baron Larrey's description is outstanding. Most of his cases followed military gunshot wounds. He first defines the terms "tetanus," "emprosthotonus," and "opisthotonus." "One can differentiate tetanus on the basis of greater or lesser intensity into acute and chronic. The first is very dangerous and usually fatal [p. 238]. . . . In complete tetanus, the limbs are stiff, the entire body becomes stiff, so that in grasping one of the extremities one can lift the body like an inflexible mass" (p. 239). Everything progresses rapidly, so that, very often, within 24 hours the patient can no longer swallow or only with the greatest difficulty. "Sometimes he is delirious; the pulse is small and rapid, a rise of fever ordinarily takes place toward evening. He loses weight under one's eye, and feels terrible pain. Stiffness increases . . . he finishes his unhappy course by the third, fourth, fifth, or seventh day" (p. 240). Larrey describes cases following various military actions but has nothing useful to suggest as to cause and no particular treatment. He thought that he had saved several patients by amputation early after symptoms appeared.

No less interesting is the account by Sir James Macgregor ("Sketch of the medical history of the British armies in the peninsula of Spain and Portugal during the late campaigns," M.-Chir. Tr., 6:381, 1815) of tetanus in the Peninsular Wars. "This very formidable disease . . . was always very prevalent among the wounded after the great battles . . . among several hundred cases . . . there are few, where this disease had made any progress, in which remedies however varied seemed to have any influence on it." He reports cases in which the effect of various therapeutic agents was obviously *post hoc*, such as one in which "the patient recovered, apparently in consequence of long continued accidental exposure to severe wet and cold. . . . The symptoms are stated to have been unusually severe. As it was impossible to think of leaving the man . . . he was carried on a bullock cart after the battalion. During the first part of the day he was drenched with rain . . . but after ascending one of the highest mountains in Gallicia the snow was knee deep, and the thermometer below 30°. The patient was exposed to this inclement weather from six o'clock in the morning till ten at night, when he arrived half starved to death, but perfectly free from every symptom of tetanus."

Other good results are attributed to laudanum and warm baths, although Surgeon Brown saw several cases at Elvas, where "opium was the favorite remedy, and every case so treated died." Venesection and purgation, of course, had their advocates. "This terrible disease is too easily distinguished to require detailed description. It occurs in every description and in every stage of wounds, from the slightest to the most formidable, from the healthy and the sloughing, from the incised and lacerated, from the most simple and most complicated. It occurs at uncertain periods; but it is remarked, that if it does not occur for 22 days from the date of the wound, the patient is safe. . . . Mr. Guthrie . . . divided the disease according to its short duration or protraction, into two species, viz., acute, and the mild, which he thought were independent of peculiarity of constitution. . . . The remedies which have been chiefly trusted to for the cure of this formidable disease are opium, mercury, wine, warm and cold bath, venesection, ipecacuanha and digitalis in large doses, enlargement of the original wound, and amputation of the limb. These have been tried alone and in various combinations, and I am obliged to confess that the whole failed, in almost every acute case of tetanus which occurred. . . . Amputation as recommended by the baron Larry [*sic*] totally failed in the fully formed disease: it was tried in many cases at Toulouse. Indeed I believe this gentleman's opinion is altered since he published the result of his experiences in Egypt. . . . I have been recently informed by Mr. Guthrie, that the baron distinctly acknowledged to him, that the loss of the French army after the battle near Dresden was principally from tetanus, when of course this practice must have been fairly tried."

All this gives a vivid impression of the doctor's helplessness in the face of a disease the cause of which was unknown, even though the clinical associations were obvious.

3. BRIGHT, [Richard]. Case of tetanus, in which quinine and stimulants were administered, very extensively, with success, Guy's Hosp. Rep., 1:111, 1836.

As we have already indicated, the medical journals at this period were full of reports of single cases of tetanus presumably cured by some special drug or procedure. The great Richard Bright fell into the same error. His case is reported with vividness and accuracy, but one doubts whether the therapy had anything to do with recovery: "W. Turner, aged 38, was admitted, under my care, into Guy's Hospital, the subject of confirmed tetanus, of four days standing. When I first saw him, he was lying on his bed, perfectly stiff, with his legs stretched out, and his feet bent almost backwards: his abdomen was hard, and unyielding as a board; all the muscles of his thighs and legs were tense: he was scarcely able to bend his fingers: his cheeks and forehead were wrinkled, and spasmodically drawn; and he could only by a great effort, open his mouth about a quarter of an inch, and imperfectly protrude his tongue. At intervals of a few minutes, severe spasms drew him backwards; and these recurred upon the least excitement, or when he made any effort to answer questions. He was covered with perspiration: pulse 100: respiration 20: tongue moist. His occupation was that of a fellmonger, or parchment-worker. He denied most positively having met with any accident, puncture, or cut, whatever; but he had one or two slight excoriations along the edges of the middle and ring fingers of his right hand, caused by the friction of a brush which he was in the habit of using, when rubbing quick-lime over the skins. These excoriations seemed nearly healed over, giving him neither pain nor uneasiness: and had it not been, that the rag with which one was covered attracted my eye, he would have made no mention of the circumstance; nor did I at the time, attach much importance to it. The day of his admission was the fifth day of his symptoms: for he stated that on the 13th he first perceived a stiffness in his jaw, which had gradually increased to the present time: but he was able to continue his work until the 16th, the day before his admission; when in walking along the street, he was seized with a sudden spasm, so severe as to throw him to the ground; and from that time the symptoms increased rapidly."

Bright then, along with his daily notes, gives the therapeutic prescriptions; for example, on August 17:

"Applicentur Cucurbitulae cruentae inter scapulas; et detrahatur sanguis ad uncias octo—Hydrarg. Submuriat, gr. iii. Opii purif., gr. i. Antimon. tartar, gr. ¼: fiat pilula, quarta quaque hora sumend. a—Habeat Decoct. Cinchonae, ℥ iss. quinae sulphat. gr. ii. Tinct. Cinchon. comp. ℨ i, secunda quaque hora."

By September 14: "Bowels regular: appetite good . . . and nothing of the complaint remains, except some rigidity of the muscles of the face."

Bright refers to a previous patient who also recovered. "To these observations I have but little to add. The treatment of the case now before us was conducted precisely on the principles here laid down; and the same combination of tonic and stimulant remedies, with calomel and opium, was adopted, as that by which the former case was brought to a successful issue. It is scarcely to be supposed that perseverance in the use of tonic remedies, with only two days' intermission for a space of twenty days—during which the patient took nearly two ounces of sulphate of quinine, and drank daily from fourteen to eighteen ounces of wine, besides taking ammonia and brandy—could have failed to produce some powerful effect upon the constitution."

4. CURLING, Thomas Blizard. A treatise on tetanus. London: J. G. & F. Rivington, 1836.

Curling's book is an admirable summary of knowledge of tetanus to date. "The following essay on Tetanus, one of a class of diseases but little understood, and exceedingly difficult of investigation, was not originally intended for publication. Having no novelties in treatment to recommend, I am induced to submit this imperfect performance to the notice of the profession in consequence of the desultory nature of the literature of this disease. . . . I have also endeavored to obtain from amongst the discrepant statements and conflicting opinions of different writers, those conclusions which their collective experience would appear to justify, and from amidst a host of remedies that have been employed, to trace to some general cause or mode of operation the salutory influence which they have been supposed to exert."

The book is based on an analysis of 128 cases of traumatic tetanus which are summarized in tabular form in an appendix, and there follows a bibliography of some 150 references, mostly to more or less contemporary case reports. The opening chapter gives, first, a definition of terms such as "emprosthotonous," "opisthotonus," "plerosthotonus," etc., and then takes up the clinical features, prognosis, and diagnosis in detail.

Chapter ii, on the pathology of tetanus, is to some extent a dead letter, as modern students agree that there are no visible lesions in uncomplicated cases. However, there are some points of historical interest. "Although the phenomena distinguishing Tetanus, are chiefly expressed in deranged action of the muscles, yet it is very generally admitted that some part of the nervous system is the source or actual seat of the disease. . . . The following appearances are often presented by the brain and its membranes . . . congestion of the sinuses; the vessels of the pia mater filled with florid blood; more or less increased vascularity of the cerebral substance; slight serous effusion between the membranes and the ventricles" (p. 45). Inflammation and disorganization of the sympathetic ganglia were also described, and "the nerves have, in several instances, been found injured and inflamed at the seat of the original wound" (p. 66). Still other lesions are described elsewhere in the body. As to the nature of the disease: "Tetanus then appears to consist in a peculiar morbid action in the tractus motorius, the intimate nature of which is altogether beyond our comprehension." Irritation, as this action is called, is sharply, and correctly, differentiated from inflammation. It appears, then, that the older observers came as near to understanding the nature of the disease as was possible without knowledge of the specific soluble toxin. Curling finally concludes: "Tetanus is a functional disease of the nervous system, that is to say, a disease unaccompanied with any perceptible lesion of structure, the nature of which, although essentially distinct from inflammation, is completely unknown. There are, therefore, no morbid changes peculiar to Tetanus, and by which it can be recognized" (p. 121).

Under "Treatment," the question of amputation (see Refs. 1, 2) is discussed at length and also the division of nerves. As to constitutional treatment, a long list of agents is critically discussed—purgatives, mercury, bloodletting, counterirritation, opium, tobacco, antimony, cold affusion, the warm bath, the vapor bath, tonics and stimulants, carbonate of iron, hydrocyanic acid, and other remedies. Curling concludes: "Perhaps for acute Tetanus, a sure and safe remedy in all cases is yet to be discovered. But if we clearly understand the indications to be fulfilled, and direct our treatment accordingly, we are infinitely more likely, as science advances, to find out this remedy, than by groping in the dark, or by disregarding the lights of experience, and stumbling where others have failed before us" (p. 206).

Not much further advance was made in the subject until the discovery of the bacillus, fifty years later.

5. NICOLAIER, Arthur. Ueber Infectiösen Tetanus, Deutsche med. Wchnschr., **10**:842, 1884.

"In the course of extensive examination of soil bacteria it appeared that implantation of certain samples of earth into mice, rabbits, and guinea pigs could elicit a symptom complex practically always lethal, featured by persistent cramplike contractions of certain muscle groups and by periodic violent extensor spasms of practically all the muscles of the body and extremities, which must be designated as tetanus." In mice in which a little earth was introduced into a "pocket" near the tail, after a latent period of 1½–2½ days, spasm of the muscles of the hind legs appeared. In the 12–20 hours before death took place, the animals showed periodic violent extensor spasms of neck and back. These spasms occurred not only spontaneously but on touching the animal, tapping the table, etc. A similar picture was produced in rabbits and guinea pigs, but not in two dogs. If the inoculation was made in the neck, the upper extremities went into spasm first. Autopsies showed no generalized lesions but in pus from the site of inoculation there were always seen "narrow long bacilli . . . which stained best with fuchsin." In several cases these bacilli were present in immense numbers. Nicolaier suggested that one was dealing with an infectious tetanus caused by micro-organisms. He thought that the presence of a fairly long incubation period was in favor of this view. He heated earth which had produced tetanus for an hour at 190° C. and found that mice injected with it remained healthy; on the other hand, filtrates of a suspension of unheated earth produced the disease. He tried to cultivate the organism with dubious success, and he was not able to isolate it in pure culture, although he stated that he had produced tetanus with the seventh generation grown on blood serum. At any rate, he concluded that "through these experiments it is shown that bacilli exist which produce tetanus by penetrating deeply into wounds." He concluded that the disease was not caused by massive growth of the bacilli through the body but that they produced locally a poison which resembled strychnine in its action. Finally, the bacilli were found in street dirt, gardens, orchards, etc.; they were not found in soil from "the woods." He raised the question of whether human tetanus is not due to contamination of wounds by soil.

As one can see, Nicolaier's studies were of fundamental importance; indeed, he discovered or sensed correctly most of the chief facts about the cause and production of tetanus. P. Fildes ("Tetanus. I. Isolation, morphology and cultural reactions of B. tetani," Brit. J. Exper. Path., **6**:62, 1925) devised a ready method for isolation of tetanus bacilli in pure culture. He found them 33 times among 70 soil specimens (cultivated and waste lands), 34 times in 200 specimens of horse feces (London stable horses), and twice in 200 specimens of human feces (hospital patients). These findings have been generally confirmed throughout the world in numerous papers.

6. CARLE and RATTONE. Studio esperimentale sull'eziologia del tetano. Communicazione preventiva, Gior. Accad. med. Torino, **32**:174, 1884.
Although numerous attempts had been made to produce tetanus in animals by injection of material from tetanus cases, Carle and Rattone seem to have been the first who were definitely successful. They stated that they would attempt to determine whether tetanus was a "neurosis" or an infectious disease. They injected into the sciatic nerve sheath of 21 rabbits a suspension of material from an acne pustule from which fatal tetanus had developed. All these animals died of the disease. Carle and Rattone were also able to pass tetanus from animal to animal by injection of a suspension of nerve from above the site of inoculation.

They concluded that (1) human tetanus is an infectious disease; (2) it can be transmitted from man to rabbit; (3) it can be transmitted from rabbit to rabbit.

7. ROSENBACH. Zur Aetiologie des Wundstarrkrampfes beim Menschen, Arch. f. klin. Chir., 34:306, 1887.

Rosenbach seems to have been the first to demonstrate bacilli of tetanus in man. He used bits of decomposing tissue from a patient with gangrene of the feet who had succumbed to the disease. Guinea pigs inoculated with this material promptly died of typical tetanus, of which he gives a beautiful description. In the pus from the human subject were found all sorts of bacteria, including bacilli resembling those described by Nicolaier (Ref. 5). Rosenbach used anaerobic methods and, like Nicolaier, was unable to isolate the bacilli in pure culture, but he produced tetanus with certain cultures. He saw and described the familiar drumstick appearance, which he recognized as due to spores. Rosenbach raised the following important questions: "Does the tetanus bacillus spread through the body?" "If so, in what manner does this spread take place?" "What relation has it to the nervous system, to the spinal cord?"

8. KITASATO, S. Ueber den Tetanusbacillus, Ztschr. f. Hyg. u. Infektionskr., 7:225, 1889.

The work of Nicolaier (Ref. 5) and of Rosenbach (Ref. 7) was soon confirmed by many writers, but, as late as 1889, Widenmann ("Beitrag zur Aetiologie des Wundstarrkrampfes," Ztschr. f. Hyg. u. Infektionskr., 5:522, 1889) cast doubt on the previous observations. He found that material from a tetanus wound in a man implanted in mice did, to be sure, produce tetanus promptly, "but in not a single case were the slender spore-bearing bacilli, designated by most authors as 'Tetanusbacilli' found." To this communication was attached an addendum by the great Carl Flügge in support of Widenmann.

Kitasato felt that to settle this question it was necessary to isolate the spore-bearing bacilli in pure culture. He found that surface growth of material from tetanus always showed a mixture of many other organisms with the "Tetanus-bacilli"; it was the consumption of oxygen by the aerobes which perhaps allowed growth of the anaerobic tetanus bacilli. Kitasato therefore heated mixed cultures at 80° C. for an hour to kill the aerobes and then planted them in an atmosphere of hydrogen. He thus obtained pure cultures of spore-bearing bacilli, which he described in detail, and with these cultures he readily produced tetanus in small animals without the addition of foreign bodies. The animals sickened in 24 hours and died in 2 or 3 days. At autopsy, hyperemia was found at the injection site but no pus or bacilli; no changes were noted in the internal organs, nor were tetanus bacilli to be isolated from them. To find out how quickly the tetanus bacilli formed a soluble toxin, the site of inoculation was excised and cauterized after various intervals. Up to an hour the animals remained well; if the excision took place after an hour, the animals all developed tetanus. Bacilli were seen at the injection site for 8–10 hours; thereafter they disappeared without leaving a trace (spurlos verschwunden). He attributed the various conclusions of different authors to variability in formation of tetanus spores; if the disease ran a quick course, there might be seen bacilli without spores, whereas spores were formed if the animal survived for a longer interval. But the bacilli were always present. Finally, Kitasato noted that even after many subcultures the bacilli were still "virulent," as were spores kept in the desiccator for several months.

The importance of this work, done in the laboratory of R. Koch, can hardly be overestimated.

9. BEHRING, [E.], and KITASATO, [S.]. Ueber das Zustandekommen der Diphtherie-Immunität und der Tetanus-Immunität bei Thieren, Deutsche med. Wchnschr., **16**:1113, 1890.

This is the classical article of Behring and Kitasato dealing with antitoxic immunity both in diphtheria and in tetanus. "The immunity of rabbits and mice which have been immunized against tetanus rests on the capability of cell-free blood serum to render harmless the toxic substances which the tetanus bacilli produce." This short sentence summarizes the principles of antitoxic immunity. More in detail the authors state: "(1) Blood from rabbits immune to tetanus possessed the property of destroying tetanus toxin. (2) This property is demonstrable also in extra-vascular blood or in its cell-free serum. (3) These properties are so persistent that they remain effective in the body of other animals, so that one can achieve outstanding therapeutic effects by blood or serum transfusions. (4) The tetanus toxin–neutralizing properties are absent in the blood of such animals as are not immune against tetanus, and if one introduces tetanus toxin into non-immune animals, it can be demonstrated after the death of the animals in the blood and other body fluids." Simple experiments supporting these theses are next described. The toxin is intensely potent: "0.00005 cc. of filtered bacteria-free 10-day culture of tetanus bacilli is enough to kill a mouse in 4–6 days." But 0.2 cc. of a mixture of 5 cc. of serum from a rabbit immune to tetanus and 1 cc. of culture—in other words, more than two hundred times the fatal dose of toxin—is harmless.

Kitasato ("Experimentelle Untersuchungen über das Tetanusgift," Ztschr. f. Hyg. u. Infektionskr., **10**:267, 1891) soon gave a more detailed account of the tetanus toxin. He explained details of filtration methods whereby the material was made absolutely bacteria-free and reported animal experiments with the filtrate in which all the findings of tetanus were reproduced. "One can now state definitely that one is dealing not with an infection but with an intoxication. Tetanus bacilli produce a substance with specific toxic action." Small animals treated with filtrate developed tetanus in at least 3 days. If they remained well until the fourth day, they did not develop tetanus. Transfer of tissues from dead animals was ineffective, but blood or pleural fluid from such animals always produced tetanus. "This proves that tetanus toxin penetrates into the blood stream." The effects of heat, drying, etc., on the potency of filtrates were next discussed and then the influence of many chemicals. Finally, Kitasato described attempts to immunize animals. It was not possible to produce immunity by accustoming the animals to increasing doses of toxin, nor could immunity be produced by injecting filtrates heated at increasing temperatures. Chickens were found refractory to tetanus, but chicken blood was ineffective as an immunizing agent.

10. BEHRING and FRANK. Experimentelle Beiträge zur Lehre von der Bekämpfung der Infectionskrankheiten. Ueber einige Eigenschaften des Tetanusheilserums, Deutsche med. Wchnschr., **18**:348, 1892.

In an interesting article Behring ("Die Blutserumtherapie bei Diphtherie und Tetanus," Ztschr. f. Hyg. u. Infektionskr., **12**:1, 1892) sketches the general principles of serum therapy. He points out that in acquired immunity the cell-free serum of the immune individual always contains protective bodies. This blood should have protective and curative value for another individual. Behring then goes into the subject in detail ("Ueber Immunisierung und Heilung von Versuchsthieren beim Tetanus," *ibid.*, p. 45) in connection with prophylaxis and cure of tetanus in small animals. He used sera developed in such animals but also horse serum prepared by Schütz ("Versuche zur Immunisierung von Pferden und Schafen gegen Tetanus," *ibid.*, p. 58). In the paper with Frank, however, he defined precisely the fatal dose of toxin for mice and demonstrated clearly the protective and curative value of the serum. They noted early that, even if treatment was begun at the very onset of symptoms, at least a thousand times as much antitoxin was needed to save the animal as to protect it and that if the disease was advanced, no amount of serum was adequate. They felt that the serum should not be used in man until the experimental facts were worked out, but they stated: "We believe that we can save people with tetanus with this serum which works a cure in mice." Kitasato ("Heilversuche an tetanuskranken Thieren," Ztschr. f. Hyg. u. Infektionskr., **12**:256, 1892), who was really working along with Behring, at about the same time published similar results. He emphasized especially the vastly greater quantity of serum necessary for cure than for prophylaxis but as yet gave no clear explanation.

11. BEHRING, [Emil Adolph]. Das Tetanusheilserum und seine Anwendung auf tetanuskranke Menschen. Leipzig: Georg Thieme, 1892.

This little book contains four articles by Behring and his associates which bring up to date all the problems of serotherapy of tetanus. The first is essentially an amplification of previous articles (Ref. 10) and it deals with estimation of the minimum lethal dose of toxin and minimal effective doses of curative sera in small animals. Behring again points out that, even with the earliest clinical symptoms, a thousand times the prophylactic dose of serum is necessary for cure, whereas, after 12 hours, a hundred thousand times the prophylactic dose is necessary and that later no amount of antitoxin suffices. He states that, since certain patients with tetanus recover spontaneously, serum therapy cannot be evaluated in individual cases but only by considering the mortality in large groups. The second article deals with the use of antitoxin in human cases of tetanus. Behring discusses the preparation of serum in horses and the general indications for its use. He critically reviews reports in the Italian literature on serotherapy and questions the validity of the claims which are made (G. Cattani, "L'Ematoterapia nel tetano," Riforma med., **2**:769, 1892; G. Tizzoni and G. Cattani, "Alcune questioni relative all'immunita pel tetano," Riforma med., **3**:495, 1892). In the third article Dr. Rotter discusses the treatment of a patient with tetanus, which he follows with a general discussion. It is pointed out that prognosis in tetanus depends on the duration of the incubation period and the speed with which clinical manifestations develop. The shorter the incubation period, the worse the prognosis. Statistics are given. These articles cover the whole subject and are definitive to date.

In modern times a good deal of skepticism has grown up as to whether antitoxin has any beneficial influence in established tetanus. F. Golla ("An analysis of recent tetanus statistics," Lancet, **2**:966, 1917) came to no definite conclusion in favor of antitoxin; and more recently R. W. Huntington, Jr., W. R. Thompson, and H. H. Gordon ("The treatment of tetanus with antitoxin," Ann. Surg., **105**:93, 1937), in an analysis of 642 cases, concluded that "relatively little has been accomplished in the specific treatment of tetanus." These observations, of course, do not apply to the prophylactic use of antitoxin.

12. MARIE, A. Recherches sur la toxine tétanique, Ann. Inst. Pasteur, **11**:591, 1897.

Marie reviews the primitive and conflicting work on what happens to tetanus toxin in the body and then takes up the subject anew. First he notes that if one determines the lethal subcutaneous dose for a rabbit, seven to eight times the amount must be given intravenously to produce a fatal effect. This made him assume that, in the first case, "a part of the toxin has followed the course of the nerve fibers and has reached the spinal cord directly." To prove this, he devised the following experiment. A fatal dose of toxin was injected directly into the sciatic nerve. On the day after inoculation the operated leg was stiff and on the following day was paralyzed with extensor contraction; by the fourth day the tetanus was generalized, and the animal died. But if one resects the second cervical nerve in a similar animal, allows the wound to heal, and then injects a fatal dose of toxin into the paralyzed paw, the animal does not fall ill. He then reports experiments to find out what becomes of toxin injected into the blood stream and concludes that it remains for a variable length of time in the blood but that, when this time has "run out," there is no evidence of toxin remaining in organs or in glandular secretions. He feels that extracts of organs from animals with tetanaus, prepared by others and alleged to be toxic, produce, if anything, immediate reactions which have nothing to do with tetanus.

Marie with V. Morax ("Sur l'absorption de la toxin tétanique," Ann. Inst. Pasteur, **16**:818, 1902) later continued his studies. He points out the specific effect of tetanus toxin on the motor neurons and attempts to determine "the mechanism of propagation of the toxin, from its point of penetration to the sensitive cell." He devised experiments which he thought proved that an injection of toxin was taken up rapidly by the local motor nerves and traveled to the ganglion cells, thus causing local tetanus. Part of the injected toxin diffused into the blood stream and was more slowly absorbed by motor nerves in general, ultimately producing generalized tetanus.

There is an immense literature on tetanus toxin which cannot be reviewed here. However, M. J. Pickett, P. D. Holford, and R. O. Germain ("Purification of high titre tetanus toxin," J. Bact., **49**:515, 1945) report purification of crude toxin by 125-fold; and L. Pillemer, R. Willter, and D. B. Grossberg ("The isolation and crystallization of tetanal toxin," Science, **103**:615, 1946) prepared crystalline material which contained 50–75 million minimum lethal doses (mouse) per mg. of N_2.

13. MEYER, Hans, and RANSOM, Fred. Untersuchungen über den Tetanus, Arch. f. exper. Path. u. Pharmakol., **49**:369, 1903.

The work described in this classical article confirms, parallels, and extends that of Marie and Morax (Ref. 12). After a review of the literature on the question of how tetanus toxin acts, the writers lay down a series of propositions with experiments to support them: "(1) After subcutaneous inoculation the poison can be demonstrated in the nerves. (2) Threatened centers in the spinal cord can be protected against the effect of tetanus toxin by blocking the afferent nerves with antitoxin. (3) Ascending spread of the poison in the spinal cord is inhibited by transection of the cord. (4) Consequences of injection of poison into nerves (tetanus occurs much more quickly than after subcutaneous injection)." They show that tetanus occurs within a few hours after intramedullary injection into the spinal cord, and they correlate the incubation period with the length of peripheral nerves in various animals. Thus the incubation period is 4 or 5 days in man or horse as against 8–12 hours in mice.

Meyer and Ransom formulated their theory of experimental tetanus poisoning as follows: "At the point of inoculation, toxin is absorbed from the lymph spaces by the endings of the motor neurones and by way of them reaches the motor spinal ganglion cells. These are thrown into a state of hyperexcitability, so that they are constantly stimulated by reflex sensory influences which are ordinarily subliminal." Thus the spasms arise. This theory was accepted without much opposition until recent years, when it was questioned, as, for example, by Abel (Ref. 17). There is much further material in this classical article which really must be studied in the original.

U. Friedemann and his associates tried to settle the controversy which had sprung up on the question of the transport of tetanus toxin by nerves. Friedemann and B. Zuger, who had been working on the general subject of "Quantitative studies on the neutralization of pathogenic agents in tissues by circulating antibodies" (J. Immunol., 36:192, 205, 219, 1939) were led to study tetanus toxin-antitoxin relationships (U. Friedemann, B. Zuger, and A. Hollander, "Investigations on the pathogenesis of tetanus. I. The permeability of the C.N.S. barrier to tetanal toxin. Passive immunity against toxin introduced by various routes," J. Immunol., 36:473; "II. The influence of section of the nerves on the neutralization of intramuscularly injected tetanal toxin by circulating antitoxin," *ibid.*, p. 485; U. Friedemann, A. Hollander, and I. M. Tarlow, "III," J. Immunol., 40:325, 1941). This work, on the whole, confirmed that of Meyer and Ransom and rendered untenable the views of Abel and his associates. The principal experiments were these: "From 5 to 80 times more circulating antitoxin is required to protect guinea-pigs from death after the intracutaneous and intramuscular than after the intravenous injection of tetanal toxin. The intramuscularly injected guinea-pigs may die despite the presence of free antitoxin in the blood." They concluded, therefore, that there was a blood barrier to the central nervous system which was impermeable to toxin and that intramuscularly injected toxin must reach the central nervous system by some other route, namely, the nerves. This position was supported by the work reported in the second communication, which showed that "section of the femoral and sciatic nerves abolishes the differences in the amounts of antitoxin required to neutralize intramuscularly and intravenously injected tetanal toxin." The third paper is a critical analysis of the literature on the whole subject. It is pointed out that it is now known that a good many viruses and chemical substances are transmitted to the central nervous system by transport along nerves, and the following final conclusions are drawn: "Tetanal toxin does not reach the central nervous system directly by way of the circulation. Tetanal toxin reaches the central nervous system by way of motor nerves. Tetanal toxin spreads within the central nervous system. Local tetanus is of central origin. Our results provide conclusive evidence for the existence of the blood central nervous system barrier."

14. PARK, William H., and NICOLL, Matthias, Jr. Experiments on the curative value of the intraspinal administration of tetanus antitoxin, J.A.M.A., **63**:235, 1914.

Realizing that clinical results with subcutaneous injection of antitoxin in established cases of tetanus were not good, Park and Nicoll experimented with intraspinal injection of antitoxin in guinea pigs which had received otherwise fatal doses of tetanus toxin. "This would seem absolutely conclusive of the superiority of the intraspinal method of giving antitoxin over the intravenous method . . . only those animals receiving antitoxin in the spine were able to survive." The writers also reported four human cases treated intraspinally who recovered. During World War I, C. S. Sherrington ("Observations with antitetanus serum in monkeys," Lancet, **2**:964, 1917) at the instigation of Bruce (Ref. 15) studied the question of the most efficacious route of injection of antitoxin into monkeys. He found a much greater number of recoveries in animals treated by the lumbar or bulbar subdural routes than by the subcutaneous or intramuscular routes. The "Tetanaus Committee" of the British army concluded that the best method of treatment "lies in the earliest possible administration of large doses of antitetanic serum by the intrathecal route" (Bruce, Ref. 15). W. M. Firor ("Intrathecal administration of tetanus antitoxin," Arch. Surg., **41**:299, 1940), working with dogs, concluded that "the intracisternal injection of antitoxin into dogs suffering from early, mild, or moderately severe tetanus yields far better results than intravenous injection. In animals with severe tetanus there is little difference in the results . . . but the difference favors the intracisternal route." Firor lists the variables which make clinical evaluation of treatment so difficult: "(*a*) length of incubation period, (*b*) interval before treatment was begun, (*c*) severity of symptoms, (*d*) details of treatment, (*e*) location of wound, (*f*) age of the patient, (*g*) the presence of other conditions which might have caused death, and (*h*) the culture of *Clostridium tetani* from the wound." J. B. Yodh ("Observations on the treatment of tetanus," Brit. M.J., **2**:589, 1932) wrote a paper which had much influence, in which he reported better results in tetanus in man if the therapy included intrathecal (intracisternal) injection of antitoxin. Nevertheless, intrathecal therapy is not advised in current textbooks, mainly because of the belief that only toxin which is freshly formed at the site of the wound is amenable to neutralization by antitoxin (Ref. 21), and such workers as H. M. Smathers and M. R. Weed ("The treatment of tetanus," Arch. Surg., **57**:291, 1948) actually found the same death rate for patients treated with and without antitoxin given intrathecally.

15. BRUCE, David. Tetanus: analysis of 1,458 cases which occurred in home military hospitals during the years 1914–1918, J. Hyg., **19**:1, 1920.

As pointed out by the early workers (Behring, Refs. 10, 11), even when incipient symptoms are present, much greater doses of antitoxin are necessary for cure than for prevention. Hence the obvious moment to give the antitoxin is shortly after the suspicious wound is incurred. Prophylactic use of antitoxin (passive immunization) was therefore heavily stressed, especially before the days of active immunization with toxoid (Ref. 16). This important analysis by Bruce shows how the incidence and mortality of tetanus fell off after prophylactic immunization was introduced into the British army in World War I.

Bruce also discusses the curative use of antitoxin after the disease is present and points out the difficulties in evaluation because of many variables. Among 1,458 cases who had had injections of antitoxin after symptoms developed, 33.5 per cent died.

The article contains much interesting material on other aspects of tetanus.

16. DESCOMBY, P. L'Anatoxine tétanique, Compt. rend. Soc. de biol., 91:239, 1924.

G. Ramon ("Anatoxine diphtérique, ses propriétés—ses applications," Ann. Inst. Pasteur, 42:959, 1928) had shown that diphtheria toxin could be rendered harmless while retaining its antigenic value by the action of formaldehyde and heat (anatoxin). Descomby used the same method with tetanus toxin with similar results. Guinea pigs withstood 5–10 cc. of such anatoxin, which before modification was fatal in doses of 1/10,000 cc. Tetanus anatoxin also had a high antigenic value. A horse, for example, after two injections of 15–20 cc. of anatoxin at intervals of 14 days became resistant to 1 cc. of a toxin, which was about thirty times the fatal dose. Ramon and Zoeller ("L'Anatoxine tétanique et l'immunization active de l'homme vis-à-vis du tétanos," Ann. Inst. Pasteur, 41:803, 1927) soon discussed in detail the theoretical and practical uses of anatoxin in man. They point out that passive immunization is transient and can be combined with active immunization with anatoxin in two doses at intervals of 20 days. They emphasize the value of active immunization in those likely to be subjected to trauma, such as military personnel, and also advise the immunization of pregnant females to protect the child against "tetanus neonatorum." In another paper Ramon and Descomby ("L'Anatoxine tétanique et la prophylaxie du tétanos chez le cheval et les animaux domestiques," Ann. Inst. Pasteur, 41:834, 1927) discuss the immunization of domestic animals. Later Ramon and Zoeller ("Sur la valeur et la durée de l'immunité conférée par l'anatoxine tétanique dans la vaccination de l'homme contre le tétanos," Compt. rend. Soc. de biol., 112:347, 1933) summarize their results and demonstrate that the sera of people immunized several years earlier may still contain enough antitoxin to neutralize up to three hundred fatal guinea-pig doses of toxin. They now advise three doses of anatoxin (1, 1.5, and 2 cc.), at intervals, to produce immunity. They also suggested "booster" doses (injection de rappel) at time of exposure (injury) to tetanus infection and found that they resulted in a great increase in the titer of antitoxin in the blood. In this country (E. M. Lincoln and C. K. Greenwald, "Active immunization of human beings with tetanus toxoid," Proc. Soc. Exper. Biol. & Med., 30:1241, 1933) similar results were obtained. D. H. Bergey ("Active immunization against tetanus infection with tetanus toxoid," J. Infect. Dis., 55:72, 1934) soon found that, as with diphtheria, anatoxin precipitation with alum resulted also with tetanus anatoxin in active preparations. F. G. Jones and J. M. Moss ("Studies on tetanus toxoid. I. The antitoxic titer of human subjects following immunization with tetanus toxoid and tetanus alum precipitated toxoid," J. Immunol., 30:115, 1936) found that two injections of alum-precipitated tetanus toxoid produced a higher immunity than did three injections of the unprecipitated toxoid. It has become customary in pediatric practice to combine several antigens for prophylactic immunization in one injection (see, e.g., J. J. Miller, J. B. Humber, and J. O. Downie, "Immunization with combined diphtheria and tetanus toxoids [aluminum hydroxide adsorbed] containing Hemophilus pertussis vaccine," J. Pediat., **24**:281, 1944). The use of active immunization became standard in the United States Army during World War II and is described by A. P. Long ("Tetanus toxoid, its use in the United States Army," Am. J. Pub. Health, **33**:53, 1943). This program was followed by the disappearance of tetanus from the army, barring a very occasional case in an unimmunized person.

An international unit for toxoid has been defined (Expert Committee on Biological Standardization, *Fifth Report* [Geneva: World Health Organization, July, 1952], p. 5 ["Technical Report Series," No. 56]).

17. ABEL, J. J., EVANS, E. A., Jr., HAMPIL, B., and LEE, F. C. Researches on tetanus. II. The toxin of the Bacillus tetani is not transported to the central nervous system by any component of the peripheral nerve trunks, Bull. Johns Hopkins Hosp., **56**:84, 1935.

Although the theories of Meyer and Ransom (Ref. 13) are generally accepted, there have been dissenting opinions. Among these, of special note are the views of J. J. Abel, the eminent Johns Hopkins pharmacologist. Abel was attracted to the problem from a general study of poisons ("On poisons and disease and some experiments with the toxin of the Bacillus tetani," Science, **79**:121, 1934). A long series of papers followed which we cannot attempt to review in detail. Suffice it to say that Abel makes a strong case on the grounds of both reasoning and experiment against the neural transmission of tetanus toxin. This, the second paper of the series, is largely a critique of the literature; it is with reference to local tetanus not resulting from neural transmission to the central nervous system that he bases a large part of his case. In another paper (J. J. Abel, B. Hampil, and A. F. Jonas, Jr., "III. Further experiments to prove that tetanus toxin is not carried in peripheral nerves to the central nervous system," Bull. Johns Hopkins Hosp., **56**:317, 1935) Abel reports that injection of toxin into the dog's sciatic nerve fails to be followed by local tetanus when a much smaller dose injected subcutaneously or intramuscularly does produce it. The fourth paper of the series ("IV. Some historical notes on tetanus and commentaries thereon," *ibid.*, **57**:343, 1936) consists of a most interesting critical review of the literature bearing on Abel's thesis. The ninth paper (J. J. Abel, W. M. Firor, and W. Chalian, "IX. Further evidence to show that tetanus toxin is not carried to central neurons by way of the axis cylinders of motor nerves," Bull. Johns Hopkins Hosp., **63**:373, 1938) summarizes and fortifies with more experiments Abel's views. He concludes: "The history of science bears testimony to the fact that it is not easy to dislodge from the mind a theory that has long been wholeheartedly accepted. We have therefore presented in this paper more arguments than might seem necessary to disprove the validity of the nerve carriage theory of tetanus toxin. . . . We have therefore reviewed critically the main arguments that have been adduced in the past in favor of the theory, and have shown that each of them may be refuted, and have given further evidence to show that tetanus toxin can be carried to the tissues of the body, whether these be the specifically reacting striated muscles and motor horn cells or structures that do not respond in a recognizable manner to the action of toxin, *only by the same mechanisms that effect the distribution of countless other drugs and poisons, namely, the blood- and lymph-vascular systems.* . . . The toxin exhibits both a central and a peripheral action, each of which may be demonstrated independently of the other. The central effect, which is characterized by reflex motor convulsions, is due to the poisoning of the motor nerve cells of the spinal cord, medulla and pons; the peripheral effect, recognized as the unremitting rigidity of voluntary muscles, results from the fixation of the toxin upon the motor end-organs." A. M. Harvey ("The peripheral action of tetanus toxin," J. Physiol., **96**:348, 1939) comes to the support of Abel with work in which modern methods of studying the transmission of the nerve impulse were used. He concludes: "These experiments afford direct experimental evidence of a peripheral action of tetanus toxin in the region of the neuromuscular junction."

We must leave the reader to study the original papers and to resolve this controversy for himself.

18. ABEL, J. J., EVANS, E. A., Jr., and HAMPIL, B. Researches on tetanus. Distribution and fate of tetanus toxin in the body, Bull. Johns Hopkins Hosp., **59**:307, 1936.

The question of how long after it is in contact with the tissues tetanus toxin is amenable to neutralization by antitoxin is paramount in planning treatment for patients. Abel and his colleagues showed that, up to a certain time, toxin which is apparently fixed in the tissues can still be neutralized by an excess of antitoxin; if administration of antitoxin is delayed too long, the toxin is not affected by it. These observations support the general feeling that therapy should be prompt and intensive.

19. COOKE, J. V., and JONES, F. G. The duration of passive tetanus immunity, J.A.M.A., **121**:1201, 1943.

The writers showed that, while passive immunization with the usual dose of 1,500 units produced immunity for only about 3 weeks, larger doses (100,000 units) conferred a much lengthier protection. They found that the antitoxin interfered with active immunization with toxoid and advised deferring such immunization for several weeks.

20. WEINSTEIN, Louis, and WESSELHOEFT, Conrad. Penicillin in the treatment of tetanus. Report of two cases, New England J. Med., **233**:681, 1945.

Following the observation (W. E. Herrell, D. R. Nicholls, and D. H. Heilman, "Penicillin: its usefulness, limitations, diffusion and detection, with analysis of 150 cases in which it was employed," J.A.M.A., **125**:1003, 1944) that penicillin inhibited the tetanus bacillus in the test tube, there appeared a brief note (R. Buxton and R. Kurman, "Tetanus: report of two cases treated with penicillin," J.A.M.A., **127**:26, 1945) on two cases which recovered in which penicillin was employed in addition to antitoxin. Weinstein and Wesselhoeft explored the matter more carefully. They reported two more patients who recovered under penicillin and antitoxin therapy, and they defined the rationale of using penicillin in tetanus: "Penicillin appears to be of the greatest value in cases of tetanus infection in which no localized areas of bacterial invasion can be detected or in which it is impossible to eradicate the focus [or foci] surgically. . . . Bacteriologic studies revealed that Clostridium tetani could no longer be isolated from wounds in these patients twenty-four hours after the first administration of penicillin." R. S. Diaz-Rivera, L. Deliz, and J. Berio-Suárez ("Penicillin in tetanus," J.A.M.A., **138**:191, 1948) reported a clinical analysis of fifty-nine penicillin-treated cases and concluded that the drug was useful, although their statistics seem inconclusive. But other observers, such as L. Lewis ("Therapeutic trial of penicillin in tetanus," Ann. Int. Med., **25**:903, 1946), working in the armed forces, could not convince himself that penicillin had any beneficial effect in tetanus.

21. FORBES, Gilbert B., and AULD, Marian. Management of tetanus, Am. J. Med., **18**:947, 1955.

A well-documented modern summary of the treatment of tetanus. The authors make the point that recovery may depend on great attention to certain details of management rather than on antitoxin. They stress the adequate use of muscle-relaxing agents, attention to keeping an open airway and preventing secondary respiratory infection, often including the use of tracheotomy, skilled use of sedatives, and the proper maintenance of fluids and electrolytes. Still other details are touched on.

Section 16

TYPHUS

Section 16

TYPHUS

ALTHOUGH typhus pretty clearly had existed in jails, armies, concentrations of people in close quarters, and crowded famine areas, the nineteenth century was well along before the disease was precisely defined. The reasons for this are not far to seek. First of all, typhus has no very characteristic localizing symptoms or signs except perhaps the rash, and this, for some peculiar reason, was often overlooked or at any rate not mentioned. Bartlett (Ref. 3), for example, tells us that "typhus fever is very generally attended with a peculiar and characteristic eruption upon the skin. . . . As to the exact frequency of the occurrence of this eruption, it is impossible to speak with entire certainty. In many cases it has probably been overlooked; and besides this, it is to be remembered that the diagnosis of typhus fever, by many who have written most extensively and most magisterially, upon the subject, has been anything but rigorous and careful. Dr. Stewart remarks, 'that the eruption of typhus was unnoticed at Edinburgh, until the attention of physicians was called to it by Dr. Peebles in 1832 . . . that, previous to a visit which Dr. Peebles made to the Glasgow Fever Hospital in the spring of 1835, the exanthem of typhus, then found to be of general occurrence, had neither been looked for, nor registered, in that institution, and was received as a new discovery' " (p. 207).

Second, there were no specific gross lesions at autopsy. There was, for example, nothing to give a definite clue, like the characteristic and invariable lesions of the small bowel in typhoid fever. The accounts of typhus were therefore vague and consisted of long rambling discussions of fever and prostration such as were typical of eighteenth-century medicine. James Carmichael Smyth's book (*A Description of the Jail Distemper as It Appeared amongst the Spanish Prisoners at Winchester, in the Year 1780* [London: J. Johnson, 1795]), for example, has as its chief claim to distinction that it was written by the father of Thackeray's stepfather. Over twenty years later, John Armstrong (*Practical Illustrations of Typhus Fever* [2d ed.; London: Baldwin, Cradock & Joy, 1818]) in his book of over three hundred pages on typhus still dealt largely with vague generalities. The terrible epidemics of 1817, 1818, and 1819 in Ireland, involving hundreds of thousands of cases, are dealt with in great detail and in more interesting fashion by F. Barker and J. Cheyne (*An Account of the Rise, Progress and Decline of the Fever Lately Epidemical in Ireland* [2 vols.; London: Baldwin, Cradock & Joy, 1821]), whose book contains a mine of descriptive material. Innumerable case reports are well documented, including mention of the exanthem. For example: "An early eruption of petechiae, which were often to be observed on the third or fourth day, or even earlier, and were visible for four or five days, was a general symptom of the disease" (1:454). But no description in any sense "modern" preceded the admirable account of Gerhard (Ref. 2).

Excellent general discussions of typhus are given by Bartlett (Ref. 3), Murchison (Ref. 4), and Curschmann (Ref. 6); a comprehensive up-to-date summary of the whole subject, with emphasis on developments in the laboratory, is that of J. C. Snyder ("The typhus fevers," *in* T. M. Rivers, *Viral and Rickettsia*

Infections of Man [Philadelphia: J. B. Lippincott Co., 1952], p. 578) with excellent bibliography. Other comprehensive bibliographies are to be found in Curschmann (Ref. 6), Murchison (Ref. 4), and A. Hirsch (*Handbuch der historisch-geographischen Pathologie* [2d ed.; Stuttgart: Ferdinand Enke, 1881], **1**:385, "Typhus exanthematicus"). The book on *Rickettsial Diseases of Man*, which consists of various papers read at a symposium in 1946 (Washington, D.C.: American Association for the Advancement of Science, 1948), contains much interesting material on typhus.

An immense amount has been written on the history of typhus; Hirsch (*loc. cit.*) and Murchison (Ref. 4) have especially good sections. Hans Zinsser's semipopular book (*Rats, Lice, and History* [Boston: Little, Brown & Co., 1935]) contains much valuable material. The story of modern research on typhus is also well summarized by P. K. Olitsky ("Hans Zinsser and his studies on typhus fever," J.A.M.A., **116**:907, 1941).

1. LOMBARD, H. C. Observations suggested by a comparison of the post mortem appearances produced by typhous fever in Dublin, Paris, and Geneva (communicated in a letter to Dr. Graves), Dublin J.M. Sc., **10**:17, 1836.

Lombard had seen in Geneva and in Paris many patients with typhoid fever, and he was quite familiar with the typical lesion of the small intestine. What was his surprise when post-mortem examinations in Ireland on what was presumably the same disease disclosed no lesions at all of the bowel. He finally began to wonder about the identity of the French and Irish "typhus," and, while their general similarity was obvious, he pointed out certain differences between the two—typhoid fever and typhus. "In the first place then the papular or measles-like eruption, which is always found in our continental typhus [typhoid fever], but which never acquires any great extent or importance, is here most remarkable both in appearance and in quantity . . . again in your fever [typhus] this rash is in bad cases mixed with true petechiae, and in many of the very malignant ones with purple blotches or *vibices*, an occurrence very rare with us. . . . Another symptom . . . which must be considered as constituting a difference, is diarrhoea, which is much less frequent, both before and during typhous fever [typhus], here than it is either in Paris or Geneva. In general it seems to me that the abdominal symptoms are less intense, and of less importance in this country than with us. . . . Another difference I wish to point out, is the highly contagious nature of the fever of this country [typhus] compared with that of the continent [typhoid]. . . . I can bring forward undeniable proofs of its transmission by contagion; but yet its transmissibility from one person to another is far less common with us than it is here."

In a second letter ("Second letter from Doctor Lombard to Doctor Graves on the subject of typhous fever," *ibid.*, p. 101) Lombard, after having toured the hospitals of England and having crystallized his thinking, says: "You have two different fevers, one highly contagious, which I may call the Irish Typhus, and in which the cephalic symptoms predominate, to the exclusion of abdominal alterations; the other which is sporadic [typhoid], and most likely not so infectious, and in which the abdominal symptoms are more predominant." Thus the explanation of this perplexity was that there was very little, if any, typhus in France or in Geneva, whereas in Ireland there was much typhus and in England both typhoid and typhus. Anyone seriously interested in the subject must actually read the two letters, since here, for the first time, typhoid and typhus fevers were clearly differentiated.

2. GERHARD, W. W. On the typhus fever, which occurred at Philadelphia in the spring and summer of 1836; illustrated by clinical observations at the Philadelphia Hospital; showing the distinction between this form of disease and dothinenteritis or the typhoid fever with alteration of the follicles of the small intestine, Am. J.M. Sc., **19**:289, 1836.

As a student in Paris, Gerhard had become thoroughly familiar with the clinical and pathological features of typhoid fever. He knew also that "the typhus fever, which is so common throughout the British dominions, especially in Ireland, is not attended with ulceration or other lesions of the glands of Peyer." He described numerous cases of typhus from the outbreak in Philadelphia in 1836 with careful autopsy reports. In a second article ("On the typhus which occurred at Philadelphia in the spring and summer of 1836," *ibid.*, **20**:289, 1837) Gerhard analyzes the clinical features. He gives a good description of the rash of typhus: "It consisted of petechiae, which in not more than six cases resembled the rose-coloured spots of dothinenteritis. . . . The petechiae appeared from the sixth to the eighth day, after the beginning of the symptoms, and disappeared from the fourteenth to the twentieth day. . . . There is a marked difference between the petechial eruption and the rose-coloured spots of typhoid fever. In typhoid fever the eruption is rare, very seldom extending beyond the abdomen and thorax; whereas in the epidemic typhus, the eruption is almost always general, extending to the limbs as well as the trunk." As to differential diagnosis: "When the disease is completely formed, the characters on which the distinction between the two forms of fevers rest, are: (1) The suffusion of the eyes . . with dusky-red aspect of the countenance. (2) The extreme stupor and inactivity of the mind even when positive delirium does not exist. (3) We also observe in typhus no constant abdominal symptom. . . . (4) If to these symptoms be added the peculiar eruption of petechiae . . . there remains hardly a possibility of error." Gerhard was sure that the typhus was very contagious.

To Gerhard, then, clearly goes the credit, after Lombard, for definitely distinguishing typhoid and typhus fevers.

3. BARTLETT, Elisha. The history, diagnosis and treatment of typhoid and of typhus fever. Philadelphia: Lea & Blanchard, 1842.

Bartlett gives the first worthwhile systematic discussion of typhus. There is a minute analysis of symptoms. The appearance of the rash "varied from the second to the thirteenth day . . . but in more than half the entire number, it appeared on the fifth or sixth day; and in three-fourths, it appeared from the fourth to the seventh day. In forty-eight cases the eruption began to decline at different periods, from the eighth to the nineteenth day" (p. 209). In a careful description of the lesions at autopsy, one notes the absence of anything specific. Bartlett, of course, could make only crude speculations as to cause. "The evidences of the contagious character of the disease are very positive" (p. 231). However, "the extreme doctrine in regard to the contagiousness of typhus is that the disease is exclusively and invariably the product of contagion. . . . This opinion is not generally entertained, and must have been always the result rather of philosophizing than of observing; for, certainly, the evidence of direct observation is altogether against this exclusive opinion." He thought it certain that the poison of typhus might be generated by "the crowding together in close unventilated apartments, amidst accumulations of personal filth, of the wretched and suffering poor" (p. 236). Under the heading of treatment he discusses bloodletting, purgatives, affusions and ablutions, stimulants and tonics, squill, camphor, opium, and emetics.

4. MURCHISON, Charles. A treatise on the continued fevers of Great Britain. 2d ed. London: Longmans, Green & Co., 1873.

The comprehensive chapter on typhus fever in Murchison's famous book occupies nearly three hundred pages. Nonetheless, there is really no material advance over Bartlett (Ref. 3) a generation before. The discussion opens with a definition: "A disease, generated by overcrowding of human beings with deficient ventilation, prevailing in an epidemic form, in periods, or under circumstances, of famine and general destitution, and communicable by contagion. Its symptoms are: More or less sudden invasion marked by rigors or chilliness; frequent compressible pulse; tongue furred and ultimately dry and brown; bowels, in most cases, constipated; skin warm and dry; a rubeoloid rash appearing between the fourth and seventh days, the spots never appearing in successive crops, at first slightly elevated and disappearing on pressure, but after the second day persistent, and often becoming converted into true petechiae; great and early prostration; heavy flushed countenance; injected conjunctivae; wakefulness and obtuseness of the mental faculties, followed, at the end of the first week, by delirium, which is sometimes acute and noisy, but ofttimes low and wandering; tendency to stupor and coma, tremors, subsultus, and involuntary evacuations, with contracted pupils. Duration of the fever from ten to twenty one days, usually fourteen. In the dead body no specific lesion; but hyperemia of all the internal organs, softening and disintegration of the heart and voluntary muscles, hypostatic congestion of the lungs, atrophy of the brain, and edema of the pia mater are common."

There follows an excellent and comprehensive section on the history of typhus, but the discussion on contagion is especially interesting. Murchison, like most others at the time, was perplexed. There seemed to be indubitable evidence of contagion, as, for example: "Persons in comfortable circumstances, and living in localities where the disease is unknown, are attacked, on visiting infected persons at a distance" (p. 82) or "Typhus is often imported by infected persons into localities free from it" (p. 83). However, there also were strong arguments for the generation of the poison *de novo*, perplexing at the time but readily intelligible in the light of carriage by a vector. Nonetheless, the rules for prevention of spread of typhus, worked out empirically, were effective in practice: isolation of patients, doing away with overcrowding, bathing patients, and destroying their clothes and bedding. The section on treatment, aside from bloodletting and the "Cold Water Treatment," consists of innumerable drugs and prescriptions which are not worth review.

5. MOREAU, L., and COCHEZ, A. Contribution à l'étude du typhus exanthématique, Gaz. hebd. de méd., **25**, 2d ser., 388, 1888.

In the case of practically all febrile diseases the bacteriological era brought attempts to define a living agent as the cause. Typhus was no exception, and, as early as 1888, Moreau and Cochez, working in Algeria, isolated from the brain, from other organs, and finally from the blood and urine of patients a bacillus whose characteristics they describe and which they put forward as the cause of typhus. A list of further claims for all sorts of organisms is given in Curschmann's treatise (Ref. 6, p. 9). Attempts to prove a bacterial cause died hard, however, and, as late as 1915, the organism of Plotz was widely accepted (Harry Plotz, Peter K. Olitsky, and George Baehr, "The etiology of typhus exanthematicus." "I. Harry Plotz: Bacteriologic studies," J. Infect. Dis., **17**:1, 1915; "II. Peter K. Olitsky: Serologic studies," *ibid.*, p. 18; "III. George Baehr, Harry Plotz, and Peter K. Olitsky: Experimental studies," *ibid.*, p. 40). In elaborate studies Plotz, with his associates Olitsky and Baehr, isolated an anaerobic bacillus with great constancy from the blood of patients with typhus; they found specific serological reactions and isolated the organism from animals which had been inoculated with it. They regarded the distemper which they produced in animals as typhus.

6. CURSCHMANN, H. Das Fleckfieber. Vienna: Alfred Hölder, 1900.

This thorough and systematic treatise by a great German clinician emphasizes how little the knowledge of typhus had advanced by the end of the century. Curschmann is too close to the old ideas to deny categorically the doctrine of generation *de novo* of the *contagium*. However, he does say that "most current investigators are of the opinion that the *contagium* is contained in the exhalations of the patient, in his expired air, in the evaporations from his skin, etc., and that it sticks to dust particles which fill the air surrounding him." This doctrine, of course, is only a step away from that of miasms. There is an admirable clinical analysis of the disease, but the pathological descriptions are inadequate and miss what were later (Ref. 13) found to be the essential lesions.

7. NICOLLE, Charles, COMTE, C., and CONSEIL, E. Transmission expérimentale du typhus exanthématique par le pou du corps, Compt. rend. Acad. d. sc., **149**:486, 1909.

Charles Nicolle ("Reproduction expérimentale du typhus exanthématique chez le singe," Compt. rend. Acad. d. sc., **149**:157, 1909) had already succeeded in infecting monkeys with blood from a typhus patient. He concluded that his experiments proved "(1) the possibility of transmitting human typhus to the chimpanzee and after passage through it to the *Macacus sinicus,* a common species; (2) the presence of the virus in the blood of man on the day of the eruption and in the blood of the chimpanzee 2 days before its appearance." After an incubation period of 25 days a febrile, prostrating disorder with rash appeared. However, monkey typhus has never been suitable for routine experimental work and was promptly superseded by the distemper produced in guinea pigs.

Nicolle, Comte, and Conseil, studying typhus in Tunis, reasoned that the disease was transmitted by the bite of an insect. "Several observed facts have led us to limit our hypothesis to the louse," such as that people bathed and freshly clothed did not get typhus, whereas those who handled the clothes did; "we know of two cases in which typhus manifestly followed the bite of a louse." Lice which had been fasted for 8 days were allowed to feed on a monkey which had been inoculated with typhus blood. The lice were then applied to other monkeys, which in due time came down with "typhus." "These experiments show that exanthematic typhus can be transmitted to the monkey by means of the body louse. The application of this finding to the etiology and prophylaxis of the disease in man is imperative." And so it indeed turned out, for this work was really the start of the great flood of modern research on typhus. Nicolle and his associates soon extended and amplified their original observations in a series of notes (C. Nicolle and E. Conseil, "Reproduction expérimentale du typhus exanthématique chez le macaque par inoculation direct du virus humain," Compt. rend. Acad. d. sc., 151:258, 1910; "Données expérimentale nouvelles sur le typhus exanthématique," *ibid.*, p. 454), and in a long article (Charles Nicolle, "Recherches expérimentales sur le typhus exanthématique entreprises à l'Institut Pasteur de Tunis pendant l'année 1909," Ann. Inst. Pasteur, 24:243, 1910; *ibid.*, 25:1, 1911) Nicolle laid emphasis on the preventive and curative properties of sera of convalescent patients and animals.

T. H. Ricketts and R. M. Wilder ("The transmission of the typhus fever of Mexico [Tabardillo] by means of the louse [Pediculus vestamenti]," J.A.M.A., 54:1304, 1910) confirmed Nicolle's results. They were more conservative, however, and pointed out that the monkey disease consisted mainly of a febrile reaction without rash and that, in passage, the infection soon died out. They demanded and furnished proof, therefore, that "typhus" really had been produced by louse bite by challenging the animals which had recovered with injections of "virulent" blood. Without exception, they remained well, and Ricketts and Wilder regarded this immunity test as essential. Ricketts and Wilder ("The etiology of the typhus fever [Tabardillo] of Mexico City: a further preliminary report," *ibid.*, p. 1373) soon made a further report. Wilder ("The problem of transmission in typhus fever," J. Infect. Dis., 9:9, 1911) a little later, after Ricketts' death from typhus, wrote a classical monograph of some ninety pages with bibliography, in which he summarized the literature and amplified the reports of his own work with Ricketts. In connection with the experimental observations, he emphasized the following points: Various species of ape were the only animals so far found susceptible. Blood for animal inoculation should be drawn from human typhus cases not later than the tenth day of fever. The course in the monkey is sufficiently characteristic to enable a positive diagnosis to be made. The disease is similar to that in man; it has an incubation period of 6–10 days. The absence of cultivable organisms in the blood and of anatomical lesions is characteristic. Leukocytosis is usually observed. One attack confers absolute immunity. The virus of typhus is non-filterable. Typhus can be transmitted to monkeys by the bites of lice and by the introduction into cutaneous scarifications of the intestinal contents of infected lice. It is indicated that the infectiousness of the virus is enhanced within the louse. Hereditary transmission of infectivity in the louse is suggested. Wilder outlined the salient points of typhus prophylaxis: (1) the destruction of lice; (2) the extermination of lice found on the bodies, clothing, or bedding of patients or of contacts; and (3) measures to minimize the danger of exposed individuals being bitten by lice.

Joseph Goldberger and John F. Anderson ("The transmission of typhus fever with especial reference to transmission by the head louse [*Pediculus capitis*]," Hygienic Lab. Bull. 86 [Washington, 1912], p. 37) soon confirmed the work of Nicolle and of Ricketts and Wilder on transmission by lice. They concluded that "(1) The body louse . . . may become infected with typhus . . . and the virus . . . is transmissible by subcutaneous injection [into monkeys] of the crushed insect or by its bite. (2) The head louse may become infected and [the disease] may be transmitted by subcutaneous injection of the crushed insect and . . . also by its bite."

8. BRILL, Nathan E. An acute infectious disease of unknown origin, Am. J.M. Sc., **139**:484, 1910.

Brill first reported "his disease" in 1898 (Nathan E. Brill, "A study of 17 cases of a disease clinically resembling typhoid fever but without the Widal reaction," New York M.J., **67**:48, 77, 1898), but his final description in 1910 was based on 221 cases. The patients were seen in New York City; they were mostly immigrants from eastern Europe. There might be a preliminary period of 3–4 days of malaise, but invasion was usually abrupt, with chill and intense headache. Headache, photophobia, apathy, and prostration increased with the temperature, which rose rapidly and remained continuously high after the first 2–3 days. The rash usually appeared about the sixth day, first on abdomen and back, and then spreading elsewhere. The face, however, was uninvolved. The rash was dull red, very slightly raised, and did not disappear on pressure. On about the twelfth day the fever usually dropped rapidly, the rash faded, and symptoms cleared. Convalescence was rapid. The spleen was usually palpable; the leukocyte count varied usually from 9,000 to 10,000 but might be higher.

Brill ("Pathological and experimental data derived from a further study of an acute infectious disease of unknown origin," Am. J.M. Sc., **142**:196, 1918) soon reported further studies. Although he suspected the disease of being typhus, he was thrown off by his inability to transmit it to monkeys, and in fatal cases no characteristic lesions were found. Brill's disease aroused great interest among doctors, and discussions were lively as to its nature.

The studies of J. F. Anderson and J. Goldberger ("The relation of so-called Brill's disease to typhus fever: an experimental demonstration of their identity," Hygienic Lab. Bull. No. 86 [1912], p. 25), however, showed that Brill's disease could be transmitted to monkeys which were then immune to a subsequent infection with virulent blood of the same strain and were also immune to infection with blood from Mexican typhus. Monkeys recovered from an infection with Mexican typhus fever were found immune to subsequent infection with material from "Brill's" disease. Hence the writers concluded that European typhus (Brill's disease) and Mexican typhus were one and the same disease. H. Zinsser ("The varieties of typhus virus and the epidemiology of the American form of European typhus fever [Brill's disease]," Am. J. Hyg., **20**:513, 1934) pointed out that, whereas the strains of virus producing the two forms of typhus were closely related, they were not identical. They might be regarded as "slightly divergent variants of the same stock." He concluded, further, that cases of Brill's disease represented recrudescences of old infections originally acquired in European foci, which in louse-infected communities might give rise to new epidemic outbreaks.

9. NICOLLE, Charles, CONSEIL, E., and CONOR, A. Le Typhus expéri-
mental du cobaye, Compt. rend. Acad. d. sc., **152**:1632, 1911.

"When one inoculates several guinea pigs with variable quantities (8, 6, 4, 3,
2 cc.) of blood from a typhus patient, some of the animals die in a few days
with loss of weight and hypothermia; these are the ones which receive the
larger doses. The others, contrariwise, inoculated with smaller amounts, show
no apparent symptoms—at the most, a transient loss of weight. However, if one
takes the temperature of these guinea pigs which show nothing objectively, one
finds that in certain animals, not in all, there is a fever for several days comparable to that which is shown by monkeys inoculated with the same blood and
with more overt typhus." The specificity of this reaction was soon confirmed
by others. John F. Anderson ("The reaction of the guinea-pig to the virus of
typhus fever," J.M. Research, **30**:467, 1914) found that many guinea pigs had
a natural immunity to a first injection of typhus blood from human cases, although only 4.7 per cent failed to react to an inoculation of virulent guinea-pig
typhus blood.

However, this test has become a standard procedure in typhus work, and it
was depended upon by Wolbach, Todd, and Palfrey (Ref. 13) in their important studies in the Polish epidemic in 1920. They review the literature[1] and give
a comprehensive account of the clinical and pathological features of the guinea-
pig disease. P. K. Olitsky ("Definition of experimental typhus fever in guinea
pigs," J.A.M.A., **78**:571, 1922) defines the guinea-pig disease precisely, and the
subject is also reviewed by John C. Snyder ("The typhus fevers" *in* Rivers, *op.
cit.*, p. 587).

10. FRAENKEL, Eugen. Ueber Fleckfieber und Roseola, München. med.
Wchnschr., **61**:57, 1914.

It occurred to Fraenkel to seek the causal agent of typhus in the skin lesions. He
excised bits of the exanthematous skin without anesthesia and fixed and stained
the material. He described a lesion quite different from that found in the rose
spots of typhoid fever; he found thickenings of the walls of small vessels which
were due "to infiltration not with leukocytes, but with mononuclear cells." He
described these cells in detail and also changes in the vessel wall. He decided
that "in fact, a peculiar lesion of the small arteries is the essential feature of the
skin lesion," and he concluded by suggesting that similar lesions might be found
in internal organs. In a later paper Fraenkel ("Zur Fleckfieberdiagnose," *ibid.*,
62:805, 1915) gave a further description and noted that one saw "swelling and
necrosis of the intima and marked swelling of the adventitial and periadventi-
tial cells." Fraenkel regarded the lesions as specific and capable of giving a
definite diagnosis. His work was soon confirmed, and changes were described in
various internal organs. The extensive literature is reviewed in Wolbach, Todd,
and Palfrey's report (Ref. 13), and the general subject of the pathology of
typhus is considered in the elaborate monograph by W. Ceelen ("Die pathologische Anatomie des Fleckfiebers," in *Ergebn. d. allg. Path. u. path. Anat.*

---

[1] Curiously enough, these writers refer to the 1909 paper of Nicolle, Comte, and
Conseil (Ref. 7) and to the 1910 papers of Ricketts and Wilder (Ref. 7) as first showing the susceptibility of the guinea pig. Actually, these papers deal only with monkeys,
and the first reference to guinea pigs is the 1911 paper of Nicolle, Conseil, and Conor
(Ref. 9).

[Wiesbaden, 1919], p. 307), which contains a comprehensive bibliography. Wolbach, Todd, and Palfrey (Ref. 13) give a minute account of the lesions and picture beautifully masses of *Rickettsia* in the cells of blood-vessel walls. An authoritative summary of the subject is also given by S. Burt Wolbach in "The pathology of the rickettsial diseases of man," in *Rickettsial Diseases of Man* (Washington: American Association for the Advancement of Science, 1948), p. 118.

11. WEIL, E., and FELIX, A. Zur serologischen Diagnose des Fleckfiebers, Wien. klin. Wchnschr., **29**:33, 1916.

Weil and Felix, in the course of examining cultures from typhus patients, grew from the urine of V., a Rumanian physician, a micro-organism which was not agglutinated by sera from typhoid, paratyphoid A and B, or dysentery cases. It was, however, agglutinated by the patient's own serum in a dilution of 1:200. The organism turned out to be a Gram-negative bacillus. Tested with typhus sera, it was agglutinated in all of thirty-three cases in dilutions of 1:25 to 1:500. The agglutinins reached their peak at the time the eruption appeared, remained up about 14 days, and then fell rapidly. Weil and Felix concluded that "in this bacterium we have found an aid in diagnosis of typhus." A little later Felix ("Die Serodiagnostik des Fleckfiebers," *ibid.*, p. 873) pointed out that the two strains isolated by Weil and Felix (X_1 and X_2) were being widely used in the diagnosis of typhus. Weil and Felix soon isolated another strain from urine of a typhus patient (X_{19}), which made the diagnosis of typhus "much easier and more certain." Felix concluded: "The highly specific agglutination reaction with X_{19} occurs earlier and in higher dilution than with the previously used strain X_2."

We cannot review the immense amount of work subsequently done on this subject but refer the reader to Kenneth Wertman's review ("The Weil-Felix reaction," in *Rickettsial Diseases of Man*, p. 184). In the same monograph C. J. D. Zarafonetis ("The serological reactions in the rickettsial diseases of man," p. 178) and Joseph E. Smadel ("Complement fixation and agglutination reactions in rickettsial diseases," p. 190) review the whole subject of serological reactions in typhus, with bibliographies.

12. DA ROCHA-LIMA, H. Beobachtungen bei Flecktyphuslaüsen, Arch. f. Schiffs- u. Tropen-Hyg., **20**:17, 1916.

Going on the presumption "no lice, no typhus fever," Da Rocha-Lima sought a causal agent in the louse. "In the first smears from infected lice . . . I was struck by a prodigious number of bacillus-like bodies which stained pinkish with Giemsa's stain." These were obviously not normal constituents of the louse, since they were absent in controls. They were found chiefly in the alimentary canal. It was not possible to grow them on the ordinary bacteriological media. Da Rocha-Lima succeeded in infecting guinea pigs with minute amounts of suspensions of intestinal contents. The "organisms" were also present in the salivary glands. Whether these were the bodies seen by Ricketts and Wilder (Ref. 7) and by S. von Prowazek ("Aetiologische Untersuchungen über den Flecktyphus in Serbien 1913 und Hamburg 1914," Beitr. z. Klin. der Infectionskr., **3**:5, 1914) is uncertain. Both Ricketts and Von Prowazek died of typhus in the course of their investigations. Da Rocha-Lima's definitive paper ("Zur Ätiologie des Fleckfiebers," Centralbl. f. allg. Path. u. path. Anat., 1916 Beiheft zu Band **27**, p. 45, 1916) soon appeared, in which he made a definite claim for his organism as the cause of typhus and gave it the name of *Rickettsia prowazeki* in honor of the investigators who succumbed to the disease. He now demonstrated and pictured the organisms in the epithelial cells of the alimentary tract, in which "a lively multiplication takes place, and only in a narrow zone of protoplasm near the nucleus." He again showed a regular coincidence of *Rickettsia* in the louse, with its infectivity for guinea pigs. Various other time and temperature relationships were worked out. In a later paper (F. Munk and H. da Rocha-Lima, "Klinik und Aetiologie des sogen. 'Wolhynischen Fiebers' [Werner-Hissche Krankheit]." II. H. da Rocha-Lima, "Ergebnis der ätiologischen Untersuchungen und deren Beziehungen zur Fleckfieberforschung," München. med. Wchnschr., **64**:1422, 1917), Da Rocha-Lima fortified his previous conclusions and distinguished *Rickettsia prowazeki* from other similar organisms in diseased and healthy lice. The definitive observations of Wolbach, Todd, and Palfrey (Ref. 13), however, settled to the satisfaction of everyone the role of *Rickettsia* as the cause of typhus. H. Plotz, J. E. Smadel, T. F. Anderson, and L. A. Chambers ("Morphological structure of *Rickettsia*," J. Exper. Med., **77**:355, 1943) studied and pictured the appearance and structure of *Rickettsia* as revealed by the electron microscope.

13. WOLBACH, S. Burt, TODD, John L., and PALFREY, Francis W. The etiology and pathology of typhus. Cambridge, Mass.: Harvard University Press, 1922.

This volume, a landmark in the history of the subject, represents work done by a commission sent to Poland in 1920 to study typhus. As the writers say in their Introduction, they amplified and consolidated rather than made fundamentally new discoveries. Thus they improved the methods of collecting, caring for, and feeding lice; they made very careful clinical studies; they proved beyond question the specificity of *Rickettsia prowazeki* for typhus by having *Rickettsia*-free lice feed on typhus patients and then producing the disease in guinea pigs by inoculation of infected louse viscera; they made definitive studies of the guinea-pig disease and its pathological anatomy; and they studied with the greatest care and pictured the pathology of typhus in man. They conclude that typhus is a disease of small blood vessels and that the parasite localizes almost exclusively in the vascular endothelium. "The reaction to the parasite is shown primarily by degenerative changes, giving rise to thromboses in blood vessels, and by a proliferative reaction on the part of endothelium [p. 200]. . . . As there is no specific stain for *Rickettsia prowazeki* the following criteria must be satisfied: (1) the size, (2) morphology, (3) staining reactions must correspond with those of *Rickettsia prowazeki* in sections of lice, and (4) they must be present in vascular endothelial cells *in situ* in relation to the lesions of typhus."

14. COX, Herald R., and BELL, E. John. Epidemic and endemic typhus: protective value for guinea-pigs of vaccines prepared from infected tissues of the developing chick embryo, Pub. Health Rep., **55**:110, 1940.

Cox ("The preparation and standardization of rickettsial vaccines," in *Rickettsial Diseases of Man*, p. 203) reviews the long story of the development of vaccines against typhus. He tells how living and attenuated live vaccines turned out to be dangerous and the difficulties of obtaining sufficient quantities of *Rickettsia* from lice for commercial use of killed vaccine. It was the development by Cox ("Use of yolk sac of developing chick embryo as medium for growing *Rickettsia* of Rocky Mountain spotted fever and typhus groups," Pub. Health Rep., **53**:2241, 1938), of a method for growing *Rickettsia* in large numbers which solved the problem. From infected tissues of developing chick embryos Cox and Bell prepared vaccines "that will protect most of the test-guinea pigs against epidemic (European) typhus." Mass production methods were soon developed. R. S. Ecke *et al.* ("The effect of Cox-type vaccine on louse borne typhus fever," Am. J. Trop. Med., **25**:447, 1945) found that, while typhus did occur in the vaccinated, the course was milder and only an occasional patient died. A. G. Gilliam ("Efficacy of Cox-type vaccine in the prevention of naturally acquired louse borne typhus fever," Am. J. Hyg., **44**:401, 1946) came to somewhat similar conclusions. Finally, J. F. Sadusk, Jr. ("Typhus fever in the United States Army following immunization: incidence, severity of disease, modification of clinical course and serological diagnosis," J.A.M.A., **133**:1192, 1947), discussed the extensive army experience. From January, 1942, to December, 1945, only 64 cases of epidemic typhus occurred in the armed forces. Sadusk feels that, while the incidence may not be reduced, the severity of attack is much diminished and mortality practically eliminated.

    15. YOUNGMANS, A., SNYDER, J. C., MURRAY, E. S., ZARAFONETIS, C. J. D., and ECKE, R. S. The therapeutic effect of para-aminobenzoic acid in louse borne typhus, J.A.M.A., **126**:349, 1944.

These workers first described beneficial effects from large doses of para-aminobenzoic acid in louse-borne typhus if treatment was started in the first week of illness. J. C. Snyder *et al.* ("Further observations on the treatment of typhus with para-aminobenzoic acid," Ann. Int. Med., **27**:1, 1947) reported further on the curative action of this drug in typhus. They give details of administration and emphasize the importance of starting the treatment early and of "attaining promptly and maintaining . . . a concentration of the drug in the blood above 10 mg. per 100 cc. for *R. prowazeki*." However, at present (1952), one of the wide-spectrum antibiotics (Refs. 16, 17) is considered the drug treatment of choice (J. C. Snyder in Rivers, *op. cit.*, p. 595).

    16. WONG, Sam C., and COX, Herald R. Action of aureomycin against experimental rickettsial and viral infections, Ann. New York Acad. Sc., **51**:290, 1948.

Wong and Cox found that aureomycin possessed marked therapeutic activity against the virus of typhus in embryonated hen's eggs, mice, and guinea pigs. Guinea pigs receiving massive doses of virus were protected by aureomycin, if the drug was given very early, against any symptoms, but the animals developed no antibodies. With small doses of virus, aureomycin protects against symptoms, and the animals develop no antibodies, nor are they immune. "These findings indicate a quantitative relationship between the dosage of infecting agent and the dosage and time of administration of aureomycin." Soon after, J. C. Snyder *et al.* ("Experimental studies on the antirickettsial properties of terramycin," Ann. New York Acad. Sc., **53**:362, 1953) found that terramycin has antirickettsial properties against *R. prowazeki* in chick embryos and mice; and, finally,

J. E. Smadel and E. B. Jackson ("Chloromycetin, an antibiotic with dermo-therapeutic activity in experimental rickettsial and viral infections," Science, **106**:418, 1947) found chloramphenicol effective in *R. prowazeki* infections of eggs and of mice.

17. SMADEL, J. E., LEON, A. P., LEY, H. L., and VARELA, G. Chloromycetin in the treatment of patients with typhus fever, Proc. Soc. Exper. Biol. & Med., **68**:12, 1948.

The experimental work on the newer antibiotics in egg and guinea-pig infections with typhus virus (Ref. 16) were soon followed by trials in man. Smadel and his group obtained favorable results in a few patients treated with chloromycetin by mouth. E. H. Payne, E. A. Sharp, and J. A. Knaudt ("Treatment of epidemic typhus with chloromycetin," Tr. Roy. Soc. Trop. Med. & Hyg., **42**:163, 1948) soon reported the treatment of twenty-two patients with the same drug both intravenously and orally: "The favorable effects of treating typhus (epidemic) with chloromycetin appear rapidly and the patient usually enters convalescence within 3 days." A little later E. B. Schoenbach ("Aureomycin therapy of re-crudescent epidemic typhus [Brill's disease]," J.A.M.A., **139**:450, 1949) reported a case of typhus treated on the sixth day with aureomycin by oral and intramuscular routes with prompt clinical improvement.

Thus the experimental results seem to be confirmed in man.

18. Control of communicable diseases in man: An official report of the American Public Health Association, p. 203. 1955.

In this outline are given in detail authoritative directions for prevention of epidemic (louse-borne) typhus, indicating the use of insecticides, delousing, immunization, etc. The technique of prevention is also well discussed, with graphic illustrations, in War Department Technical Bulletin (TB Med., No. 218), *Epidemic (Louse-borne) Typhus* (Washington, April 17, 1946).

SYPHILIS: PART I. FROM JOHN HUNTER TO DISCOVERY OF THE TREPONEME (1905)

Aneurysm	Ref. 30
Bismuth	Ref. 36
Clinical and general	Refs. 1, 2, 3, 5, 7, 11, 12, 17, 19, 22, 24, 26, 40
Congenital	Refs. 3, 11, 16, 27, 35
Discovery of spirochete	Ref. 43
Hutchinson's teeth	Ref. 23
Incubation period	Refs. 13, 22, 27
Inoculation	Refs. 10, 12, 18, 19, 22
Iodide	Ref. 9
Paresis	Ref. 31
Pathology	Refs. 20, 25, 33
Syphilis of nervous system	Refs. 21, 28, 37, 43
Syphilis and public health	Refs. 34, 41
Syphilitic aortitis	Ref. 39
Tabes dorsalis	Refs. 14, 29, 32
Transmission to animals	Ref. 42
Treatment	Refs. 6, 7, 11, 12

Section 17

SYPHILIS: PART I

IT IS not our purpose to take up in this bibliography the vast literature on the history of syphilis. For this phase of the subject the reader may be referred to such scholarly works as those of Iwan Bloch (*Der Ursprung der Syphilis* [Jena: Gustav Fischer, Part I, 1901; Part II, 1911]), of Gaston Vorberg (*Ueber den Ursprung der Syphilis* [Stuttgart: Julius Püttman, 1924]), and of Karl Sudhoff (*Aus der Frühgeschichte der Syphilis* [Leipzig: J. Barth, 1912]). An excellent brief account in English is that of William Allen Pusey (*The History and Epidemiology of Syphilis* [Springfield: Charles C Thomas, 1933]).

We shall begin rather with John Hunter in the late eighteenth century and attempt to give in this instalment the key references which trace the development of the subject until the discovery of the spirochete. The problem is difficult because nearly everyone of importance who wrote on syphilis produced a large book, mostly copied from previous writers, in which lay buried a few grains of new knowledge. However, one can trace from Hunter's primitive ideas on the identity of gonorrhea, chancroid, and syphilis a gradual realization, by astute clinical observation and by inoculation and confrontation experiments, that these were three different diseases. Along with this came more accurate classification of the clinical stages of syphilis, the timing of the incubation period, and study of the anatomy of the lesions. We shall trace the realization which gradually dawned in the last quarter of the nineteenth century of the role of syphilis in tabes and paresis and in aneurysm. One marvels how clinicians unarmed with knowledge of the spirochete, without the Wassermann reaction, and without spinal fluid examination were able to detect these relationships at all. On the whole, though, things moved very slowly, and practically no advance in treatment was made until the discovery of the arsphenamines.

It is impossible to begin to list even all the major titles; we have tried to select books or articles in which an outstanding contribution was made. For detailed bibliography one should refer to the monumental work of J. K. Proksch (*Die Literatur über die venerischen Krankheiten* [3 vols.; Bonn: Peter Hanstein, 1889–1900]).

1. HUNTER, John. A treatise on the venereal disease. London, 1786. (Numerous editions during the next fifty years. We quote from the first American edition [Philadelphia: Parry Hall, 1791].)

Modern discussion of syphilis may be said to begin with John Hunter. Hunter's great name and reputation were so influential that his work dominated the field for decades and few dared write on venereal disease without deferring, or at least referring, to him. His book ran through many editions and was translated into French and German. Actually, Hunter confused and held back the subject for two generations. Great as he was as a surgeon, his observations and ideas on syphilis were hopelessly inadequate. He accepted a preconceived doctrine that two different diseases could not coexist in a patient ("it appears to me, beyond a doubt, that no two actions can take place in the same constitution, nor in the same part, at one and the same time" [p. 2]), and consequently he believed that there was only one venereal disease, which manifested itself in three ways: as gonorrhea, chancre, or lues venerea. Whether the first manifestation was a gonorrhea or a chancre depended, Hunter thought, on the type of surface upon which the poison fell. In addition, he believed, correctly, that there were many non-specific (syphiloid) genital ulcers which could be mistaken for the true venereal disease. Often the test of whether the lesion disappeared under mercury was the only way, he claimed, of identifying syphilis.

"A chancre has commonly a thickened base," said Hunter (p. 195), but on the whole his description is not at all precise. So, too, as to incubation period. Hunter stated that, on the whole, the chancre "is rather longer in appearing than gonorrhea" (p. 198), but he gave the time as 24 hours to several weeks. Hunter thought the surest method of treating a chancre was by destruction or excision (p. 208) and that, if this was done promptly, there was but "little danger of the constitution being infected" (p. 209). But, as one could not be certain, "it would be prudent to give some mercury internally as well" (p. 209). And later: "In every case of a chancre, let it be ever so slight, mercury should be given internally; even in those cases where they were destroyed on their first appearance. It should in all cases be given the whole time of the cure, and continued for some time after the chancres are healed; for as there are perhaps few chancres without absorption of the matter, it becomes absolutely necessary to give mercury to act internally, in order to hinder the venereal disposition from forming" (p. 219). Here Hunter was certainly sound. "The immediate consequence of the local diseases, gonorrhea and chancre, which is called bubo, as also the remote or lues venerea, arise from the absorption of recent venereal matter" (p. 231).

We are especially concerned with Part VI, chapter i, "Of the Lues Venerea." This Hunter called "the constitutional part of venereal disease" in consequence of the poisonous matter being absorbed (p. 262). From this point on, however, his description of later lesions is for the most part obscure, inadequate, and based on a fanciful theory of the whole situation, although he had some idea of the stages of syphilis: "The parts that are affected by this form of the disease when in its early stage or appearance, which I have called first in order, are the skin, tonsils, nose, inside of the mouth and sometimes the tongue. When in its later state, the periosteum, fasciae, and bones come into action and these I call second in order of parts" (p. 281). But he by no means really differentiated secondary and tertiary lesions.

"Mercury in the lues venerea, as in the chancre, is the great specific, and hardly anything else is to be depended upon" (p. 307), said Hunter, and then he continued with a long discussion of preparations, quantity, and mode of administration, with a description of their actions and effects. It is easy to see how hopeless accurate evaluation of any therapeutic agent in syphilis had to be until much more was known about the fundamentals of the disease.

John Hunter was essentially a practical man. He did badly in school and never learned Latin or Greek, at that time considered essential for a gentleman's education. He got into medicine by way of his beautiful anatomical dissections and undoubtedly became a skilled and resourceful surgeon. His very precision in making observations, however, seems to have interfered, as it sometimes did in the case of the great Virchow, with sound reasoning. Hunter thought in terms of humors; his medical outlook was oriented to the past rather than to the newer points of view so well emphasized by the brilliant French clinician-pathologists.

Hunter's confused ideas about syphilis and venereal disease in general may be brought out by a few quotations from his book:

"I divide sympathy into two kinds; universal and partial."

"Universal sympathy is, an infection wherein the whole constitution sympathizes with some sensation or action. Partial sympathy is, an infection wherein one or more distinct parts sympathize with some local sensation, or action" (p. 11).

"The following case is an instance of a gonorrhoea producing a lues venerea. . . . To account for these two very different effects of the same poison it is only necessary to observe the difference in the mode of action of the parts affected when irritated let the irritation be what it may. . . . The poison then being the same in both cases, why do they not always happen together in the same person? For one would naturally suppose, that the gonorrhoea when it has appeared, can not fail to become the cause of a chancre, and that this when it happens first, must produce a gonorrhoea" (p. 16). "The venereal disease also becomes often the immediate cause of other disorders, by calling forth latent tendencies to action. This does not happen from its being venereal, but from its having destroyed the natural actions so that the moment the venereal action and disposition is terminated the other takes place" (p. 24). "It has been observed before, that there are three forms of the venereal infection, gonorrhoea, chancre, and the lues venerea, which various forms I have endeavoured to account for. As they all three arise from the same poison, and as the two first depend only on a difference in the nature of the parts, and the lues venerea on another circumstance which has been explained, it would be natural to suppose that one medicine, whatever it be, would cure all forms of this disease. But we find from experience, that this does not hold good; for one medicine, that is mercury, cures only the chancre and the lues venerea, and the gonorrhoea is not the least affected by it" (p. 304). Apparently, this observation did not suggest to Hunter that gonorrhea was a distinct disease. In other passages, some of which we have quoted above, Hunter seemed to sense dark glimmerings of the truth.

The overwhelming evidence of contact as a precursor of syphilis led Hunter and physicians generally to believe that the poison of the disease was communicable from person to person. Hence students of venereal disease for several decades centered their attention on (1) the clinical differentiation of the various venereal lesions; (2) attempts to distinguish them by inoculation of their products into the skin or genital organs of the same people or occasionally of others; (3) an analysis of the sequence of events, i.e., relation of primary to later lesions; and (4) the question of whether mercury was necessary for the cure of syphilis, and, if so, how the drug should be used.

2. BELL, Benjamin. A treatise on gonorrhoea virulenta and lues venerea. 2 vols. Edinburgh: James Watson & Co., 1793.

Bell was the first clearly to differentiate gonorrhea from syphilis. "The opinion which I have ventured to support, of the difference between the matter of Gonorrhoea and that of Lues Venerea, will no doubt be censured by many"

(1:x). "It is well known that Lues Venerea can certainly be cured by mercury only; and the opinion respecting the existence of a specific contagion of Gonorrhoea, arising from this obvious and marked difference in the method of cure, appears to be fixed and established by the following facts. The symptoms and consequences of Gonorrhoea are perfectly different from those which take place in Lues Venerea. Both diseases have appeared, at different periods, in the same countries; and in some instances have remained distinct and uncombined for a great length of time" (1:2). "That the symptoms of the two diseases are different is universally known. A particular detail of such as are peculiar to each, will be given in the ensuing chapters. At present . . . Gonorrhoea . . . is admitted to be, in almost every instance, a local affection and it very rarely contaminates the general habit of body: while Lues Venerea is a disease of the constitution arising from the absorption of venereal virus from any part of the surface of the body, but most frequently from the genitals" (1:3).

Although this was written shortly after Hunter's first edition, few seemed to pay attention until Bell's opinion was reaffirmed by Hernandez (Ref. 4) and, on the basis of inoculation experiments, by Ricord (Ref. 12). The story of this controversy is well told and documented in Rollet's book (Ref. 22, p. 70).

In Volume 2 Bell gives a clear and readable account of syphilis, far superior, we think, to Hunter's. "When Lues Venerea is not interrupted in its progress by the use of mercury or other remedies, the following is the order in which the symptoms commonly appear, viz. chancres; buboes; ulcers and inflammation of the throat; ulcers in the mouth, and nose; eruptions or blotches on the surface of the body; ulcers in different parts; nodes, and swellings in the periosteum, bones, and tendons; excrescences about the anus; swellings of the testes; loss of hair from all parts of the body; blindness, loss of hearing, and other anomalous symptoms" (2:12). Bell probably confused "soft chancre" with syphilitic primary lesion, since he speaks of it as often appearing almost immediately after contact.

Half of Volume 2 is devoted to therapy. "One of the most certain effects of mercury is, that it acts as a cure for venereal disease" (2:185). There is a long discussion of just how mercury should be used and at what time. "The preparations of mercury are very numeous: upwards of five hundred might be enumerated" (p. 215). The problems of the toxic effects of mercury are discussed, and the fact that inadequate therapy might be followed by severe later symptoms led to the usual confusion in its use. As late as 1839, one even finds a book entitled *Practical Observations Showing that Mercury Is the Sole Cause of What Are Termed Secondary Symptoms,* by P. J. Murphy (London: John Churchill, 1839).

3. BERTIN, M. Traité de la maladie vénérienne chez les enfants nouveau-nés, les femmes enceintes et les nourrices etc. Paris: Gabon, 1810.

Bertin's book was recognized by the Academy of Medicine of Paris as of great importance because his work was based on personal observation of a large number of patients. This seems to be the first systematic treatise on congenital syphilis. It begins with a critical chapter on previous work. Bertin then outlines the methods whereby congenital syphilis is acquired. He believes that there are three: infection of the fetus at the time of conception, infection during gestation, and infection during passage through the birth canal. The clinical descriptions of congenital syphilis are inadequate from the modern standpoint, but each manifestation is documented by a number of case reports. Chapter xvi on the treatment of pregnant women is of special interest. "In treating the pregnant woman, one often cures the mother and child at the same time . . . if the mother is not admitted too far along in her pregnancy." The backbone of therapy was mercury by inunction or by mouth; the details of administration are discussed at great length. This book, with all its inadequacies, is a definite landmark in the study of congenital syphilis.

4. HERNANDEZ, J. F. Essai analytique sur la non-identité des virus gonorrhoïque et syphilitique. Paris: J. J. Paschoud, 1812.

This book was "crowned" by the Société de Médecine of Bezançon for work on the following question: "To determine by experiment and conclusive observation whether there is an identity of the virus of gonorrhoea and of syphilis; whether one can give rise to the other; and whether the treatment suitable for one applies to the other." These questions Hernandez answers systematically in chapters headed as follows: "Gonorrheal Infection Always Has Gonorrhea for an Effect, and Never a Chancre"; "Gonorrheal Infection Always Gives Rise to Gonorrhea"; "Gonorrhea Occurs without Chancre or Syphilitic Ulcer in the Urethra"; "The Virus of Gonorrhea Does Not Produce Chancre"; etc. The argument is inexorably followed through the book of 350 pages.

5. SCHMIDT, Johann Adam. Vorlesungen über die syphilitische Krankheit und ihre Gestalten. Vienna: Bey Kupfter & Wimmer, 1812.

This little book may be mentioned as an example of the state of knowledge about syphilis in Germany in the early nineteenth century. The author leans heavily on Hunter. He recognizes the incubation period before the chancre and the second incubation period before generalized manifestations. However, he confuses "tripper" and chancre, again following Hunter. There are dark gropings to extract from clinical observations some rules about the progress of the disease and "clinical immunology." There is, of course, no allusion to cardiovascular or nervous system syphilis. Half the book deals with the "ins and outs" of mercurial therapy, which at the time was elevated almost to a discipline of its own.

6. CARMICHAEL, Richard. Observations on the symptoms and the specific distinctions of venereal diseases; interspersed with hints for the more effectual prosecution of the present enquiry into the uses and abuses of mercury in their treatment. London: Longman, Hurst, Rees, Orme & Brown, 1818.

This book is important, first, because Carmichael strongly supported Bell as regards the distinction of syphilis and gonorrhea (p. 5) and also because he was a prominent figure in the current dispute as to whether mercury was advisable at all in the therapy of syphilis. The toxic effects of heavy mercurial treatment were often obvious, and some thought that the late symptoms of syphilis might be due to mercury (Ref. 2). "With respect to the material point in the present investigation . . . my experience enables me decidedly to affirm, that if the papular eruption, or its accompanying symptoms do not return in a patient *who has not used mercury* after a lapse of a few weeks, he may be considered as perfectly well; but on the contrary, *if he has employed that medicine,* the disorder may return after an interval of many months" (p. 22).

This observation becomes clear in the light of modern immunological knowledge of syphilis.

7. BACOT, John. A treatise of syphilis, in which the history, symptoms and methods of treating every form of that disease are fully considered. London: Longman, Hurst, Rees, Orme & Brown, 1829.

This valuable book begins with a critical summary of contemporary views on the venereal disease problem. The opening chapters give a comprehensive review of the history of syphilis, and the third, of special importance, is entitled "Modern Doctrines of Syphilis Examined." Here contemporary views, beginning with Hunter, are carefully analyzed and compared. The upshot of all this is that there was great uncertainty in the classification of venereal disease and that syphilis and gonorrhea were usually considered due to the same poison. The primary lesion was recognized but was obviously often confused with non-syphilitic phagedenic and pyogenic ulcers. So, too, the bubo was accepted as a satellite of the primary lesion, but the frequency of suppuration indicates that other than syphilitic glandular swellings might be present. The later lesions were skin eruptions, sores in the throat, bone lesions, especially of the palate, nose, and cranium, and iritis. No hint of cardiovascular or nervous system syphilis is given; in fact, the author states: "There is no reason to believe that the viscera are ever subject to the attacks of syphilis" (p. 82).

The usual bitter discussions of just how mercury should be used and to what extent it is specific are critically gone into. "It is vain to attempt to form any rational theory as to the mode in which mercury operates in the cure of syphilis; to relate all the strange imaginations that ingenious men have thought fit to make public on this subject would only waste our time. . . . If mercury cannot be called a specific in the cure of this disease, it at least approaches as nearly to that character as any medicine can be said to do in any complaint whatsoever" (p. 256). Of special importance was the question which was raised at the time of whether mercurial treatment was of any value at all and whether patients did not do just as well with no "specific therapy." During the Peninsular Wars, English physicians learned that the Portuguese got good results with no special therapy, and Mr. Rose, an army surgeon, returning from Portugal (p. 49), "adopted the only rational plan—that of putting the question to the test of experiment, discarding all preconceived notions, and looking solely at the natural progress of the disease itself. The results of these experiments, made in the hospital of the Coldstream regiment of guards were given to the world in 1817" ("Observations on the treatment of syphilis, with an account of several cases of that disease, in which a cure was effected without the use of mercury, by Thomas Rose, Esq., A.M.," M.-Chir. Tr., **8**:349, 1817; also "Observations on the treatment of the venereal disease, without mercury," by G. J. Guthrie., Esq., M.-Chir. Tr., **8**:550, 1817; see also Carmichael [Ref. 6]). Mr. Rose found that he could cure all "genital ulcers" without mercury, and he as well as many other observers then followed the patients for the incidence of secondary manifestations. These were less common in those treated with mercury, but most of the patients seemed to remain well, although they really were not followed long enough to prove anything by modern standards. These early purposeful experiments are of interest in view of the modern observations of Bruusgaard and others.

The usual perplexities of syphilitic children being born of apparently healthy mothers are encountered.

The book is so full of important and interesting material that complete review would be unduly long; no serious student of syphilis, however, should fail to study it in detail.

8. HACKER, Heinrich August. Literatur der syphilitischen Krankheiten von Jahre 1794 bis mit 1829. Leipzig: J. F. Gleditsch, 1830.

This invaluable bibliography contains nearly a thousand references. After each there is a brief paragraph giving the substance of the material. The book seems essential for any intensive study of the period. (Hacker later continued his bibliography: *Neueste Literatur der syphilitischen Krankheiten* [vom 1830–1838] *nebst Nachträgen zu früheren Jahren* [Leipzig, 1839].)

9. [Dr. WALLACE]. Hydriodate of potash in syphilis, Lancet, 1:743, 1836.

Wallace refers to 124 cases of "secondary" syphilis which he treated with potassium iodide with great success. "When first admitted he kept the ward awake all night . . . by his roaring out with the agonizing pains in his bones . . . he says he now rests comfortably."

This is said to be the first claim for benefit from iodide in syphilis, although, according to Lancereux (Ref. 26), there were some preliminary attempts by Lugol and others. Lancereux (Ref. 26, p. 700) also summarizes the prompt confirmation of the value of iodides by numerous other workers. See also William Wallace, "Treatment of the venereal disease by the hydriodate of potash or iodide of potassium," Lancet, 2:5, 1836.

10. WALLACE, [William]. Clinical lectures and remarks delivered on diseases of the skin, venereal disease, and surgical cases at the skin infirmary, and at the Jervis Street Hospital, Dublin, Lancet, 2:534, 615, 1836–37.

To Wallace are attributed the first purposeful observation on inoculation of material from various syphilitic lesions into healthy people. A scrutiny of the experiments leaves one, however, somewhat dissatisfied. The cuticle was removed by friction from an area the size of a shilling, and material from the syphilitic lesion was applied on a piece of lint. Variable responses occurred, but in some of the cases, after initial infection and healing, later breakdown again took place. "The local specific effects which result from the inoculation with the matter of the primary pustule, and of the pustular bubo, commence almost immediately. . . . The local specific effects which result from inoculation with the matter of secondary pustule, as well as with the matter of the different varieties of exanthematic syphilis, do not occur for some weeks after inoculation." In Berkeley Hill's book (*Syphilis and Local Contagious Disorders* [London: James Walton, 1868]) is found (p. 62) a table of thirty more cases of experimental inoculation of syphilis which the writer found acceptable. How confused this branch of the subject became may be guessed from the book by Heinrich Auspitz (*Die Lehre vom syphilitischen Contagium* [Vienna: W. Braumüller,

1866]), in which all the inoculation experiments in the literature are quoted and analyzed.

11. COLLES, Abraham. Practical observations on the venereal disease and on the use of mercury. London: Sherwood, Gilbert & Piper, 1837.

While this work is known mainly for the observations on congenital syphilis (see below), which at the present time are usually formulated as Colles' law, it presents many other phases of syphilis of equal interest and importance. Colles' primary object was a defense of mercurial therapy—a procedure long in use but at the time in disfavor in some quarters—but incidentally there are taken up various clinical and immunological aspects of the disease. Colles gives credit to Hunter (Ref. 1) for first clearly recognizing the orderly temporal relationships of the manifestations of syphilis, but he realizes that only a beginning has been made in the study of the natural history of the disease. Difficulties still encountered today—namely, that patients do not stay under the observation of the same physician during their entire course and that the clinical picture is soon modified by treatment—are pointed out, and the need for group study is stressed. However, the descriptions of primary lesions both genital and extra-genital, the various eruptions, the lesions of the mucous membranes and of bone, and especially the congenital manifestations are outstanding. "Modern writers on the venereal disease have bestowed much pains in observing and arranging, in a nosological order, the varieties of cutaneous eruptions which form a part of secondary syphilis. . . . I should think the subject might still deserve a continuance of that zeal . . . were I convinced that each form of these eruptions constituted a distinct species in the disease. I fear, however, that any superstructure raised upon this hypothesis, will not stand the test of time, as I do not believe that these eruptions can be considered as characteristic of distinct and different forms of syphilis" (p. 175).

Colles devoted himself to a lesser extent than many of the contemporary writers to attempts to demonstrate the contagiousness and autoinoculability of syphilis. He reports observations which clearly show, however, that secondary, as well as primary, sores are infectious and further that people who apparently have been cured of the disease and who present no clinical manifestations may nonetheless infect their marital partners and produce syphilitic children. ". . . As long as such cases were confined to mechanics and persons in an humble rank of life, I could not bring myself to believe implicitly in their reports but when I found some occurring in the higher walks of life, and when the husbands proved to be men of acknowledged and known veracity, I could no longer withhold my assent [p. 263]. . . . But there are cases in which the foetus in utero has been infected under circumstances so strange, and so difficult to explain, that nothing short of actual observation could induce us to allow the fact. The circumstances to which I allude are these:—The father of the child has had primary symptoms six or eight months before his marriage; for these he has been treated by mercury . . . and his surgeon has . . . dismissed him as perfectly cured." Syphilitic children are born, although "both parents continue, all this time, to live in the enjoyment of perfect health; no trace of disease is to be discovered in either" (p. 266).

The discussion of therapy is of especial interest because of incidental observations on immunity, most of which have been substantiated a hundred years later by experimental methods. Colles recognized the futility of trying to eradicate the disease by local treatment of the chancre. "I have known a chancre completely cut out on the first or second day after its appearance; yet the occurrence of secondary symptoms was not prevented" (p. 77). He also noted that inguinal bubo was not a barrier to the spread of the disease (p. 98). Of particular importance are the observations on modification of the course of syphilis by treatment, and especially the recognition that inadequate therapy might be followed by violent symptoms. "Too frequently are the powers of the constitution so lowered by this indiscriminate use of mercury, that it is no longer able, as it were, to exhibit the eruptive fever, but it seems to be prematurely sunk into that weakened state which attends the latest stages of Syphilis" (p. 6). ". . . And yet at this day it must be admitted that many cases have resisted its use [mercury], –and further, that often where it did not cure, it considerably aggravated the sufferings of the patients" (p. 321). "When we inquire into the time at which the secondary disease has succeeded to the first inoculation, we shall find it to differ in different individuals, and we shall also find that it is influenced by the previous treatment of the primary symptoms. Where these have been treated on the nonmercurial plan we generally observe that the secondary symptoms are late in appearing, and that they are also preceded by less previous disturbance of the system; but when mercury has been used for a short time only, or has been discontinued as soon as the chancre had healed, we shall find in such cases that the secondary symptoms will appear more early" (p. 120).

Contemporary treatment, aside from mercury, consisted of sarsaparilla, acids, alkalies, sea bathing, and sea air. Colles rated all these as of dubious value and was a strong advocate of mercury. He stressed the importance of full doses by inunction, usually until salivation or diarrhea was attained, and also emphasized the need of rest and general upbuilding during or before the treatment in depleted patients. There is no indication, however, that he recognized the need for further therapy after clinical symptoms had disappeared.

Turning, now, to the question of infection in mother and child, it may be recalled that "Colles' law," as usually formulated, states that a non-syphilitic mother may nurse her obviously syphilitic child without acquiring any lesion. It has been implied that Colles believed the father to be syphilitic under these circumstances and that he had infected the child, whereas the mother was not syphilitic at all but had acquired some mysterious sort of protection against infection from her diseased offspring. There is not the slightest suggestion, however, from Colles' actual statement that he had any such idea at all; indeed, most of the mothers in the cases actually cited were known to have had syphilis, if they were not actually under treatment at the time. Colles simply wonders why the mother, despite the fact that she is syphilitic, gets no chancre of the nipple, whereas the non-syphilitic wet nurse does. "It is a curious fact that I have never witnessed nor ever heard of an instance in which a child deriving the infection of syphilis from its parents has caused an ulceration in the breast of its mother" (p. 285). And later: "One fact well deserving our attention is this: that a child born of a mother who is without any obvious venereal symptoms . . . will infect the most healthy nurse, whether she suckle it, or merely handle it or dress it; and yet this child is never known to infect its own mother, even though she suckle it while it has venereal ulcers of the lips and tongue" (p. 304).

Finally, one should mention Colles' important observations on non-venereal transmission of syphilis. "Those who are acquainted with the very scanty furniture of an Irish cabin, will readily comprehend with what facility and rapidity the disease can be propagated in this manner; but to others it may be necessary to say, that the family are quite satisfied with the possession of one single spoon, and the stock of cups and cans is nearly as scanty. Exposed thus to the double risk of contracting this infection when sleeping or taking nourishment, we cannot be surprised at finding three or four, in a family of six children, all at the same time infected."

12. RICORD, Ph. Traité pratique des maladies vénériennes ou recherches critiques et expérimentales sur l'inoculation appliquée à l'étude de ces maladies. Paris: De Just Rouvier & E. Le Bouvrier, 1838.

Ricord criticizes the "error, ignorance, or bad faith of most of those who have reported the innumerable observations on inoculation of syphilis which have been made since the time of Hunter" (1) to prove the existence of a specific cause of syphilitic diseases: the venereal virus; (2) to distinguish, among them, diseases apparently similar; (3) to establish the differences which exist between primary infection and general intoxication; (4) with reference to therapy, either to prove the efficacy of prophylactic agents or to modify by a new infection a first old and stubborn syphilitic infection or by adding the syphilis to a disease in itself incurable to cause it to yield to special treatment; (5) and, finally, to consider syphilis from the hygienic and medicolegal standpoints (p. 2).

The first part of the book (pp. 5–198) is devoted to a systematic critique of the contemporary literature on these subjects. Many writers denied the inoculability of chancre and, following Hunter, regarded syphilis and gonorrhea as the results of the same virus. Ricord's own ideas are summarized as follows (p. 40): "The Chancre during its period of ulceration is always re-inoculable [in the same individual]; the bubo of absorption is always re-inoculable; the pustule of inoculation can be reproduced indefinitely by its pus; the pus of non-ulcerative urethritis is non-inoculable." Ricord was obviously dealing mostly with non-syphilitic venereal lesions. The differentiation of gonorrhea and venereal ulcers was, however, Ricord's chief contribution, and it was documented by numerous detailed clinical experiments in the second part of the book (pp. 199–531). He also clearly recognized primary, secondary, and tertiary stages (p. 644). Ricord attempted animal inoculation; dogs, rabbits, guinea pigs, cats, and pigeons were used unsuccessfully, and he concluded that the disease was specific for man. He recognized extra-genital chancres and believed that the disease was not necessarily venereal.

The third portion of the book deals with therapy. Ricord evidently had a strong feeling for public health matters, and he devotes a section to prevention. He urges the thorough examination of prostitutes every three days, not superficially but with the speculum. Hygienic and cleansing methods are indorsed for both men and women.

As to actual therapy, Ricord first states that the "primary syphilitic ulcer can often heal without any treatment" (p. 547), but nonetheless he insists that "the chancre in its beginning imperiously demands abortive therapy. . . . I submit in support of this precept that there is no authentic observation of ulcers which, destroyed within the first five days after infection, have been followed by secondary symptoms" (p. 548). He discusses excision and cauterization (p. 549). Ricord was evidently confused about the whole question of mercury. People apparently got well without it and never again had recognizable trouble; others developed secondary syphilis in spite of early use of mercury. Many symptoms in syphilitics were at the time blamed on mercury. The result of all this led to a rather conservative recommendation, and "antiphlogistic" treatment was advised along with mercury as the initial step for secondary manifestations (p. 616). Mercury should be given in the "confirmed type of syphilis." "Mercury is certainly not a specific, but it is the most certain and most powerful remedy" (p. 623). He believed that salivation, emphasized as important by many writers, was not useful, since it interrupted the course of treatment (p. 627). Details of methods of using mercury are given (p. 623). Tertiary manifestations occur a long time after the primary infection and may be hard to recognize (p. 643). They include deep "tubercles" of the skin and mucous membranes, "osteocopic" pains, periostitis, and gummatous tumors. In summary, Ricord was a keen and honest observer, but he was overwhelmed by the complexity of the lesions he dealt with. His great contribution was the insistence that syphilis and gonorrhea were different diseases, although he was not really the first to make this claim (Refs. 2, 4).

He went a step further than most others in differentiating secondary and tertiary lesions. However, he had a very confused idea of the mechanism of secondary lesions. He thought the virus of syphilis went to local glands through the lymphatics and thence to the body generally through the blood, producing skin lesions, but he insisted that no secondary lesion was contagious or "inoculable" (pp. 162 ff., 477 ff.). He believed that tertiary lesions were also not contagious (p. 644). In fact, he thought that the farther the virus was from the primary lesion, the more it was modified and lost its specificity (p. 645). Finally, Ricord thought that the primary lesion began as a pustule without incubation period.

13. CAZENAVE, P. L. Alphée. Traité des syphilides ou maladies vénériennes de la peau. Paris: Labé, 1843.

The writer clearly defines the incubation period: "In summary, the time which elapses without any morbid local or general manifestation from the moment of the infecting contact until the results of infection appear; this time, I say, is a true incubation period, during which general poisoning takes place, and which is followed inevitably by the specific phenomena of syphilis" (p. 147).

14. ROMBERG, Moritz Heinrich. Lehrbuch der Nervenkrankheiten des Menschen. Berlin: A. Drucker, 1846. (English translation of the 2d ed. by Edwin H. Sieveking, M.D. [2 vols.; London: New Sydenham Society, 1853].)

Chapter 49 contains Romberg's classical description of tabes, in which he emphasizes diminution of muscle sense, numbness of feet, swaying on standing with eyes closed (Romberg's sign), insecurity of gait, especially in the dark, urinary difficulty, girdle sensation, lightning pains in legs, etc. There is a fairly good gross anatomical description of the cord lesion. Romberg emphasizes the slow, inexorable course.

D. Argyll Robertson ("On an interesting series of eye symptoms in a case of spinal disease with remarks on the action of belladonna on the iris, etc.," Edinburgh M.J., **14**:696, 1869) described a frank case of tabes (without naming it as such) in which he noted: "I found both pupils contracted to little more than pin-points. . . . I could not observe any contraction of either pupil under the influence of light but on accommodating the eyes for a near object, both pupils contracted." There follows a scholarly discussion of the pathological physiology of the condition. Argyll Robertson pursued the subject further in another paper ("Four cases of spinal myosis; with remarks on the action of light on the pupil," *ibid.*, **15**:487, 1869).

At about the same time J.-M. Charcot ("Sur quelques arthropathies qui paraissent dépendre d'une lésion du cerveau ou de la moelle épinière," Arch. de physiol. norm. et path., **1**:161, 1869; **2**:129, 1869) gave a beautiful description of tabetic arthropathy in a number of people with frank locomotor ataxia. Interestingly enough, he stated that syphilis, among other things, had nothing to do with this trouble.

W. Erb ("Ueber Sehnenreflexe bei Gesunden und bei Rückenmarkskranken," Arch. f. Psychiat., **5**:792, 1875) and C. Westphal ("Ueber einige Bewegungs-Erscheinungen an gelähmten Gliedern," Arch. f. Psychiat., **5**:803, 1875) simultaneously described the knee jerk and its aberrations in disease. Westphal (p. 819) stated: "The knee-jerk is constantly absent in patients with the frank clinical picture of tabes dorsalis" (Westphal's sign).

A good review of the history and general features of tabes is to be found in "Syphilis of the Nervous System," in D'Arcy Power and J. Keogh Murphy, *A System of Syphilis* (London: Henry Frowde, 1910), **4**:319, chap. x.

15. RICORD, Philippe. Traité complet des maladies vénériennes: clinique iconographique d. l'hôpital des vénériens. Paris: J. Rouvier, 1851.

This beautiful atlas with numerous large color plates of venereal lesions is justly famous. We do not find a single picture, however, which seems typical of an uncomplicated primary syphilitic chancre. Since many lesions are described as appearing a very few days after contact, one wonders whether most of them were not "soft" non-syphilitic ulcers, which seemed extremely prevalent at the time.

16. DIDAY, P. Traité de la syphilis des nouveau-nés et des enfants à la mamelle. Paris: V. Masson, 1854.

This thoughtful, well-reasoned book is a landmark in the history of congenital syphilis. Every conceivable question is taken up and discussed, if not answered. There are excellent descriptions of the clinical features and comprehensive discussions of prognosis and therapy. Diday inclines to the view that the mother of a syphilitic child is herself usually, but not always, syphilitic and that early treatment, first, of the syphilitic mother and then of the child itself with mercury and iodides is in order. An apparently healthy child born of syphilitic parents should be treated.

17. BASSEREAU, P. I. A. Léon. Traité des affections de la peau symptomatiques de la syphilis. Paris: J.-B. Baillière, 1852.

This is one of the first books devoted to a careful analysis of syphilitic skin lesions, but Bassereau was also noteworthy for discovering, by the method of confrontation, the duality of soft and hard (syphilitic) ulcers. "If one confronts all the subjects who have had chancre followed by constitutional syphilis with the subjects who communicated the contagion to them or with those to whom they have transmitted it, one finds that all these subjects, without exception, have had chancres followed by constitutional 'accidents.' Never among them has the chancre limited itself to a purely local action. . . . If, on the contrary, one confronts the subjects who have chancres which have not led to any symptoms of general syphilis with the people who have infected them or whom they have infected, one finds that these, without exception, have chancres which have limited their action to the point of first contamination" (p. 197).

18. CLERC, F.-F. Considérations nouvelles sur le chancre infectant et le chancroid, Union méd., **9**:509, 1855.

Clerc found that if one inoculated people with tertiary or with primary syphilis with material from a syphilitic chancre, one would fail to produce a lesion in the vast majority of cases, whereas if one used material from chancroidal ulcer, one could succeed in practically every case. Thus he definitely differentiated the two diseases.

19. FOURNIER, Alfred. Leçons sur le chancre professées par le Docteur Ricord. Paris: A. Delahaye, 1858.

The writers were struck by the differences between the effects of various primary sores—some were followed by constitutional manifestations, whereas others never were. This suggested that these were different diseases of different causation. They distinguished soft chancre (chancroid) and syphilitic chancre. "The inoculability of the pus secreted is the sign absolute" of the non-syphilitic sore. The indurated slow ulcer, on the other hand, is syphilitic and is followed by constitutional phenomena—secondary and tertiary. They did not, however, regard the secondary lesions as contagious, although they could be transmitted by heredity (p. 134). Their great conclusion was that the two diseases were the results of entirely different viruses. There is an immense amount of detailed discussion and numerous case reports which do not always clarify the issue, because of difficulty in making a definite differential diagnosis of hard and soft chancres and because of uncertainty about the significance of later lesions.

As to therapy, the writers believed that all chancres were at first a *local* disease before a constitutional "spread" took place. In this early stage they advised (during the first four days) cauterization. This doctrine was based on the fact that they had never seen constitutional symptoms following chancre (see Ref. 11) destroyed before the fifth day (p. 207). If the chancre was seen later, then the treatment was that of the constitutional diathesis—mercury. An indurated primary lesion always called for mercurial therapy. They did not favor pushing mercury to the point of salivation—"The curative action of mercury is generally suspended when the marked symptoms appertaining to this drug are produced" (p. 214). "Six months of mercury followed by three of iodide, such is the medication, gentlemen, which gives the most sustained cures in the enormous majority of cases" (p. 221). The book concludes (p. 223) with a precise summary of the difference between soft and hard chancres, including emphasis on re-inoculability of soft chancre and absence of inoculability of hard syphilitic sores.

20. VIRCHOW, R. Ueber die Natur der constitutionell syphilitischen Affec-
tionen. Berlin: G. Reimer, 1859; also in Virchows Arch. f. path. Anat.,
15:217, 1858.

This book must be mentioned in the bibliography because of the universal recognition it met with for years and because of its author's great name. Actually, one
finds little of exceptional value in it. The remarks are based on gross morbid
examinations, and it is questionable whether all the lesions were syphilitic.
Under the heading of "Syphilis of the Heart," for example, one finds a description of a lesion designated as aneurysm (not of the aorta, but of the heart)
which is clearly due to infarction of the muscle and not to syphilis. The book is,
however, a milestone in the study of syphilis from the standpoint of emphasizing how widespread the lesions may be.

21. GROS, Léon. Des affections nerveuses syphilitiques. Paris: A. Delahaye,
1861.

This book of nearly five hundred pages deals comprehensively with syphilis of
the central nervous system. The conclusions which are formulated at the end of
the book in 89 statements are based on reports of 269 cases from the literature ,
which are given in abstract. Many of these were undoubtedly syphilitic but
probably not all; the writer based the diagnosis on history and other manifestations of syphilis and the response to specific therapy. The cases are divided into
"affections without appreciable lesion," "convulsive neuroses," "paralytic neuroses," "asthma," and "troubles of intelligence." Some of the latter patients may
have been paretics.

Some of the conclusions are (I) nervous affections can develop at any period
of constitutional syphilis; (II) these affections may involve . . . sensibility, motility, or intelligence; (III) they may stimulate all sorts of other (non-syphilitic)
affections.

It is obvious that, with the means at hand, correct diagnosis could not be
made in every case, but the problem of central nervous system syphilis is clearly defined.

22. ROLLET, J. Recherches cliniques et expérimentales sur la syphilis, le
chancre simple et la blennorrhagie. Paris: J.-B. Baillière et fils, 1861.

Rollet's book is much more modern in tone than any of the preceding monographs. He regards the following points as established: Gonorrhea is a specific
disease (p. 8). Simple ulcer of the genitals is repeatedly reinoculable in the
same individual; it is not syphilitic (p. 10). Syphilitic chancre is never reinoculable in the patient who has it, although it is transmissible to others (p. 14).
Syphilitic chancre cannot be inoculated in anyone who has syphilis, no matter in
what stage (p. 12). Several chancres may develop at the same time but never
successively (p. 12). True syphilitic chancre may occur in the mouth, on the
nipple, or elsewhere (pp. 13, 242, 248). Of the three "venereal" diseases—
gonorrhea, chancroid, and syphilis—the last, because of its multiple situation
and its variable mode of transmission, is certainly the least venereal of the three
(p. 14). The incubation period of syphilis varies from 9 to 42 days, average 25
(p. 15). The syphilitic chancre rests on a hard base, which feels like a lump of
rubber or cartilage (p. 16). Secondary syphilis always follows a true syphilitic
chancre, never any other venereal disease (p. 18). The incubation period of

secondary syphilis varied from 12 to 128 days, average 52 days after the first appearance of the chancre (p. 18). Cauterization of a syphilitic chancre does not prevent secondary lesions (p. 23). Various venereal diseases may coexist accidentally (p. 31). The virus of syphilis is not only in the chancre but spreads through the blood to every tissue in the body; the contagious principle of gonorrhea and chancroid is confined to the local lesion (p. 46). Secondary syphilis is definitely contagious (p. 237), as everyone before Hunter believed. Secondary syphilis transmitted to another person produces a *primary chancre* (p. 310).

There is a comprehensive chapter on methods of contagion between nurses and infants and a discussion of medicolegal questions.

Rollet believed that chancre could be produced by inoculation of syphilitic blood (p. 344) and that syphilis could be transmitted by smallpox vaccination (p. 351). As to treatment, he thought that cauterization of a chancre, even when it first appeared, would not prevent secondaries (p. 516). The chapter on mercurial therapy is of special interest. Rollet attributed the use of mercury to Arabic physicians of the sixteenth century. He analyzed the literature on the non-mercurial treatment of syphilis (p. 567), a method which spread like an epidemic all over Europe between 1817 and 1840. Rollet also discussed "syphilization," a term which was currently in vogue (p. 576). He credited Wallace (Ref. 9) with introducing potassium iodide as a therapeutic agent (p. 580). As to the actual use of mercury and iodides, Rollet individualized. Some cases were easy to cure; some difficult (p. 584). He did not believe in pushing the drugs until severe symptoms (salivation) appeared. He thought it important to support the general condition with cod-liver oil and other measures.

The book is especially valuable for its historical summaries.

23. HUTCHINSON, Jonathan. Clinical lecture on heredito-syphilitic struma: and on the teeth as a means of diagnosis, Brit. M.J., **1**:515, 1861.

In connection with a child aged eleven with an ulcer on the tibia, Hutchinson makes the diagnosis of congenital syphilis on the basis of the teeth. "Remember that it is the permanent set only which show any peculiarities." "The central upper incisors are the test-teeth. . . . You may neglect all the others. . . . The teeth are short and narrow. Instead of becoming wider as they descend from the gum, they are narrower at their free edges than at their crowns, their angles having been as it were rounded off. In the center of their free edges is a deep vertical notch."

24. WILKS, Samuel. On the syphilitic affections of internal organs, Guy's Hosp. Rep., **9**:3d ser., 1, 1863.

This much quoted paper is mainly of negative value, since many of the cases— of disease of the liver, for example—are doubtful and since lesions of the aorta are not mentioned except the case of a prostitute with "abdominal aneurysm." There was no concept at the time, however, of syphilitic arteritis in the modern sense.

25. LANGHANS, Th. Beiträge zur normalen und pathologische Anatomie der Arterien, Virchows Arch. f. path. Anat., **36**:187, 1866.

In this intensive description of the histology of arteries by the use of modern histological methods we find what we believe may be an account of syphilitic aortitis, although the author does not associate the process with syphilis (p. 220).

26. LANCEREUX, E. Traité historique et pratique de la syphilis. Paris: J.-B. Baillière et fils, 1866.

This volume of some eight hundred pages is a landmark in the literature of the subject. It is especially noteworthy because of the detailed references to the literature. Lancereux clearly distinguished the stages of syphilis. There is an elaborate discussion of the incubation period, which he regarded as the first stage of the disease. He found it to be 24 days, more or less. The period of "local eruption" is the time from the first appearance of the chancre until the first general manifestations. The various clinical types of chancre and associated adenopathy are described in detail. The secondary lesions appear 40–50 days after the appearance of the chancre, and they affect especially the superficial layers of skin and mucous membranes and usually leave no scars. They "consist of a chronic hyperemia accompanied sometimes by a serous or purulent exudate but never by the production of the connective tissue masses called gummata" (p. 117). There are, however, "superficial" invasions of organs such as muscles, bones, eyes, and joints, with headaches and fever. These lesions are all discussed in minute detail, as are those of the tertiary stage, the feature of which is gummata, destructive in contrast to secondaries. In the several hundred pages on gummata, one looks with interest at the sections on cardiovascular and central nervous system syphilis. Gummatous myocarditis is described, but nothing which can be reconciled with syphilitic aortitis. So, too, with the nervous system there is no mention of tabes or paresis, although there are described many inflammatory lesions the exact nature of which is not clear.

There is an interesting discussion on the outcome of syphilis and the question of whether it is ever cured (p. 525). There is a long section on congenital syphilis, and a clear distinction is drawn between "hâtive" and "tardive" types.

As to the actual cause of syphilis, Lancereux felt that it was something in the clear secretion of the chancre, that pus was less contagious. The virus in the secondary stage was in the blood and was then communicable. Contagion might be any sort of contact not necessarily venereal. As to therapy, mercury was in use by medieval Arabian physicians as a treatment for skin disease and was used for syphilis first about 1497. The work on iodides is reviewed (p. 700). Other components of antisyphilitic therapy are discussed.

It is seen, then, that syphilis had come a long way from Hunter. It was now definitely recognized as a specific contagious disease. The various stages and incubation periods were clearly defined. The lesions were classified, although treatment did not progress further for fifty years. It was recognized that primary and secondary lesions would communicate the disease to others but were not re-inoculable on the same person. Central nervous system syphilis was diagnosed, and there were the beginnings of realization that tabes dorsalis was syphilitic.

27. PARROT, J. Sur une pseudo-paralysie causée par une altération du système osseux chez les nouveau-nés atteints de syphilis héréditaire, Arch. de physiol. norm. et path., 4:319, 1872.

"This work is a contribution to the pathology of the newborn and very young infants. We propose to make known a state which simulates paralysis and of which the cause is a lesion of bone due to congenital syphilis." This important condition is described at length, and there is a beautiful colored plate. The original article is reprinted in Parrot's book (*La Syphilis héréditaire et la rachitis* [Paris: G. Masson, 1886]), together with various other articles on congenital syphilis.

28. HUEBNER, O. Die luetische Erkrankung der Hirnarterien. Leipzig: F. C. W. Vogel, 1874.

Of the various monographs of the time on the subject of cerebrovascular syphilis, this one is outstanding. It begins with a comprehensive historical summary and then gives abstracts of all the reported fatal cases with autopsy, including three of the author's own. Next comes a section on the anatomy of syphilitic arterial disease. One looks in vain for a description, in the case of the aorta, of anything resembling syphilitic mesoartitis; the lesions are described as mainly in the intima. Associated gummata are also described, and the lesions are differentiated from ordinary atheroma. The physiology of occlusion of syphilitic arteries is then gone into, and finally the symptomatology, the striking features of which are headache followed by a hemiplegia or other cerebral accident. The occurrence at an early age is emphasized. Under therapy, mercurial inunctions and large doses of potash are advised. This is a comprehensive summary of the subject, from which any remarks about tabes or paresis are conspicuously absent.

29. FOURNIER, Alfred. De l'ataxie locomotrice d'origine syphilitique, Ann. de dermat. et syph., 7:187, 1875–76.

On the basis of past history of syphilis in patients with locomotor ataxia, Fournier felt sure that syphilis was a cause of the disease in certain cases. He did not, however, look on tabes as an absolutely specific disease, and he was not clear whether syphilis acted as a "predisposing factor" or whether the lesion was actually syphilitic.

Fournier was not, however, the first to notice the association of syphilis with tabes. As long ago as 1859, [G.] Duchenne ("De l'ataxie locomotrice progressive," Arch. gén. de méd., 1: [5th ser., Vol. 13], 417, 1859) said: "Several subjects have undergone a constitutional syphilitic infection," and he clearly raised the question of whether syphilis was not the cause of tabes.

Actually, the relation of syphilis to tabes was being discussed on all sides at about this time on the basis of the frequency of a positive history. Thus E. Vulpian (*Maladies du système nerveux: maladies de la moelle* [Paris: O. Doin, 1879], p. 245) states: "There are really few patients with locomotor ataxia who have not had, several years before the first symptoms of this affection, an infecting chancre and secondary syphilitic accidents." W. Gowers ("Syphilitic neurosis," Brit. M.J., 1:303, 1879) felt the same and pointed out, as had others, the futility of conventional antisyphilitic therapy. W. Erb ("Zur Pathologie der Tabes dorsalis," Deutsches Arch. f. klin. Med., 24:1, 1879) has a comprehensive article with review of both sides of the literature and a thorough discussion of the relation of syphilis to tabes. He was puzzled by the fact that "syphilitic" and "non-syphilitic" instances of tabes could not be differentiated, and he did not grasp the point that in the latter group the syphilitic infection was unrecognized. Gowers later ("Syphilis and locomotor ataxy," Lancet, **1**:94, 1881) wrote again on the subject with even greater confidence. He was inclined to think that the cases following obvious syphilis and those in which there was no history were nonetheless all the same—probably syphilitic. No case of tabes was met with earlier than seven years after the syphilitic infection. Erb ("Ueber die aetiologische Bedeutung der Syphilis für die Tabes dorsalis," Tr. Internat. Med. Congr., London, **2**:32, 1881) summarized the whole subject once more at the International Medical Congress. It is interesting that the eight eminent men who discussed Erb's paper, almost without exception, were skeptical as to the close relation of syphilis to tabes.

Finally, Fournier in a book of nearly four hundred pages (*De l'ataxie loco-notrice d'origine syphilitique* [Paris: G. Masson, 1882]) analyzed every aspect of the subject and concluded: "Major conclusion: Treat early syphilis long and energetically to prevent the serious manifestations of a later stage, to prevent especially one of its most 'redoubtable' manifestations, tabes" (p. 396).

As late as 1910, however, tabes and general paresis are spoken of as "para-syphilis"—"the term given by Fournier to those diseases of which syphilis is essentially the cause but which are not directly the result of the syphilitic virus" (see F. W. Mott, "Syphilis of the nervous system," in D'Arcy Power and J. Keogh Murphy, *A System of Syphilis* [London: Henry Frowde, 1910], **4**:186).

30. WELCH, Francis H. On aortic aneurism in the army and conditions associated with it, M.-Chir. Tr., **41**:59, 1876.

In a comprehensive article Lewis A. Connor ("Development of knowledge concerning role of syphilis in cardio-vascular disease," J.A.M.A., **102**:575, 1934) reviews the early work on the relation of syphilis to cardiovascular disease. There are a few hints as to a relation of aneurysm to syphilis, but credit for describing a specific aortic lesion associated with aneurysm and for insisting on the syphilitic nature of the process clearly goes to Welch. Working with autopsy material from the army, he described two forms of aortic disease, one a general form with which people do not die and the second a specific form associated with aneurysm, leading to early death.

"The deduction arrived at may be placed in the form of two propositions. . That the aneurismal tumors are associated with, and preceded by, a diseased condition of the contiguous layers of the intimal and middle coats of the vessel—a tissue growth terminating in degeneration—which, by impairing the elasticity and contractility of the walls, allows of their expansion and dilatation under the tension of normal arterial blood pressure. . . . 2. . . . that the structural growth is in the major number of instances associated with syphilis and in minor degree with rheumatism and alcoholism as causations: hence it follows that . . . the means for the prevention of the aneurismal tumour must be essentially directed toward elimination of the special exciting agencies."

31. FOURNIER, A. De la pseudo-paralysie général d'origine syphilitique, Progr. méd., Paris, **5**:761, 1877.

It is impossible to assign to any one man the definite recognition of paresis and tabes as syphilitic. In this lecture by Fournier he points out that many have raised the question without proof. His own point is that "true general paresis" is not syphilitic but that a distinguishable, although similar, "pseudo-general paresis" *is* syphilitic. The evidence rests largely on one case, which is reported in detail; Fournier thought that he could make definite clinical and anatomical distinctions. He gave his method of treating central nervous system syphilis with alternating courses of mercury and iodide in another article ("Traitement de la syphilis du cerveau [leçon clinique]," Bull. gén. de thérap., **96**:1, 1879) and he reviewed still elsewhere (*La Syphilis du cerveau* [Paris: G. Masson 1879], p. 333) the whole question of paresis and syphilis. There is also a large casuistic literature made up of individual case reports which are very hard to interpret, as, for example, that of F. Esmarch and W. Jessen, "Syphilis und Geistesstörung," Allg. Ztschr. f. Psychiat., **14**:20, 1857.

32. BERGER, Oscar, and ROSENBACH, Ottomar. Ueber die Coincidenz von Tabes dorsalis und Insufficienz der Aortenkleppen, Ber. klin Wchnschr., **16**:402, 1879.

In a brief communication the authors point out the association of tabes dorsalis and aortic insufficiency; nothing is said about syphilis. They never observed any other valve lesions with tabes, and the patients were in the late thirties to fifties. So, too, Babinski ("Des troubles pupillaires dans les aneurismes de l'aorte," Bull. et mém. Soc. Méd. d. hôp. de Paris, **18**:1121, 1901) reports two women with aneurysm, aortic insufficiency, irregular fixed pupils, and diminution of knee jerks. In the discussion Marie stated: "We know that aortic lesion are common in tabetics."

33. CORNIL, V. Leçons sur la syphilis. Paris: J.-B. Baillière et fils, 1879

Although this is a general treatise on syphilis, the original part of the work, as the author says in the Preface, is the histological study of the lesions. Beginning with chancre, he goes through every sort of syphilitic lesion with gross and microscopic descriptions and with a series of plates. One looks in vain for any description of aortic syphilis or tabes.

34. FOURNIER, Alfred. Syphilis et mariage. Paris: G. Masson, 1880.

Social consciousness in regard to the dangers of syphilis developed early among European physicians (Ref. 12), but it remained for the great French syphilographer Fournier to embody all the doctrines about syphilis and marriage in this book of nearly three hundred pages. He saw clearly that the longer the time which had elapsed since infection (3–4 years as a minimum) and the more thorough treatment given, the safer it was for a person to marry. The disaster which could ensue for the patient, partner, and children are so clearly brought out that for the next generation they were common knowledge and the dire results of syphilis and marriage were a not uncommon topic in the lay literature (cf. A. Conan Doyle, "The third generation," in *Round the Red Lamp* [London: Methuen & Co., 1894]).

35. FOURNIER, Alfred. La Syphilis héréditaire tardive. Paris: G. Masson 1886.

In this monumental book, Fournier sets the stage for all time with reference to late hereditary syphilis, that is, syphilis occurring at least 3 years—often much later—after birth. Fournier groups the findings as follows: (I) constitution habitus, facies; (II) retardation, imperfections, arrest of physical development

(III) cranial and nasal deformities; (IV) bony deformities of the trunk and limbs; (V) cicatricial stigmata of the skin and mucous membranes; (VI) ocular lesions; (VII) lesions and troubles of the auditory organ; (VIII) dental malformations; (IX) testicular lesions. Whether all the lesions here described are really syphilitic or not one cannot say, but Fournier delineated and defined the subject.

36. BALZER, M. F. Expériences sur la toxicité du bismuth, Compt. rend. Soc. de biol., **1**:9th ser., 537, 1889.

Balzer, as a preliminary to its use in syphilis, reported toxicity studies with subcutaneous injections of various bismuth preparations (citrate of bismuth and ammonia) in dogs. He believed that it would be necessary to follow the excretion of bismuth in the urine and warned against sudden signs of intoxication, especially stomatitis.

Bismuth was not actually used in the treatment of syphilis until 1921 (R. Sazerac and C. Levaditi, "Traitement de la syphilis par le bismuth," Compt. rend. Acad. d. sc., **173**:338, 1921).

37. ERB, W. I. Ueber syphilitische Spinal-Paralyse, Neurol. Centralbl., **11**:161, 1892.

In this article Erb describes the syphilitic spastic spinal paralysis which bears his name today. A perusal of the article, however, leaves one unconvinced as to the exact nature of the disorder. He points out as differential features from "spastic spinal paralysis" that there are very active tendon reflexes but relatively little spasticity, that the bladder is often affected, and that there is some disturbance of sensibility. This all seems vague, however, and his main point is the history of syphilis in every case. A study of Erb's former article on spastic paralysis ("Ueber die spastische Spinal-Paralyse," Virchows Arch. f. path. Anat., **70**:241, 293, 1877) shows no convincing difference between the cases described there and those in the later paper, although in connection with the first he states definitely that syphilis played no part. Just what Erb was really dealing with it is now impossible to say, especially as many cases of the "syphilitic" syndrome do not have positive serology and no spirochetes are found at autopsy.

38. JARISCH, Adolph. Therapeutische Versuche bei Syphilis, Wien. med. Wchnschr., **45**:722, 1895.

"The present findings are based on an observation which has surely been made by many syphilologists but which to my knowledge has heretofore not been appraised; I mean the observation of a reaction whereby in the first days of mercurial inunctions for syphilitic roseola there is an exaggeration of the clinical manifestations." He thought that this reaction was connected with the more rapid involution of the lesions. Jarisch goes on to speculate about the mechanism of the reaction and to report some cases. K. Herxheimer and Krause a few years later ("Ueber eine bei syphilitischen vorkommende Quecksilberreaction," Deutsche med. Wchnschr., **28**:895, 1902) describe the phenomenon more in detail. They point out the conversion of a syphilitic roseola to an erythema multiforme-like eruption with rapid clearing and also describe constitutional reactions—fever, glandular enlargement, and headache. They emphasize the diagnostic value of the reaction and speculate about its nature.

39. DÖHLE. Ueber Aortenerkrankung bei Syphilitischen und deren Bezie hung zur Aneurismenbildung, Deutsches Arch. f. klin. Med., **55**:190 1895.

The clear definition of a specific syphilitic lesion of the aorta as a prerequisite of aneurysm clearly belongs to Döhle. His paper begins with a statement that the occurrence of aortic disease in syphilitics is a well-known fact but that the lesions found at autopsy have not been regarded as specifically syphilitic. He quotes the case first described by himself ("Ein Fall von eigentümlicher Aorten erkrankung bei einem Syphilitischen," Inaug. disst., Kiel, 1885) and now add two more. There are several illustrations showing well the corrugated, barklike appearance of the ascending aorta. The histology is described in detail and the following conclusions are drawn: "(1) Syphilitic inflammation of the aorta i macroscopically recognized by starlike, scarred puckerings of the inner surface In addition, there may be a thickening of the intima (chronic endarteritis). The depressions are caused by diffuse and gummatous inflammation in the media and the adventitia, which lead to formation of scarred connective tissue. (2 The inflammatory changes in the media make possible the formation of aneu rysms."

The work of Döhle and others from the Pathological Institute at Kiel on th subject was not generally accepted, and finally Arnold Heller, the chief of th laboratory, was stimulated to speak himself on the subject at a meeting of th German Pathological Society ("Ueber die syphilitische Aortitis und ihre Bedeu tung für die Entstehung von Aneurismen," Verhandl. d. deutsch. path. Ge sellsch., Berlin, **1**:346, 1899) in support of his pupils. Heller's remarks are fol lowed by a paper on similar changes in the aorta in general paresis (Straul "Ueber die Veränderungen der Aortenwand bei progressiver Paralyse," Ver handl. d. deutsch. path. Gesellsch., Berlin, **1**:351, 1899).

The remarks of Heller and Straub were followed by a general discussion, i which the speakers were thoroughly disbelieved and castigated by most of th outstanding pathologists of Germany—Ponfick, Hansemann, Baumgarten, Zieg ler, Orth, Chiari, and Babes. Not a voice was raised in agreement.

However, by 1903, at the meeting of the same society, H. Chiari ("Ueber di syphilitischen Aortenerkrankungen," Verhandl. d. deutsch. path. Gesellsch Berlin, **6**:137, 1903), in a review of the subject, somewhat grudgingly admitte that the Heller school was correct. "If we take the results of this material, w come to the conclusion that this form of aortitis can be caused by syphilis. C. Benda ("Aneurisme und Syphilis," Verhandl. d. deutsch. path. Gesellsch Berlin, **6**:164, 1903) in a long "Korreferat" came to the same conclusion, whic has never since been in doubt. Good summaries of the whole subject are thos of Fahr ("Zur Frage der Aortitis syphilitica," Virchows Arch. f. path. Anat **177**:508, 1904) and of W. T. Longcope ("Syphilitic aortitis: its diagnosis an treatment," Arch. Int. Med., **2**:15, 1913).

40. NEUMANN, Isidor. Syphilis. Vienna: Alfred Hölder, 1899.

This large volume, from the Nothnagel system, gives an authoritative revie of knowledge of syphilis at the turn of the century. It is of interest how litt progress had been made in fifty years. That had to wait for the discovery of th spirochete and the Wassermann test.

Neumann points out that, as yet, no causal organism had been identified and that it had not been possible to transmit the disease to an animal. Primary, secondary, and tertiary stages are described, and a fourth stage consisting of cachexia, amyloid, marasmus, phthisis pulmonalis, etc., but not of aneurysm or tabes. Many of the lesions described are obviously not syphilitic, such as "syphilis of the stomach," "syphilitic" arteritis, "gummata" of lung, etc.

The question of syphilis of blood vessels is reviewed, and the relation to aneurysm is described, but no specific syphilitic mesaortitis is recognized. Aneurysm of the ascending and thoracic aorta is regarded as syphilitic in about 50 per cent of the cases, with rheumatism, alcoholism, and other things as causes of the rest. A tabetic form of syphilis is recognized, but, just as Fournier thought twenty-five years previously, syphilitic tabes is just one form of a non-specific disease.

41. FOURNIER, Alfred. Prophylaxie de la syphilis. Paris: J. Rueff, 1903.

By this time the Academy of Medicine, justly aroused by the "terrible morbidity" of syphilis, appointed a commission to study the question of prevention. This volume of over five hundred pages is the result. Modes of contagion and of prevention are gone into in the greatest detail, and there are chapters on instructing the youth on the venereal peril, control of prostitution, etc.

42. METCHNIKOFF, É., and ROUX, É. Études expérimentales sur la syphilis, Ann. Inst. Pasteur, **17**:809, 1903.

The authors review the meager literature on claims of transmission of syphilis to animals. The elaborate article of E. Klebs (Arch. f. exper. Path. u. Pharmakol., **10**:161, 1879) is referred to, although a reading of it leaves one unconvinced that Klebs transmitted anything. One must remember that, before the discovery of the spirochete, one had only clinical appearances to go by. Metchnikoff and Roux describe the case of one monkey in which they produced, by inoculation of material from a human chancre, a lesion of the vulva which was pronounced a chancre by Fournier and other experts. It seems to us probable that the writers did transmit syphilis to this animal. They conclude, among other things, that infection causes a prompt immunity, since a second inoculation 5 days after the first failed to produce a lesion. Others soon got to work on the same problem, including A. Neisser ("Meine Versuche zur Uebertragung der Syphilis auf Affen," Deutsche med. Wchnschr., **3**:1309, 1904), who was able to produce lesions in chimpanzees. Neisser and others, at this time when serum therapy was so much in vogue, hoped to obtain a therapeutic serum—a hope which, of course, failed. Neisser (*Die experimentelle Syphilisforschung* [Berlin: Julius Springer, 1906]) gives an authoritative review of the whole subject. The early work was soon amplified after the discovery of the spirochete (Ref. 44) and the serodiagnostic tests, so that immense activity took place among investigators of experimental syphilis.

43. RAVAUT, Paul. Étude cytologique du liquide céphalo-rachidien chez les syphilitiques, Ann. de dermat. et syph., **4**:4th ser., 1, 1903.

At the meeting of February 14, 1902, of the Medical Society of the Hospitals of Paris, F. Widal ("Cytologie du liquide céphalo-rachidien des syphilitiques," Bull. et mém. Soc. méd. d. hôp. de Paris, **19**:3d ser., 118, 1902) stated that various observers in his clinic had found a lymphocytosis in the spinal fluid of tabetics, paretics, and syphilitics with severe headaches. It remained for Ravaut, however, to study systematically the fluid of syphilitics, to confirm and amplify the above observations, and to point out that lymphocytosis in patients with no overt clinical findings might indicate an asymptomatic central nervous system syphilis and might be the precursor of an overt outbreak of neurosyphilis.

44. SCHAUDINN, Fritz, and HOFFMANN, Erich. Vorläufiger Bericht über das Vorkommen von Spirochaeten in syphilitischen Krankheitsprodukten und bei Papillomen, Arb. a. d. k. Gsndhtsamte, Berlin, **22**:527, 1905.

A commission was appointed to search for living organisms in syphilitic lesions. A happy choice of Schaudinn, a highly qualified bacteriologist, was made, with Hoffmann, a fine clinician and syphilologist, to work with him. In smears both from the surface and from the depths of primary untreated lesions, as well as from glands, spirochetes were demonstrated; those characteristic of syphilis were very "pale," slender, and showed many small angulations. Schaudinn named them *Spirochaeta pallida* in contrast to other coarser forms found on the genitalia —*S. refringens*. The organisms were first seen in fresh preparations but stained fairly readily with aniline dyes. The spirochetes were *not* found in papillomata.

The story of the events leading up to the discovery of the spirochete is vividly told by Metchnikoff ("The Microbiology of Syphilis," in D'Arcy Power and J. Keogh Murphy, *A System of Syphilis* [London: Henry Frowde, 1908], **1**:43).

SYPHILIS: PART II. FROM THE DISCOVERY OF THE TREPONEME (1905)

Arsenical chemotherapy	Refs. 6, 7, 10, 12, 26
Bismuth therapy	Ref. 18
Cerebrospinal fluid	Ref. 15
Course of untreated syphilis	Refs. 25, 36
Cultivation of spirochete	Ref. 8
Fever therapy	Ref. 13
General	Ref. 31
Immunity in syphilis	Refs. 16, 17, 19, 20, 22, 24, 35
Neurosyphilis	Refs. 9, 11, 13, 14
Penicillin in syphilis	Refs. 30, 32, 35, 37
Public health and syphilis	Ref. 27
Serodiagnostic tests	Refs. 4, 5
Spirochetes in lesions	Refs. 2, 3, 14
Transfusion syphilis	Ref. 28
Transmission to animals	Refs. 1, 3, 16
Treatment	Refs. 6, 7, 10, 11, 12, 13, 18, 21, 23, 26, 29, 30, 32, 36, 37
Treponema immobilization test	Ref. 33
Tryparsamide	Ref. 21

With the great discoveries made in syphilis during the first decade of the century—transmission to animals, identification of the spirochete, the Wassermann test, and Salvarsan—the entire aspect of the disease underwent a change. To clinical intuition and experience were added precise methods of study and rational control of therapy. The literature pursued several lines; to the old clinical studies were added those of experimental syphilis in animals, isolation of the spirochete from human lesions, serodiagnostic tests, immunity in syphilis, and arsenical chemotherapy. Finally, a new era dawned with the discovery that penicillin was treponemacidal, and at long last there seems to be a real prospect of eliminating syphilis as a significant disease. We have tried to refer to the important key articles along these various lines. For a comprehensive bibliography, however, reference is made to the annual reviews of syphilis in the Archives of Internal Medicine, of which the nineteenth has recently appeared (H. Beerman, I. L. Scharnberg, L. Nicholas, and L. Katzenstein, "Syphilis: review of recent literature," Arch. Int. Med., **95**:256, 1955).

1. METCHNIKOFF, É., and ROUX, É. Études expérimentales sur la syphilis, quatrième mémoire, Ann. Inst. Pasteur, **19**:673, 1905.

This is the writers' fourth and final report on transmission of syphilis to monkeys. "In 22 chimpanzees inoculated with virus of diverse origin we have not a single failure to report; all presented definite syphilitic manifestations. The incubation period varied from 15 to 49 days; on the average, it has been 30 days." Meanwhile, Schaudinn had discovered the spirochete, and the writers succeeded in demonstrating the parasite in most of their monkeys with experimental syphilis.

A comprehensive discussion of monkey syphilis is that of Albert Neisser (*Beiträge zur Pathologie und Therapie der Syphilis* [Berlin: Julius Springer, 1921]).

2. SCHAUDINN, Fritz, and HOFFMANN, Erich. Ueber Spirochaetenbefunde im Lymphdrüsensaft Syphilitischer, Deutsche med. Wchnschr., **31**:711, 1905.

Schaudinn's first announcement of the discovery of the spirochete (Fritz Schaudinn and Erich Hoffmann, "Vorläufiger Bericht über das Vorkommen von Spirochaeten in syphilitischen Krankheitsprodukten und bei Papillomen," Arb. a. d. k. Gsndhtsamte, **22**:527, 1905) was followed by innumerable reports of search for the organism in various syphilitic tissues. Schaudinn and Hoffmann again stress the difference between a dark, readily stainable and a pale, difficultly demonstrable spirochete—the latter presumably the cause of syphilis. In this paper they report finding spirochetes in eight instances of enlarged inguinal glands in cases of early syphilis. In another paper the same writers ("Ueber Spirochaete pallida bei Syphilis und die Unterschiede dieser Form gagenüber anderen Arten dieser Gattung," Berl. klin. Wchnschr., **42**:673, 1905) discuss further (with an illustration) the difference between *Spirochaeta pallida* and

S. refringens. By this time they had demonstrated *pallida* not only in primary lesions but in the spleen (puncture, autopsy) and liver of a child dead of congenital lues. All these findings were soon confirmed by B. Kiolemenoglou and Felix v. Cube ("Spirochaete pallida [Schaudinn] und Syphilis," München. med. Wchnschr., **52**:1275, 1905), although it is of interest that in the same journal a few weeks later there appeared an article (J. Siegel, "Neue Untersuchungen über die Aetiologie der Syphilis," p. 1321) in which a flagellate was found in primary lesions and lymph nodes and was put forward as the cause—*Cytorryctes luis.* Meanwhile, as acute an observer as C. Fraenkel ("Ueber das Vorkommen der Spirochaete pallida bei Syphilis," München. med. Wchnschr., **52**:1129, 1905) lent his support to Schaudinn and Hoffmann. Rille ("Ueber Spirochaeten-befunde bei Syphilis," **52**:1377, 1905) reviews the accumulating literature and adds confirmatory observations of his own, as does H. Ploeger ("'Die Spirochäten bei Syphilis," München. med. Wchnschr., **52**:1381, 1905). C. T. Noeggerath and R. Staehelin ("Zum Nachweis der Spirochaete pallida im Blut Syphilitischer," München. med. Wchnschr., **52**:1481, 1905) claimed to have demonstrated S. *pallida* in centrifuged blood of a patient with secondary syphilis. In view of later proof of transfusion syphilis (Ref. 28), this may have been correct. Ploeger ("Ueber Spirochäten bei Syphilis," München. med. Wchnschr., **52**:2394, 1905) describes the demonstration of S. *pallida* in skin lesions of syphilis.

From this time on, there were innumerable reports on the findings of spirochetes in various organs.[1] A full bibliography of the earlier literature is found in S. Sobernheim, "Syphilisspirochäte," in W. Kolle and A. von Wassermann, *Handbuch der pathogenen Mikroorganismen* (2d ed.; Jena: Gustav Fischer, 1913), **7**:812, whereas more recent work is summarized in a later edition of the same treatise (3d ed.; 1930), **7**: Part I, 31).

A vast amount of work has been done on the morphology and life-cycle of the spirochete (see, for example, E. V. De Lamater, R. H. Wiggall, and M. Hannes, "Studies in the life cycle of spirochetes," J. Exper. Med., **92**:239, 247, 1950).

3. BERTARELLI, E. Ueber die Transmission der Syphilis auf das Kaninchen, Centralbl. f. Bakt., **41**:320, 1906.

Following the transmission of syphilis to monkeys by Metchnikoff and Roux and the discovery of the parasite, innumerable attempts were promptly made to transmit syphilis to all sorts of animals. Claims and denials were abundant. Bertarelli was the first definitely to transmit syphilis to rabbits, a feat of great importance, since rabbit infection has been used extensively in studying problems of immunity in syphilis. Bertarelli ground up material obtained from the center of a "syphiloma" and rubbed it into the lightly scarified cornea of a rabbit. Inoculation was made on January 31; on February 10 a slowly progressive lesion of the cornea appeared. On February 13 the eye was removed and showed "myriads" of spirochetes which had the characteristics of *pallida*.

---

[1] Much of this work was done with the dark-field technique. See E. Friedberger and H. Reiter, "Die allgemeinen Methoden der Bakteriologie," in Kolle and Wassermann, *Handbuch der pathogenen Mikroorganismen* (2d ed.; Jena: Gustav Fischer, 1912), **1**:305; and Hideyo Noguchi, *Laboratory Diagnosis of Syphilis* (New York: Paul B. Hoeber, 1923), pp. 251 ff.

4. WASSERMANN, A., NEISSER, A., and BRUCK, C. Eine serodiagnostische Reaction bei Syphilis, Deutsche med. Wchnschr., **32**:745, 1906.

Jules Bordet and Octave Gengou ("Sur l'existence de substances sensibilatrices dans la plupart des sérums antimicrobiens," Ann. Inst. Pasteur, **15**:289, 1901) clearly defined the complement-fixation reaction, using bacterial suspensions as antigens. There is no suggestion that they thought of using complement fixation in syphilis, perhaps because no antigenic suspension of the causal agent was available. Actually, they thought at first of complement fixation as a therapeutic method. A. Wassermann and C. Bruck ("Experimentelle Studien über die Wirkung von Tuberkelbacillen-Preparaten auf den tuberculöserkrankten Organismus," Deutsche med. Wchnschr., **32**:449, 1906) began their complement-fixation work, giving full credit to Bordet, by attempting to demonstrate tuberculin in tuberculous organs. A little later, in the present paper, they applied the method to syphilis. They used, as antigen, materials presumably rich in spirochetes, namely, extracts of organs (liver) of children or fetuses with congenital syphilis, the placentas of mothers with secondary syphilis, extracts of primary lesions or of condylomata lata or of organs or bone marrow of syphilitic monkeys. "The practical importance of these findings is obvious. We are in the position to determine, on the one hand, whether a human serum or an immune serum contains specific antibodies against the 'incitor' of syphilis, and we can determine whether a particular organ harbors syphilitic substances. . . . But it would be of the greatest diagnostic and therapeutic importance if one could regularly demonstrate syphilitic material or antibodies in the circulating blood of syphilitics." This hope was soon realized by the authors with A. Schmidt ("Weitere Mitteilungen über den Nachweis spezifischluetischen Substanzen durch Komplementverankerung," Ztschr f. Hyg. u. Infektionskr., **55**:451, 1906), although they got only 49 positive reactions among 257 "certain" syphilitics. At about the same time, Wassermann with F. Plaut ("Ueber das Vorhandensein syphilitischer Antistoffe in der Cerebrospinalflüssigkeit von Paralytikern," Deutsche med. Wchnschr., **32**:1769, 1906) employed the complement-fixation reaction on the spinal fluid of 41 paretics, with positive result in 32. Fluids from controls were negative. Ladislaus Detre ("Ueber den Nachweis von spezifischen Syphilis-Antisubstanzen und deren Antigenen bei Luetikern," Wien. klin. Wchnschr., **19**:619, 1906) published a few weeks after Wassermann and confirmed his findings. Wassermann at first clearly regarded the test as immunologically specific; in this he was to be disappointed (Ref. 5).

5. LANDSTEINER, K., MÜLLER, R., and PÖTZL, O. Zur Frage der Komplementbindungsreaktion bei Syphilis, Wien. klin. Wchnschr., **20**:1565, 1907.

Wassermann had thought of his reaction as a test for a specific syphilitic substance, but this view was soon to be questioned. Leonor Michaelis ("Die Wassermannsche Syphilisreaktion," Berl. klin. Wchnschr., **44**:1103, 1907) found that normal liver, as well as syphilitic liver, gave positive complement fixation with serum of syphilitics, although the test was usually weaker with the former. Landsteiner and his associates found that alcohol extracts of normal organs, such as guinea-pig heart, served as an adequate antigen for fixing complement with sera of syphilitics. This led to an era of lively speculation on the nature of the antibody in syphilitics, with the conclusion that the reaction was at any rate *clinically* specific. Landsteiner also opened the question of false positive tests (Ref. 34) by finding that the sera of animals infected with *Trypanosoma gambiense* fixed complement. C. Levaditi and T. Yamanouchi ("Le Séro-diagnostic de la syphilis," Compt. rend. Soc. de biol., **63**:740, 1907) also found that alcoholic extracts of liver, as well as suspensions of sodium taurocholate and glycocholate, served as antigens, and they concluded that a positive test was not brought about by specific antibodies in the usual sense but that this fact did not lessen the practical value of the procedure. Carl H. Browning, John Cruickshank, and Ivy M'Kenzie ("Constituents concerned in the Wassermann reaction, with special reference to lecithin and cholestrin," J. Path. & Bact., **14**:484, 1909–10) showed that the addition of cholesterol to Wassermann antigens had a fortifying effect which made them more sensitive.

From this point on, an immense literature on the Wassermann reaction and on other serodiagnostic tests (flocculation) for syphilis has developed which is summarized in a number of books, of which these are important: H. Noguchi, *Serum Diagnosis of Syphilis and the Butyric Acid Test for Syphilis* (Philadelphia and London: J. B. Lippincott Co., 1910); R. L. Kahn, *The Kahn Test: A Practical Guide* (Baltimore: Williams & Wilkins Co., 1928); Harry Eagle, *The Laboratory Diagnosis of Syphilis* (St. Louis: C. V. Mosby Co., 1937); Josephine Henrichson, *Modern Serologic Tests for Syphilis* (Ven. Dis. Inform. Suppl., No. 14 [1941]). Eagle's book is especially useful because of its full theoretical discussion of the reactions and its bibliography.

6. EHRLICH, Paul, and HATA, S. Die experimentelle Chemotherapie der Spirillosen. Berlin: Julius Springer, 1910.

The name of Paul Ehrlich is inextricably bound up with the great modern era of chemotherapy of syphilis. In this book Ehrlich tells the story of the development of knowledge—how he had always thought that the key to chemotherapy was the finding of drugs which had a special affinity for chemoreceptors of the parasite rather than for those of the host; how he became interested in arsenic compounds, the first of which were ineffective or toxic; and, finally, how in animal experiment, first, with trypanosomes and spirilloses and finally with syphilis, dioxydiaminoarsenobenzol—the 606th compound developed and tested—yielded definite beneficial results. Ehrlich distributed small amounts of the material to various clinicians and clinics for trial; at the end of the book (p. 161) is a list of papers which had appeared up to October, 1910, on the practical use of the compound. At first, it was given in one dose of 0.3 gm. intramuscularly. Lesions melted away, and treponemes were seen to disappear rapidly from chancres. Later it was found to be more effective intravenously. In order to keep the record straight, we must correct the statement often made that Ehrlich claimed to extirpate the infection completely with one injection. He definitely did not, but he aimed in that direction. "I advise, therefore, that at present we should not use up our strength in looking for new compounds but should concentrate on improving the method of use, careful increase of dosage, antisepsis, repetition of the treatment, and the finding of ancillary measures to increase the potency of the drug so that we can always come closer to the principle of the therapia magna sterilisans."

Preceding Ehrlich's discussion is the report of Hata's experiments with 606 in syphilis of the eye and scrotum of rabbits which were completed before the clinical trials. These experiments are conclusive—and we quote part of one:

"X-28-11   Whole cornea opaque, great development of blood vessels. Weight 3,050 gm. Injection of 0.01 gm. Salvarsan per kilo of animal intravenously.

4-11   Clouding materially less; pupil well seen, two small vessels.

10-11   Cornea entirely clear.

30-12   Entirely clear."

A somewhat romanticized, but vivid, account of Ehrlich and his work is that of Martha Marquart (*Paul Ehrlich* [New York: Henry Schuman, 1951]).

7. NEISSER, A., and KUZNITZKY, E. Ueber die Bedeutung des Ehr-lich'schen Arsenobenzols für die Syphilisbehandlung, Berl. klin. Wchnschr., **7**:1485, 1910.

It is difficult now to appreciate the furor which arose over the prospect of curing syphilis quickly and surely with "606." The German *Wochenschrifte* and a little later journals in other countries were soon filled with brief reports on the results of therapy. Neisser's paper is one of the most important early ones. "In brief, there is no doubt about the eminent action of Arsenobenzol on syphilitic processes. The most outstanding effects of mercury and iodides are surpassed." Neisser was reserved about occasional failures and thought that perhaps the dose had been too small or that the syphilitic process was in an avascular area. "We must advise every syphilitic . . . to seek the new medicine." Meanwhile, L. Michaelis ("Ueber die Anwendung des Ehrlich-Hata'schen Syphilismittels in neutraler Suspension," Berl. klin. Wchnschr., **7**:1401, 1910), the physical chemist, had devised a method for neutralizing the drug so as to render the intramuscular injection painless. Later in the year Michaelis ("110 Fälle von Syphilis, behandelt nach Ehrlich-Hata," *ibid.*, p. 1695) reported extensive clinical trials. Interestingly enough, Michaelis avoided the intravenous route because he believed the drug to be insoluble at the practically neutral reaction of the blood. In regard to the permanence of effect, Michaelis now had three cases which relapsed. Meanwhile, C. Fraenkel and C. Grouven ("Erfahrungen mit dem Ehrlichen Mittel '606,'" München. med. Wchnschr., **57**:1771, 1910) had a death after intravenous injection, to which Ehrlich himself ("Bietet die intra-venöse Injection von '606' besondere Gefahren?" München. med. Wchnschr., **57**:1826, 1910) replied, suggesting that it was not the intravenous route but a hypersensitivity on the part of the patient which was responsible.

Apparently, there were no reports on the actual use of "606" in America at this time because, at the suggestion of the editor, Samuel J. Meltzer ("Dioxydi-aminoarsenobenzol or '606,' Ehrlich's newest remedy for syphilis," New York M.J., **92**:371, 1910) wrote a general article on the subject: "No matter what qualifications the present statements may have to undergo, this great fact is well assured—a single injection of a synthetically made compound is capable of completely sterilizing the diseased animal body in a very short time. . . . If reports continue to hold what they promise, syphilis could be eradicated from civilized humanity in two or three decades. What a hope, what a dream!" The first British paper was that of James McIntosh and Paul Fildes ("The theory and practice of the treatment of syphilis with Ehrlich's new specific '606,'" Lancet, **2**:1684, 1910). They emphasized the rapid disappearance of spirochetes, and they concluded: "The importance of the observation lies in the probability that cases of syphilis can be rendered practically non-infective in a day or two. If this be true Ehrlich will have swept away the scourge of 2000 years. . . ."

These papers bring out the optimistic temper of the times as regards a quick cure for syphilis.

In the Zeitschrift für Chemotherapie for 1912 (Vol. **1**, Part II, Referate) are to be found comprehensive reviews of the American, French, Russian, British, and Italian literature to date on Salvarsan therapy.

8. NOGUCHI, Hideyo. Cultivation of pathogenic Treponema pallidum, J.A.M.A., **57**:102, 1911.

Noguchi criticized the previous attempts of others to grow pathogenic treponemes in the test tube. He described a method of his own whereby he claimed to have accomplished such growth, and with two of these culture strains he produced typical syphilis in the rabbit by intra-testicular inoculation. This note was promptly amplified by a longer article ("A method for the pure cultivation of pathogenic Treponema pallidum [Spirochaeta pallida]," J. Exper. Med., **14**:99, 1911) with beautiful and convincing plates. Noguchi later ("A method for cultivating Treponema pallidum in fluid media," J. Exper. Med., **16**:211, 1912) described a method for obtaining pure cultures in fluid media, which, however, was not suitable for growth of spirochetes when "they are admixed with contaminating bacteria."

The spirochete is, however, very difficult to grow, and methods have never been adapted for routine practical work. Spirochetes are usually preserved in syphilitic rabbits, from whose lymph nodes they can be readily obtained. W. Kolle and H. Schlossberger ("Die Persistenz der Syphilisspirochäte in Mäusen während langer Zeiträume," Deutsche med. Wchnschr., **54**:129, 1928) found that mice which had been inoculated 1½–16½ months previously still harbored spirochetes in lymph glands, spleen, blood, and brain, as demonstrated by inoculation of other animals with these materials.

9. ELLIS, Arthur W. M. Secondary syphilitic meningitis, J.A.M.A., **53**:1263, 1912.

It was Paul Ravaut ("Les Réactions nerveuses tardives, observé chez certains syphilitiques traités par le Salvarsan," Presse méd., **20**:181, 1912) who raised the vexed question of whether secondary syphilitic meningitis, often with cranial nerve involvement (*neurorécidives*), was not promoted by Salvarsan. Ellis reviewed the entire literature on early syphilitic meningitis, reported 6 cases of his own carefully studied, and concluded: "The contention that Salvarsan predisposes in any way to development of disease of the nervous system has not yet been established," and he advised further intensive therapy. A critical discussion of the subject is to be found in Max Nonne, *Syphilis und Nervensystem* (3d ed.; Berlin: S. Karger, 1915), pp. 796 ff.

10. GENNERICH, [W.]. Die Resultate der Abortivbehandlung der Syphilis mit Salvarsan bezw. kombinierter Behandlung, Ztschr. f. Chemotherap., **1**, Part II, 69, 1912.

The initial hope of the complete cure of syphilis by one dose of "606" (Ref. 6) was soon to be disappointed. By 1912 Gennerich, for example, was giving courses of eight injections at 4-day intervals, in some cases followed by a few weeks of iodides and then more Salvarsan, without extirpating the infection. It was soon found that the best chance of a quick cure was in seronegative primary patients but that in late cases such a result was not to be expected. Homer F. Swift and A. W. M. Ellis ("The intensive treatment of syphilis," J.A.M.A., **59**:1251, 1912) emphasized the same point and advised combination therapy of Salvarsan *and* mercury, by the use of which "the relative number of 'cures' has materially increased." "A reliable rule to follow is four or five intravenous injections of from 0.3 to 0.5 gms. . . . with or followed by a course of insoluble mercury intramuscularly. After the mercury Salvarsan should again be repeated."

The position is summarized editorially in the Journal of the American Medical Association ("The present position of salvarsan in syphilis," **59**:1295, 1912).

11. SWIFT, Homer F., and ELLIS, Arthur W. M. The direct treatment of syphilitic diseases of the central nervous system, New York M.J., **96**:53, 1912.

Swift and Ellis, working at the Rockefeller Institute and stimulated by Flexner's direct application of serum to the subarachnoid space in meningitis, conceived the idea of a similar procedure in neurosyphilis. In preliminary experiments with monkeys (Arthur W. M. Ellis and Homer F. Swift, "The effect of intraspinous injections of Salvarsan and Neosalvarsan in monkeys," J. Exper. Med., **18**:428, 1913) they found that even small amounts of Salvarsan were excessively irritating, as had others in the literature, which is reviewed. They resorted, therefore, to intravenous injection of Salvarsan, following which the patient was bled and 30 cc. of serum diluted with saline were injected intraspinally. They found that the serum of patients treated with Salvarsan had an increased spirocheticidal action (Swift and Ellis, "A study of the spirocheticidal action of the serum of patients treated with Salvarsan," *ibid.*, p. 435), and they also believed that their patients were improved. This was the so-called "Swift-Ellis" treatment which had a tremendous vogue and was a precursor of many variations of intraspinal therapy, all now obsolete.

12. SCHREIBER, E. Ueber Neosalvarsan, München. med. Wchnschr., **59**:905, 1912.

By this time, various shortcomings of the old Salvarsan were recognized. Ehrlich had now brought out his 914th compound, which was commercially designated as "Neosalvarsan." The principal claim for the new drug was that it was less toxic than the old. Schreiber concludes that the advantages of Neosalvarsan are "(1) its easy solubility at absolutely neutral reaction; (2) it is better tolerated and can therefore be given in larger doses; (3) its effect is at least as good as that of the old Salvarsan; (4) the material lends itself better to intramuscular injection."

13. JAUREGG, Wagner v. Über Behandlung der progressiven Paralyse mit Bacterientoxinen, Wien. klin. Wchnschr., **25**:61, 1912.

Fever therapy in syphilis, especially in late neurosyphilis, has been such an important factor in treatment that it deserves mention in the bibliography. Wagner v. Jauregg as early as 1888 ("Ueber die Einwirkung fieberhafter Erkrankungen auf Psychosen," Jahrb. f. Psychiat., **7**:94, 1887) noted that, in the case reports on so-called recovery from progressive paralysis, suppurative lesions were prominent in the history and probably were a factor in healing. The present report deals first with treatment of paresis by a mercury-iodide "cure" together with old tuberculin. In many cases there was a satisfactory remission. These results were confirmed by A. Pilcz ("Beiträge zur Lehre von progressiven Paralysen," Jahrb. f. Psychiat., **25**:97, 1904). However, at that time it was thought that suppuration was the important factor. Wagner v. Jauregg gradually laid more emphasis on fever than on suppuration and got good results by treatment with injections of staphylococcus vaccine in increasing doses, with which he stressed both suppuration and fever.

Pursuing these ideas further, it occurred to Wagner v. Jauregg to induce malaria purposefully as a source of fever ("Die Behandlung der progressiven Paralyse and Tabes," Wien med. Wchnschr., **71**:1106, 1210, 1921). The use of malaria became a huge discipline in itself, all phases of which are authoritatively reviewed by J. E. Moore (Ref. 29, p. 374).

Many other methods of inducing fever had their proponents and their vogue: foreign protein therapy (M. M. Kunde, George W. Hall, and F. J. Gerty, "General paralysis: the effect of nonspecific protein therapy on the blood and spinal fluid," J.A.M.A., **89**:1304, 1927 [literature]); physical measures such as diathermy (Clarence A. Neymann and S. L. Osborne, "The treatment of dementia paralytica with hyperpyrexia produced by diathermy," J.A.M.A., **96**:7, 1931); hot baths (Jay F. Schamberg and Hsien-Wu Tseng, "Experiments on the therapeutic value of hot baths with special reference to the treatment of syphilis and some physiologic observations," Am. J. Syph., **2**:337, 1927; H. G. Mehrtens and P. S. Pouppirt, "Hyperpyrexia produced by baths," Arch. Neurol. & Psychiat., **22**:700, 1929; Jay F. Schamberg and A. M. Rule, "Studies of the therapeutic effect of fever in experimental rabbit syphilis," Arch. Dermat. & Syph., **14**:243, 1928).

14. NOGUCHI, Hideyo, and MOORE, J. W. A demonstration of Treponema pallidum in the brain in cases of general paralysis, J. Exper. Med., **17**:232, 1913.

Although by this time no one doubted the essentially syphilitic nature of paresis on the basis of history, blood Wassermann test, and spinal fluid changes, it remained for Noguchi clearly to demonstrate the presence of treponemes. In the brains of twelve of seventy cases of "undoubted" general paralysis, treponemes were demonstrated by a modification of the Levaditi silver method and are pictured in the article. Noguchi soon amplified his findings ("Additional studies on the presence of Spirochaeta pallida in general paralysis and tabes dorsalis," J. Cutan. Dis., **31**:543, 1913) and reported the demonstration of treponemes in about one-fourth of two hundred cases of paresis and tabes. Noguchi's work was promptly confirmed by M. M. G. Marinesco and M. J. Minea ("Présence du Treponema pallidum dans un cas de méningite syphilitique associée à la paralysie générale et dans la paralysie générale," Bull. Acad.

de méd., Paris, **69**:235, 1913) but in only one of twenty-four cases of general paralysis.

15. ELLIS, Arthur W. M., and SWIFT, Homer F. The cerebrospinal fluid in syphilis, J. Exper. Med., **18**:162, 1913.

Swift and Ellis, after reviewing the literature, report systematic studies of the spinal fluid in 113 cases of syphilis of all types. Pressure, cell counts, globulin, and Wassermann were all done. Of special importance was the finding in several interesting cases of secondary syphilis of slightly increased cell count and globulin. They conclude with these now well-recognized recommendations: "The diagnosis of any syphilitic condition of the central nervous system is not complete without an examination of the spinal fluid, and in the treatment of these conditions repeated examinations of the fluid furnish the best guide to therapy. A negative Wassermann reaction in the blood is no evidence that the nervous system is not affected and every patient with increased cells, globulin, or a positive Wassermann reaction in the spinal fluid needs active antisyphilitic treatment. No patient who has been infected with syphilis can conscientiously be discharged as cured until the spinal fluid has been examined and found normal, even though he remains free from signs and symptoms and has a persistently negative Wassermann reaction in the blood." Authoritative discussions of the spinal fluid in neurosyphilis with a review of the literature are those of Max Nonne in *Syphilis und Nervensystem* (2d ed.; Berlin: S. Karger, 1909), pp. 607 ff.; and of Bernhard Dattner, *The Management of Neurosyphilis* (New York: Grune & Stratton, 1944).

16. BROWN, Wade H., and PEARCE, Louise. Experimental syphilis in the rabbit. I. Primary infection of the testicle, J. Exper. Med., **20**:475, 1920.

Parodi (Umberto Parodi, "Ueber die Uebertragung der Syphilis auf den Hoden des Kaninchens," Centralbl. f. Bakt., **44**:428, 1907) inserted a small bit of a syphilitic papule under the tunica vaginalis of the testis of a rabbit on May 11. On June 9 the animal was killed, and a round-cell infiltration and numerous spirochetes were found under the microscope. This method of testicular inoculation has become a standard one in studying syphilitic infection and immunity. The extensive early work on the rabbit is fully summarized by P. Uhlenhuth and P. Mulzer ("Beiträge zur experimentellen Pathologie und Therapie der Syphilis mit besonderer Berücksichtigung der Impf-Syphilis der Kaninchen," Arb. a. d. k. Gsndhtsamte, **44**:307, 1913) in a classical monograph which includes numerous experiments of their own on every phase of experimental syphilis in rabbits and monkeys.

Brown and Pearce made elaborate studies of experimental rabbit syphilis, but this paper is especially important as the first of a long series on experimental infection and immunity, many of which are to be found in the Journal of Experimental Medicine for 1920–22.

17. BROWN, Wade H., and PEARCE, Louise. A note on the dissemination of Spirochaeta pallida from the primary focus of infection, Arch. Dermat. & Syph., N.S., **2**:470, 1920.

The question of how quickly the virus of syphilis spreads after inoculation is an old one which vexed the early therapists in deciding whether excision of chancre prevented general dissemination of the disease. Brown and Pearce studied this point by excising at various intervals after scrotal inoculation the inguinal lymph nodes of rabbits and testing for spirochetes by injecting the excised nodes into other animals. In a series of twenty-three animals tested at intervals of from 2 to 5 days after inoculation, it was uniformly found that spirochetes were present in the regional lymph nodes, an indication of definite spread of the organisms even before the appearance of the primary lesion. Furthermore, as early as 1 week after injection, blood withdrawn from the heart contained enough spirochetes to produce syphilis when injected into the testes of other rabbits. Finally, despite excision of the scrotum and testes 48 hours after inoculation, all the animals developed syphilitic lesions. "It would appear, therefore, that for practical purposes, there is no appreciable time during which a syphilitic lesion can be regarded as confined to the focus of entry."

18. SAZERAC, R., and LEVADITI, C. Traitement de la syphilis par le bismuth, Compt. rend. Acad. d. sc., **173**:338, 1921.

The writers, after having experimented with sodium and potassium bismuth tartrate in experimental syphilis of rabbits ("Action du bismuth sur la syphilis et sur la trypanosomiase du Nagana," *ibid.*, **172**:1391, 1921), report five cases of syphilis treated with this preparation by intramuscular injection. There was rapid (2–3 days) disappearance of spirochetes and healing of the lesions in about a week. Gummata also healed and became scarred. Bismuth immediately became popular, and innumerable preparations, soluble and insoluble, were thrown on the market. The subject is summarized in Moore (Ref. 29, p. 134) with bibliography. Perhaps the most important American work on the subject was that of Hanzlik and his associates (P. J. Hanzlik and H. G. Mehrtens, "Comparative excretion and absorption of different bismuth products," Arch. Dermat. & Syph., **22**:861, 1930; P. J. Hanzlik, H. G. Mehrtens, C. Gurchot, and C. C. Johnson, "Iodobismitol," J.A.M.A., **98**:537, 1932; see also W. F. von Oettingen, "The absorption, distribution and excretion of bismuth," Physiol. Rev., **10**:222, 1930).

After having a tremendous vogue and having practically replaced mercury in the treatment of syphilis, bismuth is now, in the penicillin era, little used.

19. KOLLE, W. Experimentelle Untersuchungen über die "Abortivheilung" der Syphilis, Deutsche med. Wchnschr., **48**:1301, 1922.

The problems of immunity in syphilis which perplexed the older clinicians are not yet fully solved today. It is impossible to refer in detail to the huge literature; all we can do is to pick out certain key pieces of work.

Kolle set himself the problem of finding out whether it was possible to achieve a biological cure of experimental syphilis in rabbits, and, if so, how long after infection one might begin treatment and still produce a cure. He had found that infected untreated rabbits could not be "reinfected" after 90 days, whereas the earlier reinoculation was practiced, the more frequently reinfection was possible. He concluded that a syphilitic man is, like the rabbit, proof against reinfection because he still harbors spirochetes. But if some balance is upset, syphilitics may suffer years later from the renewed activity of their own organisms (gummata). Kolle assumed reinfection to be evidence of biological cure with extirpation of all spirochetes. He treated rabbits with experimental syphilis with three large doses of Salvarsan 3, 15, 20, 25, 30, 45, 60, 90, and 120 days after infection. After an interval of over 90 days had elapsed in each animal, he applied the test of complete cure by attempting to reinoculate. The results were striking. Up to 45 days after the original infection it was usually possible to sterilize the animal, but after 45 days only an occasional rabbit developed chancre on later reinoculation. These experiments had great repercussions on human therapeutic practice. It is of interest that the older clinicians had observed that partial treatment might be worse than none and that they often advised that the "secondaries" be allowed to appear before therapy was started with mercury. In other words, if complete sterilization is possible by early intensive treatment, it should be conscientiously practiced, but partial subcurative therapy in the early stages might simply interfere with development of the patient's own immunity and therefore be worse than none. These experiments on the importance of early intensive therapy influenced clinical practice for years to come.

Meanwhile, Wade H. Brown and Louise Pearce ("Superinfection in experimental syphilis following the administration of subcurative doses of Arsphenamine or Neoarsphenamine," J. Exper. Med., **33**:553, 1921) came to somewhat different conclusions: "namely, that subcurative treatment of animals with marked primary lesions of the testicles altered their resistance to such an extent as to render them susceptible to a second cutaneous infection without having effected a cure of the original infection."

Along this line Brown and Pearce ("Experimental production of clinical types of syphilis in the rabbit," Arch. Dermat. & Syph., **3**:254, 1921) found that, by modifying the course of the infection, as, for example, by castration or subcurative therapy, whereas the syphilitic lesions as a rule remained localized in the controls, almost all the "treated" animals showed generalized lesions involving eye, mucous membranes, periosteum, bone, and skin. The conclusion seemed justified that the ordinary progress of syphilis is bound up with immunity reactions which are capable of modification by spontaneous or by externally regulated influences. Such considerations as these are obviously most important in therapy.

20. PEARCE, Louise, and BROWN, Wade H. A study of the relation of Treponema pallidum to lymphoid tissues in experimental syphilis, J. Exper. Med., **35**:39, 1922.

Having demonstrated (Ref. 17) the wide dissemination of spirochetes in rabbits before clinical signs appear, Brown and Pearce made studies to determine their possible persistence in animals which had spontaneously recovered and had remained well for considerable periods of time. They excised popliteal lymph nodes from these animals and reinjected the emulsified glands into the testes of other rabbits. Six rabbits were studied which had been infected for 7–51 months and in which the clinical latent period was of at least 3 months' duration. In the excised nodes of all these animals it was possible to demonstrate spirochetes capable of producing disease. From these facts it may be concluded that rabbits which have recovered from clinical syphilis may harbor virulent spirochetes almost indefinitely, even though no further manifestations of infection occur.

21. BROWN, Wade H., and PEARCE, Louise. Tryparsamide, its action and uses, J.A.M.A., **82**:5, 1924.

The properties of this drug were first described by W. A. Jacobs and Michael Heidelberger ("Chemotherapy of trypanosome and spirochete infections. I. *N*-phenylglycine-amide-*p*-arsonic acid," J. Exper. Med., **30**:417, 1919). Differing from the arsphenamines in being a pentavalent instead of a trivalent arsenic compound, it appeared to be of very low toxicity and could be given to animals in large doses (Wade H. Brown and Louise Pearce, "Chemotherapy of trypanosome and spirochete infections, biological series. I. The toxic action of *N*-phenylglycine-amide-*p*-arsonic acid," J. Exper. Med., **30**:417, 1919) until retrobulbar neuritis was found to be a fairly frequent result (L. L. Sloan and A. C. Woods, "The effect of tryparsamide on the eye: a clinical study of the objective ocular reaction," Am. J. Syph., **20**:583, 1936). In the present paper Brown and Pearce give a critical summary of the actions and uses of the drug. Meanwhile, W. F. Lorenz, A. S. Loewenhart, W. J. Blackwenn, and F. J. Hodges ("The therapeutic uses of tryparsamide in neurosyphilis," J.A.M.A., **80**:1487, 1923) emphasized its special value in neurosyphilis. The drug is fully discussed in Moore's book (Ref. 29).

22. CHESNEY, Alan M., and KEMP, Jarold E. Studies in experimental syphilis. III. Further observations on the possibility of cure of syphilis in the rabbit with arsphenamine, J. Exper. Med., **43**:17, 1925.

The elaborate studies of Chesney and his associates followed those of Brown and Pearce (Ref. 16). Chesney found that syphilitic rabbits can be treated with arsphenamine in such a manner as to render the lymph nodes incapable of transmitting the infection to normal rabbits, even if treatment is begun late in the course of the disease. Those treated late in spite of apparent cure were almost uniformly refractory to a second infection. Chesney felt, contrary to earlier ideas, that this refractory state could be explained by the existence of acquired immunity which persists after abolition of the disease rather than by the persistence of first infection.

Chesney summarized his views on immunity in syphilis (Alan M. Chesney, "Acquired immunity in syphilis," Am. J.. Syph., **14**:289, 1930) as follows: "I think of acquired immunity in syphilis as a state of resistance which evolves comparatively slowly and at its best is not always complete, general in its distribution but imparted to some tissues more than to others . . . but not necessarily dependent upon the persistence of infection for its maintenance."

Chesney and Kemp ("The curability of syphilis," J.A.M.A., **88**:905, 1927) later emphasized the method of inoculating rabbits with lymph nodes from human patients as a test for cure.

Chesney summarizes the whole question of immunity in syphilis to date in his monograph of 1926 (Ref. 24).

23. MOORE, Joseph Earle, and KEIDEL, Albert. The treatment of early syphilis. I. A plan of treatment for routine use, Bull. Johns Hopkins Hosp., **39**:1, 1926.

At the end of the nineteenth century a feeling grew up among syphilologists that it was important to continue treatment after clinical manifestations had disappeared, in order to obtain a real cure. This feeling became a conviction when it was found that a single dose of Salvarsan did not necessarily cure and when it was felt that reversal of Wassermann reaction was an obligatory criterion. Treatment became longer and longer; doctors began to insist on a full year, and innumerable treatment schedules were devised. Moore and Keidel pointed out that full curative treatment was especially necessary in early syphilis, whereas in late syphilis it was more important to control the presenting lesions. They developed an organized definitive plan of therapy, consisting essentially of 70 weeks of continuous therapy with alternating courses of arsphenamine and bismuth. This general plan of therapy remained in vogue until the advent of penicillin. They summarized their principles as follows:

"That treatment shall be *continuous*, consisting of courses of arsphenamine alternating with courses of mercury by inunction (or of insoluble bismuth salts intramuscularly) plus potassium iodide, that treatment be carried out under full serological control, that treatment shall be prolonged without intermission for one year after the blood and spinal fluid have become and have remained completely negative."

Interestingly enough, just before penicillin became available, there was under study (H. T. Hyman, L. Chargin, J. L. Rice, and W. Leifer, "Massive dose chemotherapy of early syphilis by the intravenous drip method," J.A.M.A., **113**:1208, 1939) a quick method of cure of early syphilis by continuous intravenous infusion of arsphenamine in dextrose at the rate of 1,500 cc. of 5 per cent glucose containing 1 gm. of arsphenamine in 15 hours. The co-operating clinics of New York and midwestern groups ("Massive arsenotherapy for syphilis," J.A.M.A., **126**:554, 1944) reviewed the therapeutic results in 4,351 cases and found a satisfactory outcome in 85–90 per cent of primary syphilis and 70 per cent of secondary syphilis.

24. CHESNEY, Alan M. Immunity in syphilis, Medicine, **5**:375, 1926.

Before the discovery of the spirochete it was recognized that reinfection in syphilis was very infrequent, and certain other crude facts of immunity were dimly sensed. However, no sooner had transmission of the disease to animals been achieved and the causal organism been demonstrated than there appeared a great flood of work on experimental syphilis and immunity. Early important summaries of much of this material are to be found in A. Neisser, *Beiträge zur Pathologie und Therapie der Syphilis* (Berlin: Julius Springer, 1911). The monograph of Chesney is, however, a landmark, definitive to date. A late authoritative review of the subject is that of C. Bruck, "Immunität bei Syphilis," in W. Kolle and A. von Wassermann, *Handbuch der pathogenen Microorganismen* (Jena: Gustav Fischer, 1930), **7**:155. Harold J. Magnuson wrote an excellent recent summary: "Current concepts of immunity in syphilis," Am. J. Med., **5**:641, 1948.

25. BRUUSGAARD, E. Ueber das Schicksal der nicht spezifisch behandelten Luetiker, Arch. f. Dermat. u. Syph., **157**:309, 1929.

The early-nineteenth-century physicians often questioned the value of mercurial treatment of syphilis, but they had no adequate follow-up of their untreated cases. Bruusgaard reports on patients first seen in the clinic between 1889 and 1910 who received no specific therapy. Although lesions occurred in some patients at all stages of the disease, it was surprising that in many individuals "resistance factors" sufficed "not only to hold the infection in check but to fully overcome it." Bruusgaard's actual figures were approximately as follows: no clinical or serological evidence of disease, 25 per cent; dead of other causes than syphilis, 25 per cent; positive serology only, 15 per cent; syphilis of skin, mucous membrane, or bone, 12 per cent; cardiovascular syphilis, 12 per cent; neurosyphilis, 9.5 per cent. Moore and his group (J. E. Moore, H. N. Cole, P. A. O'Leary, J. H. Stokes, U. J. Wile, T. Parran, Jr., and L. J. Usilton, "Cooperative clinical studies in the treatment of syphilis," Ven. Dis. Inform., 13:351, 1932) also estimate that spontaneous "cure" occurs in 25–35 per cent of untreated syphilitics, whereas in another 25–35 per cent all that is demonstrable is a positive Wassermann reaction. J. J. Peters, J. H. Peers, S. Olansky, J. C. Cutler, and G. A. Gleeson ("Untreated syphilis in the male Negro," J. Chronic Dis., 1:127, 1955) emphasize the frequency of cardiovascular and neurosyphilis at autopsy in untreated male Negroes. The subject is well summarized by Hugh J. Morgan, "The prognosis of syphilis," J.A.M.A., 112:311, 1939.

It is of interest that Danholt and his colleagues (N. Danholt, E. G. Clark, and F. Gjestland, "The Oslo-study of untreated syphilis: a re-study of the Boeck-Bruusgaard material concerning the fate of syphilitics who receive no specific treatment: a preliminary report," Acta dermat.-venereol., 34:34, 1954) have recently restudied Bruusgaard's material.

26. TATUM, A. L., and COOPER, G. A. An experimental study of mapharsen (meta-amino para-hydroxy phenyl arsine oxide) as an antisyphilitic agent, J. Pharmacol. & Exper. Therap., 50:198, 1934.

This drug, described by Ehrlich (Ref. 6), was revived by Tatum and Cooper, thoroughly tested in animals, and recommended for clinical trial. They point out that mapharsen is a pure chemical, whereas the arsphenamines are chemical mixtures which vary with each lot and therefore require biological assay. Mapharsen became popular enough to replace the arsphenamines in the treatment schemes of many American clinics. Mapharsen as well as other arsenicals are thoroughly discussed in J. E. Moore's book (Ref. 29).

27. STOKES, John H., and GARNER, Vaughan C. Public health problems: methods and policy in the control of syphilis, Am. J.M. Sc., 194:578, 1937.

We cannot, in this bibliography, go into the public health aspects. This authoritative review is to be mentioned, however, as an introduction to this phase of the subject.

28. REIN, Charles R., WISE, Fred, and CUKERBAUM, Alfred R. The control and prevention of transfusion syphilis, J.A.M.A., 111:13, 1938.

The authors refer to the first reported case of transfusion syphilis (John A. Fordyce, "Some problems in the pathology of syphilis," Am. J.M. Sc., 149:781, 1915) and point out that, while only 68 proved cases of syphilis transmitted by transfusions have been reported, the total number is obviously greater. They make a plea for rigid serological tests on all donors.[2] In these cases following transfusion there is no visible primary lesion, but the first clinical manifestations are "secondaries."

29. MOORE, Joseph Earle. The modern treatment of syphilis. 2d ed. Springfield: Charles C Thomas, 1941; also 1st ed., 1933.

In this monumental book of nearly seven hundred pages Moore discusses authoritatively and in detail every facet of the treatment of syphilis in the pre-penicillin era. Extensive bibliographies are given. The book is a definite landmark in the history of the subject.

30. MAHONEY, John F., ARNOLD, R. C., and HARRIS, A. Penicillin treatment of early syphilis: a preliminary report, Ven. Dis. Inform., **24**:355, 1943; also Am. J. Pub. Health, **33**:1387, 1943.

The writers decided to try penicillin in syphilis "after limited animal experimentation indicated that penicillin possessed some spirocheticidal activity." Four patients with primary lesions were treated with 25,000 units of the drug intramuscularly at 4-hour intervals night and day for 8 days. The chancres all became dark-field-negative within 16 hours. Various serological tests rapidly became negative. It was of interest that during the first 8 hours of therapy the patients complained of malaise and headache and had slight elevations of temperature. The lesions became painful, and the regional lymph nodes were enlarged and tender. Mahoney's observations were promptly confirmed by C. W. Barnett (Arthur L. Bloomfield, Lowell A. Rantz, and William M. M. Kirby, "The clinical use of penicillin," J.A.M.A., **124**:627, 1944), who reported similar results in 7 cases of early syphilis. Mahoney (J. F. Mahoney, R. C. Arnold, Burton L. Sterner, A. Harris, and M. R. Zwally, "Penicillin treatment of early syphilis. II," J.A.M.A., **126**:63, 1944) soon reported a follow-up study of their original patients, and in 1946 the Committee on Medical Research of the National Research Council and the United States Public Health Service issued a joint statement ("The treatment of early syphilis with penicillin," J.A.M.A., **131**:265, 1946), in which it was pointed out that there were some treatment failures, especially in those treated late and in those treated with a total of only 600,000 units as against 2,400,000 units of penicillin.

31. STOKES, John H., BEERMAN, Herman, and INGRAHAM, Norman R., Jr. Modern clinical syphilology—diagnosis, treatment, case study. 3d ed. Philadelphia and London: W. B. Saunders Co., 1944.

A tremendous treatise which covers the entire field of clinical syphilis up to the penicillin era.

32. MOORE, Joseph Earle. Penicillin in syphilis. Springfield: Charles C Thomas, 1946.

The early reports were followed by a flood of studies of such dimensions that, by 1946, Moore felt impelled to summarize them, together with his own con-

---

[2] Yet this obviously does not replace careful history and physical examination. We have seen one case in which transfusion from a man in the primary seronegative stage transmitted a violent syphilitic infection to the recipient—his father.

clusions, in book form. This compilation is definitive to date and deals with penicillin in every stage of syphilis, with extensive bibliographies. By 1953 the same writer (J. E. Moore, "The changing pattern of syphilis, 1941–1953," Am. Int. Med., **39**:644, 1953) was able to state that "penicillin, first introduced into the treatment of syphilis in 1943, has now completely replaced arsenic, bismuth and mercury in all stages of syphilis." A. C. Curtis, D. K. Kitchen, P. A. O'Leary, H. Ratner, C. R. Rein, A. G. Shoch, L. W. Shaffer, and U. J. Wile ("Penicillin treatment of syphilis," J.A.M.A., **145**:1223, 1951) also summarize methods and results of penicillin therapy in various stages of syphilis.

33. NELSON, Robert A., Jr., and MAYER, Manfred M. Immobilization of Treponema pallidum in vitro by antibody produced in syphilitic infection, J. Exper. Med., **89**:369, 1949.

As a tool for studying immunity in syphilis, the writers sought a serological test more specific than the usual complement-fixation or precipitin tests for "reagin." They were able to extract from the testes of rabbits with acute syphilitic orchitis a heavy suspension of motile treponemes. By adding appropriate quantities of serum from syphilitic people and animals, together with complement, most of the treponemes were rendered immobile in the dark field, in contrast to normal sera, which in control tests did not interfere with the motility of treponemes. They feel that this procedure—the treponemal immobilization test—is a test for specific syphilitic antibody. Nelson and his associates soon published further studies (A. S. Khan, R. A. Nelson, Jr., and T. B. Turner, "Immunological relationships among species and strains of virulent treponemes as determined with the treponemal immobilization test," Am. J. Hyg., **53**:296, 1951; R. A. Nelson, Jr., H. E. C. Zhentlin, J. A. Diesendruck, and P. G. M. Austin, Jr., "Studies on treponemal immobilizing antibodies in syphilis; incidence in serum and cerebrospinal fluid in human beings and absence in 'biologic false positive' reactors," Am. J. Syph., **34**:101, 1950; R. A. Nelson, Jr., and J. A. Diesendruck, "Studies on treponemal immobilization antibodies in syphilis. I. Techniques of measurement and factors influencing immobilization," J. Immunol., **66**:667, 1951). Nelson's work was soon confirmed by others (J. L. Miller, M. H. Slatkin, R. R. Feiner, J. Portnoy, and A. B. Cannon, "Treponemal immobilization test, reliability of results for the diagnosis of syphilis," J.A.M.A., **149**:987, 1952), who found no false positives with the test, but an occasional negative "after a certain time in patients who have had syphilis, particularly if adequate treatment was given in the early stages." J. L. Miller, M. H. Slatkin, M. Brodey, H. L. Wechsler, and J. H. Hill ("Studies with the treponemal immobilizing test," J.A.M.A., **154**:1241, 1954) report an extensive experience with the test, and they emphasize its specificity and value in ruling out false positives. It is improbable that this valuable test will soon be available for "routine" use. However, it is invaluable as a tool for immunological studies and is obtainable in many places for special human cases. A clear, simple statement about the procedure is made by C. W. Barnett, "The treponemal immobilization test in the diagnosis of syphilis," Stanford M. Bull., **9**:205, 1951.

34. MOORE, J. E., and MOHR, C. F. Biologically false positive serologic tests for syphilis: type, incidence, and cause, J.A.M.A., **150**:467, 1952.

Ever since the early days of the Wassermann test it has been known that false positive tests might be obtained. Moore and his associates have recently made systematic studies of this phenomenon and have designated as biologically false positives those which were not due to technical errors. They distinguish between "acute" and "chronic" BFP reactors. The "acute" variety is a temporary phenomenon which occurs especially in connection with various acute infectious diseases and usually disappears spontaneously within 6 months. The "chronic" variety, on the other hand, is not associated with any evident acute cause, and the standard serodiagnostic test remains positive indefinitely. This type has recently been comprehensively dealt with by Moore and Lutz (Joseph Earle Moore and W. Beale Lutz, "The natural history of systemic lupus erythematosus: an approach to its study through chronic biologic false positive reactors," J. Chronic Dis., 1:297, 1955).

35. HOLLANDER, David H., TURNER, Thomas B., and NELL, E. Ellen. The effect of long continued subcurative doses of penicillin during the incubation period of experimental syphilis, Bull. Johns Hopkins Hosp., 90:105, 1952.

The introduction of penicillin made necessary a re-evaluation of immunity factors in connection with penicillin therapy. In this important study, for example, it was found that subcurative doses of penicillin prolonged the incubation period. In some rabbits the incubation period was prolonged up to 2 weeks by means of subclinical infection, but then "the evolution of the syphilitic infection after termination of treatment was in general similar to that observed in untreated animals. . . . Wholly symptomless infection was not observed. Rabbits were either cured, or subsequently developed clinically recognizable lesions." The implication is clear that in man it is better to waste some penicillin than to give too little in both prophylaxis and therapy.

36. BARNETT, C. W., EPSTEIN, Norman N., BREWER, A. Frank, KOCH, Richard A., and BEIRNE, Gilbert A. The effect of treatment in latent syphilis, Arch. Dermat. & Syph., 69:91, 1954.

It has long been a question whether specific therapy was advantageous in latent syphilis. Barnett first wrote philosophically on the subject (C. W. Barnett, "Why treat latent syphilis?" Stanford M. Bull., 2:51, 1944; "The effect of treatment on the prognosis of late latent syphilis," J. Insur. Med., 4:7, 1949; H. L. Blum and C. W. Barnett, "Prognosis in latent syphilis," Arch. Int. Med., 82:393, 1948). In the present paper, however, he and his group reported results of therapy in 2,470 patients treated with metal chemotherapy and 231 treated with penicillin. Barnett introduced the novel idea of determining the effectiveness of treatment by the incidence of clinical progression per century of patient observation. By this method of calculation it was shown that progression was less in those who received much treatment with metals than in those who received little. Penicillin did not completely prevent progression.

37. WILLCOX, R. R. A W.H.O. study of treatment schedules for early syphilis in use throughout the world, Bull. World Health Organ., 10:579, 1954.

A world-wide questionnaire was sent out to syphilis clinics, inquiring about their current methods of treating early syphilis. Two hundred and seventy-seven replies were received from 55 countries, giving particulars of 294 schedules. A total of 65.3 per cent of the participants used penicillin alone, and 28.9 per cent used it in combination with other drugs. Penicillin alone was used especially in North American clinics. The paper is full of interesting details and charts, which must be consulted. James K. Shafer, Lida J. Usilton, and Eleanor V. Price ("Long-term studies of results of penicillin therapy in early syphilis," Bull. World Health Organ., 10:563, 1954) came to the conclusion in a follow-up study that 4,800,000 units of penicillin were desirable for the treatment of early syphilis, and, at the sixth year following penicillin treatment, satisfactory results were recorded in 98–99 per cent of the patients with primary and secondary syphilis. J. K. Shafer and C. A. Smith ("Treatment of early infectious syphilis with $N_1 N'$-dibenzylethylenediamene dipenicillin G, Bull. World Health Organ., 10:619, 1954) also found that 2,500,000 units of this depository penicillin in one injection seemed to prove equally as effective as 4,800,000 units of procaine penicillin and aluminum monostearate (P.A.M.) for the treatment of early syphilis.

38. HARDY, Paul H., Jr., and NELL, E. Ellen. Specific agglutination of Treponema pallidum by sera from rabbits and human beings with treponema infections, J. Exper. Med., 101:367, 1955.

The writers refer to the work of T. B. Turner ("Protective antibodies in the serum of syphilitic rabbits," J. Exper. Med., 69:867, 1939), who first demonstrated, by neutralization experiments in rabbits, the development of *specific* immunity in treponemal infections. Turner's method was, however, too complicated and cumbersome for general use. Hardy and Nell were able to prepare suspensions of *Treponema pallidum* suitable for specific agglutination studies and capable of being stored for months. By means of such studies they demonstrated true syphilitic antibodies different from "non-specific" Wassermann antibody. This test, like the treponemal immobilization test (Ref. 33), is highly specific.

MALARIA

Anemia	Ref. 5
Avian malaria	Ref. 13
Etiology	Refs. 6 through 9; 11, 12; 14 through 16
Exoerythrocytic cycle	Refs. 46, 50
Fertilization of parasite	Refs. 23 through 35
Flagella	Refs. 19, 23, 24, 29
General	Refs. 1, 2, 18, 22, 34, 39, 53
Immunity	Refs. 32, 52
Inoculation malaria	Refs. 10, 12, 38
Melanemia	Refs. 1 through 5
Modern chemotherapy	Refs. 40, 41, 44, 47, 51, 53
Mosquito	Refs. 21; 25 through 27; 29 through 31; 33, 39
Parasite	Refs. 7 through 9; 11, 12, 14, 16, 20, 48

(*Continued on following page*)

Pathology	Refs. 1, 2, 4, 48
Prevention	Refs. 28, 32, 35, 36
Quinine	Refs. 2, 43
Staining of parasites	Ref. 17
Transmission	Refs. 21; 25 through 27; 29, 31, 39

THE present section, like the one on tuberculosis, has presented great difficulties; the literature is overwhelmingly immense, many items are relatively inaccessible in Italian journals, and there are numerous offshoots into epidemiology, preventive medicine, protozoölogy, and pharmacology. As in previous chapters, our guide has been the fact that this bibliography is compiled primarily for clinicians with general interests, such as medical students and internists. No apology is made, therefore, for slighting certain phases of the subject, such as the public health aspects and some questions of immunity and of chemotherapy which the limits of space (and reason) make necessary. No doubt many significant papers have been entirely overlooked.

It should be recalled also that the two important decades, 1880–1900—from the discovery of the parasite by Laveran to the culmination of Ross's work—was an era of bitter controversy, of disputed claims of priority, and even of accusations of frank plagiarism between the "Roman School" and first Laveran and later Ross. In Ross's memoirs (Ref. 39) there is even a chapter headed "Roman Brigandage." We have tried to deal fairly with this dispute, although it is easy to see how Laveran and Ross felt themselves ill-used.

The striking clinical features of the intermittent fevers have given them an ancient and honorable medical history which has not been adequately dealt with by many writers. We have not attempted, therefore, to go back of modern times, that is to say, earlier than the nineteenth century.

For thorough discussions of every phase of the subject, one should consult the monumental work on "malariology" edited by Mark F. Boyd (Philadelphia and London: W. B. Saunders Co., 1949). There are seventy chapters, each by an authority in the field, with comprehensive bibliographies. Good reference lists to the older literature are to be found in Laveran (Ref. 11), Marchiafava and Bignami (Ref. 18), Mannaberg (Ref. 20), Thayer and Hewetson (Ref. 22), and Ross (Refs. 36, 39).

1. BAILLY, E. M. Traité anatomico-pathologique des fièvres intermittentes. Paris: Gabon & Cie, 1825.

Reference is frequently made in the early literature to Bailly's book, mainly because of the pathologic studies, and he is often given credit for describing the characteristic malarial pigmentation of various organs. Actually, the text is long and discursive, and the clinical pictures are too vague to have any useful meaning. There are numerous case reports with gross autopsy findings. These are not very satisfactory; in the "pernicious" intermittent fevers, arachnitis is a frequent diagnosis, often with "splenitis" or "gastroenteritis." The typical slaty or black pigmentation of the organs is mentioned only in passing; no special significance was attributed to it, and, at best, in an occasional case an organ was spoken of as dark (*foncé*) or grayish black (*gris-noirâtre*). In summary, the book serves best as a contrast for the advances in knowledge soon to come.

Bailly was familiar with the use of quinine sulfate but thought of it as "a specific sedative for the abdominal nervous system" (p. 426).

2. MAILLOT, F. G. Traité des fièvres, etc. Paris: J.-B. Baillière, 1836.

Maillot's book, eleven years after Bailly's, shows a good deal of advance. The disease observed in France, Corsica, and Africa is now recognizable as malaria; the clinical descriptions are excellent. However, there is as yet no precise differentiation of tertian and quartan or of other types. The deep pigmentation of organs is definitely noted; in one case the liver was chocolate-colored, as was the spleen in seven cases (p. 285). In five instances of the comatose type the brain had a blackish tint (p. 287). However, there was still no orderly synthesis of these observations and no realization that they had any special significance. Quinine was used along with other febrifuges; Maillot noted that where 5 grains of quinine sulfate were ineffective, 20 grains might prevent further paroxysms.

3. CHARCOT, J.-M. De la mélanémie, altération du sang par des granules et des corpuscules de pigment, Gaz. hebd. de méd., 4:659, 1857.

Pigmentation of certain viscera, especially spleen, liver, bone marrow, and brain, the mechanism of which is now clear, was long ago widely noted as an empirical fact in connection with intermittent fevers. We have already mentioned the observations of Bailly (Ref. 1) and of Maillot (Ref. 2). Richard Bright in his *Reports of Medical Cases* ([London: Longman, Rees, Orne, Brown & Green, 1831], Vol. 2, Case CI, p. 217, Pl. XVII) pictured a section of a brain which was "almost the color of black lead." Although this case is often quoted in the literature on malarial melanosis, there is no satisfactory evidence for such a diagnosis.

Meckel, a psychiatrist, is generally credited with being the first to note that brown pigmentation of organs in malaria was associated with an accumulation of pigment in the blood. His case report (Heinrich Meckel, "Ueber schwartzes Pigment in der Milz und dem Blute einer Geisteskranken," Allg. Ztschr. f. Psychiat., 4:198, 1847) is, however, difficult to interpret. The patient had no clinical evidence of malaria and died in a psychotic state, with weakness, edema, and ascites. The brain was chocolate-colored, the capillaries were full of pigment granules, and the spleen was "very large" and dark brown. Meckel thought the pigment was formed in the spleen, whence it entered the blood. He performed various chemical tests but did not identify the pigment. Later ("Körnigen Farbstoff in der Milz und im Blute bei Wechselfieberkranken," Deutsche Klin., 2:551, 1850) he pursued the whole matter further and brought more evidence that certain kinds of pigmentation of blood and viscera are characteristic of malaria. He now thought that the pigment came from blood which had been altered in the capillaries. Virchow went a step further ("Zur pathologischen Physiologie des Bluts," Virchows Arch. f. path. Anat., 2:587, 1849) in reporting an autopsy on a case of intermittent fever in which he described pigment *in* blood cells which he thought were leukocytes. Whether or not any of these observers saw malarial parasites is hard to say; at any rate, they had no inkling of their nature.

In Charcot's excellent article, modern in tone, is given an authoritative summary of current understanding of melanemia. The following facts were accepted: Melanemia (literally, "black blood") of marked degree occurred only in association with intermittent fevers. The pigment was brown or black, in small or large clumps, sometimes free in the blood or in organs but more often in cells or "corpuscles," which were regarded as leukocytes, not as red cells. There was enlargement of the spleen of variable degree, less so of the liver. These and other organs often showed marked darkening; sometimes they looked black. The pigment was recognized as being related to the coloring matter of blood, and there was more when the number of red cells was greatly diminished. The association of acute comatose types of fever with plugging of the capillaries by innumerable "corpuscles" filled with pigment was clearly recognized, and the failure of quinine in some of these cases was thought to be explained by this. Hemorrhages from plugged capillaries were described. The exact relation of pigment to symptoms was not clear. Cachexia with dropsy and skin pigmentation was occasionally noted. Albumin and casts (Bright's disease) were observed in some cases. Pigmented corpuscles were seen in the blood of *living* people— often ten to fifteen to a "field of the microscope"; these were not thought to be red cells, although the decrease in red cells was recognized.

Where and how the pigment was formed were unknown; there was no idea of a parasite and no understanding of phagocytosis by fixed tissue cells in organs. Charcot insisted that the pigmentation was not a primary disease; but he thought that the study of these phenomena "should perhaps one day form an important chapter in the general history of malarial intoxication."

One wonders why none of the many workers on the subject suspected the presence of parasites. Poor microscopes, lack of staining methods, and study mainly of post-mortem material may be the explanation.

4. FRERICHS, Friedrich Theodor von. Klinik der Leberkrankheiten, chap. viii, Veränderungen der Leber bei Intermittens, p. 325. Braunschweig: F. Vieweg & Sohn, 1858.

Frerichs, the great German physician of the mid-nineteenth century, gave a detailed and authoritative description, with beautiful plates, of the pathology of malaria. For Frerichs, all the lesions were probably the consequence of the melanemia. He described the pigment granules free in cells supposed to be leukocytes and in large cells probably of reticuloendothelial origin which he believed were lining cells of splenic sinuses. Frerichs thought that in malaria, as a result of febrile hyperemia, the normal tendency of red blood cells to be destroyed in the spleen was greatly exaggerated, with massive pigment formation from excess of hemoglobin (*blutroth*) liberation. This in turn was carried to the liver and thence to other organs. Why melanemia did not occur in other fevers with splenomegaly was a puzzle. Frerichs' descriptions were authoritative because they were based on autopsies made by him during the study of an epidemic of intermittent fever in Silesia in 1854–55.

5. KELSCH, A. Contribution à l'anatomie pathologique des palustres endémiques, Arch de physiol. norm. et path., **11**, 2d ser., 690, 1875.

Although the occurrence of anemia in malaria had long been known, Kelsch seems to have been the first to make systematic blood counts during life. He observed initial rapid declines, often of as many as 1,000,000 cells a day, with less rapid later changes. He noted the extremely low counts in some cases of chronic paludism. The old discussions of melanemia are again gone through, but Kelsch did not get much further than Frerichs (Ref. 4). Again there was no suggestion of parasites. He thought that the pigment came from some obscure destruction of blood throughout the body, not only, or primarily, in the spleen. Even in the year when parasites were described (1880), the same absence of correct interpretation prevailed (Kelsch, "Contribution à l'histoire des maladies palustres: de la mélanémie," Arch. gén. de méd., **146**:385, 1880).

6. KLEBS, E., and TOMMASI-CRUDELI, C. Einige Sätze über die Ursachen der Wechselfieber und die Natur den Malaria, Arch. f. exper. Path. u. pharmakol., **11**:122, 1879.

The history of many infectious diseases, such as scarlet fever, influenza, poliomyelitis, and others, is that all sorts of bacteria were at first assigned a causal role. As one was shown not to be the true agent, another was blamed, and this error might be repeated many times before the true etiology was established. This was so with malaria; the early literature on bacterial claims is reviewed by Laveran (Ref. 11, 1891, pp. 1 ff.) and by Thayer (Ref. 22, p. 5). However, the findings of Klebs and Tommasi-Crudeli, supported by the authority of Klebs's name, seemed so plausible that they were generally accepted; nearly twenty years later, long after the discovery of the parasite, an editorial article appeared in one of the leading English medical journals stating the causal role of the bacillus of Klebs as a settled fact (Thayer, Ref. 22, p. 7).

Klebs and Tommasi-Crudeli, in brief, claimed that they could extract from the earth of malarial regions and from the air near the ground bacteria which directly or in subculture, when injected into rabbits, produced a febrile illness with an intermittent type of fever resembling malaria, enlarged spleen, and, at autopsy, "abundant black pigment in the spleen as in people ill with malaria." They classed the organism as a bacillus and named it *Bacillus malariae*.

Klebs seemed to have all the necessary controls, and it is hard to understand how he could have erred so badly. A few months later (E. Klebs and C. Tommasi-Crudeli, "Studien über die Ursache des Wechselfiebers und über die Natur der Malaria," Arch. f. exper. Path. u. Pharmakol., **11**: 311, 1879), the earlier brief statement was elaborated into a tremendous article of eighty-eight pages in which the details of the experiments leading to the same conclusions were given.[1] It is of interest to note the large number of workers, including such men as Marchiafava, who thought that they had confirmed Klebs and Tommasi-Crudeli. Cuboni and Marchiafava, for example, began their paper on "New studies on the nature of malaria" (Arch. f. exper. Path. u. Pharmakol., **13**: 265, 1881): "Knowledge of the parasitic nature of malaria has received the most brilliant confirmation through the recent work of Klebs and Tommasi-Crudeli."

7. [LAVERAN]. Presentation by M. Colin of a manuscript entitled "Note sur un nouveau parasite trouvé dans le sang de plusiers malades atteints de fièvre palustre," Bull. Acad. de méd., **9**: 1235, 1880.

[1] In 1924 I recorded in my diary an anecdote told me by Professor Kraus during a visit to Berlin: "He [Kraus] began to speak of the malarial treatment of paresis and from this got on to malaria. It appears that before the discovery of the parasite, Klebs joined an Italian commission and did some field work, returning with earth from the Roman Campagna. From this he grew a bacillus about which there was great excitement and which was regarded as the possible causal agent. Klebs inoculated two rabbits and left them overnight with two assistants (one of whom I suspect was Kraus), who were to watch and take their temperature. The assistants got a jug of beer and played Skat and finally went to sleep, and in the morning found the rabbits frozen to death. Klebs, then, in his lecture, much excited, said he couldn't demonstrate the temperature curves of the rabbits because they had died in the night *of malaria!*"

It is difficult to say who first saw the malarial parasite. In systematic treatises various persons are mentioned whose descriptions of pigmented cells or bodies in the blood may have actually concerned the parasite, but primitive microscopes and inadequate technical methods without stains leave one quite uncertain. The bodies pictured by Virchow, for example (Ref. 3), bear no definite resemblance to the plasmodia.

The actual discovery must be credited to Laveran. The popular notion, however, that, as he gazed into his microscope, the parasites were immediately evident and the whole matter clear is far from the actual record. Laveran's first communication was presented by proxy at the meeting of November 23 of the Academy of Medicine by M. Léon Colin, who stated that he had the honor to present for M. le docteur Laveran, stationed at the military hospital at Constantine (Algiers), a manuscript entitled "Note on a new parasite found in the blood of several patients sick with malaria." The drawing which Laveran submitted is not reproduced, but three types of "elements" are described in the blood: "(1) These are elongated, cylindrical, slightly curved like a crescent, showing in their center a spot made up of blackish granulations; (2) other round bodies, volume a little less than that of the red blood cells, sometimes immobile, sometimes moved by long tentacles which are attached to their borders; (3) round elements much larger than the preceding, doubtless because of swelling of the cells by imbibition of serum."

Colin went on to say in tactful terms that he doubted that these bodies were parasites, partly because of the non-contagiousness of malaria, and he proposed that a commission be set up to pass on the validity of similar future studies. One can see that Laveran was to have a rough road.

At the meeting of the academy of December 28, M. Léon Colin again had a paper to present for M. Laveran entitled "A second note relative to a new parasite found in the blood of patients ill with malaria" ("Deuxième note relative à un nouveau parasite trouvé dans le sang des malades atteints de la fièvre palustre," Bull. Acad. de méd., **19**:1346, 1880). The communication consists, however, mainly of a blast by M. Colin to the effect that Laveran's "parasites" were probably only leukocytes which had ingested pigment, a phenomenon common in the melanemia of malaria. Laveran, evidently on the defensive, now requested of the commission the aid of an expert histologist, M. Kiener of Val-de-Grâce, which in civil life was Laveran's own university.

8. LAVERAN, A. De la nature parasitaire des accidents de l'impaludisme, Compt. rend. Acad. d. sc., **93**:627, 1881.

This time, at the meeting of October 24, 1881, of the Academy of Sciences, Laveran spoke for himself: "There are present in the blood of malaria patients parasites which present themselves under the following aspects." He described four varieties: (1) elongated crescentic bodies, (2) spherical, pigmented cells with filaments three or four times the diameter of a red cell in length, (3) spherical, pigmented bodies of irregular form, which, however, are not pigmented leukocytes, (4) smaller spherical, slightly pigmented bodies, some only one-sixth the diameter of a red cell. "The living nature of the spherical bodies inclosing mobile grains of pigment and armed with mobile peripheral filaments is unquestionable." Laveran also noted pigment granules and pigmented white cells in the blood. He stated that he had now studied nearly two hundred patients with malaria. Most of those who showed no parasites had been treated with quinine. Parasites were found in no other disease. He noted that the parasites were most likely to be found shortly before the paroxysm of fever but that in stubborn cases they were there all the time. He thought that between bouts of fever the parasites resorted to internal organs, especially liver and spleen. He noted in autopsies on malignant cases how the internal capillaries were packed with pigmented bodies. He concluded: "Attacks of malaria are produced by the introduction into the blood of parasites which appear in the various forms herewith described; it is because quinine kills these parasites that it cures malaria."

9. [RICHARD, E.]. Sur la parasite de la malaria, Compt. rend. Acad. d. sc., **94**:496, 1882.

Although Laveran's name now stands out, one must picture the tremendous ferment of activity which went on in the study of malaria in the 1880's. For the most part, doctors were skeptical or downright hostile to Laveran's claims. There were those who adhered to a bacterial cause like the bacillus of Klebs (Ref. 6); there were those who believed spores or molds were the etiological agent; and many still held to bad air or swamp emanations and did not believe in a *contagium vivum* of any sort. One can picture the patient hours spent at the microscope by faithful students, as a "wild surmise" dawned that they might be looking at a living parasite. One of the earliest supporters of Laveran was his friend Richard, who worked in the hospital at Philippeville (Algeria), where there was much malaria. Richard read this paper before the Academy of Sciences on February 20, 1882. The same remarks were published in the Gazette médicale de Paris in the issue for May 20, 1882 (**4**:252). Richard confirmed and strongly supported the discovery of the parasite, which Laveran had named *Oscillaria malariae* because of the dancing appearance of the pigment granules. He examined fresh blood, unstained, and emphasized the fact, still true, that this is the best way to study the motility of the parasite. He differed with Laveran in one important point. Laveran thought that the parasite was on the cell; Richard was sure that it was *in* the red cell, in which "it develops like a weevil in a lentil." He described the growth of the parasite at the cost of the host cell until it was finally surrounded by a mere veil. Filaments were then thrust forth and finally the parasite burst from its "shell."

10. GERHARDT, C. Ueber Intermittens-Impfungen, Ztschr. f. klin. med., **7**:372, 1884.

Inoculation malaria, later to become an everyday procedure in the treatment of paresis (Ref. 38), seems to have been first attempted by Gerhardt. A hypodermic syringe full of blood from the thirty-seven-year-old Brewer G. with intermittent fever was injected subcutaneously into the thirty-nine-year-old hysterical B. S. on August 11, 1882. On August 22 there were chill and fever and splenic enlargement. The fever subsided after quinine. Gerhardt later repeated the procedure in another case. Nothing is said of parasites in this report, and there were no bacteriologic studies. After the parasite was recognized, attempts at transmission by inoculation were soon made; the early literature is well summarized by Thayer and Hewetson (Ref. 22, pp. 35 ff.) and very completely by Ross (Ref. 36, pp. 66 ff.).

11. LAVERAN, A. Traité des fièvres palustres avec la description des microbes du paludisme. Paris: O. Doin, 1884.

In 1881, after the appearance of his first paper (Ref. 7), Laveran summarized the findings in a brief monograph entitled *Nature parasitaire des accidents de l'impaludisme. Description d'un nouveau parasite trouvé dans le sang des malades atteints de fièvre palustre* (Paris: O. Doin, 1881). He continued, however, to work energetically on the subject, fighting a hard battle to convince others of the correctness of his views, which were later embodied in his book of 1884 dealing with every phase of malarial fever. In the Preface he stated that it was in studying the mode of formation of the well-known pigmented elements in malarial blood that he was led to discover their parasitic nature. He continued somewhat nostalgically "On November 6, 1880, . . . I demonstrated for the first time the presence of mobile filaments which adhered to the pigmented bodies and the living nature of which could not be in doubt. At this very moment I had the intuition that I was in the presence of the true parasites of malaria and everything I have done since has confirmed this impression." No indication of this sudden and dramatic revelation is given in his original reports (Refs. 7, 8). This book went through many editions in the next thirty years. Another important monograph appeared later (*Du paludisme et de son hématozoaire* [Paris: G. Masson, 1891]), which was translated into English by J. W. Martin (*Paludism, by Dr. A. Laveran* [London: New Sydenham Society, 1893]). There is an excellent historical introduction. Although Richard (Ref. 9) believed that the parasites were intracellular, Laveran sitll felt that "our knowledge of the structure and composition of the blood-corpuscle in man makes it difficult for us to understand how these parasites can enter them. The probability is that they simply adhere to the corpuscles by pressing upon them. What makes this supposition more likely to be true is that the parasitic elements are often found in the blood in a free state" (p. 16). The latter statement is, of course, erroneous. Laveran recognized some difference between the parasites in various types of malaria: decolorization of red cells in tertian, in contrast to quartan; diminution in size of parasitized red cells in quartan fever; and differences in segmentation in tertian and quartan fever. He was not certain that crescents were restricted to any special type of fever, as others had claimed. Although he quoted Golgi as believing that there are different races of malarial parasites, in the excellent plate at the end of the book all types—segmenters, flagellates, and crescents—are mixed together. Every phase of the disease, including prophylaxis and therapy, is discussed, and there is a section on avian malaria.

12. MARCHIAFAVA, Ettore, and CELLI, Angelo. Nuove ricerche sulla infezione malarica, Arch. per le sc. med., **9**:311, 1885. (A German translation of the manuscript was published simultaneously: "Neuere Untersuchungen über die Malariainfection," Fortschr. d. Med., **3**:39, 1885.)

Marchiafava's name has become so exalted in the history of malaria that it becomes important to analyze his work critically. Marchiafava stubbornly supported the etiological role of Klebs and Tommasi-Crudeli's "malaria bacillus," long after Laveran reported his work (Refs. 7, 8). Marchiafava and Celli in 1882 denied the parasitic nature of Laveran's bodies, although Laveran went to

Rome and gave a demonstration of their presence in local cases[2] of malaria (Ref. 11, 1884, p. viii, and 1891, p. 48). In 1883 Marchiafava and Celli ("Die Veränderung der rothen Blutscheiben bei Malariakranken," Fortschr. d. Med., 1:573, 1883) hedged. Without any mention of Laveran, they described what obviously were malarial parasites. "What now is the meaning of these bodies which we see [in malaria] within the red cells? Are they a regressive metamorphosis, or are they foreign elements which have entered the cells? At the present time we lean to the latter interpretation and presume that we are concerned with a parasite . . . however, none of this can be settled definitely as yet. We hope to clear the matter up by further work; meanwhile, the first-mentioned possibility that we may be dealing only with a regressive metamorphosis of red cells is still to be considered." This is evasive, to say the least. Laveran further said (Ref. 11, 1891, p. 48): "In a letter dated Rome, April 9, 1884, M. Marchiafava makes it clear that he and his collaborators have reached conclusions very different from mine. . . . 'We believe that the pigmented forms which you [Laveran] have described are nothing but degenerated and pigmented red cells. . . .' There can be no doubt on this point . . . four years after the publication of my work . . . they thought that the parasite of paludism was a micrococcus."

It would be interesting if one could reconstruct the medical politics of the time. Klebs and Tommasi-Crudeli were big names. The latter was head of the bacteriologic institute in Rome; Marchiafava worked in the same institution. There must have been great pressure to take sides in this controversy with a relatively insignificant doctor from Val-de-Grâce.

However, by 1885, Marchiafava and Celli seem to have been suddenly committed to a parasitic cause for malaria. Marchiafava had become an expert on stained smears, and, turning now to fresh preparations, he laid special emphasis on small ring forms which might be ameboid and which contained no pigment. He also described larger pigmented forms, for the discovery of which, as well as crescents, he gave credit to Laveran. In four among forty-two cases carefully studied, the flagella (*filaments mobiles*), also seen by Laveran, were noted. The activity of the flagella is vividly pictured. Marchiafava and Celli pointed out that filaments were not seen in stained blood. There is also a description of what seem to be segmenters and segmentation, although the drawing of *scissione* ("division") is inaccurate and pictures a cell containing innumerable closely packed granules. Flagella and crescents were seen much less often than the other cells but were constantly present in pernicious fever. Marchiafava and Celli raised the question of whether segmenters gave rise to a new generation of parasites and begged the question about the significance of filaments other than that they were living bodies. They felt certain that the small ameboid bodies were parasites which entered the red cells and destroyed them.

They went on to describe attempts at transmission by injecting into a volunteer about 1 cc. of blood freshly drawn from a malaria patient. The fact that they produced "typical" malarial fever, found the characteristic bodies in the blood, and made them and the fever go away with quinine—"all these circumstances make our hypothesis that these are living forms probable."

Finally, efforts were made to cultivate the parasite on ordinary bacteriologic

---

[2] Marchiafava and Celli described this visit and denied that Laveran had demonstrated the parasites (Arch. ital. biol., 9:308, 1888).

media. In most cases the cultures remained sterile. "In others one obtained culture products which were morphologically identical with the initial forms [of the parasite]. . . . The multiplication of these bodies was especially evident in slide cultures of malarial blood."

It is obvious, then, that Marchiafava and Celli were still unclear about the significance of their findings and, in essence, did little more than confirm Laveran's findings.

A little later Marchiafava and Celli ("Studi ulteriori sulla infezione malarica," Arch. per le sc. med., **10**:185, 1886; German translation from the manuscript in Fortschr. d. Med., **3**:787, 1885) elaborated their previous observations. They emphasized the small non-pigmented ameboid forms as their own discovery and followed them through to segmentation, which they thought was a method of multiplication, to be followed by the invasion of the red cells by the liberated granules. They insisted that pigment was a product of the transformation of hemoglobin. It was in this paper that they suggested the name "plasmodium" or "hemoplasmodium," biologically unsound but later universally adopted.[3] In this paper also the feud between Laveran and Marchiafava became overt. We cannot give the details of the controversy further, but Laveran's side is summarized in his book on *Paludism* (Paris: G. Masson, 1891), pp. 48 ff.

13. DANILEWSKY, B. Zur Parasitologie des Blutes, Biol. Centralbl., **5**:529, 1885–86.

Danilewsky, under the heading of "The Hematozoa of Birds," enumerated three forms. The description of the third form—clear rings which assume a spherical shape when more developed—could hardly have been anything else than "bird malaria." No analogy to the parasites of human malaria is suggested.

Many varieties of malaria in birds were later described; they have been of immense importance in the development of knowledge of the disease. The epoch-making observations of MacCallum on fertilization (Ref. 24) and of Ross on the cycle in the mosquito (Ref. 27) were made with bird malaria. Finally, during the second World War, innumerable potential antimalarials were screened by means of their effect on malaria of ducks.

14. COUNCILMAN, W. T., and ABBOTT, A. C. A contribution to the pathology of malarial fever, Am. J.M. Sc., **89**:416, 1885.

Although the prevalence of malaria in Italy and North Africa stimulated the early work of French and Italian observers, interest was soon aroused in this country. The foreign reports had hardly appeared, before enthusiastic young American physicians began to study the subject in those regions of the eastern seaboard where malaria was prevalent. However, most of this work was done in a spirit of confirming or disproving those foreign observations which were the subject of active controversy. Councilman and Abbott described in meticulous detail the lesions in two patients dead of "comatose malaria." They described the intense pigmentation of the organs and the small cerebral vessels choked with pigmented hyaline masses as if they were outlined in ink. The writers discussed the controversy as to a bacillary or protozoal cause and, like many early

[3] For a full discussion of nomenclature see Sir Gordon Covell, P. F. Russell, and N. H. Swellengrebel, *Malaria Terminology* ("Monograph Series" [Geneva: World Health Organization, 1953]).

writers, begged the question. "We confess our inability to say what these hyaline bodies are."

In the same year Councilman ("Certain elements found in the blood in cases of malarial fever," Tr. A. Am. Physicians, **1**:89, 1886) presented a critical discussion of the whole subject at the Association of American Physicians. "What the real nature of this body is—whether it is a parasite and the cause of malaria . . . time and further investigation will show." In the discussion Osler said: "I am not prepared to give a positive opinion as to the nature of these bodies. They look to me more like vacuoles or areas of hyaline transformation than definite organisms." One year later Councilman had described and accepted the parasites as the cause of malaria, and he clearly related different forms of the parasite to different clinical types of disease; "where the crescentic or elongated masses are found he has either some form of remittent [not intermittent] fever or malarial cachexia" ("Further observations on the blood in cases of malarial fever," M. News, **50**:59, 1887).

Another early American student who did important work was Sternberg, who reviewed the literature and described confirmatory observations of his own. He was inclined to accept the parasites as the cause of malaria (George M. Sternberg, "The malarial 'germ' of Laveran," M. Rec., **29**:489, 517, 1886).

Finally, there should be mentioned the later studies of Osler ("The haematozoa of malaria," Brit. M.J., **1**:557, 1887), who observed the parasites, now related them to malaria, and discussed their diagnostic value.

Many other Americans at about this time contributed useful studies on malaria, but they made no fundamental advances. All this work is reviewed by Laveran (Ref. 11) and by Thayer (Ref. 22).

> 15. GOLGI, Camillo. Sull'infezione malarica, Arch. per le sc. med., **10**:109, 1886; abstract in German by Carl Günther, Fortschr. d. Med., **4**:575, 1886.

As everyone came to accept the parasitic cause of malaria, it was natural to inquire whether the different forms of fever were caused by special types of plasmodia. Laveran (Ref. 11, 1884, p. 196) said that "one could raise the question of whether in the intermittent fevers the nature of the parasitic elements varies with the type of fever." He came, however, to no definite conclusion. Golgi took the first step toward distinguishing different types of parasites when he observed that in the quartan fevers prevalent in Pavia it took the whole length of the clinical cycle for the parasites, which developed in orderly fashion, to reach the segmented stage. He also observed that segmentation preceded a paroxysm and that immediately thereafter the parasites seemed to disappear from the blood, only to return as the cycle was renewed. *He did not, however, in this paper positively claim that there was a special race of parasites in quartan fever*, although his pictures show beautifully that the segmenters always consisted of less than twelve merozoites. Golgi stated that the ameboid non-pigmented forms were probably distinct from the pigmented forms, although in a later paper (Ref. 16) he denied this.

A little later Golgi ("Ancora sulla infezione malarica," Gazz. d. osp., **7**:419, 1886; German abstract, Fortschr. d. Med., **4**:692, 1886) extended these meticulous observations to tertian fevers. The findings were analogous to those in quartan fever, as far as an orderly development of the parasitic cycle is concerned; the differences between quartan and tertian parasites are well described. Golgi did not, as yet, positively assert that these were immutably different species.

16. GOLGI, Camillo. Sul ciclo evolutivo dei parasiti malarici nella febbre terzana, Arch. per le sc. med., **13**:173, 1889. (German translation: Ueber den Entwickelungskreislauf der Malaria Parasiten bei der Ferbris tertiana, Fortschr. d. Med., **7**:81, 1889.)

By 1889 Golgi had clearly settled the fact that the various clinical forms of malaria were caused by distinct races of parasites. The well-known differences between the parasites of tertian and quartan fevers are systematically summarized. He noted that the early forms of tertian were more motile than quartan and that there was less early pigment formation; he observed the rapid decolorization of the red cells in tertian and the difference in number of segments in the two forms; he saw that the quartan merozoites were larger than the tertian and that the quartan parasites had larger pigment granules. He also described bodies which may well have been sexual forms. In addition, he said: "We now have reason to speak of still a third variety of malaria which is linked with the presence of the crescent-like bodies of Laveran." He noted the resistance to quinine of these bodies and pointed out the "irregular development" of the younger forms in this sort of (estivo-autumnal) malaria. The article is a classic and must be read in detail.

It is of interest that, as late as 1891, Laveran denied the existence of several parasites and, indeed, of more than one form of malaria. "In 1884 I reached the conclusion that the different forms under which the hematozoa of malaria present themselves belong to one and the same polymorphous parasite; since then I have always defended this opinion" (Ref. 11, 1891, p. 126).

The cycle of estivo-autumnal fever was worked out by Marchiafava and Celli, whose preliminary report appeared in Riforma med., **5**:1281, 1889, and by Canalis, Riforma med., **5**:1443, 1889. The proof of a separate species was given by other Italian investigators (Tito Gualdo and Enrico Antolisei, "Inoculazione delle forme semilunari di Laveran," Riforma med., **5**:1640, 1889), who gave a paretic person 2 cc. of blood intravenously from a patient whose blood contained crescents. The recipient developed malaria with crescents.

An immense amount of further work on the details of the parasitic cycle in relation to clinical events was carried out in the next few years, largely by the Italian school. These papers are reviewed in detail by Thayer and Hewetson (Ref. 22).

17. ROMANOWSKY, D. Zur Frage der Parasitologie und Therapie der Malaria, St. Petersburg med. Wchnschr., **15**:297, 307, 1891.

No sooner had the parasites been generally accepted as living bodies than many workers began to study the details of their structure. The early work is reviewed by Thayer and Hewetson (Ref. 22, p. 45). Romanowsky in this paper described the staining methods which still bear his name and reported important histologic studies of the malarial parasite.

An authoritative modern discussion is to be found in *Manual for the Microscopic Diagnosis of Malaria in Man,* by Aimee Wilcox (National Institutes of Health Bull. 180 [2d ed., rev.; Washington, D.C.: Federal Security Agency,

Public Health Service, 1950]). Both technical matters, such as the preparation of films, and the finer microscopic appearances of various forms of parasite are described.

18. MARCHIAFAVA, E., and BIGNAMI, A. Sulla febbre malariche estivo-autumnali. Roma: E. Loescher, 1892. (English translation by J. Harry Thompson [London: New Sydenham Society, 1894].)

Following the original work of Marchiafava and Celli (Ref. 12), there was an immense resurgence of malarial study by the "young Roman" group of physicians. To be mentioned are Celli, Bignami, Bastianelli, Grassi, Feletti, and others. We cannot list the numerous papers, but their work dealt with the significance of the various parasitic bodies, the life-cycle of the parasites, their relation to the course of the disease, the effects of quinine upon them, and clinical classification and description of the various fevers in relation to the type of parasite involved.

Most of this work was summarized in this important book of Marchiafava and Bignami. They clearly described the different species of parasites and emphasized the spherical forms as the important part of the cycle, whereas Laveran had stressed the mobile filaments as the completed parasite. They perceived the relation between liberation of the "spores" by segmentation and the paroxysm; related the crescents to estivo-autumnal fever but thought that they were degenerated forms of the parasite; studied in detail the relation of quinine to inhibition of the parasite at various stages of the cycle; described accurately the malignant and comatose forms; and related them to plugging of the cerebral vessels by parasite-containing red cells. They had no idea of the sexual cycle and no inkling of the real meaning of crescents and flagella. There are excellent illustrations of parasites. This book is a storehouse of knowledge of the whole subject to date.

19. SAKHAROFF, N. Recherches sur les hématozoaires des oiseaux, Ann. Inst. Pasteur, 7:801, 1893.

There had been great dispute as to the significance of the flagella of malarial parasites. Some, especially the Italian school, thought of them as degenerative dying forms; to others they seemed to be active bodies which must fulfil some important purpose. Sakharoff noted that the flagella of "crow malaria" contained nuclear material. "In our opinion the exit of chromatic filaments from the parasite and their energetic movements in their free state in the blood plasma are facts which could be of general significance in cellular biology."

This was soon to be verified by the observations of Simond (Ref. 23) and of MacCallum (Ref. 24) and elaborated many years later by MacDougall (Ref. 49).

20. MANNABERG, Julius. Die Malaria Parasiten. Vienna: A. Hölder, 1893. (English translation by R. W. Felkin [London: New Sydenham Society, 1894].)

This scholarly book gives an authoritative summary to date of the knowledge of the malarial parasite based on Mannaberg's own work and on a comprehensive review of the literature. Mannaberg pointed out the widely differing views on crescents and, on the basis of morphology, thought it likely that they were concerned with reproduction. From inoculation experiments in which the type of parasite in the injected blood was almost always found in the disease which was produced, he concluded that each parasite is a true species which does not undergo a transformation into other forms; there was a definite relation between the species of parasite and the type of fever. He had no idea how the disease was transmitted and was puzzled by the varying length of the incubation period. There are detailed descriptions of the parasites at all stages of the cycle and beautiful plates of both stained and fresh preparations.

21. MANSON, Patrick. On the nature and significance of the crescentic and flagellated bodies in malarial blood, Brit. M.J., **2**:1306, 1894.

The story of the association of the mosquito with malaria is of great interest. One wonders over and over again how the causal relation could have been missed in view of the close association of mosquitoes with the circumstances of the disease.

King, in a much-quoted paper (A. F. A. King, "Insects and disease—mosquitoes and malaria," Pop. Sc. Month., **33**:644, 1883), without any reference to the parasite, gave an orderly argument in favor of the mosquito as the transmitting agent. This is based on analogy to other mosquito-transmitted diseases—filariasis and perhaps yellow fever—and on the association of mosquitoes with malaria. King, of course, did not know just how such transmission was brought about. Laveran (Ref. 11, 1891, p. 147) remarked that "perhaps these insects [mosquitoes] play a role in the propagation of malaria as they do in filariasis," but he pursued the idea no further. Similarly, others had mentioned more or less casually the possibility of insect transmission, but no one seemed inclined to perform any purposeful experiments until Manson. There is a good review of the early literature in Nuttall's monograph (Ref. 30, pp. 75 ff.).

Manson's paper seems to be the first in which any really impressive claim was made. Manson described and emphasized the forms later known to be gametocytes, described exflagellation, and reasoned clearly that the crescents and analogous spherical forms as well as flagella must have something to do with the propagation of the malarial process outside the human body. As there was no evidence that the parasites left the body in the excreta or through the skin, since the disease could be transmitted by injection of blood from malaria patients and since filariasis, a disease in many ways analogous to malaria, had been proved to be transmitted by the mosquito, Manson concluded that malaria also must be transmitted either by the mosquito or by some other suctorial insect. He postulated a cycle in the mosquito but thought that it was not worth speculating further when experimental work could easily be done; this he hoped someone would achieve in the proper area, such as India. Manson's argument clearly included the flagella as an active and essential part of the cycle produced only outside the human host, and not as a degenerative stage of the parasite, as the Italian school held (Ref. 18). Manson did not know what happened in the mosquito or how the parasite returned to man; he did not state that it must be by mosquito bite but at first rather thought it was by way of ingestion of water contaminated by infected mosquito larvae.

22. THAYER, William Sidney, and HEWETSON, John. The malarial fevers of Baltimore, Johns Hopkins Hosp. Rep., **5**:3, 1895.

This monograph is the first comprehensive and authoritative American work on malaria.[4] There is a thorough review of the literature, with a bibliography of 359 references dealing with all the early experimental work. The authors' own meticulous clinical and parasitological observations are next presented, and finally the classical drawings of malarial parasites by Max Broedel are here reproduced for the first time. Supplementary to this report is Thayer's *Lectures on the Malarial Fevers* (New York: D. Appleton & Co., 1897). These works are definitive to date and still make exciting and valuable reading.

> 23. SIMOND, P.-L. L'Évolution des sporozoaires du genre Coccidium, Ann. Inst. Pasteur, **11**:545, 1897.

Simond, working with *Coccidium oviforme*, concluded that the flagellate bodies are male sexual forms. He did not actually observe conjugation but paved the way for MacCallum's work (Ref. 24). "The mobile stage of *Coccidium* gives the most rational explanation of the flagella of malaria . . . we should recognize the possibility of conjugation necessary for the production of a resistant form."

> 24. MacCALLUM, W. G. On the flagellated form of the malarial parasite, Lancet, **2**:1240, 1897.

In this brief paper MacCallum, working with the malaria of crows (Halteridium), vividly described the formation of flagella and their conjugation with other sexual forms. "The granular forms lie quiet beside the nuclei and shadows of the red blood corpuscles which lately contained them, but are soon seen to be approached by the flagella which, having torn themselves away from the hyaline organism from whose protoplasm they were formed, struggle about among the corpuscles—one of them plunges its head into the sphere and finally wriggles its whole body into that organism." This epoch-making observation was confirmed in the case of a woman with estivo-autumnal fever and finally resolved the numerous erroneous speculations of previous observers as to the significance of flagellated forms.

This paper was preceded by a brief note in the Johns Hopkins Hospital Bulletin describing conjugation ("On the haematozoan infection of birds," **8**:235, 1897), in which MacCallum gave Opie credit for describing the hyaline and granular sexual forms and for suggesting that the hyaline bodies gave rise to flagella (see E. L. Opie, "On the haemocytozoa of birds," J. Exper. Med., **3**:79, 1898). In a later paper ("On the haematozoan infections of birds," J. Exper. Med., **3**:117, 1898), MacCallum described the process of flagella formation and conjugation in much more detail, with a good drawing of the process. He had no idea, however, of the subsequent fate of the fertilized cell and made no mention of the mosquito. An analysis of previous views of the significance of flagellation is a useful part of this paper.[5]

---

[4] The book by George M. Sternberg, *Malaria and Malarial Diseases* (New York: W. Wood & Co., 1884), is definitely premodern in tone, and there is no mention of the parasite which Laveran had described four years previously.

[5] It is of interest that in historical accounts and in bibliographies (see, for example, F. H. Garrison and L. T. Morton, *Medical Bibliography* [London:Grafton & Co., 1943], pp. 267–68) the name of E. L. Opie is often coupled with that of W. G MacCallum in this discovery. Both were medical students working at the same time on avian malaria under the supervision of W. S. Thayer. Both presented their observations at the same

25. ROSS, Ronald. Observations on a condition necessary to the transformation of the malaria crescent, Brit. M.J., **1**:251, 1897.

Ross threw himself into the controversy between Manson and Bignami (Amico Bignami, "Le Ipotesi sulla biologia dei parasiti malarici fuori dell'uomo," Policlinico, **3**:320, 1896) on the significance of crescents and of exflagellation. The Italian school, as we have said, looked on this as a degenerative involutional process; in other words, the flagellum was a dying form. Manson, on the other hand, thought that the crescents and flagella represented a vital stage in an extra-corporeal cycle of the parasite. Exflagellation presumably did not occur in human circulating blood but only after the blood had been altered in some fashion. Ross showed that if mosquitoes fed on a patient whose blood contained many crescents, there was a rapid change within the insect from crescent to sphere to exflagellation. In this paper he went no further in elucidating the cycle in the mosquito.

26. ROSS, Ronald. On some peculiar pigmented cells found in two mosquitos fed on malarial blood, Brit. M.J., **2**: 1786, 1897.

In this paper Ross went a step further. In mosquitoes fed on patients whose blood contained many crescents, he later found peculiar pigmented cells which suggested the presence of a parasitic stage. The specimens were sent to authorities in England; no one was certain, but Manson wrote: "Considering the peculiar groupings of the pigment in many instances, a grouping that forcibly recalls what one sees in the living malaria parasite, and the distinctness and regularity of the outlines of the bodies, I am inclined to think that Ross may have found the extra-corporeal phase of malaria."[6]

27. [ROSS]. The role of the mosquito in the evolution of the malarial parasite: the recent researches of Surgeon-Major Ronald Ross, I.M.S., Lancet, **2**:488, 1898.

---

meeting of the Johns Hopkins Hospital Medical Society on November 16, 1896, and their preliminary findings were published in the Johns Hopkins Hospital Bulletin (**8**:51, 1897). Neither then nor later, however, did they publish jointly, and Opie to all intents seems to have disclaimed the fertilization idea when he wrote: "After a while individual flagella not infrequently become detached and float away, continuing their active serpentine movements. After persisting for some time the flagella become less active and finally disappear, by exactly what process can not be said in every case" ("On the haemocytozoa of birds," J. Exper. Med., **3**:95, 1898). Can it be that these brilliant medical students disagreed and that Opie did not accept, at least at the time, MacCallum's observation?

[6] In reading textbook accounts of these transactions (for example, P. F. Russell, L. S. West, and R. O. Manwell, *Practical Malariology* [Philadelphia: W. B. Saunders Co., 1946], p. 11), one gets the impression that Ross suddenly saw a parasite developing in the mosquito and that he "had no doubt that he was looking at the malaria parasite." Nothing could be more misleading. Ross's ideas evolved gradually and painfully in the course of immense labor. "It would of course be absurd to attempt final conclusions as yet," "they seem to open the question of their being indeed the form of haemamoeba we are in search of," "the parasitic nature of the cells cannot finally be accepted until certain facts as to structure, sporulation and so on have been demonstrated" are phrases which Ross used in his paper. The whole story is vividly told in Ross's memoirs (Ref. 39, pp. 225 ff.).

At the meeting of the British Medical Association, Manson reported the latest news of Ross's investigations on bird malaria (Proteosoma) in India. Ross had found that the pigmented bodies (Ref. 26) progress to "coccidia," which penetrate the stomach of the mosquito and protrude into the celom. "The coccidia now burst and . . . germinal vermicules which had been formed in its interior are set free in the body, blood and tissues of the mosquito. Then came . . . the discovery of those vermicules in the veneno-salivary glands of the mosquito." Finally, Ross allowed mosquitoes to feed on infected birds and a few days later permitted these insects to bite birds whose blood was "void of any parasite infection." The birds became infected, and their blood was charged with parasites. "Thus the analogy between bird and human infection has only to be proved to establish that the mosquito is a carrier of malaria and an infector of man." The modest wording does not convey the full import of Ross's epochal clarification of the malarial cycle in the mosquito and the proof that the parasite was conveyed to man by bite and not by infected water.

This report was amplified a little later by a communication by Ross to the British Medical Journal ("Mosquitos and malaria," **1**:432, 1899); for Ross's other numerous communications on his discoveries the reader is referred to the bibliography given in his memoirs (Ref. 39).

While Ross is clearly responsible for tracing the cycle in the mosquito from gametocyte through to the salivary gland, he did not himself observe fertilization in the stomach blood of the mosquito, as Schaudinn did later (Ref. 35), and he did not have an opportunity personally to produce malaria in volunteers with human strains, as Manson did (Ref. 29), or to study the cycle of a human parasite in the mosquito until 1899 (Ref. 31).

28. ROSS, Ronald. The possibility of extirpating malaria from certain locations by a new method, Brit. M.J., **2**:1, 1899.

Laveran as early as 1891 (Ref. 11, p. 147) remarked: "Mosquitoes always abound in malarial regions and one notes that soil drainage which suppressed the fevers, also suppresses the mosquitoes. . . . Perhaps these insects play a part in the propagation of malaria as they do in filariasis." He pursued the matter no further at the time.

But no sooner had the spread of malaria by the mosquito been proved than men of wide vision began to think about mass preventive measures. It is almost unbelievable how resistant physicians in general were to these ideas, as well as the bureaucrats without whose support nothing could be done. Ross, a pioneer in malaria control, told vividly about these difficulties in his memoirs (Ref. 39). In the present paper he discussed measures for eliminating the types of mosquito which carry malaria by draining and otherwise getting rid of the fresh-water pools in which they bred. This method of malaria prevention—mosquito control—has, of course, been of immense importance in the subsequent history of the subject. Koch, on the other hand (Ref. 32), was doubtful about the feasibility of eliminating mosquitoes but, on the basis of his work in Africa, proposed giving quinine to everyone infected with malaria, especially in the chronic cases with no fever, to prevent the mosquitoes from ingesting parasites. Manson (Ref. 29) laid emphasis on screening.

It is impossible in this bibliography to list all the important work on preventive and other public health measures in malaria. The brilliant work of Ross in Sierra Leone, the triumphs of Gorgas in Havana and in the Canal Zone, the useful efforts in the South Pacific in World War II require an extensive bibliography of their own (but see Ref. 36).

29. MANSON, Patrick. Experimental proof of the mosquito-malaria theory, Brit. M.J., **2**:949, 1900.

It is hard now to appreciate the general resistance in 1900 to belief in the mosquito theory of malaria transmission. Although A. Bignami ("The inoculation theory of malarial infection," Lancet, 2:1461, 1541, 1898) claimed in 1898 to have transmitted human malaria in Italy by mosquito bite, many people were unconvinced. In Manson's classical demonstration, infected mosquitoes were sent from Rome to London and there allowed, on August 29, to bite a volunteer (Manson's son), who developed typical malaria on September 13, with tertian parasites in the blood, and who was cured by quinine.[7] Conversely, Drs. Sanborn and Low and Signor Terzi set up a mosquito-proof hut in an intensely malarial spot in Italy and lived in it from July to September without acquiring malaria, "in marked contrast to their neighbors who were all of them either ill with fever or had suffered malarial attacks." Manson drew important conclusions from these experiments as to malaria control and prevention.

30. NUTTALL, George H. F. On the role of insects, arachnids and myriapods as carriers in the spread of bacterial and parasitic diseases of man and animals: a critical and historical study, Johns Hopkins Hosp. Rep., **8**:1, 1900.

This is a valuable review of parasites in relation to disease, including malaria, with useful bibliography of early work on mosquitoes and mosquito control.

31. GRASSI, Battista. Studi di uno zoologa sulla malaria. Rome: Tipografia della R. Accademia dei Lincei, 1900; also 2d ed., 1901.

This classical monograph, handsomely printed, with beautiful color plates, deals with the work to date of the "Roman school" on every phase of malaria in relation to mosquitoes. The book has been bitterly attacked by Ross (Ref. 39) and others on the grounds of plagiarism. The Italians certainly took advantage of the fact that Ross had not had the opportunity to follow the cycle of *human* strains of malarial parasites in the mosquito to belittle his work.[8] However, we must let the individual reader adjudicate this dispute,[9] and, at any rate, the book is a storehouse of valuable information on mosquito transmission.

32. KOCH, R. Zusammenfassende Darstellung der Ergebnisse der Malaria Expedition, Deutsche med. Wchnschr., **26**:781, 801, 1900.

[7] This story is vividly retold in Ross's memoirs (Ref. 39, p. 417), and there is a complete summary of all the early mosquito inoculations in Ross, Ref. 36, pp. 77 ff.

[8] A note in the British Medical Journal (**2**:608, 1899) entitled "The cultivation of the malarial quartan parasite in Anopheles" is a report of a telegram from Ross in Africa stating that he had studied the quartan cycle in the mosquito.

[9] For a fair appraisal of the claims of Ross and of the Italian school see George H. F. Nuttall, "On the question of priority with regard to certain discoveries upon the etiology of malarial diseases," Quart. J. Micr. Sc., **44**, Part I, 429, 1900.

Koch, working in New Guinea, was one of the first to emphasize splenomegaly as an index of the degree of malarial infection in a locality. He found it most common in children three to six years old who had had no evidence of active malaria for 2–3 years. By the time these children were fourteen to fifteen years old, the splenic tumor was no longer palpable; other evidence of malaria had also disappeared. Koch thought all this due to an immunity reaction. Ross (Ref. 36, p. 127) discussed the matter systematically and introduced the term "average spleen index." This has turned out to be very important from the epidemiologic and immunologic standpoints.

33. GILES, George M. Handbook of the gnats or mosquitos. London: J. Bale Sons & Danielsson, 1900; also 2d ed., rewritten and enlarged, 1902.

During the whole of Ross's work on transmission, the definition of the varieties of mosquito which were carriers of malaria presented one of the great difficulties. Mosquito classification in various areas was still inadequate, and Ross did not at first speak of *Anopheles* or *Culex* but described the insects as gray or brown, dapple-winged, and so forth. It was the gradual evolution of the work of many students which led to the conclusion that only certain strains of *Anopheles* were capable of transmitting malaria.

Giles's elaborate book was one of the early treatises in which mosquitoes were systematically described and those which transmitted malaria were identified. During the whole history of malaria studies it has been necessary to appraise the type of mosquito at fault in various regions where the disease was encountered. A key to the mosquitoes of the Australasian region was issued early in World War II (K. L. Knight, R. M. Bohart, and G. E. Bohart [Washington: National Research Council, Division of Medical Sciences, 1944], issued by the Office of Medical Information). A list of malaria-transmitting anophelines is given in C. F. Craig and E. C. Faust, *Clinical Parasitology* (4th ed.; Philadelphia: Lea & Febiger, 1945), p. 642; in P. F. Russell, L. S. West, and R. O. Manwell, *Practical Malariology* (Philadelphia: W. B. Saunders Co., 1946), p. 587; and in T. T. Mackie, G. W. Hunter, and C. B. Watt, *A Manual of Tropical Medicine* (2d ed.; Philadelphia: W. B. Saunders Co., 1954), p. 294.

34. ROSS, Ronald. Malarial fever, its cause, prevention and treatment. London: Longmans, Green & Co., 1902.

Although most of the principal facts about malaria were known by 1900, people in general were reluctant to accept the mosquito theory of transmission and its epidemiologic implications.

This little book by Ross is a classic. In simple terms all the fundamental knowledge about the disease ("containing full details for the use of travellers, sportsmen, soldiers, and residents in malarious places") is set forth, with special emphasis on the public health aspects, proper methods of using quinine, and so forth. "But there is no longer any reason at all why we should suppose that the infection of malaria rises from water or soil. . . . *It is not the germ which rises from stagnant water; it is the carrier of the germ which does so*" (author's italics). The book did a great deal toward education of the public about malaria.

As early as 1900, Ross (J. Soc. Arts, **49**:17, 1900) read a vigorous paper on malaria and mosquitoes. It concludes with a strenuous plea for the government to apply the obvious preventive measures for malaria: "In my opinion the period of probation has been completed and the time for action has arrived. Nothing will stimulate public action in this matter so much as will the authoritative support of our principal men of science."

35. SCHAUDINN, Fritz. Studien über Krankheitserregende Protozoen. II. Plasmodium vivax (Grassi und Feletti) der Erreger des Tertianfiebers beim Menschen, Arb. a. d. k. Gsndhtsamte, **19**:169, 1903.

In this thorough monograph on the life-cycle of the tertian parasite, Schaudinn gave a minute and vivid description of fertilization in blood withdrawn from the stomach of mosquitoes who had fed on a patient with clinical malaria, thus amplifying the work of MacCallum (Ref. 24) and of Ross (Ref. 25). There are plates illustrating graphically the various stages of the process.

In this communication Schaudinn also described sporozoites (from mosquito bite) actively penetrating and invading the red cells. This work has never been confirmed, but belief in Schaudinn's observations held back for many years work on the exo-erythrocytic cycle (Refs. 46, 50).

36. ROSS, Ronald. The prevention of malaria. London: John Murray, 1910.

This is a comprehensive discussion of every phase of malaria prevention, definitive to date. There are contributions by a number of authorities in addition to Ross. A recent authoritative summary is that of Sir Gordon Covell, "Current research toward a global control of malaria," New England J. Med., **249**:125, 1953.

37. BASS, C. C., and JOHNS, Foster M. The cultivation of malaria plasmodia (Plasmodium vivax and Plasmodium falciparum) in vitro, J. Exper. Med., **16**:567, 1912.

From the time of the discovery of the parasite, attempts at cultivation have been made. These early efforts, in spite of some claims of success, were all clearly failures. A number of interesting experiments were, however, made on survival of the parasites in leeches which had fed on malarial patients. O. Rosenbach ("Die Conservierung lebender Malariaparasiten," Berl. klin. Wchnschr., **28**:839, 1891) believed that such parasites remained alive at least 48 hours. N. Sacharoff ("Ueber den Einfluss der Kälte auf die Lebensfähigkeit der Malariaparasiten," Centralbl. f. Bakt., **15**:158, 1894) found parasites still motile in leeches which had fed 7 days before. Thayer and his associates confirmed these findings (Ref. 22, *Lectures*, p. 27).

Bass in 1911 had made a preliminary note ("A new conception of immunity," J.A.M.A., **57**:1534, 1911) on his cultivation work, but this is the definitive report. The technique is given in full. "In successive cultures the asexual parasites grow, segment, and form rosettes, which burst and give rise to merozoites, many of which enter new red blood cells in exactly the same manner as they do in the body of man." It was important that *Plasmodium vivax* and *P. falciparum* cultivated in identical fashion remained distinct. The subject was carried further, and its difficulties and complexities were discussed by W. Trager ("Studies on conditions affecting the survival in vitro of a malarial parasite [*Plasmodium lophurae*]," J. Exper. Med., **74**:441, 1941, and "Studies on the extracellular cultivation of an intracellular parasite [avian malaria]," *ibid.*, **92**:349, 1950). Geiman and his associates (Q. M. Geiman, C. B. Anfinsen, R. W. McKee, R. A.

Ormsbee, and E. G. Ball, "Studies on malarial parasites. VII. Methods and techniques for cultivation," J. Exper. Med., **84**:583, 1946) also have a valuable paper on the problem of cultivation. F. Hawking reviewed attempts to grow malarial plasmodia in tissue culture ("Tissue culture of plasmodia," Brit. M. Bull., **8**:16, 1951). The upshot of all this work is that, as yet, there is no simple, reliable method of cultivating human malarial parasites through successive generations.

38. WAGNER-JAUREGG. Die Behandlung der progressiven Paralyse und Tabes, Wien. med. Wchnschr., **71**:1106, 1210, 1921.

The early inoculation experiments (Refs. 10, 12) were carried out purely to determine the transmissibility of malaria. Wagner-Jauregg, however, introduced inoculation malaria as a means of causing therapeutic fever in general paresis. While the subsequent huge literature (authoritatively reviewed by J. E. Moore, *The Modern Treatment of Syphilis* [2d ed.; Springfield, Ill.: Charles C Thomas, 1941], pp. 374 ff.) deals largely with the results of treatment, valuable data have also been accumulated on the natural history of inoculation malaria (for example, Warrington Yorke and J. W. S. McFie, "Observations on malaria made during treatment of general paresis," Tr. Roy. Soc. Trop. Med. & Hyg., **18**:13, 1924), and its value in the study of immunologic questions and as a means of testing therapeutic agents has been widely explored. N. Kopeloff ("Inoculation malaria: sexual and asexual strains," Am. J.M. Sc., **197**:800, 1930), for example, noted that, after 7 months of transfer through patients, a strain began to lose its capacity to produce gametocytes and became asexual. A condensation of Wagner-Jauregg's article soon appeared in English ("The treatment of general paresis by inoculation of malaria," J. Nerv. & Ment. Dis., **55**:369, 1922).

39. ROSS, Ronald. Memoirs, with a full account of the great malaria problem and its solution. London: John Murray, 1923.

In the course of these fascinating memoirs Ross tells the intimate story of his malaria research. During the years in which this work was done (*ca.* 1895–1900) Ross was a bitter, disappointed man. He had to work under the most adverse conditions, he was frustrated over and over again by an incredibly stupid bureaucracy, and, when the discovery was finally made, presumably reputable scientists tried to steal his glory, and a skeptical public was inert to the tremendous sanitary implications. Ross was essentially an idealist and a humanitarian. His discovery thrilled him not as a biologist but because it indicated the way to elimination of a dread disease. As he pointed out, he was a sanitarian rather than a zoölogist. The book is a mine of source material and should be read by everyone interested in malaria or public health.

40. SINTON, J. A., and BIRD, W. Studies on malaria, with special reference to treatment: plasmoquine in the treatment of malaria, Indian J.M. Research, **16**:159, 1928.

Plasmochin (pamaquine), a synthetic quinoline derivative, had been described as an antimalarial drug in 1926 by Schulemann and others (Weiner Schulemann and Guglielmo Mennini, "Plasmochin, ein Synthetisches gegen die Malariainfection wirksames Chinolin-Derivat," Arch. Schiffs- u. Tropen-Hyg., **30**:59,

1926, Beih. 3). At that time the importance of differentiating the action on the erythrocytic and on the exoerythrocytic stages of the parasite was not well understood, and, as the suppressive and preventive actions of the drug were not outstandingly better than quinine and there were important toxic symptoms, its use was not pushed. Sinton and Bird first clearly demonstrated the action of plasmochin in preventing relapses, that is, in producing radical cure. Sinton, J. Smith, and D. Pottinger continued these studies ("Studies in malaria with special reference to treatment. XII. Further researches into the treatment of chronic benign tertian malaria with plasmoquine and quinine," Indian J.M. Research, **17**:793, 1930) and showed that, in situations where the relapse rate was 70 per cent or more in patients treated with quinine only, the addition of plasmochin reduced the relapses to 30 per cent or less. Other reports to the same general effect were those of S. James, W. Nicol, and P. Shute ("The prevention of malaria with plasmochine," Lancet, **2**:341, 1931); of H. Most, C. Kane, P. Lavietes, I. London, E. Schroeder, and J. Hayman ("Combined quinine-plasmochin treatment of vivax malaria: effect on relapse rate," Am. J.M. Sc., **212**:550, 1946), working with Pacific strains of vivax; and of R. Berliner, D. Earle, J. Taggart, W. Welch, C. Zubrod, P. Knowlton, J. Atchley, and J. Shannon ("Studies on the chemotherapy of human malarias. VII. The antimalarial activity of pamaquine," J. Clin. Investigation, **27**:Part 2, 108, 1948) with experimentally induced *vivax* and *falciparum* malaria. Here again pamaquine had a relatively feeble suppressive effect, even in maximal doses. If the schizogenous cycle was interrupted by quinine, then the curative (antirelapse) effect was evident in *vivax* malaria.

41. MAUSS, H., and MIETSCH, F. Atebrin, ein neues Heilmittel gegen Malaria, Klin. Wchnschr., **12**:1276, 1933.

The writers discuss the composition and properties of Atabrine (quinacrine U.S.P.), which was soon recognized as a valuable antimalarial. Early trials (F. M. Peter, "Ueber die Wirkung des Atebrin gegen natürliche Malariainfection," Deutsche med. Wchnschr., **58**:533, 1932; L. E. Napier and B. M. Das Gupta, "Atebrin: synthetic drug for treatment of malaria," Indian M. Gaz., **67**:181, 1932; R. Green, "Report on 50 cases of malaria treated with Atebrin," Lancet, **1**:826, 1932) did not fully answer the question of whether Atabrine was fundamentally superior to quinine, although it has recently been claimed that Atabrine gives more prompt and effective control of parasitemia and symptoms and promotes longer intervals until relapse (Harry Most and Joseph M. Hayman, Jr., "Relative efficiency of quinacrine [Atabrine] and quinine in treatment of acute attacks of vivax malaria," Am. J.M. Sc., **211**:320, 1946). A shortage of quinine during World War II led to renewed study of Atabrine. It was shown that its chemotherapeutic activity was a simple function of the plasma concentration ("Plasma quinacrine concentration as a function of dosage and environment: a joint report of the Armored Medical Research Laboratory, Fort Knox, Kentucky, and the Commission on Tropical Diseases, Army Epidemiological Board, Preventive Medicine Service, Office of the Surgeon General, United States Army," Arch. Int. Med., **78**:64, 1946). This work led to more intelligent dosage schedules for suppression and therapy of acute attacks. The failure to prevent relapses (radical cure), the development of more effective drugs, and the occurrence of severe toxic symptoms have led to its displacement. The violent skin reactions are described in a series of articles in the Bulletin of the U.S. Army Medical Department (4:653, 687, 724, 725, 1925).

42. EATON, Paul. Susceptibility of red cells to malaria, Am. J. Trop. Med., 14:431, 1934.

The question has often been raised of why malarial parasites do not multiply until every blood cell is infected. Eaton offered an explanation of this in a case of inoculation malaria (presumably tertian) when he found that the parasite seemed only to invade the reticulocytes (young cells). He presumed that schizonts, which do not infect, are promptly phagocytosed. This work was amplified by R. Hegner ("Relative frequency of ring-stage plasmodia in reticulocytes and mature erythrocytes in man and monkeys," Am. J. Hyg., 27:690, 1938), who found that tertian parasites mostly invaded young cells but that quartan and *falciparum* parasites were found mainly in mature red cells. The exact meaning of all this work is not clear. It is of interest that R. Craick ("The erythrocyte in malaria," Lancet, 1:1110, 1920) had found that stippled red cells resulting from ingestion of lead were prone to invasion by *P. vivax*.

43. HAGGIS, A. W. Fundamental errors in the early history of cinchona, Bull. Hist. Med., 10:417, 1941.

For some three hundred years, until the development of quinacrine, cinchona bark or its alkaloids were the only effective therapy for malaria; history owes quinine an unrepayable debt, even though in the last ten years it has been largely replaced by more effective drugs (Refs. 40, 47, 51, 53). Haggis, in an important study, seems to disprove the traditional view that the Countess of Chinchon introduced the remedy into Spain when she returned with her husband from Peru. The full history of the terms "cinchona" and "quina-quina" is discussed.

At the date when this bibliography begins, the use of Peruvian bark in intermittent fever was common knowledge. The subsequent literature is vast. The quinine alkaloids were extracted by Pelletier and Caventou in 1820 ("Recherches chimiques sur les quinquinas," Ann. chim. et phys., 15:289, 1820) and have been generally used since then. Considerations of the action of quinine important to the clinician are reviewed by Laveran (Ref. 11, 1891, p. 183), by Thayer and Hewetson (Ref. 22), and by Ross (Ref. 36), and a more modern summary is that of Erwin E. Nelson, "Cinchona and its alkaloids in the treatment of malaria," in *A Symposium on Human Malaria* (Washington: American Association for the Advancement of Science, Smithsonian Institution Building, 1941), p. 255. The realization that quinine, even in large doses, could not be depended on for radical cure of malaria became clear when it was found that it failed to eliminate the extra-erythrocytic cycle of the types of malignant *vivax* infection seen in the South Pacific in World War II (Ref. 46).

44. TEMKIN, Owsei, and RAMSAY, Elizabeth. Antimalarial drugs. Washington: National Research Council, Division of Medical Sciences; issued by the Office of Medical Information, 1944.

At the beginning of World War II, quinine was still the standard remedy for malaria, and Atabrine was the only other known drug which had any noteworthy effect. The shortage of the supply of quinine due to enemy action and the realization that neither quinine nor Atabrine was effective in completely eradicating the disease and preventing relapses led to a frantic search for new antimalarials; and thousands of prospective compounds were developed and tested. Out of this work came the new drugs which are effective in both suppression and eradication. An idea of the "antimalarial drugs" situation in 1944 is obtained from this monograph, "intended to give the general background of present knowledge of the treatment of malaria by drugs under existing war conditions."

It should be emphasized that the few references on chemotherapy which we are able to include in this bibliography give no idea of the thousands of papers dealing with the effects of antimalarials. Authoritative reviews to date are that of J. A. Shannon, "Study of antimalarials and antimalarial activity in human malarias," Harvey Lect., **41**:43, 1945–46, and that of N. Hamilton Fairley, "Malaria. Lecture II. Chemotherapy," Brit. M.J., **2**:891, 1949.

45. ASH, J. E., and SPITZ, Sophie. Pathology of tropical diseases: an atlas, "Malaria," p. 206. Philadelphia and London: W. B. Saunders Co., 1945.

This is an authoritative account, with beautiful plates, of the pathology of malaria. For a full description of the microscopic anatomy with extensive bibliography, consult William H. Taliaferro and H. W. Mulligan, *The Histopathology of Malaria with Special Reference to the Function and Origin of the Macrophages in Defence* ("Indian M. Research Memoirs," [Calcutta, 1933]).

46. FAIRLEY, N. Hamilton. Chemotherapeutic suppression and prophylaxis in malaria, Tr. Roy. Soc. Trop. Med. & Hyg., **38**:311, 1945.

The idea of an exo-erythrocytic phase in human malaria was "in the air" in the 1940's, and Fairley's work brought strong indirect evidence. The failure of such drugs as quinine, which eliminate trophozoite-transmitted (inoculation) malaria, to prevent relapses and produce permanent cure suggests that quinine-resistant forms must be elsewhere in the tissues than in the blood. Fairley also showed by subinoculation experiments that *vivax* sporozoites injected by mosquito bite disappeared from the blood, to reappear 9 days later; he presumed that they were developing outside the circulation. Further elaborate and most instructive observations by Fairley and his associates on the results of subinoculations and the effect of drugs under various conditions ("Researches on Paludrine [M. 4888] in malaria," *ibid.*, **40**:105, 1946; and "Sidelights on malaria in man obtained by subinoculation experiments," *ibid.*, p. 621, 1947) were made in the next few years; but it remained for Shortt and Garnham (Ref. 50) actually to demonstrate the pre-erythrocytic tissue stage in man.

Fairley also presumed that, in contrast to *vivax*, P. *falciparum* has only a short-lived tissue stage; there is a brief pre-erythrocytic stage but no subsequent exo-erythrocytic stage. Radical cure can therefore be achieved by drugs such as quinine, Atabrine, and chloroquine, which have only a suppressive effect in *vivax* malaria. Fairley's important summary of the whole problem should also be consulted (Ref. 52).

The early views on relapses are discussed in Ross's book (Ref. 36, p. 108). Some of these theories were that relapse was due to inadequate quinine therapy or temporary "encystment" of parasites in internal organs, whence they "broke out," or that crescents kept infection going. Ross believed that "rallies" were due to extensive destruction of parasites by some immune process; when this flagged, parasites "escaped" and relapse occurred. Many traumatic factors, such as cold, fatigue, illness, or excessive alcohol, might be precipitating circumstances. C. F. Craig, the great American malariologist ("A study of latent and recurrent malarial infection and the significance of intracorpuscular conjugation in the malarial plasmodia," J. Infect. Dis., **4**:108, 1907) thought that "intracorpuscular conjugation" produced a resting stage of the plasmodia resistant to quinine, which later gave birth to young plasmodia, thus causing a relapse. This view was widely accepted. The true explanation of relapses was not fully understood until the exo-erythrocytic stage of the parasite in man was worked out (Ref. 50).

47. MOST, H., LONDON, I. M., KANE, C. A., LAVIETES, P. H., SCHROEDER, E. F., and HAYMAN, J. M. Chloroquine for treatment of acute attacks of vivax malaria, J.A.M.A., **131**:963, 1946.

Chloroquine, a 4-amino-quinoline derivative, turned out to be one of the most effective of the new synthetic antimalarials developed during the war. Its properties were described in a statement approved by the Board for Coordination of Malarial Studies ("Activity of a new antimalarial agent Chloroquine [S.N. 7618]," J.A.M.A., **130**:1069, 1946). In clinical trials, Most and his associates found it superior to quinine and quinacrine in acute attacks of *vivax* malaria. This finding was generally accepted, but Pullman and his associates soon showed that the relapse rate after treatment with quinine, quinacrine, and chloroquine was about the same, 90 per cent or over (T. N. Pullman, C. Branch, Jr., A. S. Alving, C. M. Whorton, R. Jones, Jr., and L. Eichelberger, "Comparison of chloroquine, quinacrine [Atabrine] and quinine, in the treatment of acute attacks of sporozoite-induced *vivax* malaria [Chesson strain]," J. Clin. Investigation, Vol. **27**, No. 3, Part 2, p. 46, 1948). Hence the drug did not produce radical cure, but it is an important survivor of the vast number of potential antimalarials tested.

48. Symposium on biochemistry of malarial parasites, Fed. Proc., **5**:390, 1946.

Although the subject is outside the scope of this bibliography, those interested will find here several papers which deal authoritatively with this part of the subject.

49. MacDOUGALL, Mary Stuart. Cytological studies of plasmodium: the male gamete, J. Nat. Malaria Soc., **6**:91, 1947.

The significance of the sexual forms gradually became clear through the work of MacCallum (Ref. 24) and others (Ref. 23). It is of interest that chromosomes seem now to have been definitely demonstrated in the various sexual forms. Many interesting and important details are brought out in this paper by MacDougall.

50. SHORTT, H. E., and GARNHAM, P. C. C. The pre-erythrocytic development of Plasmodium cynomolgi and Plasmodium vivax, Tr. Roy. Soc. Trop. Med. & Hyg., **41**:785, 1948.

Although an exo-erythrocytic cycle in bird malaria had been described as early as 1936 and in monkey malaria later (for review of the subject see C. G. Huff and F. J. Coulston, "The development of Plasmodium galenaceum from sporozoite to erythrocytic trophozoite," J. Infect. Dis., **75**:231, 1944), the human exo-erythrocytic cycle was first reported in a brief note by H. E. Shortt, P. C. C. Garnham, G. Covell, and P. G. Shute, "The pre-erythrocytic stage of human malaria, Plasmodium vivax," Brit. M.J., **1**:547, 1948. The findings are described in more detail in the present paper. It is pointed out that, after "inoculation" malaria, there is really no incubation period, whereas, after infection by mosquito bite, there is a "clear cut incubation period varying in length according to the species of parasite." It is also noted that inoculation malaria can be promptly eradicated by drugs, whereas "after sporozoite inoculation [by mosquito] the disease will make its appearance sooner or later in spite of the drug." All this strongly suggested a different sequence of infection with merozoites and sporozoites.

A volunteer was bitten by a huge number of anopheles infected with *P. vivax* and was also given an intravenous injection of an emulsion of infected mosquito salivary glands. Seven days later *liver* biopsy showed "plasmodial masses studded with chromatin particles" which were interpreted as merozoites. Interesting immunologic implications of the extra-erythrocytic cycle are also discussed.

Shortt, Fairley, Covell, Shute, and Garnham ("Pre-erythrocytic stages of Plasmodium falciparum," Tr. Roy. Soc. Trop. Med. & Hyg., **44**:405, 1951) later described the pre-erythrocytic stage of *Plasmodium falciparum* in two volunteers. Liver biopsies on the fourth, fifth, and sixth days after inoculation showed beautifully the pre-erythrocytic schizonts in parenchymal cells.

For a summary of the pertinent literature leading up to the whole question of the pre-erythrocytic and extra-erythrocytic cycle in man see N. Hamilton Fairley's penetrating review (Ref. 52) and P. C. C. Garnham's authoritative summary, with literature, "Exo-erythrocytic schizogony in malaria," Trop. Dis. Bull., **45**:831, 1948. For a brief discussion see the recent article by P. C. C. Garnham, "The life history of the malaria parasite" in *Lectures on the Scientific Basis of Medicine*, **2**:323 (London: Athlone Press, 1954). Thus the sequence has been established in *vivax* malaria of the erythrocytic cycle (in man), the cycle in the mosquito, the pre-erythrocytic cycle in man, erythrocytic cycle again, followed by exo-erythrocytic cycle in tissues.

51. ALVING, A. S., CRAIG, Branch, JONES, Ralph, Jr., WHORTON, C. Merrill, PULLMAN, Theodore N., and EICHELBERGER, Lillian. Pentaquine (Sn-13, 276), a therapeutic agent effective in reducing the relapse rate in *vivax* malaria, J. Clin. Investigation, Vol. **27**, No. 3, Part 2, p. 25, 1948.

In a search for agents which might have a more potent curative effect, the authors (*ibid.*, p. 34) had conducted clinical trials with eighteen analogues of pamaquine. Pentaquine seemed most promising. The drug was tested in volunteers infected with *vivax* malaria. While its effect in suppressing fever and parasitemia was not significantly different from quinine alone or quinine and pentaquine administered concurrently, only one among thirty subjects suffered a relapse. Pentaquine was thought to be somewhat more effective than pama-quine in producing radical cure. This work has been confirmed by others, in-cluding L. T. Coggeshall and R. A. Rice ("Cure of chronic vivax malaria with pentaquine," J.A.M.A., **139**:437, 1949) and B. Straus and J. Gennis ("Evalu-ation of pentaquine as a cure of relapsing vivax malaria," Bull. New York Acad. Med., **24**:395, 1948; "Radical cure of relapsing vivax malaria with pentaquine-quinine: a controlled study," Ann. Int. Med., **33**:1413, 1950).

52. FAIRLEY, N. Hamilton. Malaria, with special reference to certain ex-perimental, clinical and chemotherapeutic investigations, Brit. M.J., **2**:825, 1949.

Innumerable observations on resistance and immunity may be culled from the early writings. King (Ref. 21), for example, noted the resistance of African Negroes to malaria and thought that the pigmentation which gradually devel-oped in white skins as the disease became chronic was a desirable event which indicated increased resistance. Laveran (Ref. 11, 1891, p. 175) recognized the fact that "cures called spontaneous, that is, without the use of quinine, are not rare." He believed, following Metchnikoff, that phagocytosis of parasites by leukocytes and macrophages was the essential factor in immunity. Koch's re-marks (Ref. 32) are also of interest.

Modern views on immunity are summarized by L. T. Coggeshall ("Immunity in malaria," Medicine, **22**:87, 1943), but the position of the extra-erythrocytic phase in immunity is more fully developed by Fairley in this lecture and by P. C. C. Garnham and H. E. Shortt ("Demonstration of a persisting exo-erythrocytic cycle in Plasmodium cynomolgi and its bearing on the production of relapses," Brit. M.J., **1**:1225, 1948). These workers believe that the "anti-parasitic defence mechanism" of the host is directed against the erythrocytic cycle and not against pre-erythrocytic or exo-erythrocytic forms, which seem to be protected against destruction by their situation in the liver cells. They think that there is a "specific cellulo-humoral response" to red cell invasion by the erythrocytic parasites. Clinical immunity does not mean that every parasite is permanently cleared from the blood. The parasites actually seem to be de-stroyed in various internal organs. The relations of latency and relapse to immunity, especially when the situation is modified by therapy, therefore be-come excessively complicated. Another interesting phase is specificity of im-munity to species or even to strains. This question is discussed by Coggeshall (*op. cit.*), and active work, summarized by Young (Ref. 54), is at present going on.

53. GENNIS, Joseph, STRAUS, Bernard, KENNEY, Michael, and KLEIN, Bernard. The use of primaquine for the treatment of malaria in Korean veterans, Am. J. Med., **17**:223, 1954.

Primaquine, still another quinoline derivative, was recently discussed in a com-prehensive report to the Council on Pharmacy and Chemistry ("Status of prima-quine," J.A.M.A., **149**:1558, 1952). Gennis and his associates described the use of this compound in Korean war veterans with *vivax* malaria. One hundred and one patients were treated, with only one relapse. There were four recurrences (return of fever in less than 1 month after therapy). The writers advise, therefore, combined therapy with chloroquine for its suppressive effect, with primaquine for radical cure. This seems to be the most effective treatment today for malaria.

Table 1 illustrates the development of drug therapy as outlined in References 47 and 51.

TABLE 1

	Suppression of Symptoms (Prophylaxis)	Cure of Clinical Attack	Radical Cure (Prevention of Relapse)
Quinine..........................	+	+	0
Quinacrine (Atabrine)	++	++	0
Chloroquine⎫	+++	+++	0
Paludrine ⎰			
Plasmochin (pamaquine)..........	±	±	+
Pentaquine......................	±	±	++
Primaquine,.....................	±	±	+++

This table is an oversimplification and doubtless will soon be modified by further work as new antimalarials are constantly being tested. Meanwhile, the subject of chemotherapy is brilliantly reviewed by N. Hamilton Fairley, "Malaria. Lecture II. Chemotherapy," Brit. M.J., **2**:891, 1949.

54. YOUNG, Martin D. Malaria during the last decade, Am. J. Trop. Med. & Hyg., **2**:347, 1953.

This is a review of important recent contributions.

AMEBIC DYSENTERY

Amebic brain abscess	Ref. 17
Amebic granuloma	Ref. 27
Amebic liver abscess	Refs. 1, 2, 9, 10, 11, 13, 18, 19
Chemotherapy	Refs. 24, 26
Clinical	Refs. 1, 2, 5, 10, 11
Cultivation of amebae	Ref. 16
Cysts	Refs. 12, 14
Experimental amebiasis	Refs. 8, 12, 20, 21, 25
General	Refs. 1, 2, 10, 11
Histology	Refs. 7, 11
Latent amebiasis	Refs. 16, 23
Parasitology	Refs. 4, 5, 6, 7, 8, 10, 11, 13, 16
Toxicity of emetine	Ref. 22
Treatment with emetine	Ref. 19
Treatment with ipecac	Refs. 3, 18

Section 20

AMEBIC DYSENTERY

THE subject of amebic dysentery and amebiasis is systematically covered in a wide variety of textbooks and monographs. Leonard Rogers' *Dysenteries, Their Differentiation and Treatment* (London: Henry Frowde, 1913) gives an authoritative discussion with an excellent historical review and a good selected bibliography. Other recent books of note are those by C. F. Craig, *The Etiology, Diagnosis, and Treatment of Amebiasis* (Baltimore: Williams & Wilkins Co., 1944); by H. H. Anderson, W. L. Bostick, and H. G. Johnstone, *Amebiasis, Pathology, Diagnosis, and Chemotherapy* (Springfield, Ill.: Charles C Thomas, 1953) with extensive references to the recent literature; and by E. C. Faust, *Amebiasis* (Springfield, Ill.: Charles C Thomas, 1954), which gives a concise outline of the subject. Books on the parasitology of amebiasis suitable for the general reader are those of C. Dobell, *The Amoebae Living in Man* (London: John Bale, Sons & Danielsson, Ltd., 1919), and of C. Dobell and F. W. O'Connor, *The Intestinal Protozoa of Man* (London: John Bale & Danielsson, Ltd., 1921). A somewhat more comprehensive treatise is that of M. Hartmann and C. Schilling, *Die pathogenen Protozoen* (Berlin: Julius Springer, 1917).

1. ANNESLEY, James. Researches into the causes, nature and treatment of the more prevalent diseases of India, and of warm climates generally. 2 vols. London: Longman, Rees, Orme, Brown & Green, 1828.

One cannot neglect, in the bibliography of amebic dysentery, Annesley's two monumental folio volumes. This is indeed a magnum opus. The author says in his Preface: "To this end he has sedulously watched disease throughout its course; and when it proved fatal, compared the symptoms while living with the appearances after death" (p. xiv). This is the keynote of the book, which deals less with vague speculations than with descriptions of observed facts. The elaborate section on hepatic abscess (1:516) first gives a general discussion, followed by case reports. "It [hepatic inflammation] frequently supervenes to the insidious inflammation of the substance of the liver, which often accompanies, if it does not actually occasion, a particular variety of dysentery." As to dysentery (2:151, chap. v) he says: "In the observations which we shall have to make on this very important and prevalent disease, we shall, first, consider it in its simpler or less complicated forms; we shall next treat of that variety which is characterized by attendant disorder of the liver; and afterwards offer some remarks on the chronic forms of the disease, and on the scorbutic dysentery which is occasionally met with in intertropical practice" (1:151). He gives an excellent description of acute dysentery, but whether bacterial or amebic, one cannot be sure. Section II deals with "Hepatic Dysentery or Dysentery Complicated with Disease of the Liver," and this is almost surely amebic. "Hepatic dysentery assumes various forms or modifications: it is sometimes acute, but much more frequently sub-acute and chronic" (1:197). Like other observers at the time, Annesley was confused about the relation of dysentery and liver abscess; he was uncertain which came first and which was the cause of the other. His speculations on the cause of dysentery are disappointing, in contrast to his description of cases.

"The influence of the moon in the production of dysentery, as well as of fevers, has been much discussed. . . . That dysentery and fever are both observed to supervene in a manner well calculated to authorize a belief in sol-lunar influence, cannot be denied by any experienced practitioner" (2:247). "On the subject also of the infectious nature of dysentery, much has been advanced. As the disease is met with in warm climates, it seldom or never proves contagious" (2:249). Treatment consisted of bleeding, purgation, and various medicines, among which ipecac is mentioned without special emphasis. The volume concludes with a series of beautiful colored plates of diseased bowels. Those of the liver (Vol. 1) in many cases picture indubitable amebic abscesses.

William Twining's book, *Clinical Illustrations of the Most Important Diseases of Bengal* (Calcutta: Baptist Mission Press, 1832), published a few years later, covers essentially the same ground and contains little that is new concerning dysentery.

2. PARKES, E. A. Remarks on the dysentery and hepatitis of India. London: Longman, Hunt, Rees & Orme, 1846.

Parkes, working in the Indian army medical service, had plenty of opportunity to study dysentery, and this book illustrates very well the rudimentary state of knowledge of the disease at the halfway mark of the century. Nothing was known as to cause. "I shall pass over this difficult subject rapidly, as the causes of dysentery are as undetermined as its pathology" (p. 131). There are mentioned the following: "all acid agents, suppression of secretions rapidly accomplished, epidemic states of the atmosphere, and alterations of blood." As to the great frequency of dysentery in India, Parkes says that, discounting all other possible causes, "there still must remain to be accounted for an unusual proneness in the mucous membrane of the large intestines to be acted upon by exciting causes" (p. 132). "Perhaps no individual ever can have during a lifetime opportunities of accurately studying all the varieties of dysentery,—its complications with remittent fever, with cholera, with gastro-enteritis, and with typhus,—its union with scurvy and purpura, with several kinds of hepatitis, with delirium tremens, with pancreatic and spleen diseases . . . its numerous chronic states, depending on various stages of alteration, hypertrophy, ulceration, or otherwise, of the colonic and cecal solitary glands, and thickening of the intestinal coats" (p. 137). The association of dysentery with hepatic abscess is clearly recognized, but it is not known which causes the other or, indeed, which really comes first. "The causes of primary hepatitis, meaning by that term the low insidious suppurative form, generally in an advanced stage, complicated with dysentery, are much more obscure. The first opinion which claims our attention is that which refers the disease to the action of external heat" (p. 229). Under treatment, stress is laid on depletion—bleeding—plus a great variety of medicines. Parkes does point out, however, that the "large doses of ipecacuanha, viz. from 30 grs. to 1 dr. are much more efficacious" than smaller doses (p. 145). Parkes's objective descriptions of clinical cases and autopsies are, however, refreshing in the midst of otherwise arid material.

Finally, how much of Parkes's dysentery was bacillary and how much was amebic remains a puzzle. There had been little progress since Annesley's vast monograph in 1828 (Ref. 1).

3. DOCKER, E. S. On the treatment of dysentery by the administration of large doses of ipecacuanha, Lancet, **2**:113, 1858.

We cannot trace in detail the introduction of ipecac into the treatment of tropical dysentery. Apparently, the drug was in common use, however, in India by the beginning of the nineteenth century. Docker, working in Mauritius, seems, however, to deserve the credit for using ipecac in really large and effective doses. "Out of upwards of fifty cases of dysentery I lost but one (in four years the mortality ranged from ten to eighteen percent)." He points out the "ineffectiveness" of the small amounts commonly employed. "I give it in doses ranging from ten to ninety grains. . . . In all constitutions, robust as well as delicate, under all circumstances, the result is the same. In the very worst cases . . . after the whole range of remedies has been tried in vain, the disease running its course swiftly and surely to a fatal issue, ninety grains of ipecacuanha have been given, and forthwith the character of the disease, or, I should rather say, the character of the *symptoms* has been entirely changed; for the disease itself is literally cured, put a summary stop to, driven out." Striking illustrative cases are presented.

4. LAMBL, Wilhelm. Mikroscopische Untersuchungen der Darm-Excrete, Vrtljschr. f. d. prakt. Heilk., **1**:1, 1859.

Lambl is usually mentioned as the first observer concerned with amebae in the stools. In this paper, however, which deals in detail with the character of the stools in disease, no mention is made of amebae, nor is anything resembling them shown in the illustrations. Under the heading of "Intestinal Parasites," only larger parasites, such as tapeworms, are mentioned. In Lambl's second communication (I. Theil: *Beobachtungen und Studien aus dem Gebiete der pathologischen Anatomie und Histologie* [Prague: Friedrich Tempsky, 1860]) he was no more definite, as his illustration (reproduced in Stilwell, *op. cit.*) shows. Whatever the bodies pictured may be, they are certainly not amebae.

5. LÖSCH, F. Massenhafte Entwickelung von Amoeben im Dickdarm, Virchows Arch. f. path. Anat., **65**:196, 1875.

The famous case of Lösch is supposed to be the first well-described instance of amebic dysentery. It concerned J. Markow, a peasant who was taken sick in St. Petersburg, in the summer of 1871, with a stubborn diarrhea which persisted for several months. The story is that of relapses and remissions until his death in the hospital after a period of nearly 3 years. The stools were largely pus, blood, and mucus, but at times they were profuse and watery. The patient became weak, pale, and edematous, and death occurred on April 12, "with the picture of severe anemia and general exhaustion." It is of interest that Professor Eichwald, because of the anemia, suggested a transfusion, which was performed on February 11 by Dr. Roussel "with the apparatus constructed by him, and 9 ounces of blood drawn from the median cephalic vein of a strong healthy man were injected directly into the cephalic vein of the upper arm of the patient." Right after this transfusion a chill occurred, lasting half an hour, followed by a feeling of heat. The temperature rose in three hours to 40.1° but by evening fell to 38.5°. "The stools showed in large numbers, as many as 60 to 70 or more per field, some free, some enclosed in mucus, large cell-like structures which were immediately to be recognized as parasites, in fact amebae, because of their peculiar motility." While the amebae were for a long time a constant finding, from March 11 on, "despite the greatest care, no more amebae were demonstrated throughout his course." A beautiful description of the parasites is given, dealing with structure, size, motility, nucleus, etc. Lösch does not, however, emphasize the presence of red blood cells in the parasites: "Aside from the nucleus, the vacuoles and the granules, one observes not uncommonly in the protoplasm various formed particles taken up from the outside . . . bacteria, vibrios, chains of mycothrix, cocci, and exceptionally larger elements such as red and white blood corpuscles." Lösch suggests the name *Amoeba coli* because the colon seemed to be its principal site and because it was unlike any hitherto described ameba. The pictures given in his Plate X are excellent; again the absence of red cells in the parasites is striking. The autopsy findings were those of an advanced cicatricial colitis; the lower ileum was also involved. "The thickening and swelling of the mucous membrane of the colon depended, as microscopic examination showed, mainly upon an inflammatory infiltration of the submucosa."

Lösch, after trying numerous medicaments, decided to use quinine because he found that a solution of quinidine, 1–5,000, in vitro killed the amebae in 1 minute, at least they became motionless, round, and granular. Lösch used the quinine in a clyster, 20 gm. to the pound of water, after which the amebae disappeared from the stools for several days but soon reappeared. This observation was, however, the start of chemotherapy for amebiasis, although all the early efforts were with solutions used locally rather than systematically.

Lösch analyzed the case in relation to the amebae and concluded: "One must therefore assume that Markow sickened first with dysentery and that only later did the amebae enter the bowel and grow there, and there maintained the inflammation."

Is this suggestion of Lösch correct? It must be admitted that the clinical features—a sporadic case in a cool climate, the long duration with remissions and exacerbations, the character of the stools, the final disappearance of the amebae—suggest ulcerative colitis rather than amebic dysentery. However, the huge numbers of amebae are hard to explain in any other than a causal role, even though the paucity of ingested red cells is striking.

Lösch also reports some experiments in which he fed to dogs or injected into the rectum stools from the patient. Three of four experiments were "entirely negative." The results in the fourth are hard to interpret. Globules of mucus adhering to particles of formed stool contained many amebae some days after inoculation. The animal did not seem ill and was sacrificed on the eighteenth day. There were three superficial ulcerations in the rectum. It is impossible to say whether Lösch really produced amebic dysentery; but subsequent writers usually found dogs refractory to the experimental disease.

The exact interpretation of Lösch's case is therefore not entirely clear.

6. KARTULIS, [S.]. Zur Aetiologie der Dysenterie in Aegypten, Virchows Arch. f. path. Anat., 105:521, 1886.

Kartulis was evidently alert to the possibility of amebae in stools because he raised the question in connection with certain bodies which he found ("Ueber Riesen-Amöben[?] bei chronischer Darmentzündung bei Aegypter," *ibid.*, 99:145, 1885) in the stools of a boy who had had dysentery several months previously. It is obvious from the description and the drawing that these bodies, queried by Kartulis himself, are not amebae at all. But a year later Kartulis unequivocally described amebae which were found "in every case of undoubted dysentery. In no cases [of other disease] could I find amebae." There is a splendid description of the organisms which leaves no doubt as to their nature, although Kartulis mentions slight differences between his and Lösch's (Ref. 5) amebae. Kartulis went beyond Lösch in describing amebae in stained sections of bowel. Alcoholic solutions of methylene blue and gentian violet were especially suitable. The parasites were seen most abundantly in fresh ulcers. "In several preparations the amebae were present in such numbers that the whole submucosa seemed full of them." "Their form in sections is usually round or oval." Kartulis was unable to cultivate the amebae. He found them dead in 24 hours, and in sugar or salt water they died in a few hours. In hanging drop they survived for 12 hours. Introduction into the colons of two guinea pigs and one rabbit was without result. The amebae were found in all stages of dysentery. "That the amebae must be accepted as the cause of tropical dysentery seems definite on the basis of what has been reported. But how the organisms enter and succeed in developing in the colon is hard to explain." Kartulis' work is impressive, and he clearly established amebae as the cause of dysentery, although his finding of their invariable presence in dysentery and invariable absence in other diseases is perhaps to be questioned. Later N. G. Masiutin ("Ob amoebakh kak tchougeiadnykh tolotiakh kislok," Vrach., **10**:557, 1889;[1] German abstract: "Ueber die Amoeben als Parasiten des Dickdarms," Centralbl. f. Bakt., **6**:451, 1889) found amebae similar to those of Lösch in five cases of various bowel disturbances, including one of "typhoid" fever. For this reason he doubted the primary etiological role of amebae but suggested that they entered the body in drinking water, multiplied, and were a factor in keeping up a disease process caused by some other agent. Like his predecessors, he prescribed clysters of various substances, of which he regarded quinine as the most effective in extirpating the amebae and allowing the disease process to subside. Kartulis ("Ueber weitere Verbreitungsgebiete der Dysenterie-Amoeben," Centralbl. f. Bakt., **7**:54, 1890) disputed Masiutin's doubts about the causal role of amebae and reported two cases of dysentery, which he examined on a visit to Greece, in the discharges of which the same amebae were found as those he had seen in Egypt. He thought that Masiutin's observations simply widened the field of symptom complexes which could be produced by these amebae. One gets the picture of the doubts and speculations of the early observers as to the true role in disease of these animalcules.

7. KOCH, Robert. Bericht über die Thätigkeit der zur Erforschung der Cholera im Jahre 1883 nach Egypten und Indien entstandten Kommission, Arb. a. d. k. Gsndhtsamte, Vol. **3**, Anlage VI, p. 63, 1887.

Koch made careful autopsies as early as 1883 not only on cholera patients but on people dead of other diseases; there were five instances of dysentery, two of which were complicated by liver abscess. "There were found in the bases of fresh ulcers [in the colon], in addition to innumerable bacteria, peculiar ameba-like structures." These bodies were seen only in sections of the ulcers or in material taken from them rather than in the stools, a fact which indicated to

[1] I am indebted to Mrs. A. Hoen for the correct transcription of this title from the original Russian.

Koch "a close relation to disease." Amebae were also seen in the capillaries near a liver abscess. Koch was evidently the first to recognize amebae in stained sections of tissue, but he does not seem to have pursued the matter further himself, although Kartulis, his pupil, acknowledged Koch's influence (Ref. 6).

8. HLAVA, Jaroslav. O úplavici předběžné sdělení, Časop. lék. cesk., **26**:70, 1887. (Abstract by Kartulis, Centralbl. f. Bakt., **1**:537, 1887.)

We have not seen the original article which is described in the interesting paper by G. G. Stilwell ("Amoebiasis: its early history," Gastroenterology, **28**:606, 1955), together with the error which Kartulis made in his abstract in setting down O. Uplavici (on dysentery) as the author's name. Hlava had sought for bacteria in the stools of dysentery patients, but, as he had convinced himself that no constant bacterial form was present, he looked for amebae. In sixty cases, partly sporadic, partly endemic, he always found amebae in the fresh stools. He injected ameba-containing stools into the rectums of seventeen dogs, with two positive results; of six cats, with four positive results; and of a number of rabbits, chickens, and guinea pigs, with no reaction. Since dysentery was transmissible to cats, the writer concluded that the ameba was the cause of dysentery. Finally, he reports a case with giant amebae with which he infected a cat and again recovered giant amebae from it. These observations were carried on in Prague, not in the tropics, and one cannot help feeling some reservations about them. It is, however, of interest that cats or at least kittens have turned out to be the most satisfactory animals for experimental amebiasis.

In setting the record straight about Dr. Hlava, one should refer to C. Dobell's article, "Dr. O. Uplavici (1887–1938)," Parasitology, **30**:239, 1938, where this comedy of errors is fully explained.

9. KARTULIS, [S.]. Zur Aetiologie der Leberabscesse. Lebende Dysenterie-Amoeben im Eiter der dysenterischen Leberabscesse, Centralbl. f. Bakt., **1**:681, 1887.

"The constant finding of amebae in every case of dysentery impelled me to look for them in the liver abscesses which complicate this disease." Amebae were found in all of twenty cases. Kartulis reports an instance in which the abscess had ruptured into the pleura; the patient died shortly after thoracotomy. The pus at autopsy from an intact liver abscess showed the amebae "practically in pure culture." Bacterial cultures were made in four cases, and various organisms were obtained. Kartulis regarded these as secondary invaders which entered with the amebae. A little later ("Ueber tropische Leberabscesse und ihr Verhältniss zur Dysenterie," Virchows Arch. f. path. Anat., **118**:97, 1889) he discussed critically the whole subject of tropical liver abscess in relation to dysentery. He concluded: "From what has been said it seems probable that in Egypt amebae play an etiological role in the genesis of dysenteric liver abscess and that pyogenic bacteria, probably originating in the gastro-intestinal tract, cause idiopathic liver abscess."

There is an immense literature on hepatic amebiasis which we cannot review further; the reader is referred to sections on the subject in all the books to which reference is made in the introduction. Recently, however, N. J. Conan, Jr. ("The treatment of hepatic abscess with chloroquine," Am. J. Med., **6**:309, 1949) recommends chloroquine as a specific; his work is confirmed by W. A. Sodeman,

A. A. Dolvinen, E. M. Gordon, and C. M. Gillikin, "Chloroquine in hepatic amebiasis," Ann. Int. Med., **35**:331, 1951.

10. OSLER, William. On the Amoeba coli in dysentery and in dysenteric liver abscess, Bull. Johns Hopkins Hosp., **1**:53, 1890.

Osler was the first on this side of the Atlantic to describe amebae in dysentery and liver abscess. "Dr. B., age 29, resident in Panama for nearly six years . . . had a chronic dysentery . . . he began to have an irregular fever with occasional chilly sensations and sweats, to lose flesh and to have a very sallow complexion. . . . He had six or eight mucoid stools with traces of blood daily." Liver abscess was diagnosed and evacuated surgically. Osler found in the pus "in large numbers the amoebae which Kartulis had described. . . . The material was taken at once to the Pathological Laboratory where Prof. Welch and Dr. Councilman confirmed the observation. . . . After the operation the dysenteric symptoms did not abate in the slightest; he continued to have from eight to sixteen movements daily." Osler then gives a detailed description of the amebae, drawings of which are reproduced for the first time in Stilwell's article (Ref. 8). Osler concluded: "It is impossible to speak as yet with any certainty as to the relation of these organisms to the disease. The subject is deserving of extended study, and a point of special interest will be the determination of their presence in the endemic dysentery of this country."[2] Shortly after, Lafleur ("Demonstration of Amoeba coli in dysentery," Bull. Johns Hopkins Hosp., **1**:91, 1890) reported a case of dysentery in a sailor on a steamship sailing between Baltimore and Bremen "in which the Amoeba coli had been found in the stools, and exhibited the living parasite under the microscope." The patient had been in the tropics in 1880. A third case was soon reported by Simon ("Abscess of the liver, perforation into the lung; Amoeba coli in sputum," Bull. Johns Hopkins Hosp., **1**:97, 1890). The patient had been in the West Indies in 1883 but was quite well when there. He developed diarrhea and cough, and "on the day of admission the expectoration was noticed to be a peculiar rustry, reddish-brown color purulent and resembling anchovy sauce. Actively moving amoebae were found in it, a fact which at once called attention to the bowels and to the liver. . . . Our attention would never have been called to his actual condition by the character of the stools. As they looked perfectly healthy, with simply adherent mucus, we should probably have regarded the case as one of pleurisy." The atmosphere at Johns Hopkins, thus, was ripe for the work of Councilman and Lafleur (Ref. 11).

From now on, there are various confirmatory reports of the presence of amebae in dysentery and liver abscess. They are carefully reviewed by Councilman and Lafleur.

[2] On March 20, Osler wrote to Musser as follows: "We have been much excited over Kartulis' amoebae which we have found in a liver abscess from a case of dysentery —a Dr. from Panama. They are most extraordinary & striking creatures & take one's breath away at first to see these big amoebae—10–20 times the size of a leucocyte—crawling about in the pus. The movements are very active & in one case kept up for 10 hours. I get a fresh stock of pus from the drainage tube every day so if you could run down some eve. we could look for the creatures in the morning. . . . Keep an eye on your Blockley dysenteries as it would be most interesting to find similar bodies in our dysenteries" (Harvey Cushing, *The Life of Sir William Osler* [Oxford, 1926], **1**:326).

11. COUNCILMAN, W. T., and LAFLEUR, H. A. Amoebic dysentery, Johns Hopkins Hosp. Rep., **2**:395, 1891.

This monograph of some hundred and fifty pages, stimulated by the cases seen at Johns Hopkins (Ref. 10), is indeed a landmark in the study of the subject. "In this article we propose to consider a disease which is characterized by definite pathological lesions, and is separated not only by its destructive pathological anatomy, but also by its aetiology and clinical history from other affections of the intestines with which it has hitherto been classed under the general name of dysentery." Councilman and Lafleur were therefore the first unequivocally to define amebic dysentery as a specific disease and, indeed, to give it a specific name and to rename its causal agent *Amoeba dysenteriae*. They give a detailed description of the parasites and emphasize the presence in them of red blood cells, "as many as six or eight having been seen in a single amoeba." They describe and picture the appearance of dead amebae stained in various ways. They report fifteen cases of amebic dysentery and give a classical clinical analysis of every feature of the disease. The section on hepatic abscess is specially important, and they point out the frequency of this complication in patients who have no overt dysentery. In short, modern study has added little to this definitive analysis. As to therapy, "Ipecacuanha was administered in case VIII after the manner recognized by surgeons in India," and in other cases "quinine was given by mouth, on theoretical grounds rather than from empirical evidence as to its value." Clysters of quinine as well as of bichloride of mercury, 1:5,000 or 1:3,000, were employed in two cases, and each injection was retained for 10–15 minutes. "The results achieved are not brilliant but warrant a more extended trial. This much can be said, that quinine injections do destroy amoebae in the contents of the bowel, but whether they reach and destroy the amoebae in the tissues is an open question." The section in which the pathological lesions are meticulously described is one of the outstanding features of this monograph. The writers thought that the amebae produced a necrosis of tissue and exercised a solvent effect on the intercellular substance. "The ulceration is produced by infiltration of the submucous tissue and necrosis of the overlying mucous membranes, the ulcer in consequence having the undermined form. Frequently in addition to the ulcers there is infiltration of the submucous tissue without ulceration. In all of these lesions unless complicated by the action of bacteria there is absence of the products of purulent inflammation." "These abscesses [of the liver] differ in their anatomical features from those produced by other causes. The chief difference is found in the absence of purulent inflammation, the abscess being caused by necrosis, softening and liquefaction of the tissue. In these liver abscesses the amoebae are not associated with any other organism." "This is the form of dysentery which has been commonly called tropical dysentery." There are numerous reproductions of microscopic sections of the lesions and colored drawings of stained amebae showing their structure. There is a bibliogaphy of 98 pertinent titles.

In short, this monograph is a definitive account of the disease to date which has hardly been superseded today.

12. QUINCKE, H., and ROOS, E. I. Ueber Amoeben-Enteritis, Berl. klin. Wchnschr., **30**:1089, 1893.

Quincke and Roos made notable contributions to the subject. They were the first to describe cysts: "Of special importance is the encysted condition of the amebae. These forms are considerably smaller, have a diameter of 10–12 μ, a much sharper, if not definitely doubled, contour; they appear shiny, transparent, and show the nucleus very unclearly." "Very noteworthy is the great *Haltbarkeit* of these encysted forms; in the moist chamber as well as in the stools they could still be recognized after 20 days but not after 4–8 weeks." Whereas the vegetative forms injected into the rectum of kittens caused dysentery, they were harmless when given by mouth; on the other hand, the cysts produced disease when fed. Another important finding was the discovery of other amebae in the bowel definitely different from those associated with severe dysentery. "There are similar but milder forms of endemic dysentery; the parasite causing them (*Amoeba coli mitis*) is different from the *Amoeba coli* of Lösch and is not pathogenic for kittens. One ameba often found in healthy people and doubtless harmless (*A. intestinalis vulgaris*) is probably different from both." A little later, Roos ("Zur Kentniss der Amoebenenteritis," Arch. f. exper. Path. u. Pharmakol., **33**:389, 1894) pursued the subject further. He reports elaborate observations on production of dysentery in cats by rectal instillation of material containing amebae and by introducing cysts into the stomach. On the other hand, no disease was produced by stools containing *A. coli mitis*. "According to our experiments, infection with the parasites probably results from the ingestion of cysts of amebae by mouth." This work was later confirmed by R. P. Strong and W. E. Musgrave ("Preliminary note regarding the etiology of the dysenteries in Manila," Rep. of the Surg. Gen. of the Army, Washington, 1900, p. 251). Quincke and Roos therefore opened the way to the discovery of the mode of transmission of amebic dysentery.

Meanwhile, there appeared a comprehensive review by A. Schulberg ("Die parasitischen Amöben des menschlichen Darmes," Centralbl. f. Bakt., **13**:598, 654, 701, 1893) with a subtitle of "Critical Review of the Development of Current Knowledge." Schulberg analyzes the conflicting claims in the literature with regard to the pathogenicity of amebae found in the bowel, with a bibliography of some fifty titles.

13. KRUSE, W., and PASQUALE, A. Untersuchungen über Dysenterie und Leberabscess, Ztschr. f. Hyg. u. Infectionskr., **16**:1, 1894.

In this tremendous communication of 149 pages on amebic dysentery and liver abscess, Kruse and Pasquale reported confirmation of much of the earlier work, as well as many experiments in which the disease was successfully transmitted to kittens. They used pus from liver abscesses and produced dysentery in three experiments. "In two of these three experiments pus was used which the microscope and culture showed was completely sterile apart from the amebae." Thus they made the important observation that amebae alone could produce dysentery without the associated activity of bacteria, as many had insisted. Indeed, at the time the view was prevalent that amebae were "opportunists" which took advantage of existing lesions to invade and aggravate them. Thus as keen an observer as George Dock ("Observations on the Amoeba coli in dysentery and abscess of the liver," Texas M.J., **6**:419, 1891), after finding amebae in a variety of apparently poorly related conditions, concluded: "We have no reason for ascribing pathogenic powers to the parasite, though the evidence is such that it offers a promising field for future investigations."

14. HUBER. [Demonstration of dysentery amebae], Deutsche med. Wchnschr., **29**:267, 1903.

"Further I would like to call attention to one important finding . . . namely small, delicate, spherical cysts which I must conclude are encysted forms of the amebae. Every time when the patient's stool became hard and the amebae disappeared, these cysts appeared, and when a relapse occurred and amebae were again present in the stools, the cysts disappeared. . . . Furthermore, I have been able to infect animals per os with such cyst-containing stools. The cysts found by me are distinguished from those of the ordinary ameba which Schaudinn has exactly described. Unstained, the nucleus is very hard to recognize. In stained preparations the nucleus is more prominent as a delicate chromatin-poor ring. . . . On occasion one finds two or four nuclei."

With this classic description Huber amplified that of Quincke and Roos (Ref. 12). He pursued the subject further in a more comprehensive article, "Untersuchungen über Amöbendysenterie," Ztschr. f. klin. Med., **67**:262, 1909.

15. SCHAUDINN, Fritz. Untersuchungen über die Fortpflanzung einiger Rhizopoden (vorläufige Mittheilung), Arb. a. d. k. Gsndhtsamte, **19**:547, 1903.

Fritz Schaudinn, the great discoverer of the spirochete of syphilis, erred badly in his interpretation of the life-cycle of amebae, as he had in his studies of the invasion of red cells by sporozoites in malaria. Part of his work, on the vegetative forms of amebae, was sound, and he coined the name *Amoeba histolytica.* "I choose to call them *Entamoeba histolytica* because of their capacity to destroy tissue." But he went wrong in his interpretation of encystment and his belief that he had demonstrated multiplication by sporulation. Schaudinn's authority confused the subject for many years; the details of the story are given in Stilwell's article (Ref. 8).

16. MUSGRAVE, W. E., and CLEGG, Moses T. Amebas: their cultivation and etiological significance. Manila: Bureau of Government Laboratories, October, 1904.

Musgrave and Clegg first review the conflicting literature on attempts to grow amebae outside the body. They succeeded with various strains on a medium the base of which was agar, sodium chloride, and extract of beef, provided that the amebae were grown in symbiosis with pure cultures of bacteria which favored their development. "Amebas are the etiologic factors in the disease generally known as amebic dysentery, and by following the methods described in this paper, such amebas may be grown on artificial media, and the disease reproduced in monkeys and man by the ingestion of these cultures. Amebas may be reclaimed by culture from the stools or the intestinal ulcers." The authors concluded: "All amebas are or may become pathogenic. This proposition, pending a complete solution of the problem, is the only safe one to adopt from the standpoint of public health in the Tropics." Musgrave and Clegg also introduced the term "amebiasis." "The term amebiasis, which has been introduced in this article, denoting an infection with amebas, is comparable in its application to filariasis, trypanosomiasis, uncinariasis, etc. It is not open to the objections so frequently offered to 'amebic dysentery,' 'amebic enteritis,' and the other names usually given to the disease." Musgrave ("Intestinal amoebiasis without diarrhoea," Philippine J. Sc., **5B**:229, 1910) later reported patients who had died of various conditions, mostly unrelated to amebic infection and usually without bowel symptoms, but who at autopsy showed "characteristic amoebic lesions." Such symptoms as abdominal "aching," flatulence, constipation, distention, and loss of weight were noted in some patients. "When we come to study the clinical phenomena shown by this class of cases, it is seen that there is nothing specific or definite in any one, or in all the findings, except the one of the presence of amoebae in the stools."

E. L. Walker ("A comparative study of the amoebae in the Manila water supply, in the intestinal tract of healthy people, and in amoebic dysentery," Philippine J. Sc., **6B**:259, 1911) had been working on the problem of amebae for some years. "It has been my experience . . . that if the character of both the trophozoite and the cyst be taken into consideration, they can always be separated into species having well defined morphological characteristics." He was able to confirm Musgrave and Clegg in so far as it was possible to cultivate amebae by their methods, but only non-pathogenic amebae were derived from the Manila water supply. "The amoeboid organisms parasitic in the intestinal tract of man belong to a distinct genus, *Entamoeba*. . . . The entamoebae are strict or obligatory parasites and are incapable of multiplication outside the body of the host. They cannot be cultivated on Musgrave and Clegg's medium." Walker emphasized the morphological differences between *Entamoeba histolytica* and the harmless *E. coli*. "The infection with *Entamoeba histolytica* may persist for an indefinite period after the symptoms of amoebic dysentery have disappeared, during which time the resistant encysted entamoebae may be passed in large numbers in the stools and constitute an important source of infection to others. Such persons are 'carriers' of amoebic dysentery, comparable to the 'carriers' of typhoid fever or cholera. The prophylactic measures for the prevention of amoebic dysentery are sufficiently indicated by the preceding conclusions; they are identical with those required for prevention of other specific infectious diseases of the intestinal tract, like typhoid fever and cholera." There are reproductions of excellent drawings of the various types of amebae. The importance of Walker's observations cannot be overestimated.

While the work of Musgrave and Clegg was not generally accepted, D. W. Cutler ("A method for the cultivation of *Entamoeba histolytica*," J. Path. & Bact., **22**:22, 1918) described a method "by which *E. histolytica* can be maintained in culture for several months. These cultures, if inoculated into cats, produce dysenteric lesions of the intestines." He found that cysts could be produced in cultures by omitting to subculture for 4 or 5 days. W. C. Boeck and J. Drbohlav ("The cultivation of Endamoeba histolytica," Am. J. Hyg., **5**:371, 1925) later also claimed to have cultivated pathogenic amebae and to have produced lesions in kittens with culture material. They were unable, however with their method to produce encystment. The work of Cutler has been sharply criticized by C. Dobell (*The Amoebae Living in Man*, p. 70). A summary of the whole problem of cultivation of amebae is to be found in Anderson, Bostick and Johnstone (*op. cit.*, pp. 346 ff.).

17. KARTULIS. Gehirnabscesse nach dysenterischen Leberabscessen, Centralbl. f. Bakt., **37**:527, 1904.

Kartulis reviews the meager literature on brain abscess occurring in association with dysentery and reports two cases of his own in which he found amebae both in the pus and in sections of the wall. The subject is reviewed in detail by J. A. Orbison, N. Reeves, C. L. Leedham, and J. M. Blumberg, "Amebic brain abscess: review of the literature and report of five additional cases," Medicine, **30**:247, 1951. This article has a bibliography of 82 titles.

18. ROGERS, Leonard. The prevention and treatment of amoebic abscess of the liver, Philippine J. Sc., **5B**:219, 1910.

Rogers was the first to insist on the value of ipecac in the treatment of amebic hepatitis and abscess of the liver. He points out that 86 per cent of a large series of liver abscesses were sterile as far as bacteria were concerned, although in a few cases "numerous cocci and bacteria are found." "Lastly, I would urge that every patient operated on for amoebic-liver abscess should be given a course of full doses of ipecacuanha as soon as possible, with the view to healing the ulcers in the large bowel, which have originated the hepatic trouble and are often latent and give rise to no symptoms."

19. ROGERS, Leonard. The rapid cure of amoebic dysentery and hepatitis by hypodermic injections of soluble salts of emetine, Brit. M.J., **1**:1424, 1912.

Rogers briefly tells the story of ipecac in the history of medicine. "The Brazilian root was first brought to Europe by Piso in 1658, and was successfully used by Helvetius in the treatment of Louis XIV, and sold as a secret remedy to the French Government." Turning, however, to emetine, Magendie and Pelletier ("Sur l'émétine et sur les trois espèces d'ipecacuanha," J. gén. de méd., **59**:223, 1817) extracted an alkaloid from various types of ipecac; the ligneous internal part of brown ipecac, psycotria emetica, contained, for example, 1.15 parts of "emetine." This material taken by mouth in 1- or 2-gm. doses produced vomiting, just as did ipecac. Six to 12 gm. killed a dog. Finally, the authors advised giving emetine in a sort of camomile tea, in which "it is agreeable even to infants." The academy approved the report and thought "emetine" worthy of further clinical study, although no results were reported in tropical dysentery. H. B. Paul and A. J. Cownley ("The chemistry of ipecacuanha," Pharm. J. & Tr., **53** [3d ser., Vol. **24**], 61, 1893) showed that the "emetine" of earlier workers was really a mixture of several alkaloids. It was many years later before E. B. Vedder ("A preliminary account of some experiments undertaken to test the efficacy of the ipecac treatment of dysentery," Bull. Manila M. Soc., **3**:48, 1911), using cultures of non-pathogenic amebae, showed that both ipecac and emetine killed the organisms in the test tube. Some preparations of emetine were effective in dilutions of 1:200,000. Vedder concluded: "I would state my belief that the ipecac treatment of dysentery caused by protozoa should not on light grounds be set aside in favor of any other, but that in using this treatment great care should be taken to make sure that the dysentery is truly caused by protozoa and is not bacillary, and also to obtain an ipecac that is shown by critical analysis to contain its proper amount of emetin, and when this is not possible, to insist upon obtaining the Brazil root." It is to Rogers, however, that credit clearly goes for introducing the use of hypodermic injections of emetine in the treatment of amebiasis. Three brilliantly successful cases are reported. Rogers ("Further experience of the specific curative action in amoebic disease of hypodermic injections of soluble salts of emetine," Brit. M.J., **2**:405, 1912) soon reported twelve further cases of various types of amebic dysentery and liver abscess cured by emetine. "We have, then, in my method of the subcutaneous injection of soluble salts of emetine a specific treatment of amoebic hepatitis and amoebic dysentery, which is so rapidly beneficial in the latter as to be also of great diagnostic value between that and other causes of the passage of blood and mucus in the stools. Yet, strange to say, this remarkable remedy—probably the most specific in the whole range of medicine, not excluding quinine and salvarsan—has for long been thrown away by those who pinned their faith on ipecacuanha sine emetina."

This paper really opened the modern era of chemotherapy of amebiasis; like similar efforts in other fields, it was destined to be to some extent a disappointment, since it was soon discovered that emetine was often inadequate to extirpate fully the infection, so that relapses were prone to occur. Rogers also devotes a chapter in his book (*op. cit.*, p. 117) to ipecac and emetine in amebic dysentery.

Emetine was soon combined with iodine and bismuth (E.B.I., emetine bismuthous iodide) and was first tried on man in 1916 by G. C. Low and C. Dobell ("Three cases of Entamoeba histolytica infection treated with emetine bismuth iodide," Lancet, **2**:319, 1916; see also G. C. Low, "Emetine bismuth iodide in amoebic dysentery, amoebic hepatitis, and general amoebiasis," Lancet, **1**:482, 1917). It seemed more effective than emetine in eradicating cysts and in treating the chronic tissue stages of the disease and is still widely used in England.

20. WALKER, E. L., and SELLARDS, A. W. Experimental amoebic dysentery, Philippine J. Sc., ser. B, **8**:253, 1913.

Walker and Sellards set about to prove that amebae really were the cause of "amebic" dysentery, by reproducing the disease experimentally. The results of these elaborate investigations are quite clear. First, Walker re-emphasizes the necessity in practice of distinguishing the harmless *E. coli* from the pathogenic *E. histolytica* in the stools of patients. The differential features of both the motile stage and the encysted stage are clearly listed in tabular form. Volunteers were then fed cysts of the various strains. Those who ingested *E. coli* developed no disease, whereas dysentery was produced in some of those who received *histolytical* cysts. Furthermore, many of these who did not develop clinical dysentery became "carriers." Walker and Sellards drew the important final conclusion that *E. histolytica* was, to all intents and purposes, the sole cause of amebic dysentery and that therefore exact diagnosis was of the utmost importance. They also emphasized that vegetative forms did not survive outside the body but that cysts were the important element in transmission of the disease. Consequently, the recognition of "carriers" of cysts was the key to intelligent public health preventive measures.

As to treatment, this important statement is made: "The evidence . . . points to the conclusion that the ordinary routine treatment with ipecac, while efficient in relieving attacks of dysentery and in causing the entamoeba to disappear temporarily from the stools, frequently does not kill all of the entamoeba in the intestine; consequently the patient is liable to a relapse of the dysentery."

21. SELLARDS, A. W., and BAETJER, W. A. The propagation of amoebic dysentery in animals and the recognition and reproduction in animals of atypical forms of the disease, Am. J. Trop. Med., **2**:231, 1914.

Sellards and Baetjer summarize their work on experimental amebic dysentery. Employing the device of injecting the stools containing amebae from acute attacks of dysentery directly into the cecum of kittens, they succeeded in producing amebic infection in nearly 100 per cent of the animals and in propagating the disease through eleven generations. They produced acute fatal infections, chronic infections with relapses and liver abscess, and carriers. They succeeded in increasing the virulence of the infection on repeated passages, in contrast to the usual reports of attenuation. Their work was of great importance insofar as Sellards and Baetjer developed a valuable experimental tool. H. H. Dale and C. Dobell ("Experiments on the therapeutics of amoebic dysentery," J. Pharmacol. & Exper. Therap., **10**:399, 1917) established amebic dysentery by injecting material high into the colon through a glass nozzle. They studied the effect of emetine on the experimental disease. "Experimental dysentery in kittens was refractory to all kinds of treatment. Neither the ipecacuanha alkaloids, nor other substances having a powerful action on the amoebae in vitro, could cure the infection or definitely modify its course." They therefore concluded that the theory of direct amebicidal action of emetine on the parasite was no longer tenable.

In this connection one should not fail to mention the early systematic experiments on production of amebic dysentery in cats and kittens by F. Kovács ("Beobachtungen und Versuche über die sogenannte Amoebendysenterie," Ztschr. f. Heilk., **13**:509, 1892). Incidentally, his paper opens with one of the best reviews we have found of early work on the relation of amebae to dysentery.

22. LEVY, R. L., and ROWNTREE, L. G. On the toxicity of various commercial preparations of emetine hydrochloride, Arch. Int. Med., **17**:420, 1916.

In this important study the writers review the earlier literature and report several new cases of emetine poisoning. Bowel and cardiac disturbances are described. In animals they were able to produce ventricular fibrillation confirmed by the electrocardiograph. They point out that toxic effects are largely the result of overdosage and that intravenous injection is usually unnecessary. "One third of a grain three times a day for a week or ten days is usually a safe dosage." S. Dack and R. E. Molostok ("Cardiac manifestations of toxic action of emetine hydrochloride in amebic dysentery," Arch. Int. Med., **79**:228, 1947) have recently reviewed the subject, as have G. Klatstein and H. Friedman ("Emetine toxicity in man," Ann. Int. Med., **28**:892, 1948). The latter paper contains a comprehensive bibliography.

Earlier papers of interest on ipecac poisoning are those of D. Duckworth ("Observations upon the action of ipecacuanha and its alkaloid emetia," St.

Barts. Hosp. Rep., **5**:218, 1869), who reviews previous experiments and reports observations on the gross effects of the drug in animals, and of von Podwyssotzki ("Beiträge zur Kentniss des Emetins," Arch. f. exper. Path. u. Pharmakol., **11**:231, 1879), who made a systematic study of the drug, using classical pharmacological technique. His description of the action on the exposed frog heart with progressive irregularity until "finally the entire heart remains in an exquisite paralytic diastolic standstill" is very vivid.

> 23. THOMSON, J. G. Human entamoebiasis in temperate zones, J. State Med., **33**:563, 1925.

Musgrave (Ref. 16) had already introduced the idea of "amoebiasis" and of "carriers." The concept rapidly gained acceptance, and it was soon found that amebae could be found frequently in apparently healthy persons outside the "tropics." Thomson gives an elaborate table of reports on the incidence of amebae in people, some of whom had never been out of the temperate zone. "It can be said . . . that an amoebic infection is, in the majority of instances, an insidious disease of such a mild character as to pass unnoticed by the patient, and while it may be true that a 'contact carrier' may remain apparently healthy all his life, there is no method of accurately telling what pathological lesions are produced except in the post-mortem room." W. M. James ("Diagnosis of intestinal amebiasis," J.A.M.A., **89**:1469, 1927) points out the difficulty of accurate diagnosis of intestinal infection with *histolytica* and also gives figures on incidence. C. A. Kofoid ("Statistical summary of persons examined for protozoa and worms, etc., *Twenty-ninth Biannual Report of the State Board of Health of California* [Sacramento, 1926], p. 93) gives the widely quoted figure of 13.1 per cent incidence of *Endamoeba dysenteriae* among some sixteen hundred "healthy" people. J. F. Kessel and V. R. Mason ("Protozoan infection of the human bowel," J.A.M.A., **94**:1, 1930) arrived at a similar figure in the Los Angeles County Hospital. An especially valuable review of this whole subject is that of W. C. Boeck, "Survey of 8,029 persons in the United States, for intestinal parasites, with especial reference to amoebic dysentery among returned soldiers," Hyg. Lab. Bull., No. 133 (Washington, 1923), p. 1. At any rate, it is clear that there exists a widespread incidence of bowel infestation with these parasites, a far cry from the original view that there existed only vegetative forms associated with acute dysentery.

> 24. REED, A. C., ANDERSON, H. H., DAVID, N. A., and LEAKE, C. D. Carbarsone in the treatment of amebiasis, J.A.M.A., **98**:189, 1932.

For a decade after its introduction by Rogers (Ref. 19) emetine had no serious contenders in the field of therapy of amebiasis, although it was soon realized that relapses were common and that complete cure was effected in only 28–70 per cent of the cases (Ref. 20). Serious toxic effects also turned out to be not uncommon (Ref. 22). Attention was therefore soon turned to other drugs which might be useful, and in subsequent years innumerable preparations have been tried which cannot all be reviewed here. For the earlier literature the reader is referred to the review by O. Willner, "Remedies recently introduced in the therapy of amoebiasis," Medicine, **6**:341, 1927, and to the excellent paper by C. D. Leake, "Chemotherapy of amebiasis," J.A.M.A., **98**:195, 1932. Later reviews are those of G. A. Martin *et al.*, "Comparative efficacy of amebicides and antibiotics in acute amebic dysentery," J.A.M.A., **151**:1055, 1953, and of H. E. Hamilton, "Treatment of amoebiasis," Arch. Int. Med., **94**:612, 1954.

Carbarsone (4-carbamino-phenyl arsonic acid) is one of the few earlier drugs which have stood the test of time. Reed and his associates report a careful clinical study with good results. "More closely than any other drug now exploited does carbarsone meet the requirements of an ideal antiamebic agent. It is clinically nontoxic in effective doses; it may conveniently be administered orally without interference with the patient's usual routine; it has no untoward side actions and it is comparatively cheap."

Hamilton's review (*op. cit.*) is especially helpful in bringing out the confused state of the subject at present. He points out that, with single drugs, relapse rates have been disappointingly high and that the tendency now is to use two or three agents in combination or succession. He notes that the drugs effective in clearing the bowel infection—bowel phase—must be distinguished from those more effective against the parasites deep in the tissues—tissue phase. The drugs primarily effective against the tissue phase are chloroquine, emetine, and quinacrine. Of these, chloroquine (see N. J. Conan, "Chloroquine in amebiasis," Am. J. Trop. Med., **28**:107, 1948) seems at present most safe and efficient. Hamilton also lists the drugs effective against the bowel phase, of which di-iodo-hydroxyquinoline is quite satisfactory. The point of all this, however, is clear. There is as yet no entirely satisfactory drug, nor is there agreement among various observers as to which is the best. The subject is still in a state of flux.

25. SCHWARTZWELDER, J. C. Experimental studies on *Endamoeba histolytica* in the dog, Am. J. Hyg., **29**:89, 1939.

Much work has been done in the attempt to define the mode of infection by the parasite. Schwartzwelder reviews the literature and reports his own observations on excystation in dogs, which occurred both in the ileum and in the large intestine. "The time required to bring about the process varied from 1.5 to 4.5 hours following oral inoculation with cysts." The details of invasion of the bowel by the excysted amebae are reviewed and discussed by W. M. James, "Human amoebiasis due to infection with *Entamoeba histolytica*," Ann. Trop. Med., **22**:201, 1928.

26. McHARDY, G., and FRYE, W. W. Antibiotics in management of amebiasis, J.A.M.A., **154**:646, 1954.

It was inevitable, with the advent of the antibiotics, that they should be tried in amebiasis, and there are numerous papers reporting trials with one or another agent. This work is reviewed by McHardy and Frye, who concluded that, of the broad-spectrum antibiotics, oxytetracycline (Terramycin) is the drug of choice, since in the literature only 8.5 per cent of relapses were reported among 435 treated cases. "Hepatitis, hepatic abscess, and other extracolonic amebic involvements are not benefitted by treatment with the antibiotics evaluated."

27. SPICKNALL, C. G., and PIERCE, E. C., II. Amoebic granuloma, New England J. Med., **250**:1055, 1954.

The first description of "amebic tumors" is usually attributed to Kartulis (*Dysenterie* [Vienna: Alfred Hölder, 1896], p. 60), but an inspection of his article does not make it clear that he saw localized tumors which could be, for example, confused with cancer. H. Gunn and N. J. Howard ("Amebic granuloma of the large bowel," J.A.M.A., **97**:166, 1931) review the early references and introduce the term "amebic granuloma," which is now widely accepted. "The pathologic process consists in persistence of an isolated chronic ulcer with progressive erosion of the wall of the bowel. In response to the amebic ulceration and secondary infection, large amounts of edematous fibrous granulation tissue appear. . . . These granulomas may be easily mistaken for carcinoma, for they give symptoms, physical signs and radiologic appearances that may be identical with those produced by carcinoma." Spicknall and Pierce, however, give a definitive review of the subject with a bibliography of 125 titles. The main point is the frequency of a lesion in the cecal region and the likelihood of its being confused with acute appendicitis, abscess, or tumor.

Section 21

INFLUENZA

THE bibliography of influenza presents an extremely difficult problem. Before the pandemic of 1918, there was great confusion on the clinical side; since the "discovery" of the virus (1933), a vast literature has accumulated dealing with the complexities of transmission, of immunity, of multiple strains, of the constitution of the virus, and many other phases of the subject. A long list could readily be compiled, for example, of articles that deal only with the size of influenza virus particles. In a bibliography of this sort, therefore, designed primarily for students and clinicians, it has been necessary to confine ourselves mainly to the first or to early articles on each phase of the subject; this procedure may be regarded as an excuse for incompleteness, but the purpose has been to induct our readers into the subject as a whole rather than to pinpoint special aspects.

Comprehensive bibliographies are to be found in the following works:

HIRSCH, AUGUST. *Handbook of Geographical and Historical Pathology*, 1:41. London: New Sydenham Society, 1883.
LEICHTENSTERN, O. "Influenza." In NOTHNAGEL, *Specielle Pathologie und Therapie*, Vol. 4, Part I. Vienna: Alfred Hölder, 1896.
JORDAN, EDWIN O. *Epidemic Influenza: A Survey*. Chicago: American Medical Association, 1927.
THOMSON, D., and THOMSON, R. "Influenza." In *Annals of the Pickett-Thomson Research Laboratory*, Vol. 10. Baltimore: Williams & Wilkins Co., 1934.
For references to the modern experimental study of influenza see the article by Horsfall *in* RIVERS, THOMAS M., *Viral and Rickettsial Infections of Man*, p. 382. Philadelphia: J. B. Lippincott Co., 1952.

It is not our purpose to try to disentangle the early vague and uncertain accounts of epidemics of respiratory disease. The occurrence, however, of sharp and widespread outbreaks of a disorder of brief duration featured by sudden onset, great prostration, and "catarrhal" symptoms makes it probable that many of these actually were influenza. Lists of such epidemics or pandemics going back many centuries are given in the monographs by Hirsch and by Leichtenstern, and firsthand descriptions may be read in Theophilus Thompson's compilation, *Annals of Influenza, etc.* (London: Sydenham Society, 1852).

The origin of the term "influenza" is obscure. Leichtenstern—later often quoted—states that the word comes from the Italian *influenza di freddo*, or the influence of cold. In general, however, the word "influence" in this sense has been used more with reference to the stars or the planets than to atmospheric effects. Dr. Thomas Glass of Exeter, for example, is quoted in the *Annals of Influenza* (p. 101) as saying: "Physicians imputed the Epidemic Catarrhous Semi-Pestilential Fever to the influence of the stars; whence the Italians gave it the name of Influenza." Furthermore, in many of the earlier accounts the word seems to be used not as a specific name but as a general designation—as one spoke of a "flux" or of a "fever." Thus Dr. Molyneux in 1694 (*Annals of Influenza*, p. 24) says: "So general did this influenza rage that few or none escaped." By the end of the eighteenth century, however, the term "influenza" was used in much the same sense as today, to designate a distinct disorder.

In the pandemic of 1918–19 the violent disease had such fixed clinical characteristics as to be easily recognized. Since then, however, most outbreaks have not been very severe, and it has often been impossible to differentiate, on clinical grounds alone, mild "influenza" from a severe "common cold" or from other minor respiratory infections. This difficulty has greatly complicated studies of the etiology and ecology of influenza.

1. PARKES, Edmund A. Influenza, *in* A system of medicine, ed. J. Russell Reynolds, 1:28. 2d ed. London: Macmillan & Co., 1870.

Although there are innumerable clinical descriptions of influenza in the older literature, they usually consist of a catalogue of various symptoms without any real appreciation of a specific disease entity. The occurrence, in epidemics or pandemics, of fever, great prostration, respiratory, and other complaints is emphasized in varying degree. Whether or not Charles Lamb, for example, was suffering from postinfluenzal asthenia when he wrote the following in 1824 (*The Letters of Charles and Mary Lamb*, ed. E. V. Lucas [London: J. M. Dent & Sons, 1935], 2:413) we leave to the reader to guess: "Do you know what it is to succumb under an insurmountable day mare—an indisposition to do anything, or to be anything—a total deadness and distaste—a suspension of vitality—an indifference to locality—a numb soporifical good for nothingness—did you ever have a very bad cold with a total irresolution to submit to water gruel processes?"

The first clinical description we have found which seems to show any real understanding of the disease is that of Parkes: "The symptoms of Influenza are compounded of two conditions—a general fever of determinate duration and a marked and evidently specific affection of the mucous membrane of the nose, mouth, throat and respiratory tract, which has also a determinate course." The symptoms "last for four or five days usually—sometimes they continue ten or twelve days but this is generally when pneumonic complication supervenes." "A punctiform redness of the mucous membrane of the palate, something like the eruption of measles, has been lately described by Tigri [A. Tigri, "Sul grippe," Ann. Univ. de med., Milano, 102:667, 1867] and considered to be pathognomonic." Parkes sensed that influenza was not simply an indefinite "catarrhal" disease but a disorder of fixed and specific characteristics.

2. PFEIFFER, R. Vorläufige Mittheilungen über die Erreger der Influenza, Deutsche med. Wchschr., 18:28, 1892.

Although it is now known that the bacillus of Pfeiffer is not the cause of influenza, its etiological role was considered to be settled for so many years that the important articles dealing with the subject should be included in the bibliography. It must be remembered that Pfeiffer was a topflight bacteriologist. He was a colleague and friend of Robert Koch, Flügge, and Kolle. He did outstanding work in cholera, typhoid fever, and other diseases. He worked in one of the best-equipped institutions in the world for the study of infectious diseases. His integrity was unquestioned, and his work had to be taken seriously.

In this brief communication Pfeiffer reports the results of his studies in thirty-one cases of influenza, six with autopsy. In every case he found in the bronchial secretions a "certain bacillus." "In uncomplicated cases of influenza these rods were present in pure culture and usually in tremendous numbers." Furthermore, they were found only in influenza patients. He describes the morphology of the organism, the staining reactions (Gram-negative), and the difficulties of artificial culture. This convincing array of evidence was amplified in the next paper.

3. PFEIFFER, R. Die Aetiologie der Influenza, Ztschr. f. Hyg. u. Infektionskr., 13:357, 1893.

In this comprehensive paper Pfeiffer amplifies his brief preliminary report (Ref. 2). The constant finding of the "influenza bacillus" in cases of influenza is reiterated, and the necessity of a hemoglobin-containing medium for successful growth is pointed out. Inoculation experiments in monkeys are interpreted much more conservatively than those of Blake and Cecil nearly thirty years later (Ref. 5). The paper is a model of careful work by an experienced investigator, and, as one reads it, it is easy to see why the Pfeiffer bacillus was almost universally accepted as the cause of influenza until the pandemic of 1918. Even then and for reasons identical with Pfeiffer's, many experienced students of infectious disease still believed firmly in the etiological role of the Pfeiffer bacillus (see E. L. Opie, J. Small, F. G. Blake, and T. M. Rivers, *Epidemic Respiratory Disease* [St. Louis: C. V. Mosby Co., 1921]).

However, Pfeiffer probably confused the situation by regarding hemoglobinophilic bacteria isolated from diseases other than influenza as pseudo-influenza bacilli.

4. LEICHTENSTERN, O. Influenza, in Nothnagel, Specielle Pathologie und Therapie, Vol. 4, Part I. Vienna: Alfred Hölder, 1896.

No student of influenza can afford not to be familiar with this classical monograph. Based largely on the pandemic of 1890, it is definitive to date and takes up in great detail every aspect of the subject.

5. BLOOMFIELD, Arthur, and HARROP, George A., Jr. Clinical observations on epidemic influenza, Bull. Johns Hopkins Hosp., 30:1, 1919.

During the pandemic of 1918, Bloomfield and Harrop were able to study carefully the clinical phenomena in a closed group of young people. They were struck by the fact that epidemic influenza was a disease of highly fixed characteristics, like measles, chickenpox, or other disorders of probable viral origin. They emphasized (a) typical onset with a group of constitutional symptoms, (b) a striking erythema of the head and upper body, (c) a typical enanthem, (d) diffuse inflammation of the upper air passages, (e) fever of determinate duration, (f) leucopenia, and (g) a remarkable tendency to secondary bacterial infection in the lungs. To this might be added a curious and unexplained profound prostration quite out of proportion to what is usually seen in other infections.

Although at the time the influenza bacillus was generally accepted in America as the cause of the 1918 pandemic (Ref. 3), Bloomfield and Harrop could not believe that an organism so ubiquitously found as a saprophyte in interepidemic times could suddenly cause a specific disease of such highly fixed characteristics. Furthermore, in the Baltimore outbreak as well as elsewhere, influenza bacilli frequently were not isolated (S. E. Howard, "Bacteriological findings in epidemic influenza," Bull. Johns Hopkins Hosp., **30**:13, 1919). After casting doubt on the role of the Pfeiffer bacillus as the primary cause of influenza, the writers stated: "It is probable that the actual virus is as yet unidentified," a prediction which was verified in 1933 (Refs. 9, 10). At about the same time, the case against the influenza bacillus was clearly stated by F. T. Lord, A. Scott, and R. N. Nye ("Relation of the influenza bacillus to the recent epidemic of influenza," J.A.M.A., **72**:188, 1919). On the other hand, as late as 1920, prominent workers, such as F. G. Blake and R. L. Cecil ("The production of an acute respiratory disease in monkeys by inoculation with Bacillus influenzae," J.A.M.A., **74**:170, 1920) believed that they had produced influenza in monkeys by buccal or nasal instillation of cultures of *B. influenzae*. Some of their conclusions were: "The disease appears to be identical with influenza in man." "It seems reasonable to infer that 'B. influenzae' is the specific cause of influenza." All this will give the reader some idea of the active dispute as to etiology which followed the 1918 pandemic. The extensive contemporary literature is reviewed by Jordan (*op. cit.*).

Bloomfield (Bull. Johns Hopkins Hosp., **33**:172, 1922) later discussed the general significance of the influenza bacilli. He analyzed the evidence that these organisms, which were not present in over 20 per cent of normal throats before the pandemic of 1918, became widespread during and for 2 years after the pandemic but by 1921 were again found in less than 20 per cent of healthy people. Since the influenza bacilli isolated from patients were found to be a group of immunologically distinct varieties (see W. H. Park, J.A.M.A., **83**:318, 1919) and since they were frequently obtained from the respiratory passages of patients with diseases other than influenza, such as measles (A. W. Sellards and E. Sturm, "The occurrence of the Pfeiffer bacillus in measles," Bull. Johns Hopkins Hosp., **30**:331, 1919), it appeared that certain disorders, especially influenza, promoted an associated infection or infestation with the influenza bacillus group but that these organisms were not the cause of the primary disease. An analogous situation was worked out by R. E. Shope ("The influenzas of swine and man," Medicine, **15**:453, 1936), who showed that in swine influenza there was an association of a virus (the primary cause) with swine influenza bacilli.

At any rate, it seems clear that pandemic influenza in some way promotes great prevalence of the Pfeiffer bacillus in the respiratory passages of the general population.

6. DOUGLAS, Beverly. The reaction of the leucocytes in epidemic influenza, Bull. Johns Hopkins Hosp., **30**:338, 1919.

Careful total and differential leukocyte counts were made during the pandemic of 1918, and the frequency of marked leukopenia was pointed out. Fifty per cent of Douglas' group had leukocyte counts of under 5,000. Ten per cent had counts of less than 3,000. In a comparable group of mild non-pandemic cases studied by Doull and Bahlke (Ref. 19) only 23.2 per cent had counts under 5,000.

Douglas' paper seems to be the first systematic study of this important diagnostic sign.

7. MacCALLUM, W. G. The pathology of the pneumonia following influenza, J.A.M.A., **72**:720, 1919.

During and after the pandemic of 1918–19 an extensive and confusing literature on the pathological anatomy of influenza accumulated. The cause of influenza being as yet unknown, it was impossible to distinguish the fundamental lesions of the disease from those produced by the secondary invaders so abundant and so invariably present in the respiratory tract. We believe that credit is due to MacCallum for sensing a basic lesion, even though vaguely, apart from the secondary bacterial bronchopneumonias. "But now it appears that streptococci and influenza bacilli may in precisely similar ways be governed . . . it seems unnecessary to ascribe one type of lesion to the streptococcus and another to the influenza bacillus." MacCallum described quite distinctly the interstitial changes in the lung now known to be characteristic of virus pneumonitis of various kinds. The whole subject is elaborated and extensively pictured in his monographs ("The pathology of the pneumonia in the United States Army camps during the winter of 1917–18," Johns Hopkins Hosp. Rep., Vol. **20**, Fasc. 1 [Baltimore, 1920], and "Pathological anatomy of pneumonia associated with influenza," *ibid.*, Fasc. 2 [1921]). Another outstanding pathologist reviewed the subject later (E. L. Opie, "The pathological anatomy of influenza," Arch. Path. & Lab. Med., **5**:285, 1928), but it was necessary to wait for the experimental production of influenza in animals (Refs. 10, 11) to define the uncomplicated lesions. No accounts can be found of fatal influenza uncomplicated by secondary lesions of bacterial origin.

8. ROSENAU, Milton J. Experiments to determine mode of spread of influenza, J.A.M.A., **73**:311, 1919.

The question of how influenza spreads through the population had always been under active dispute. In the early days authorities divided themselves into "contagionists" and "non-contagionists." The former thought that an infective agent was transmitted from case to contact; the latter believed rather that some "miasm" was widely diffused, probably through the air, so that large groups were simultaneously attacked. A. Biermer, for example, an astute observer whose account of influenza as early as 1854 is a masterpiece (in R. Virchow [ed.], *Handbuch der speciellen Pathologie und Therapie* [Erlangen: Ferdinand Enke, 1854], **5**:592), argued against contagion. He was impressed by the frequency with which people living in intimate contact with patients failed to acquire the disease, and he thought that outbreaks of influenza were often too explosive to be explained by person-to-person contact. After the 1890 pandemic, when everyone believed the Pfeiffer bacillus was the cause of influenza, it was assumed that the disease was spread by rapid dissemination of these organisms. However, there were still many contradictions in the observed epidemiological facts, so Rosenau during the 1918 pandemic planned the rigorous tests described in this paper. Even though the results were negative, they are of the greatest importance. The procedure was as follows: The donors were patients in the first to third day of typical epidemic influenza. The volunteers were healthy young men who, as far as could be told, had not had influenza. There was no reason to think they were all immune. Nasal washings from the donors were sprayed and instilled into the throats of the volunteers. Swabs from the donors were rubbed directly over the pharynges of the volunteers. When these methods failed to produce any disease the following drastic experiment was carried out:

The volunteer was led up to the bedside of the patient; he was introduced. He sat down alongside the bed of the patient. They shook hands, and by instructions, he got as close as he conveniently could, and they talked for five minutes. At the end of the five minutes the patient breathed out as hard as he could, while the volunteer, muzzle to muzzle (in accordance with his instructions, about 2 inches between the two), received this expired breath and at the same time was breathing in as the patient breathed out. This they repeated five times, and they did it fairly faithfully in almost all the instances.

After they had done this for five times, the patient coughed directly into the face of the volunteer, face to face, five different times. After one volunteer had had this sort of contact with the patient, talking and chatting and shaking hands with him for five minutes, and receiving his breath five times, and then his cough five times directly in his face, he moved to the next patient whom he had selected and repeated this, and so on, until this volunteer had had that sort of contact with ten different cases of influenza, in different stages of the disease, mostly fresh cases, none of them more than 3 days old.

This experiment was repeated at various times and in various locations. In no case was an illness in any way resembling influenza produced. The full protocols are given in Bulletin No. 123 from the Hygienic Laboratory of the United States Public Health Service, Washington, February, 1921. The importance of these negative experiments cannot be overlooked; why others (Ref. 9) were able to transmit mild interepidemic influenza by much less drastic methods remains a puzzle.

The modern philosophy of transmission is discussed in Reference 25.

9. DOCHEZ, A. R., MILLS, K. C., and KNEELAND, Yale, Jr. Studies of the etiology of influenza, Proc. Soc. Exper. Biol. & Med., **30**:1017, 1933.

Although opinion generally favored a bacterial agent as the cause of influenza at the time of the 1918 pandemic, some workers were already investigating the question of a viral etiology. Various "rudimentary" transmission experiments, presently to be discussed, suffered from uncertainty as to the identity of the disease which was produced, usually a mild general reaction, often without any respiratory symptoms. In interepidemic times it was also hard to be sure of the identity of the donor disease. H. Selter ("Zur Aetiologie der Influenza," Deutsche med. Wchnschr., **44**:932, 1918) sprayed the throats of two volunteers with a filtrate of material obtained by throat swabs. A mild illness with constitutional symptoms, slight fever, but little in the way of respiratory symptoms, resulted. The author, however, thought his observations supported a virus etiology. Similarly, C. Nicolle and C. Lebailly ("Recherches expérimentales sur la grippe," Ann. Inst. Pasteur, **33**:395, 1919) thought that they had produced an influenza-like disorder in monkeys by nasal instillation and subconjunctival injection of filtrate from throat washings of influenza patients. Two human volunteers were considered to develop influenza after subcutaneous injection of filtrate. T. Yamanouchi and his associates in a brief note from Japan ("The infecting agent in influenza," Lancet, **1**:971, 1919) believed that they had produced influenza with sputum filtrates instilled into the throat and also by subcutaneous injection. Filtrates of blood from influenza patients instilled into the noses and throats of human volunteers were also said to produce influenza. After a preliminary note ("A filterable virus as the cause of the early stage of the present epidemic of influenza," Brit. M.J., **2**:645, 1918), H. Gibson, F. Bowman, and J. Connor issued a lengthy report ("Medical Research Committee, Special Reports," No. 36 [London, 1919]) on transmission experiments with filtrates of throat secretions and blood from influenza cases to monkeys, rabbits, guinea pigs, and mice—work which later observers (Ref. 10) were unable to confirm. More convincing are the careful observations of P. Long, E. Bliss, and H. Carpenter ("Etiology of influenza," J.A.M.A., **97**:1122, 1931), who produced a disorder "characterized by fever, prostration and leukopenia" in monkeys by pharyngeal inoculation of filtrates of nasopharyngeal washings from cases of influenza. All this work is, however, difficult to interpret, especially in the light of the extensive negative transmission experiments of Rosenau (Ref. 8). Furthermore, monkeys have not been found to develop clinical symptoms from inoculation of influenza virus, nor have animals or man come down when inoculated by routes other than the respiratory tract, even though parenteral injection has led to the development of immune bodies (Ref. 12).

The work of Dochez and his associates was much more decisive. They clearly produced a respiratory disease in a volunteer inoculated intranasally with filtrates of throat washings from a case of influenza. They also succeeded in propagating an infectious agent in chick embryo medium (see Dochez, Mills, and Kneeland, "Study of the virus of the common cold and its cultivation in tissue medium," Proc. Soc. Exper. Biol. & Med., **28**:513, 1931) through many generations, after which the material again produced respiratory infection in man. Dochez found it difficult to distinguish possible influenza virus from that of the common cold. In another paper ("Studies on the virus of influenza," J. Exper. Med., **63**:581, 1936) the same writers amplified their work. Meanwhile, T. Francis, Jr., and T. P. Magill ("Cultivation of human influenza virus in an artificial medium," Science, **82**:353, 1935) reported more extensive cultivation experiments in chick embryo medium, in which virus from mouse lung, propagated for many generations, was then capable of producing disease in both mice and ferrets.

10. SMITH, Wilson, ANDREWES, C. H., and LAIDLAW, P. P. A virus obtained from influenza patients, Lancet, **2**:66, 1933.

Although Dochez's paper (Ref. 9), published a few weeks before that of Smith, Andrewes, and Laidlaw, gives convincing evidence of isolation of a filterable virus from patients with influenza, it was with the work of the latter investigators that the modern study of influenza may really be said to have begun. This paper is therefore an important landmark. Throat washings from cases of influenza seen during the 1933 epidemic in England were inoculated into various animals without success until ferrets were used. The original animals received the material both intranasally and subcutaneously. The experimental disease had an incubation period of 1 or 2 days and was featured by fever, lethargy, weakness, and catarrhal symptoms, although there was a good deal of variation. Sections of the nasal mucosa of the ferrets showed acute inflammation, often with necrosis of the epithelium (see also Ref. 16). The disease was transmitted serially to other ferrets by contact or by nasal instillation of filtrates of an emulsion of the nasal mucosa. No route of infection other than the nasal proved effective. "The infectivity of the filtrates, coupled with the fact that we failed to grow anything from the filtrate—has convinced us we are dealing with a true virus disease." Ferrets recovered from the disease were immune to subsequent infection with the same strain of virus, and the serum of ferrets recovered from the disease neutralized emulsions of the virus. Normal ferret serum had no such power. Throat washings from healthy subjects and influenza convalescents poduced no disease in ferrets, nor did the secretions from a subject with a severe common cold, Convalescent sera and some human sera in general contained neutralizing bodies against the ferret disease.

This thorough work by experts in the field was immediately acclaimed, and a vast amount of investigation followed, which confirmed the writers' findings. We cannot catalogue the huge literature which has accumulated except for the papers that bring out something fundamentally new. It was Smith, Andrewes, and Laidlaw's report, however, which led to universal agreement that influenza was a disease of viral origin. The confirmatory but independent work of Francis ("Transmission of influenza by a filterable virus," Science, **80**:457, 1934) is especially to be mentioned.

11. ANDREWES, C. H., LAIDLAW, P. P., and SMITH, Wilson. The susceptibility of mice to the viruses of human and swine influenza, Lancet, **2**:859, 1934.

The work described in the previous paper (Ref. 10) was carried further by similar methods, and it was found that a disease transmissible in series could be produced in mice lightly anesthetized, by nasal instillation of material from the lungs of infected ferrets. In the mouse, in contrast to the ferret, the principal lesion was in the lung—an area of consolidation "not unlike some of those encountered in influenzal pneumonia in man." However, I. Brightman (Am. J. Dis. Child., **52**:78, 1936) later described lesions in the lungs of ferrets inoculated with influenza washings which conform to the interstitial type of pneumonitis commonly produced by various viruses. The use of mice has been an important aid in the study of influenza virus.

12. FRANCIS, Thomas, Jr., and MAGILL, T. P. Immunological studies with the virus of influenza, J. Exper. Med., **62**:505, 1935.

Francis and Magill made the important observation that subcutaneous inoculation of rabbits and mice with influenza virus did not cause clinical disease but produced active immunity, with the appearance of antibodies in the blood. Studies of this sort later furnished the basis for attempts actively to immunize human beings (Ref. 15).

During the next few years innumerable papers appeared on various phases of immunity to influenza.

13. SMITH, Wilson, and STUART-HARRIS, C. H. Influenza infection of man from the ferret, Lancet, **2**:121, 1936.

An important step in the characterization of influenza virus was, of course, proof that the experimental disease could be transmitted back to man. In this paper there is fairly convincing evidence that "S-H" contracted influenza from a ferret sick with passage virus. Immunological studies demonstrating increase in antibodies in the patient are presented.

Francis and his associates later (Am. J. Pub. Health, **34**:317, 1944) reported on the production of influenza in man with type B virus which had been passed through eggs and ferrets for many generations.

> 14. FRANCIS, Thomas, Jr., and MAGILL, T. P. The incidence of neutralizing antibodies for human influenza virus in the serum of human individuals of different ages, J. Exper. Med., **63**:665, 1936.

The writers found that about 50 per cent of the sera of individuals of various ages with no history of influenza contained sufficient antibody *after* the first year of life to furnish complete protection to mice. These observations suggested, of course, a high degree of unrecognized infection with influenza virus. The complexities of this subject were further analyzed by E. Rickard, E. Lennette, and F. Horsfall ("Comprehensive study of influenza in a rural community," Pub. Health Rep., **55**:2146, 1940). Antibody levels against influenza A virus were determined during a non-epidemic interval among 1,101 persons from four to eighty-five years of age. Variations in titer in relation to many factors, including history of infection, resistance, etc., are discussed. The same investigators, with G. Hirst, carried the study further ("Correlation between neutralizing antibodies in serum against influenza viruses and susceptibility to influenza in man," Pub. Health Rep., **56**:1819, 1941) and showed that the level of neutralizing bodies against the homologous type was important in determining susceptibility to influenza, but there was no cross-immunity between types A and B (Ref. 18). A great many other papers which we cannot list deal with variations on this theme.

> 15. FRANCIS, Thomas, Jr., and MAGILL, T. P. The antibody response of human subjects vaccinated with the virus of human influenza, J. Exper. Med., **65**:251, 1937.

It had been shown (Refs. 10, 11) that infection of mice and ferrets took place only by the respiratory route. However, animals inoculated subcutaneously or intraperitoneally developed active resistance to infection by the respiratory route (Refs. 10, 12). Francis and Magill vaccinated human volunteers by the subcutaneous or intradermal routes with virus grown in tissue culture medium. A "good titer" of circulating antibodies effective against mouse passage virus developed. The antibodies persisted for at least 5 months. A preliminary note of this work appeared in 1936 ("Vaccination of human subjects with virus of human influenza," Proc. Soc. Exper. Biol. & Med., **33**:604).

These experiments furnished the basis for the attempts at systematic vaccination against influenza which were later made. J. Stokes and his associates, for example ("Results of immunization by means of active virus of human influenza," J. Clin. Investigation, **16**:237, 1937), working in a state colony in the presence of an oncoming epidemic of "influenza," found that among those vaccinated there was an incidence of 2.7 per cent of febrile cases as against 12.5 per cent among the controls.

Although a large amount of work on the subject was subsequently done, vaccination against influenza has never had wide success, partly because immunity is short-lived, partly because it is impossible to predict the character of the strains which cause various outbreaks, and partly because there are wide variations in antibody response of different individuals (Hirst, Rickard, Whitman, and Horsfall, "Antibody response of human beings following vaccination with influenza viruses," J. Exper. Med., **75**:495, 1942). Early reports of clinical experiences are to be found in the American Journal of Hygiene for 1945, where the entire July number is devoted to the subject. T. Francis, Jr., J. Salk, and their associates also made important observations ("Protective effect of vaccination against induced influenza," J. Clin. Investigation, **24**:536, 1945; see also Ref. 18).

16. FRANCIS, Thomas, Jr., and STUART-HARRIS, C. H. Studies of the nasal histology of epidemic influenza in the ferret, J. Exper. Med., **68**:789, 1938.

The writers made daily histological studies of the nasal mucosa of ferrets after instillation of influenza virus. They found that, by 48 hours, complete destruction of the respiratory epithelium had occurred. This was followed by deeper changes. It required several weeks for the reparative processes to be complete. Meanwhile, M. Straub (J. Path. & Bact., **45**:75, 1937) reported on the microscopic changes in the lungs of mice infected with influenza virus. The same pattern was disclosed, namely, "necrobiosis and fibrinoid necrosis of the epithelium of the respiratory and terminal bronchioles leading to a state of complete epithelial desquamation." It appears that the virus of influenza in the experimental animal and in the chick embryo (Ref. 17) localizes specifically in the respiratory epithelium and is not to be found in other accessible areas or in the blood.

If a similar lesion occurs in the deeper air passages in human influenza, as seems highly probable, many of the clinical features of the disease are explained, including the tendency to secondary infection because of the injured mucous membrane and the prolonged and distressing cough which so often follows the acute attack.

17. BURNET, F. M. Influenza virus infection of the chick embryo by the amniotic route, Australian J. Exper. Biol. & M. Sc., **18**:353, 1940.

The use of chick embryo infection has become so essential in the study of influenza that this important paper should be mentioned. The technique of egg inoculation is described. It is pointed out that the lesions affect primarily the epithelial lining of the respiratory tract, particularly within the developing lung, which contains more virus than any other organ, although large amounts are present in both amniotic and allantoic fluids (see also F. M. Burnet, "Influenza virus infection of the chick embryo lung," Brit. J. Exper. Path., **21**:147, 1940). Hirst later ("Direct isolation of influenza virus in chick embryos," Proc. Soc. Exper. Biol. & Med., **58**:155, 1945) found that, by adding penicillin to unfiltered throat washings, they could be inoculated directly into the amniotic sac without the complication of bacterial infection. Wilson Smith ("Cultivation of the virus of influenza," Brit. J. Exper. Path., **16**:508, 1935) seems, however, to have been the first to propagate influenza virus in the living chick embryo, although no lesions were to be seen in the early passages. The whole subject is reviewed by Burnet in *The Use of the Developing Egg in Virus Research* ("Medical Research Council, Special Report Series," No. 220 [London, 1936]).

18. FRANCIS, T., Jr. A new type of virus from epidemic influenza, Science, **92**:405, 1940.

During the first few years of the experimental study of influenza (Ref. 10) it was thought that there was only one type of virus. Strains isolated in England, in the United States, in Puerto Rico, and elsewhere were shown by immunological tests to be identical. H. Reimann and J. Stokes ("Epidemic infection of respiratory tract in 1938–1939; a newly recognized entity," Tr. A. Am. Physicians, **54**:123, 1939) and others had, however, studied outbreaks of respiratory disease which resembled influenza, in which convalescent sera contained no neutralizing antibodies for the viruses previously isolated. In 1940 Francis isolated from an outbreak in New York State an agent which produced the typical reactions of influenza in ferrets but which, by all existing immunological criteria, could not be the hitherto identified virus. It turned out that it was another type of influenza virus immunologically quite distinct from the original strains. Francis suggested that the new type be designated type B, in contrast to the previously defined type A. At about the same time, Magill ("A virus from cases of influenza-like upper-respiratory infection," Proc. Soc. Exper. Biol. & Med., **45**:162, 1940) also reported recovery of a virus immunologically distinct from the standard PR_8 strain (A). The diseases produced by the two types were clinically indistinguishable. In the same year, Horsfall, Lennette, and Rickard (Lancet, **2**:413, 1940) discussed the whole question of the terminology of respiratory viruses and suggested the probability that further immunologically unrelated strains would be discovered. A. Rasmussen, J. Stokes, and J. Smadel ("The army experience with influenza, 1946–1947. II. Laboratory aspects," Am. J. Hyg., **47**:142, 1948) reported on influenza in the army during 1946–47. The so-called Fort Monmouth strain of virus from this outbreak was definitely not influenza B and also had significant immunological differences from the usual strains of influenza A. Standard influenza A vaccine failed to protect against infection with the F.M. strains (see also Ref. 15). These reports illustrate the extreme complexity of the antigenic relations among various strains of influenza virus.

Francis ("Differentiation of influenza A and influenza B by complement fixation reaction," Proc. Soc. Exper. Biol. & Med., **45**:861, 1940) was able to differentiate influenza viruses A and B by means of complement fixation. W. Smith ("The complement fixation reaction in influenza," Lancet, **2**:1256, 1936) had already shown that infected mouse lungs could be used as antigen for complement fixation, and Lennette and Horsfall ("Studies on epidemic influenza virus; the nature and properties of the complement-fixing antigen," J. Exper. Med., **72**:233, 1940) were later to show that influenza virus elaborates a soluble antigen.

19. STUART-HARRIS, C. H., SMITH, W., and ANDREWES, C. H. The influenza epidemic of January–March, 1939, Lancet, **1**:205, 1940.

The clinical definition of influenza in relation to the type of virus is, of course, of great importance. Numerous papers have dealt with this subject, which is still in a confused state because of the difficulty in clinical identification of mild respiratory infections. This paper and that of F. Horsfall, R. Hahn, and E. Rickard ("Four recent influenza epidemics: an experimental study," J. Clin.

Investigation, **19**:379, 1940) may be mentioned as examples of thorough study of mild interpandemic influenza, from both the clinical and the viral standpoint. J. Doull and A. Bahlke ("Epidemic influenza: a comparison of clinical observations in a major and a minor epidemic," Am. J. Hyg., **17**:562, 1933) made a careful comparison of the clinical features of a minor epidemic (1928–29) occurring in the institution where pandemic influenza had been carefully studied in 1918–19. They concluded that, except for a lesser severity manifested especially by freedom from pneumonia, the later outbreak bore a striking resemblance to the 1918 pandemic.

20. HIRST, George K. The agglutination of red cells by allantoic fluid of chick embryos infected with influenza virus, Science, **94**:22, 1941.

When the allantoic fluid from chick embryos previously infected with strains of influenza A virus was being removed, it was noted that the red cells of the infected chick, coming from ruptured vessels, were agglutinated in this fluid. Since red cells in the allantoic fluid of chick embryos inoculated with sterile materials were not agglutinated at all, it seemed that this phenomenon might be the result of infection with influenza virus in the chick.

This fundamental observation made possible a relatively simple method for isolating and concentrating influenza virus, since the adsorbed virus can be released from the red cells and recaptured. It has also made possible a simple test for antibodies because virus neutralized by immune serum no longer agglutinates chicken red cells.

In other papers ("The quantitative determination of influenza virus and antibodies by means of red cell agglutination," J. Exper. Med., **75**:49, 1942; "Adsorption of influenza hemagglutinins and virus by red blood cells," *ibid.*, **76**:195) Hirst elaborated the whole subject and pointed out that, by testing the inhibition of red cell agglutination, one can obtain quantitative data on the titer of immune sera and also that the degree of agglutination was proportional to the concentration of virus in the test material.

Hirst also made the important observation ("Adsorption of influenza virus on cells of the respiratory tract," J. Exper. Med., **78**:99, 1943) that influenza virus was adsorbed by the cells of the excised ferret lung as well as by the lung of the living ferret.

Cultivation of virus in chick embryo and the red cell agglutination tests have made viral and immunological studies of influenza relatively simple.

21. HIRST, George K. Studies of antigenic differences among strains of influenza A by means of red cell agglutination, J. Exper. Med., **78**:406, 1943.

Hirst showed that within the group of type A influenza viruses there were strains of different antigenic patterns. It was found that certain epidemics were caused by multiple strains. The implications for vaccination against influenza virus are obvious. The subject was elaborated by T. Magill and J. Sugg ("The significance of antigenic differences among strains of the 'A group' of influenza viruses," J. Exper. Med., **80**:1, 1944). Sugg and Magill ("Significance of antigenic differences among strains of influenza A virus in reinfection of ferrets," Proc. Soc. Exper. Biol. & Med., **63**:1, 1946) later showed that ferrets immune to clinical reinfection with the same strain of virus were susceptible to another strain antigenically related to, but different from, that used for the original infection (see also Refs. 15, 18).

22. CHAMBERS, Leslie A., HENLE, Werner, LAUFFER, Max A., and ANDERSON, Thomas F. Studies on the nature of the virus of influenza. II. The size of the infectious unit in influenza A, J. Exper. Med., **77**:265, 1943.

These workers thought that they had showed, by ultracentrifugation of infected extra-embryonic fluids of the developing chick embryo, that previous estimation of the size of the virus particles (about 100 mμ) was much too large. "Electron micrographs of the isolated virus protein indicated that the predominating unit is roughly spherical in shape and has a modal particle diameter of about 11 mμ in good agreement with the sedimentation data indicating a molecular weight of about 650,000."

The matter turned out not to be so simple, however, and W. Friedewald and E. Pickels ("Size of infective particle and hemagglutinin of influenza virus as determined by centrifugal analysis," Proc. Soc. Exper. Biol. & Med., **52**:261, 1943) soon claimed that the particle size was much larger. The extensive studies of W. Stanley ("The size of influenza virus," J. Exper. Med., **79**:267, 1944) led to the conclusion that virus activity is associated with a particle diameter of about 70 mμ. J. W. Beard and his associates, working on the problem at the same time ("Ultracentrifugal, chemical and electron microscopic identification of influenza virus," Southern M.J., **37**:313, 1944), found influenza B particles to be slightly larger than influenza A particles. The ultracentrifuge, the electron microscope, and chemical analysis were all used in this work, the usual source of the virus being a concentrate obtained by adsorption on and elution from chicken red blood cells of infected amniotic fluids of chick embryos. Purification and chemical composition were further studied by C. Knight ("The preparation of highly purified PR 8 influenza virus from infected mouse lungs," J. Exper. Med., **83**:11, 1946; "The nucleic acid and carbohydrate of influenza virus," *ibid.*, **85**:99, 1947; "Amino acid composition of highly purified viral particles of influenza A and B," *ibid.*, **86**:125, 1947). R. Williams and R. Wyckoff ("Electron shadow-micrography of virus particles," Proc. Soc. Exper. Biol. & Med., **58**:265, 1945) devised a "shadow" technique of electron microscopy which gives vivid pictures of virus particles. The present consensus as a result of much further work seems to be that influenza virus particles have a diameter of about 80 mμ (see R. C. Williams, "The shapes and sizes of purified viruses as determined by electron microscopy," Cold Spring Harbor Symposia Quant. Biol., **18**:185, 1953). C. Morgan, H. Rose, and D. Moore ("Structure and development of viruses observed in the electron microscope," J. Exper. Med., **104**:171, 1956) give further data on the shape and structure of influenza virus particles.

23. CROWLEY, James H., THIGPEN, Minnie P., and RICKARD, E. R. Isolation of influenza A virus from normal human contacts during an epidemic of influenza A, Proc. Soc. Exper. Biol. & Med., **57**:354, 1944.

The question of carriers of influenza virus or of subclinical infection is, of course, of great importance. In this paper direct allantoic inoculation of throat washings from apparently healthy contacts yielded five positive results in thirteen trials. Increase in neutralizing antibodies was noted in most cases, which suggested a subclinical infection, but in three cases no significant increase in antibodies was found, so that these individuals may have been carriers without actual infection.

Others had reported (T. Francis, Jr., T. P. Magill, E. R. Rickard, and M. D. Beck, "Etiological and serological studies in epidemic influenza," Am. J. Pub. Health, **27**:1141, 1937) increase in neutralizing bodies in the sera of individuals exposed, but without apparent infection; no one had hitherto isolated virus from such cases.

24. COMMISSION ON ACUTE RESPIRATORY DISEASE, FORT BRAGG, NORTH CAROLINA. The periodicity of influenza, Am. J. Hyg., **43**:29, 1946.

It is impossible in this bibliography to refer extensively to the huge literature on the epidemiology of influenza. This report, however, seems of direct importance to the clinician. In a study of sixteen epidemics of influenza in the United States between 1920 and 1944 it turned out that influenza A occurred in a cycle of 2–3 years and influenza B in a cycle of 4–6 years. The writers speculate on the significance of this periodicity.

25. BURNET, Frank Macfarland. Some biological implications of studies on influenza viruses, Bull. Johns Hopkins Hosp., **88**:119, 1951.

This is an extremely important discussion by a great authority on the subject, which should be studied by everyone interested in influenza. The complicated problems of transmission, mechanism of infection, and immunity are analyzed against the background of virus infections in general. Almost equally useful is the chapter on influenza in Burnet's book, *Virus as Organism* (Cambridge: Harvard University Press, 1945). Burnet later summarized his views on the structure of influenza virus (Science, **123**:1101, 1956) with reference to mode of entry into the cells, structure, multiplication, etc.

POLIOMYELITIS: 1800 TO EXPERIMENTAL TRANSMISSION (1909)

A MONUMENTAL compilation sponsored by the National Foundation for Infantile Paralysis (A *Bibliography of Infantile Paralysis, 1789–1949* [2d ed.; Philadelphia: J. B. Lippincott Co., 1951]) gives a complete list of articles and books on poliomyelitis and supplants all previous less comprehensive bibliographies. However, in the survey of poliomyelitis published by the Milbank Foundation (*Poliomyelitis* [Baltimore: Williams & Wilkins Co., 1932]), there is to be found a very useful reference list of over eight hundred titles.

Valuable contemporary monographs which cover approximately the period of this bibliography are as follows:

RÖMER, P. H. *Die epidemische Kinderlähmung.* Berlin: J. Springer, 1911. English translation by H. RIDLEY PRENTICE, *Epidemic Infantile Paralysis.* London: John Bale, 1913.

WICKMAN, IVAN. *Acute Poliomyelitis.* Authorized translation by DR. J. WILLIAM J. A. M. MALONEY. New York: Journal of Nervous and Mental Disease Publishing Co., 1913.

MÜLLER, EDUARD. *Die spinale Kinderlähmung.* Berlin: Julius Springer, 1910.

PEABODY, FRANCIS W., DRAPER, GEORGE, and DOCHEZ, A. R. *A Clinical Study of Acute Poliomyelitis.* New York: Rockefeller Institute for Medical Research, 1912.

1. The various early-nineteenth-century accounts of poliomyelitis are brief, confused, and inadequate. Descriptions of the disorder are included, as a rule, in general discussions of the paralyses of childhood. Many of them deal with late stages of deformity, the original cause of which is quite unrecognizable.[1] However, those case reports which concern a child suddenly paralyzed in one or more limbs either out of a clear sky or following some sort of an indisposition may well have had to do with poliomyelitis. Modern writers credit Underwood at the turn of the nineteenth century with the first significant description of infantile paralysis. However, a scrutiny of his book (Michael Underwood, *A Treatise on the Diseases of Children, etc.* [2d American ed.; Boston: D. West, 1806])[2] yields little that is definite, although what he describes under "Debility of the lower extremities" (p. 261) may perhaps have been poliomyelitis. "But the complaint at other times . . . seems to arise from debility and usually attacks children previously reduced by fever. . . . It is a chronical, or lingering complaint, and not attended with pain, fever or any manifest disease. . . . When both [legs] have been paralytic, nothing has seemed to do any good but irons to the legs." The position was later well summarized (1855) by Duchenne (Ref. 3), who writes, with reference to the older accounts: "I must say that if one had to depend only on the de-

---

[1] Those who wish references to all the early case reports, both definite and questionable, will find them listed in the National Foundation's *Bibliography of Poliomyelitis.*

[2] The earliest edition of Underwood's book in which reference is made to this disorder appeared in 1789.

scriptions of these authors the diagnosis and prognosis of this disease of childhood would remain very uncertain [*dans une grande obscurité*]."

In sharp contrast to the professional accounts is the admirable description of his own case given by Sir Walter Scott in his autobiography (J. G. Lockhart, *Memoirs of the Life of Sir Walter Scott, Bart.* [Edinburgh: Robert Cadell, 1837], 1:14), written in 1808: "One night, I have been told, I showed great reluctance to be caught and put to bed, and after being chased about the room, was apprehended and consigned to my dormitory with some difficulty. It was the last time I was to show such personal agility. In the morning I was discovered to be affected with the fever which often accompanies the cutting of larger teeth. It held me three days. On the fourth, when they went to bathe me as usual, they discovered that I had lost the power of my right leg."

As to terminology, the first use of various designations was as follows:

Debility of the lower extremities: Underwood (1789), Ref. 1.
Essential paralysis of childhood (*paralysie essentielle de l'enfance*): Rilliet (1843), Ref. 2.
Acute anterior poliomyelitis (*poliomyelitis anterior acuta*): Erb (1847), Ref. 8.
Atrophic fatty paralysis of childhood (*paralysie atrophique graisseuse de l'enfance*): Duchenne (1855), Ref. 3.
Infantile paralysis: Terry (1855); Kennedy (1861), Ref. 2.
Infantile spinal paralysis (*spinale Kinderlähmung*): Heine (1860), Ref. 2.

It should be remembered that exact appraisal of many of the case reports in the early literature is impossible. With the etiological agent unknown, with no specific diagnostic test, and without examination of the spinal fluid, it is understandable that confusion should exist about a disease which is often abortive and which often shows irregular features.

2. HEINE, J. Beobachtungen über Lähmungszustände der unteren Extremitäten und deren Behandlung. Stuttgart: F. H. Köhler, 1840.

The work of Heine has been so much extolled—indeed, in Germany and Scandinavia his name has been attached to the disease he described (Heine-Medinsche Krankheit)—that it is difficult to make an unbiased appraisal of his observations. Heine was certainly the first to collect any considerable number of cases and to describe them carefully; he attempted to bring order into the subject, and his monograph is clear and well written. Heine believed that disease of the spinal cord was responsible for the clinical features, but he had no fatal cases in his series and made no firsthand observations of the lesions. "These phenomena lead us to the presumption that an affection of the spinal cord of irritative or congestive sort underlies the disease." He gives no indication, however, of appreciating any specific changes in the anterior horn cells. In his description of the clinical picture he emphasizes occurrence in children six to thirty-six months old and in previous good health. As initial symptoms there may be fever, "congestive and irritative" states, depression, crying, drowsiness, and difficult teething. Convulsions are frequent. In other cases convulsions, nausea, collapse, foaming at the mouth and nose, and cyanosis constitute a sudden onset. Sometimes there are no recognizable symptoms, and the paralysis is simply noticed. As observed by others, the patients rarely died and often promptly recovered, even from extensive disability. Some, however, had permanent weakness, and Heine, who was an orthopedist, gives a comprehensive account of the physical therapy and rehabilitation which are necessary. His monograph is illustrated with excellent drawings of deformities following paralysis and of braces applied to the legs. While he emphasized paralysis of the lower extremities, he also described patients with hemiplegia and paralysis of the arms.

Just what all these disorders actually were it is hard to say now. Peripheral neuritis and perhaps encephalitis may have been present in some cases. Heine certainly deserves credit for being the first to crystallize the subject. His monograph of 1840 was preceded by a more inaccessible paper ("Ueber Lähmungen, die im kindlichen Alter nach Convulsionen entstehen können und gewöhnlich von bedeutender oder peripherer Difformität der unteren Extremitäten begleitet werden," Tageblatt d. Vers. deutsch. Naturforsch. u. Aertze, 1838) and was followed by other articles ("Aufförderungen an praktische Aerzte," Schweiz. Monatschr. f. prakt. Med., **2**:269, 1857) and by his book of 1860 (*Spinale Kinderlähmung* [Stuttgart: J. G. Cotta'scher Verlag, 1860]), in which he introduced the designation "infantile paralysis" but otherwise added nothing essential to his monograph of 1840.

Other more or less contemporary accounts, some of which have been much quoted, are the following:

J. Badham reported four cases ("Paralysis in childhood," London M. Gaz., **17**:215, 1834–35) which were probably poliomyelitis, although the brief clinical descriptions are not entirely decisive. From the mélange of patients reported by C. West ("On some forms of paralysis incidental to infancy and childhood," London M. Gaz., N.S., **2**:829, 1842–43), one may select three or four who quite definitely had infantile paralysis. These very cases, however, in contrast to those caused by "disease of the brain," West regarded as representing a mild disorder due to teething or to measles with probably no organic lesion. He appears to have been unaware of Heine's work.

F. Rilliet and E. Barthez in their book (*Traité clinique et pratique des maladies des enfants* [Paris: Gearner Baillière, 1843], **2**:335), under the heading of "Essential Paralysis" discuss sudden palsies occurring in children which may perhaps have been poliomyelitis. In the one case which they report in detail, the brain and spinal cord were said to show no lesion. Rilliet later ("De la paralysie essentielle chez les enfants," Gaz. méd., Paris, **6**, ser. 3, 681, 1851) wrote systematically on the subject but added little to his previous remarks. The account of H. Kennedy ("On some of the forms of paralysis which occur in early life," Dublin J.M. Sc., **9**:85, 1850) is no less confusing and deals with superficial clinical considerations. Whether some of his cases were poliomyelitis or not it is impossible to say. Kennedy believed that there was no anatomical lesion, although he had no autopsies; indeed, none of his patients died. Kennedy did, however, suggest that the same varieties of paralysis might occur in adults: "I am satisfied there is much less difference between the paralysis of early and more advanced life than what might at first sight appear—I am sure I have seen in the adult all the forms of paralysis which it has been my wish to describe as occurring in the young." Chaussignac's description ("De la paralysie douloureuse des enfants jeunes," Arch. gén. de méd., **1**:653, 1856) does not in the slightest way resemble poliomyelitis, nor can anything useful be extracted from the lectures of C. E. Brown-Séquard (*Lectures on the Diagnosis and Treatment of the Principal Forms of Paralysis of the Lower Extremities* [Philadelphia: J. B. Lippincott & Co., 1861]). Joseph Bierbaum, a general practitioner in the town of Dorsten, has an article of ninety-nine pages ("Die Paralysen der Kinder," J. F. Kinderkr., **32**:18, 1859) which brings out very clearly the confusion that existed in the minds of doctors about the paralyses of children. "In my situation without access to libraries, it is impossible to have a wide knowledge of the literature," says Bierbaum; but nonetheless his article represents a good effort to straighten out the situation. The main difficulties were inadequate knowledge of neuroanatomy and clinical neurology, lack of fatal cases with autopsies, and the widely prevailing idea that paralysis of a limb or limbs in small children could often occur as a functional disturbance without any lesion.

In all these early accounts, as we said, one is struck by the common story of sudden complete paralysis of a limb coming out of a perfectly clear sky, the lack of fatal cases, and often complete rapid recovery of a totally disabled part. If this disease really was poliomyelitis, the clinical features and perhaps the strains of virus have clearly changed through the years—a well-known phenomenon in medicine, as witness syphilis, typhoid fever, smallpox, and many others. It should also be mentioned that the early writers for the most part regarded the paralysis as "reflex" from some source of irritation such as teething. Later, hemorrhage was often blamed. The actual lesion was not generally recognized until the 1870's (Ref. 5).

3. DUCHENNE DE BOULOGNE, [Guillaume Benjamin Armand]. Paralysie atrophique graisseuse de l'enfance. Paris: J.-B. Baillière et fils, 1855.

Aside from his achievements in neurology, Duchenne was a pioneer in medical electricity; his book *De l'électrisation localisée* is a classic and ran through many editions.[3] By studying the electrical reactions of paralyzed children, Duchenne discovered that different muscles or muscle groups were variously affected, even though shortly after the paralysis the muscles did not yet appear atrophied. He concluded, by analogy with cases of cord injury, that the lesion in infantile paralysis must also lie in the spinal cord, although he did not define the histological changes. Duchenne also gave an admirable clinical description of the disease; he noted the frequency of fever at onset, the sensory symptoms, the types of paralysis, and the late atrophies and deformities. He designated the disease "atrophic fatty paralysis of childhood" but later (see the third edition of his *Électrisation* [1871]) dropped the "fatty" and spoke simply of "atrophic paralysis of childhood." At this time he thought the disease occurred only in children and could find no more plausible cause than teething. Later (Ref. 6) he realized that the same disease affected adults. He developed electrotherapy and was able, on the basis of the degree of altered electrical reaction, to predict which muscle groups would recover most quickly. Duchenne's observations were later elaborated in a long article ("De la paralysie atrophique graisseuse de l'enfance," Arch. gén. de méd., **2**:28, 184, 441, 1864). Erb's name ("Ueber

[3] English translation of the third edition: *A Treatise on Localized Electrization, etc.*, by Dr. G. B. Duchenne, translated by Herbert Tibbits, M.D. (London: Robert Hardwicke, 1871).

Poliomyelitis anterior chronica nebst Bemerkungen über die diagnostische und pathologisch-physiologische Bedeutung der Entartungsreaction," Arch. f. Psychiat., **8**:216, 1878) is also prominently associated with interpretation of electrical reactions in cases of poliomyelitis.

4. TAYLOR, Charles Fayette. Infantile paralysis and its attendant deformities. Philadelphia: J. B. Lippincott Co., 1867.

Even in the earliest accounts of poliomyelitis, attention was directed toward treatment. As early as Underwood (Ref. 1), the need of braces for the late deformities was recognized. Heine gives a detailed discussion of this phase in his books (Ref. 2). Other measures both medical and physical, including electrical treatment, were discussed by such writers as Duchenne and Taylor.

In view of the modern Kenny treatment it is of interest to note that Taylor, as long ago as 1867, fully recognized the value of heat in general and of hot packs in particular for the first stages of the disease. "All those who have had experience in these cases have recommended the warm or hot local bath as of great value. My experience is that the value of local heat in these cases cannot be overestimated." Taylor also gives a sophisticated account of the mechanism of production of deformities, their prevention and their treatment by orthopedic methods and appliances. He noticed, furthermore, that the incidence of infantile parlysis was increasing rapidly in this country.

5. CHARCOT, J. A., and JOFFROY, A. Cas de paralysie infantile spinale avec lésions des cornes antérieures de la substance grise de la moelle épinière, Arch. de physiol., **3**:134, 1870.

It is very difficult to decide who deserves credit for first describing the nature of the spinal cord lesion in infantile paralysis. All the early reports dealt with autopsies of patients whose paralysis had occurred months to many years before death. Charcot's case, for example, concerned a girl who, at the age of six, following an indisposition of some sort, suddenly lost the use of arms and legs without sphincter disturbance or sensory loss. There was some gradual recovery in the arms but little return of power in the legs. At the time of her death, twenty years after the acute phase, there were, of course, severe atrophies and contractures. The writers described in detail the gross appearance of muscles and spinal cord; they showed in excellent drawings the atrophy of the anterior horns. They pointed out that certain muscles had become transformed into fibrous strands; others "conserved their normal bulk, but almost all the tissue was replaced by fat through which ran reddish shreds which are nothing else than muscle fibers." A section through the cord (cervical) showed that "the anterior horns are wasted and deformed. No traces of nerve cells are any longer found." Charcot correlated the degree of damage in the cord with the extent of the muscular atrophy: "The alterations which we have described are clearly nothing more than the vestiges of a pathological process whose activity is long since extinct." He doubted current views that hemorrhage or softening was the original lesion: "Why this remarkable localization in the area of the anterior horns if the neuroglia was first affected? Is it not more probable that the motor nerve cells, whose function is so specialized, were the primary seat of the disease?" This point of view was elaborated in another paper ("Groupe des myopathies de cause spinale—paralyse infantile," Rev. phot. d'hôp. de Paris, 4:1, 1872).

V. Cornil ("Paralyse infantile," Compt. rend. Soc. de biol., **5**, 3d ser., 187, 1863) had previously reported from Charcot's clinic what appears to be a dubious case. It concerned a forty-nine-year-old woman whose feet were said to have been paralyzed from the age of two years. She died of cancer of the breast. The cord lesion was described as "an atrophy of the anteroposterior tracts [*faisceux*] of the cord, with production of amyloid bodies through its extent." The case of J. L. Prevost ("Observation de paralysie infantile; lésion des muscles et de la moelle," Compt. rend. Soc. de biol., **2**, 4th ser., 215, 1865) is also unsatisfactory; the patient died at seventy-eight years of age, and the story of the childhood paralysis is obviously vague. At autopsy there was a purulent meningitis. However, many of the anterior roots were atrophic, and there was atrophy of cells of the anterior horns corresponding to the innervation of the paralyzed foot, so the case may well have been an old poliomyelitis. The much-quoted report of Lockhart Clarke and Hughlings Jackson ("On a case of muscular atrophy, etc.," M.-Chir. Tr., **32**:489, 1867), however, obviously concerns a patient with amyotrophic lateral sclerosis and not poliomyelitis.

It was not until much later (Ref. 12) that the lesions of the acute attack were described, although F. C. Turner (Tr. Path. Soc., London, **30**:202, 1879) gives an excellent and comprehensive description of the pathology of a cord from a child who died only two months after onset of paralysis. He noted that the main changes were in the anterior horns and pointed out perivascular cuffing by leukocytes.

Roger and Damaschino (Compt. rend. Soc. de biol., **23**:49, 1871) carried the subject along with anatomical studies, from which they concluded that "the characteristic alteration is a lesion of the spinal cord of which the atrophy of nerves and muscles is the result." They localized the lesion especially in the anterior horns and pointed out that "the softening is inflammatory in nature and the disease is a myelitis."

It was not, however, until the twentieth century that comprehensive descriptions of the pathology of poliomyelitis in the modern sense became available (see I. Wickman *in* M. Lewandowsky, *Handbuch der Neurologie* [Berlin: J. Springer, 1911], **2**:807).

6. DUCHENNE (DE BOULOGNE). De l'électrisation localisée, etc., pp. 437 ff. 3d ed. Paris: J.-B. Baillière et fils, 1872.

Although Kennedy (Ref. 2) and perhaps others thought that poliomyelitis could occur in adults, it was generally regarded as affecting only small children. Duchenne, however, reported quite typical cases in older people. He concluded (p. 444): "There have been no anatomical reports on cases of acute spinal paralysis of adults, but, reasoning by analogy, one reaches this conclusion. If one considers the resemblance of symptoms, course, and termination of this disorder in adults to the findings in children, where the pathology of the cord is well known, one must conclude that the same lesion will be found in adults— atrophy of the anterior horn cells of the cord."

Many papers soon followed confirming this point of view. Gombault (Arch. de physiol., **5**:80, 1873) described two supposed cases of poliomyelitis in men aged thirty-five and forty years[4] and also an instance in a girl of seventeen, who came to autopsy seven years later with a lesion practically confined to "the large motor cells of the anterior horns." M. Bernhardt ("Ueber eine der spinalen Kinderlähmung ähnliche Affection Erwachsener," Arch. f. Psychiat., **4**:370, 1873) reported several more typical cases in adults, and, from this time on, it was generally accepted that poliomyelitis was not confined to infants.

7. EISENLOHR, C. Zur Lehre von der akuten spinalen Paralyse, Arch. f. Psychiat., **5**:219, 1875.

The idea that physical strain or exposure in the early stages of poliomyelitis had a detrimental effect on the course of the disease is often set forward as a modern concept. This view was, however, emphasized in many reports as long ago as seventy-five years. Eisenlohr, for example, tells of a man of thirty-three who went home in the cool of the morning lightly clad after dancing all night (*nach einer durchtanzten Nacht*) and then developed progressive motor weakness in the lower extremities. The same point is vividly brought out by T. Althaus ("On acute anterior myelitis in the adult," Am. J.M. Sc., **75**:409, 1878). He tells of a man who was out taking exercise in a very powerful sun and toward evening took a bath in the sea. "The water felt very chilly, but he never-the-less remained about three-quarters of an hour in it. On coming out at last he felt benumbed and in the night had acute pain in the small of the back and legs." During the next day he had difficulty walking, which rapidly went on to paralysis. Bull ("Sub-acute spinal paralysis of adults," Lancet, **1**:563, 1880) also reported a patient in whom "an interesting feature of the case was the undoubted relation of the attack to exposure."

8. ERB, W. Ueber acute Spinallähmung (Poliomyelitis anterior acuta) bei Erwachsenen, etc., Arch. f. Psychiat., **5**:758, 1875.

Erb's paper is of note because here for the first time is used the term "acute anterior poliomyelitis." Erb also carried the subject forward by a brilliant clinical description of the disease, in which he points out that mild and severe cases are not essentially different disorders, as many previously had thought, but rather different phases of one spectrum. One hopes to read that he went further and sensed the abortive or non-paralytic cases, but he did not. He describes several cases in adults.

9. SINKLER, Wharton. On the palsies of children, Am. J.M. Sc., **69**:348, 1875.

Sinkler definitely noted that infantile paralysis is a summer disease. "It is in the second summer, however, that most of these cases of infantile paralysis occur." "I have carefully noted the time of year when the paralysis came on. . . . I found that two cases in March, one in April, one in May, eight in June, eleven in July, nine in August . . . forty of the fifty-seven cases were affected in the summer months." "This fact has not, to my knowledge, been remarked before." However, soon after, W. H. Barlow ("On regressive paralysis [infantile paralysis; spinal paralysis of adults]," Liverpool and Manchester M. & S. Rep.,

---

[4] One of these cases, previously described by Cuming (Dublin J.M. Sc., **47**:471, 1869), seems to us very doubtful, and the pathological report is quite inadequate to allow any conclusions.

6:1, 1878) remarked: "Of the influence of season we have strong evidence; of 53 cases . . . 27 occurred in the months of July and August." Barlow's ideas of why this was so seem fanciful now, but his facts are important. Under treatment he emphasized moist heat—"hot flannels and cloths dipped in the water, well wrung out and applied to the paralysed parts" (see Ref. 4).

Sinkler later ("Etiology of epidemic poliomyelitis," Arch. Diagnosis, 1:28, 1908) gives a useful list of all epidemics described to date.

10. STRÜMPELL, Adolph. Ueber die Ursachen der Erkrankungen des Nervensystems, Deutsches Arch. f. klin. Med., 35:1, 1884.

Even after many diseases such as tuberculosis were known to be caused by a living infectious agent, doctors still seemed reluctant to believe that central nervous system disorders might fall into a similar category. Strümpell, the great German clinician, in a general lecture on the causes of disease of the nervous system seems to have been the first to insist that poliomyelitis, as well as certain cases of "acute multiple neuritis" and acute encephalitis of children, were infectious and probably were caused by similar agents. Thus he widened the concept of poliomyelitis, the lesions of which were previously regarded as confined to the spinal cord. "All these illnesses begin rather abruptly with fever, often of considerable degree. The patients are dull, have headache, gastro-intestinal disturbances, etc." "According to present views, these are all symptoms which point to an infection of the body with an organized disease producer." The weight of Strümpell's authority was important in promoting these views, but it was, of course, the appearance of poliomyelitis in epidemic form within the next decades which made the significance of infection obvious.

In a paper appearing in the following year Strümpell ("Ueber die acute Encephalitis der Kinder," Jahrb. f. Kinderh., 22:173, 1885) pursued further the relationship between classical poliomyelitis and acute encephalitis of children. "Both disorders usually attack healthy young children. There is an acute initial stage which is hardly to be distinguished in the two conditions. Then there remains a paralysis," in one case of cerebral origin, in the other of spinal origin. Strümpell, of course, had no specific tests available, and his cerebral cases may have been various kinds of encephalitis, but he clearly widened the concept of poliomyelitis beyond the classical limits of a spinal disease. "I myself incline to the assumption that both disorders are essentially related or, indeed, identical in the sense that in both the same (perhaps infectious) agent attacks in the one case the gray matter of the cord, in the other the gray matter of the cortex." This position was confirmed by the studies of Medin and of Wickman (Refs. 14, 19).

The contemporary views on poliomyelitis are admirably summarized in Strümpell's textbook (*Lehrbuch der speciellen Pathologie und Therapie, etc.* [4th ed.; Leipzig: F. C. W. Vogel, 1877], 2:255). The role of infection as well as communicability is especially emphasized.

11. DRUMMOND, David. On the nature of the spinal cord lesion in poliomyelitis anterior acuta, or infantile paralysis, Brain, 8:14, 1885–86.

Most of the early reports on the pathology of poliomyelitis dealt with subjects who died long after the acute disease. Drummond reports a patient who died only 7 hours after the onset of symptoms, presumably of respiratory paralysis. Proof of the etiology is, of course, not absolutely complete. However, there were extensive changes especially in the anterior horns, where the "large cells formed prominent objects although they were apparently swollen, granular and rather ill-defined. . . . The cells that presented the most obvious changes were more or less surrounded with dilated and blocked capillaries and minute hemorrhages." This is the first report we can find on the pathology of poliomyelitis in the very early stage.

12. RISSLER, J. Zur Kenntnis der Veränderungen des Nervensystems bei Poliomyelitis anterior acuta, Nord. med. ark., **20**:1, 1888.

While Drummond (Ref. 11) preceded Rissler in describing the pathological changes of poliomyelitis early in the acute stage, Rissler's careful study is the first to deal with the subject in comprehensive fashion. He reports autopsies on patients who died, respectively, on the sixth and eighth days of the disease. He emphasizes the degeneration of anterior horn cells but points out variations in the severity of the lesion in different cells in the same region. He also demonstrated changes in the motor cranial nerves, as well as lesions elsewhere in the nervous system, such as the posterior horns and Clarke's columns. Rissler observed lesions outside the central nervous system, such as enlargement of spleen and lymph nodes.

A review of the most important contemporary articles on the pathology of poliomyelitis is given by G. von Kahlden ("Neuere Arbeiten über Poliomyelitis anterior acuta," Centralbl. f. allg. Path., **5**:729, 1894).

13. CORDIER, S. Relation d'une épidémie de paralysie atrophique de l'enfance, Lyon méd., **57**:5, 1888.

Although credit for first suggesting the occurrence of poliomyelitis in epidemic form is usually given to George Colmer (Am. J.M. Sc., **31**:248, 1843), one finds in his article only a brief paragraph, in which he says: "The parents told me that eight or ten other cases of either hemiplegia or paraplegia had occurred during the preceding three or four months within a few miles of their residence." Cordier, however, on the basis of thirteen cases of infantile paralysis occurring over a 2-month period (June, July) in a town of fourteen hundred people says: "In showing that the atrophic paralysis of childhood can occur in epidemic fashion these cases will show also, I hope, that this paralysis is a specific infectious disease, one might say microbial." He also concludes: "And for my part I would not hesitate to isolate [éloigner] young infants if I saw infantile paralysis appear in their neighborhood."

While there are in the early literature hints of other outbreaks, it remained for Medin (Ref. 14) to describe a frank epidemic.

14. MEDIN, O. Ueber eine Epidemie von spinaler Kinderlähmung, Verhandl. d. X. Internat. med. Kongr. (August, 1890), Berlin, **2**:37, 1891, see also Hygeia, **52**:657, 1890.

It seems improbable that the presence of so striking a disease as poliomyelitis could be overlooked; one must conclude, therefore, that poliomyelitis actually did not occur in epidemic form until the last decades of the nineteenth century. The outbreak described by Medin is the first of any large proportions (but see

Cordier, Ref. 13), and full advantage was taken by him in studying it. Ordinarily, Medin saw in Stockholm only "a few" cases each year, but in 1887 he observed twenty-nine instances of poliomyelitis between August 9 and September 23. He was convinced that the disease was infectious but doubted its contagiousness, as emphasized by Cordier. Children only were affected. The occurrence at the same time of various clinical types was noted and seemed to speak for a common etiology; these observations supported the views previously expressed by Strümpell (Ref. 10) and were of the greatest importance in widening the older concepts of the disease. Aside from classical acute poliomyelitis, there were cases with motor cranial nerve palsies, as evidenced by failure of respiratory muscles, hoarseness, difficulty in swallowing, double vision, etc., and cases with polyneuritis and with polioencephalitis. Emphasis was placed on the severity of the acute attack, which was fatal in a number of children; Medin emphasized fever, somnolence, pain, and muscle tenderness.

This study was, of course, of great significance and should be read in detail by every student; the German clinicians were sufficiently impressed later to rename the disease "die Heine-Medinsche Krankheit" (Ref. 19). But most important of all seems to be the fact that there must have been an actual change at about this time in the natural history of poliomyelitis. Previously benign (as to survival) and sporadic, epidemics from this time on have been frequent, with many acutely fatal cases.

Medin's views were elaborated by him on the basis of further experiences in 1896 (Nord. med. ark., **6**:1). This article is more accessible in a French translation ("L'État de la paralysie infantile," Arch. de méd. d. enf., **1**:257, 321, 1898). The clear description of the early phenomena, such as somnolence, intestinal symptoms, hyperesthesia, etc., is especially important. Medin widened the concept of poliomyelitis from that of a localized disease of the spinal cord to that of a generalized infection.

15. CAVERLY, C. S. History of an epidemic of acute nervous disease of unusual type, M. Rec., **46**:673, 1894.

"During the month of June, 1894, there appeared in a portion of the valley of the Otter Creek, in the State of Vermont, an epidemic of nervous disease, in which the distinctive and most common symptom was paralysis." The outbreak is described in vivid style by C. S. Caverly, of the Vermont Board of Health, and is a model of precise reporting. The outbreak was confined to a narrow region around the city of Rutland. There were over 125 cases. The clinical picture was typical of epidemic poliomyelitis as we now know it, but Caverly noted the many deviations from the standard contemporary accounts: "It is at once noticed that individual cases can be readily recognized as presenting a typical picture of poliomyelitis anterior, but that the variations from the text-book type of this disease are many and marked. Opisthotonos, eye symptoms, and hyperesthesia are out of place in the phenomena of this disease, so that the epidemic, as a whole, presents notable departures from the regular features of the disease." In some of the patients there was little or no paralysis. Dr. A. Jacobi from a written description said: "All your cases belong to the same class, cerebrospinal meningitis"; but Allen Starr and Charles L. Dana believed them to be poliomyelitis. Caverly was familiar with "Medim's [*sic*] account," and he concluded: "Under the newer pathology given of poliomyelitis, symptoms referable to the meninges and cerebral ganglia can be reasonably explained." Caverly went wrong on one important point; he considered the disease to be non-contagious.

The importance of Caverly's report rests, first of all, on his admirable description of the first epidemic of poliomyelitis in this country. Even more significant, however, is the evidence that poliomyelitis in outbreaks of this sort differs in its natural history from the classical sporadic disease. The possibility is strong that the epidemics so frequent from this time on may have been due to new or different strains of virus. Caverly later redescribed the Vermont epidemic in the Journal of the American Medical Association ("Notes on an epidemic of acute anterior poliomyelitis," **26**:1, 1896), but nothing new is added. An interesting point is that during the epidemic various domestic animals were said to have died paralyzed.

Later Joseph Collins ("Acute anterior poliomyelitis or acute spinal paralysis of children: remarks on the epidemic now prevailing in New York," M. Rec., **72**:725, 1907) gave an account of the first really large American epidemic, that in New York City in the summer of 1907. There were said to be over twenty-five hundred cases, mostly in young children. The writer had no ideas on etiology but advised lumbar puncture on the slightest suspicion. A valuable report on this epidemic, which summarizes contemporary knowledge of the whole subject, was that of a committee of the New York Neurological Society (J. Nerv. & Ment. Dis., **36**:619, 1909).

16. PASTEUR, W. An epidemic of infantile paralysis occurring in children of the same family, Tr. Clin. Soc. London, **13**:143, 1897.

Caverly (Ref. 15) thought poliomyelitis was non-contagious because it was unusual for more than one child in a household to be affected. Pasteur, however, describes an interesting family "epidemic" in which "early in June the whole seven [children] were attacked in rapid succession within the space of ten days." But the heretofore unique feature of the outbreak was that all forms of the disease occurred in this small group—some with typical paralysis, some with cranial nerve lesions, some with fever but no paralysis. The etiological unity of various clinical forms, as well as contagiousness, seemed then to be proved beyond question.

During succeeding decades, most students of the disease came to believe that it was infectious, but many doubted its communicability from person to person. L. E. Holt and F. H. Bartlett ("The epidemiology of acute poliomyelitis: a study of thirty-five epidemics," Am. J.M. Sc., **135**:647, 1908), on the basis of a careful analysis of the reported epidemics, stated: "We cannot resist the conclusion that the disease is communicable, although only to a slight degree." Even now, fifty years later, the finer details of transmission have not yet been worked out.

17. WICKMAN, Ivar. Studien über Poliomyelitis acuta, Arb. a. d. path. Inst. d. Univ. Helsingfors, **1**:109, 1905.

This, the first to be published of Wickman's important studies on poliomyelitis, is a rather ponderous treatise of some one hundred pages, dealing chiefly with the pathological changes. Wickman's main point was that the lesions were not limited to the anterior horns but were much more widespread. Item 1 of his conclusions, for example, says: "An infiltrative myelitis lies at the basis of poliomyelitis. This occurs in scattered foci and is therefore to be thought of as a disseminated myelitis. The disseminated character is especially evident in the medulla oblongata and in the brain, where in my cases changes, if sought for, were always present."

Many of Wickman's patients died early in the disease, and some ran a course like "Landry's" paralysis. Wickman did the subject good service in widening the concept of poliomyelitis, but without virus studies one cannot now be sure of the identity of all his cases.

Wickman speculated on the route of infection, whether hematogenous, lymphogenous, or along the nerves, but again his material and methods prevented him from progressing beyond the philosophical stage. His experiments with the injection of banal bacteria into the arteries of the cord have little significance in the light of modern knowledge.

18. WICKMAN, Ivar. Ueber die Prognose der akuten Poliomyelitis und ätiologisch verwandter Erkrankungen, Ztschr. f. klin. Med., **63**:362, 1907.

Wickman points out that, before the Swedish epidemic described by Medin, poliomyelitis was regarded as a disease rarely fatal, even if disability persisted. He analyzed the Swedish material and found that, among 1,025 cases, 145 patients died before the fifteenth day of the disease, a death rate of 12.2 per cent. He also points out that the mortality was higher in older children and in adults (28–33 per cent) than in younger children. These percentage figures applied only to overt paralytic cases.

19. WICKMAN, Ivar. Beiträge zur Kenntnis der Heine-Medinschen Krankheit. Berlin: S. Karger, 1907.

"With the name of Heine-Medin disease I designate a whole group of illnesses which are united because of a common etiology; indeed, they are caused by a specific virus of infectious nature. In the center of the picture stands infantile paralysis. But many cases deviate from this; they may present symptoms and signs pointing to parts of the nervous system other than the spinal cord, such as the brain, bulb, or meninges; or they may run the course of a generalized infection without demonstrable localizing signs." So begins Wickman's classical monograph, which is just as exciting as his previous report (Ref. 17) is dull. It was the occurrence in epidemics which made possible the clear recognition of these variations in the clinical picture of poliomyelitis. Wickman distinguished (1) the poliomyelitic form (classical infantile paralysis), (2) the form showing an ascending paralysis (Landry's paralysis), (3) the bulbar or pontine form, (4) the encephalitic form, (5) the ataxic form, (6) the polyneuritic form, (7) the meningitic form, and (8) the abortive forms. Thus he brought system and order to what had already been roughly recognized. A special contribution was the description of the abortive forms, although many of Wickman's cases would today be described as non-paralytic rather than abortive, since fever and general symptoms were marked. The symptoms were aches and pains, headache, hyperesthesia, diarrhea, fever, etc. It was the occurrence of paralytic forms at the same time in the brothers or sisters which made

Wickman sure that the non-paralytic forms were caused by the same agent. These findings also spoke for contagion, but his chief evidence of communicability was the tracing of successive cases in rural communities, where it was shown that contact in school, for example, was paramount in the spread of the disease. These detailed studies are of the greatest interest. Wickman was the first, then, clearly to describe epidemic spread, and thereafter no one seriously questioned the contagiousness of poliomyelitis. Wickman stated that "contact does not have to be direct. On the contrary, it often seems to be true that contact is mediated by a healthy intermediary." Thus he clearly raised the question of carriers, which, he said, are well known to be of importance in the epidemiology of various infectious diseases. As to etiology, ordinary bacteriological studies were negative in Wickman's hands, but he was convinced that there was a specific infectious agent, which was soon to be established by others (Ref. 26). Wickman tells in detail (pp. 5–9) why he feels that the name "Heine-Medin disease" is appropriate.

This monograph should be carefully read by any serious student of the disease. It is not to be confused with a later, brief summary (*in* Lewandowsky, *Handbuch der Neurologie* [Berlin: J. Springer, 1911], **2**:807) from which the English translation is taken ("Nervous and Mental Disease Monograph Series," No. 16 [New York, 1913]).

20. BUZZARD, E. Farquhar. On certain infective or toxic conditions of the nervous system, Brain, **30**:1, 1907.

Buzzard describes in great detail the pathology of a man of twenty-six years who died from respiratory failure within 24 hours of the onset of paralysis.

21. GAY, Frederick P., and LUCAS, William P. Anterior poliomyelitis: methods of diagnosis from spinal fluid and blood in monkeys and in human beings, Arch. Int. Med., **6**:330, 1910.

Primitive efforts to examine the spinal fluid in cases of poliomyelitis usually consisted in staining centrifuged material and making bacteriological cultures. Various organisms—obviously contaminants or secondary invaders, in the light of present knowledge—were seen or were grown, and cells of various sorts were described in the stained sediment. Thus F. Schultze ("Zur Aetiologie der acuten Poliomyelitis," München. med. Wchnschr., **45**:1197, 1898) saw what he believed to be meningococci. F. Engel ("Bakteriologisches Ergebniss einer Lumbalpunction bei Poliomyelitis acuta," Prag. med. Wchnschr., **25**:135, 1900) drew 30 cc. of clear spinal fluid from a boy on the sixth day of acute poliomyelitis. No cells were seen, but various bacteria grew. In F. X. Dercum's case ("Note on a case of acute poliomyelitis in which the cerebro-spinal fluid obtained by a Quincke puncture contained a diplococcus resembling the diplococcus of Sternberg," J. Nerv. & Ment. Dis., **27**:116, 1900) "a few leucocytes" were seen. Triboulet and Lippmann ("Poliomyélite antérieure aiguë: ponction lombaire; mononucléose," Bull. et mém. Soc. méd. d. hôp. de Paris, **19**:23, 1902) found that fluid drawn on the twenty-fourth day showed many "mononuclear lymphocytes" but no "polynuclears"; and L. Guinon and Paris ("Paralysie infantile avec réaction méningée," Bull. et mém. Soc. méd. d. hôp. de Paris, **20**:673, 1903) on the thirteenth day also found numerous "lymphocytes" but no bacteria. C. Achard and H. Grenet ("Paralysie infantile et lymphocytose arach-noïdienne," Rev. neurol., **11**:345, 1903) report similar findings. M. Wollstein ("A biological study of the cerebrospinal fluid in anterior poliomyelitis," J. Exper. Med., **10**:476, 1908) examined fluid from eleven cases during the first 2 weeks. In centrifuged smears, "one to three mononuclear leucocytes were found but large numbers were never present." These variable and inadequate examinations were superseded by the careful studies of Gay and Lucas, who appear to be the first to have made accurate counts of the cells of the spinal fluid in poliomyelitis, both in the monkey and in man. Counts were made in 14 cases of poliomyelitis from the second to the seventeenth day. The number of cells varied from 50 to 580 per cubic millimeter; almost all were "mononuclears" or "lymphocytes." The leucocyte counts of the blood varied from 7,800 to 17,400, usually with increase in lymphocytes.

22. LANDSTEINER, Karl, and POPPER, Erwin. "Uebertragung der Polio-myelitis acuta auf Affen, Ztschr. f. Immunitätsforsch. u. Exper. Therap., **2**:377, 1909.

This article is a landmark in the subject, since it really marks the beginning of the modern experimental study of poliomyelitis. The authors point out that, on the basis of epidemic occurrence, everyone agreed that the disease was infectious in origin. The alleged claims that animals—horses, chickens, rabbits—developed paralyses during outbreaks of human poliomyelitis are reviewed and discredited. The claims for a bacterial cause are thoroughly discussed. The writers point out that, whereas many bacteria such as meningococci, pneumo-cocci, staphylococci, streptococci, and others have been incriminated, no con-sistent findings have been obtained by various workers, and, indeed, a number of reliable observers have been unable to isolate any bacteria from spinal fluid or nervous tissues of poliomyelitis cases.[5]

Landsteiner and Popper's own experiments were not made primarily with the idea of searching for a filtrable virus but simply to see whether the disease could be transmitted to animals. They worked with emulsions of the spinal cord of a boy dead of poliomyelitis and made intraperitoneal injections into rabbits, guinea pigs, mice, and monkeys. Cultures of the material yielded no growth by the usual bacteriological methods. The rabbits, guinea pigs, and mice remained well, but the monkeys came down with typical poliomyelitis. One died 8 days after inoculation, and the spinal cord showed outspoken lesions. The second animal became paralyzed in the lower legs. Injection of material from this animal into other monkeys was ineffective, and it remained for others to transmit the disease in series. The final conclusion of the authors was: "The presumption is therefore strong that a so-called invisible virus or one belonging to the class of Protozoa is the cause of the disease."

This work was first announced on December 18, 1908, at a meeting of the Gesellschaft der Aerzte in Vienna (see "Mikroscopische Präparate von einen menschlichen und zwei Affenrückenmarken," Wien. klin. Wchnschr., **21**:1830, 1908). A tiny note to the same effect by Landsteiner ("Poliomyélite antérieure

[5] It is of interest that, as late as 1952, an article appeared in which it was claimed that streptococci were the cause of poliomyelitis (E. C. Rosenow, California Med., **76**:396, 1952).

aiguë chez le singe," Semaine méd., **28**:620, 1908) also appeared in the same year.

From the time of Landsteiner's work on transmission, almost every phase of poliomyelitis has been under controversy. Route of entry of the virus, excretion, presence in various regions, such as the bowel, nasopharynx, and lymph glands, the question of viremia—all have been subjects of lively dispute. Volumes have been written on modes of transmission and etiology, and the exact merits of various vaccines have been questioned. The subject is evidently not ripe as yet for a review such as ours; perhaps in fifty years these problems will have resolved themselves. At present, even experts in the subject disagree among themselves to such a point that it would be foolish to rush in. A comprehensive list of recent references on poliomyelitis may, however, be found in the bibliography of the National Foundation (*op. cit.*).

I am greatly indebted to my colleague, Dr. Harold K. Faber, for invaluable advice and assistance in preparing this section of the bibliography.

THE COMMON COLD

Section 23

THE COMMON COLD

THE pertinent literature on the common cold is not very extensive. First of all, a cold is, for the most part, a mild indisposition which most doctors have not thought worthy of very careful study. Second, until recent years—indeed, even now—the true infectious cold has been confused with secondary complications such as sinusitis which are not really colds at all, as well as with the results of exposure to cold—cold trauma. Later on, in the bacteriological era, the cold was blamed on almost any bacteria which could be grown from the upper air passages; it was not until the normal flora, transients, and focal carriage of bacteria were worked out in the early 1920's that it became clear that most of the previous etiological claims had dealt with members of the normal flora, and the way was clearly opened for virus studies. There seems no doubt now that the common cold can be produced by instillation of filtrates of secretions from people with colds. Beyond this the problem is still unsolved; the agents isolated by various workers have had different characteristics, and, while growth has been claimed by some in chick embryos or in culture media, no constant visible changes are reported. Aside from monkeys, no animal has definitely been infected. But with the recent immense developments in the technique of virus culture, the problem may soon be solved. For the literature to 1932 one should consult the monumental review by David and Robert Thomson, *The Common Cold* ("Annals of the Pickett-Thomson Research Laboratory," Vol. **8** [London: Baillière, Tyndale & Cox, 1932]).

1. HAYES, T. A serious address on the dangerous consequences of neglecting common coughs and colds: with successful directions how to prevent and cure consumptions. 4th ed. Dublin: L. White, 1786.

In this admirable little treatise contemporary views are well summarized. "A cold arises from the effect of cold or moist air applied to the surface of the body and lungs, from going too thinly clad or exposing the body to cold air, after having been heated by exercise; or when the pores are opened from drinking warm liquors." Hayes gives a good description of the clinical features of the common cold, in which the primary disease is well differentiated from its sequelae. One cannot be sure, of course, that all of Hayes's cases were infectious colds and not instances of cold trauma (Ref. 18).

2. WALSH, James J. The etiology of colds, M. News, New York, **82**:481, 1903.

The views of Hayes (Ref. 1) were pretty much accepted until the bacteriological era. Walsh points out that mere exposure to cold, as a rule, does not suffice to bring on "a cold." He feels that "so-called cold in the head or rhinitis ... is almost surely due to bacterial infection." Walsh's idea was that the "cold" is caused by any bacteria which happen to be present in the upper air passages, provided that resistance is lowered, usually by exposure to cold, draughts, coming out of an overheated room, etc. N. James ("Colds and the prevention of colds," M. News, New York, **86**:1123, 1905) held much the same view: "The mucous membrane of the nose and pharynx has upon its surface . . . a large number of many varieties of bacteria. When congestion . . . develops, the amount of mucus is increased and these organisms are supplied with more material to thrive upon." In general, the standard view until the 1920's, despite the work of Kruse (Ref. 3) and of Foster (Ref. 4), was that a cold trauma lowered resistance to a non-specific infection with any bacteria at hand.

3. KRUSE, W. Die Erreger von Husten und Schnupfen, München. med. Wchnschr., **61**:1547, 1914.

The modern study of the common cold really begins with Kruse's work. He was not satisfied with the causal role of ordinary bacteria and deliberately looked for a filter-passing agent. Diluted filtered secretions from a patient with a cold were instilled into the nares of thirty-six volunteers, of whom fifteen, or 42 per cent, came down with a "cold" after an incubation period of 1–4 days. Cultures of the filtered material were sterile. Kruse suggested the name "aphanozoa" ("invisible") for the whole group of filterable organisms and *A. coryzae* for those responsible for colds.

4. FOSTER, George B., Jr. The etiology of common colds: the probable role of a filterable virus as the causative factor: a preliminary note, J.A.M.A., **66**:1180, 1916.

Foster repeated and confirmed Kruse's (Ref. 3) observations in nine out of ten volunteers. His filtrates were also sterile by ordinary culture methods. Foster, using a method modified from Noguchi, thought that he was able to grow from the filtrate a tiny globoid organism. Although this finding has not been confirmed, Foster's paper remains a model of precise work. Foster later ("The etiology of common colds," J. Infect. Dis., **21**:451, 1917) reported his studies in detail. He thought that he had produced colds in volunteers with intranasal instillation of the second generation of the small anaerobic organism which he had grown in culture. Peter K. Olitsky and James E. McCartney ("Studies on the nasopharyngeal secretions from patients with common colds," J. Exper. Med., **38**:427, 1923) later confirmed the work of Kruse and of Foster on transmission but were unable to grow from filtered secretions either the globoid bodies described by Foster or any constant pathogenetic agent. On the other hand, in quite extensive experiments in which filtered nasal secretions were sprayed onto the nasal mucosa of one hundred volunteers, no convincing evidence of having produced any disease was obtained by Robert C. Robinson and Robert L. Groves ("Experimental human inoculations with filtered nasal secretions from acute coryza," J. Infect. Dis., **34**:400, 1924). These writers also give a review of the literature.

Thus, even early, there were conflicting experimental results; the clinical difficulty of being sure that a true cold had been produced and not some nonspecific irritation may have been an important factor.

5. VOORHEES, Irving Wilson. Colds—their cause and cure, Am. Med., **12**:125, 1917.

By this time the writer spoke of the cold germ or *Micrococcus catarrhalis*, although he realized that "a number of micro-organisms are usually found together and their 'team work' is so perfect that they often resist all ordinary simple remedies." Voorhees laid less stress on cold as a predisposing factor and more on contagion than on "auto-infection." "Perpetual warfare ought to be waged against those who wilfully cough and sneeze into the open without protecting the face with a handkerchief." Treatment was as effective in 1917 as in 1957, "a purgative, hot mustard footbaths, quinine and whiskey, aspirin, Turkish bath," etc., although Voorhees advised consulting a nose and throat specialist, "who can see just where the trouble is and treat it accordingly." Cleaveland Floyd ("The 'common cold' in relation to certain micro-organisms and its treatment with bacterial vaccines," Boston M. & S.J., **182**:389, 1920) went further in considering the cold as a purely bacterial infection predominantly with streptococci and pneumococci, and he advocated energetic vaccine therapy. He fell into error by not understanding that he was dealing with the normal bacterial flora of the throat, as did many other writers at the time (see A. L. Bloomfield, "The significance of the bacteria found in the throats of healthy people," Bull. Johns Hopkins Hosp., **32**:33, 1921).

   6. SCHADE, H. Beiträge zur Umgrenzung und Klärung einer Lehre von der Erkältung, Ztschr. f. d. ges. exper. Med., **7**:275, 1919.

In this comprehensive article on the influence of cold on the body, Schade points out certain definite effects on the mucous membranes of the upper air passages. These are reflex vasomotor changes which may lead to anemia or hyperemia and also to direct irritative phenomena. Schade describes very clearly a so-called "cold catarrh" which must be differentiated from a true cold (Ref. 7) and which has led to much confusion in the literature. Its features are onset during or directly after the cold trauma, with rawness and secretion. The mucous membranes may appear reddened. There is no fever, and the disturbance, which is purely local, lasts only 1 or 2 days. Schade thought that this cold catarrh might allow bacterial invasion with secondary effects. Schade in later papers ("Untersuchungen in die Erkältungsfrage," München. med. Wchnschr., **66**:1021, 1919; *ibid.*, **67**:449, 1920) pursued the matter further in seventeen thousand men at the front in World War I. J. A. Miller and W. C. Noble ("The effects of exposure to cold upon experimental infection of the respiratory tract," J. Exper. Med., **24**:223, 1916) review the experimental work on the relation of cold to infection and report experiments to the effect that respiratory infection of rabbits with *Bacillus bovisepticus* is favored by chilling. S. Mudd and S. B. Grant ("Reaction to chilling of body surface," J.M. Research, **40**:53, 1919) and S. Mudd, M. D. Goldman, and S. B. Grant ("Reactions of the nasal cavity and postnasal space to chilling of the body surface," J. Exper. Med., **34**:11, 1921) also showed that chilling of the body surface causes vasoconstriction and ischemia in the mucous membranes of the palate, pharynx, and tonsils. Finally, in a comprehensive paper Stuart Mudd, Samuel B. Grant, and Alfred Goldman ("The etiology of acute inflammations of the nose, pharynx and tonsils," Ann. Otol., Rhin. & Laryng., **30**:1, 1921) review in detail the ideas to date on the etiology of colds. Kerr and his associates later pursued the subject of the effect of cold and heat on nasal mucosa (H. J. Ralston and W. J. Kerr, "Vascular responses of the nasal mucosa to thermal stimuli with some observations on skin temperature," Am. J. Physiol., **144**:305, 1945).

7. BLOOMFIELD, Arthur. Variations in the bacterial flora of the upper air passages during the course of common colds, Bull. Johns Hopkins Hosp., **32**:121, 1921.

Bloomfield clearly defined the clinical features of the true common cold. He emphasized that the uncomplicated cold was a mild disease featured by a constitutional reaction and by local hyperemic phenomena in the upper air passages. The primary disease was to be sharply differentiated from bacterial complications, such as bronchitis, sinusitis, otitis, and also from cold trauma. He reviewed the earlier literature and pointed out how little had really been written on the disease, probably because of its lack of clear definition, and how fanciful many of the ideas of writers on the subject were.

His main contribution, however, was the making of repeated quantitative throat cultures in ten people with colds during the attack and over weeks or months thereafter. "The cultural studies . . . fail to show in uncomplicated cases any variation in the flora which would enable one to select any organism . . . as the cause of colds. On the other hand, where complications occurred pathogenic organisms were definitely associated with them . . . therefore the primary cause of colds is probably an organism as yet unknown. . . . But the primary cold, whatever its cause, alters the mucous membranes in such a way as to allow secondary bacterial invasion and consequent frequent development of local complications." G. S. Shibley, F. M. Hanger, and A. R. Dochez ("Observations of the normal bacterial flora of nose and throat with variations occurring during colds," J. Exper. Med., **43**:415, 1926) came to similar conclusions, and Y. Kneeland ("The relationship of bacteria to the common cold," Bull. New York Acad. Med., **25**:534, 1949) later reviewed the whole subject.

8. SMILEY, D. F. A study of the weekly incidence of colds in normal and in cold-susceptible groups throughout a winter, Am. J. Hyg., **9**:477, 1929.

The writer, in attempting to explain seasonal variations in the incidence of colds, found that the ordinary winter or spring epidemic of colds among college students is almost entirely limited to a specially "cold-susceptible" group of students. Daniel F. Milam and Wilson G. Smillie ("A bacteriological study of 'colds' on an isolated tropical island [St. John, United States Virgin Islands, West Indies]," J. Exper. Med., **53**:733, 1931) concluded that there was "strong evidence that environmental factors, particularly reduction in atmospheric temperature, have some influence upon the incidence of colds, although they believed that the cold was initiated by an infectious agent.

9. HILDING, Anderson. The common cold, Arch. Otolaryng., **12**:131, 1930.

Since people do not die of colds, there are few observations on the lesions. Hilding, however, did biopsies of nasal mucosa in twenty-five cases from the second hour of symptoms until the fourteenth day. He describes and pictures beautifully lesions typical of a virus, similar to those found in the turbinate bones of ferrets with experimental influenza, as shown by T. Francis, Jr., and C. H. Stuart-Harris, "Studies on the nasal histology of epidemic influenza virus in the ferret," J. Exper. Med., **68**:789, 1938. These lesions consisted of a necrosis of the superficial epithelium with submucous round-cell infiltration. The epithelium was "gradually regenerated and repaired by the growth and multiplication of the stellate cells normally found deep in the epithelium." This gradual repair no doubt accounts for the raw feeling which often persists so long after the active stages of a cold.

10. DOCHEZ, A. R., SHIBLEY, Gerald S., and MILLS, Katherine C. Studies in the common cold. IV. Experimental transmission of the common cold to anthropoid apes and human beings by means of a filtrable agent, J. Exper. Med., **52**:701, 1930.

Dochez and his associates deserve full credit for reawakening interest in the search for a virus in the common cold. They worked first with monkeys, in which they thought that they had reproduced colds by instillation into the nasal passages of filtered nasal washings from people with fresh colds. By a similar procedure, colds were produced in human volunteers in four of nine cases. They noted an abundance of pneumococci in the noses and throats of monkeys in the course of colds and thought that perhaps these grew on a "substrate of primary injury due to the filtrable agent." P. H. Long and J. A. Doull ("Etiology of acute upper respiratory infection [common cold]," Proc. Soc. Exper. Biol. & Med., **28**:53, 1930) soon confirmed Dochez's work. They not only produced colds in volunteers with nasopharyngeal washings from people with colds but accomplished serial transfers through two and four individuals. Their protocols are given in detail in a longer paper (P. H. Long, J. A. Doull, J. M. Bourn, and E. McComb. J. Exper. Med., **53**:447, 1931).

11. DOCHEZ, A. R., MILLS, Katherine C., and KNEELAND, Yale, Jr. Study of the virus of the common cold and its cultivation in tissue medium, Proc. Soc. Exper. Biol. & Med., **28**:513, 1931.

The writers found that the virus survived for 13 days in the icebox. They decided, therefore, to attempt to cultivate it. The medium, which is described in detail, contained a chick embryo hash. After twelve to fifteen subcultures at intervals of 3–9 days the material still produced colds in volunteers. The writers therefore concluded that they had successfully grown an invisible agent. These studies were elaborated and reported in greater detail by Dochez, Mills, and Kneeland ("Studies of the common cold. VI. Cultivation of the virus in tissue medium," J. Exper. Med., **63**:559, 1936). A little later the same workers ("Cultivation of the virus of the common cold in the chorio-allantoic membrane of the chick embryo," Proc. Soc. Exper. Biol. & Med., **35**:213, 1936) reported implantation of virus-containing material from a human cold on the chorio-allantoic membrane of the chick embryo and passage through a series of three eggs. Material from the third series produced a typical cold when tested on volunteers. Meanwhile, H. M. Powell and G. H. A. Clowes ("Cultivation of the virus of the common cold and its inoculation in human subjects," Proc. Soc. Exper. Biol. & Med., **29**:332, 1931) found that nasal washings from patients with colds could be grown for several generations in tissue culture and that the material then infected man in 69 per cent of trials. A little later, Morris Pollard and Coleman D. Caplovitz ("Experimental studies with the agent of the common cold," Science, **106**:243, 1947) reported transmission of cold virus in the chorio-allantoic cavity of the chick embryo and thence to man with the production of colds; and Norman H. Topping and Leon T. Atlas ("The common cold: a note regarding isolation of an agent," Science, **106**:636, 1947) told of producing colds in volunteers with seventh-passage allantoic fluid. Curiously enough, C. H.

Andrewes ("The natural history of the common cold," Lancet, **1**:71, 1949), a great expert in virology working with the British Common Cold Research Team, although he was successful in producing "experimental colds" in 60 per cent of volunteers with bacteria-free filtrates of nasal secretions from subjects with colds, was entirely unable to cultivate an agent by inoculation of embryonated hens' eggs by any route. Andrewes' very important paper takes up many other problems of the common cold. Meanwhile, Dochez, Mills, and Kneeland ("Filterable viruses in infection of the upper respiratory tract," J.A.M.A., **110**:177, 1938) reviewed the whole subject of "cold virus." They pointed out that, unlike influenza virus, it could not be established in ferrets but could in mice and that it was generally inactivated at 56° C. but well preserved in the icebox anaerobically. A perplexing aspect of the whole problem of cold viruses is that the various authors mentioned above all assigned quite different characteristics to their strains (Topping, Dochez, Andrewes, and L. T. Atlas, and G. A. Hotter, "The common cold: titration of MR-1 virus in embryonated eggs," Science, **108**:743, 1948). This suggests a multiplicity of agents. The subject is further complicated by the fact that no visible changes were seen in either culture media or chick embryos even when growth appeared to have been achieved.

12. PAUL, J. H., and FREESE, H. L. An epidemiological and bacteriological study of the "common cold" in an isolated Arctic community (Spitzbergen), Am. J. Hyg., **17**:517, 1933.

There was only a very occasional cold among the inhabitants of Spitzbergen during the winter, but the arrival of the first ship on May 23 was followed by a sharp outbreak of nearly two hundred cases in the two following weeks. This observation, which has been confirmed by similar ones with other viral infections such as measles (P. Panum, "Ueber das Verhalten einiger epidemischen Krankheiten auf Färo, Island, und in Dänemark," Verhandl. d. phys. med. Gesellsch. in Würzburg, **3**:16, 1852) leaves no doubt that the common cold is caused by a living agent. It seems clear that whatever transient protection has been conferred by last summer's colds, if any, wears off during the winter, so that a highly susceptible population is available which readily becomes infected by the new arrivals. It is of interest that among the new arrivals there may be no one with clinical infection, which suggests that carriers may introduce the virus.

There was no change in the bacterial flora of the upper air passages, as previous workers (Ref. 7) had also found. The literature on these epidemiological observations is critically reviewed by Andrewes (Ref. 14).

13. KERR, William J. The common cold, J.A.M.A., **107**:323, 1936.

Kerr questions the doctrine that "colds" are caused by a living agent. This idea was based on observations in which people who were subject to colds were placed in intimate and prolonged contact with people in the early active stages of a cold. Kerr also instilled fresh nasal secretions from people with colds into the conjunctivae of the volunteers. In no case was a cold produced. These observations are in line with common clinical experience on the acquisition of colds, and, although perhaps Kerr goes too far in questioning the need of a living agent, there may be necessary, in addition, a resistance-lowering factor (the "jolt" of Andrewes) which was absent in his experiments. Details of

Kerr's observations may be found in a paper by W. J. Kerr and J. B. Lagen ("Transmissibility of the common cold: exposure of susceptible individuals under controlled conditions," Proc. Soc. Exper. Biol. & Med., **31**:713, 1934). Andrewes (Ref. 14) later had a similar experience. These observations must mean that virus was inhaled in inadequate dosage; that some factor of lowered resistance, necessary to potentiate infection, was absent; or that virus from the donor was already inactive. Andrewes (Ref. 14) in infected volunteers found virus in nasal washings as long as 24 hours before any symptoms appeared, and P. H. Long, E. A. Bliss, and H. M. Carpenter ("A note on the communicability of colds," Bull. Johns Hopkins Hosp., **51**:278, 1932) in an observation made during an experiment on transmission to monkeys also found that a cold is transmissible during the incubation period.

14. ANDREWES, Christopher Howard. Adventures among viruses. III. The puzzle of the common cold, New England J. Med., **242**:235, 1950.

In this important summary of the work of the British Common Cold Research Unit, Andrewes points out, first, the difficulties of transmission experiments: that the cold cannot be transmitted to small animals or cultivated conveniently in the laboratory. Human volunteers are therefore necessary. Andrewes describes the complex system of quarantine of the volunteers necessary in transmission experiments. He again tells of failures to transmit any disease to a dozen or more varieties of animals—small and large. By passing washings through graded filters, a virus size of about 0.1 μ is indicated, a discouraging fact, since small-particle viruses are notably unaffected by antibiotics. Various other physical characteristics are enumerated. Andrewes reminds us that simple exposure to cold will not produce a "cold," but he raises the question of whether in certain individuals who may be chronic carriers of cold virus some types of chilling may not act as a factor which lowers resistance to autoinfection, much as happens with herpes simplex virus carriers. Such chronic carriage might explain individuals who are subject to frequent colds when their close associates have none. Many more interesting problems in the transmission of colds are discussed.

15. POWELL, H. M., SPARKS, A. L., and CLOWES, G. H. A. Further inoculation-experiments with the common-cold virus, J. Immunol., **38**:309, 1940.

In an attempt to prevent colds, the writers administered to volunteers a tissue culture virus by either the hypodermic or the intranasal route. They found this vaccine ineffective in preventing natural colds. Dochez and his group had similar experiences (Ref. 11). These findings do not seem remarkable because the spontaneous disease confers so little protection. Other failures to protect against colds are those with bacterial vaccines ("Use of vaccines for common cold, status report of the Council on Pharmacy and Chemistry and the Council on Industrial Health," J.A.M.A., **126**:895, 1944) and with penicillin (C. Kuh and M. F. Collen, "Mass penicillin prophylaxis," J.A.M.A., **140**:1324, 1949).

16. COMMISSION ON ACUTE RESPIRATORY DISEASES. Experimental transmission of minor respiratory illness to human volunteers by filter-passing agents, J. Clin. Investigation, **26**:957, 1947.

Using bacteria-free filtrates of nasopharyngeal secretions of patients with mild acute respiratory infections, these workers were able to produce two types of illness. One was coryza-like, with an incubation period of 24–48 hours; the other, after an incubation period of 5 or 6 days, was featured by sore throat and minimal nasal symptoms. In another paper the same workers showed (*ibid.*, p. 974) that a specific immunity was conferred by each type and that cross-immunity was not demonstrable.

17. TOPPING, N. H. Research on the common cold, Bull. New York Acad. Med., **25**:530, 1949.

An important review in which the writer points out that the common cold practically heads the list of unsolved problems in respiratory infection.

18. BLOOMFIELD, Arthur L. Some problems of the common cold, J.A.M.A., **144**:287, 1950.

The writer critically reviews the whole subject to date. He emphasizes the importance of distinguishing the true common cold—a viral infection—from traumatic rhinitis (cold, dust, fumes, allergic reactions, psychic), with which it is often confused. In either the true cold or traumatic rhinitis there may be secondary bacterial invasion with suppurative complications. The literature on prophylaxis and on treatment, including antibiotics and "antihistaminics," is also reviewed.

19. LOWELL, F. C., SCHILLER, I. W., ALMAN, J. E., and MOUNTANI, C. F. The antihistaminic drugs in the treatment of the common cold, New England J. Med., **244**:132, 1951.

Histamine had such a vogue in the alleged control of the common cold that this definitive paper should be mentioned. "We were unable to distinguish any effect of the three [antihistaminic] drugs, in the dosage used on the common cold that differed significantly from the placebo."

20. FINLAND, Maxwell. Antimicrobial treatment for oral and related infections. II. Antibiotic treatment of acute respiratory infections and influenza, New England J. Med., **247**:557, 1952.

Finland gives a critical analysis of the value of antibiotics in the prevention and treatment of the common cold. He concludes that "none of the antimicrobial agents have been unequivocally demonstrated to have a favorable effect" but that they may prove useful for complications due to ordinary bacteria.

21. ANDREWES, C. H., CHAPRONIÈRE, Donna M., GOMPELS, Annette E. H., PEREIRA, H. G., and RODEN, A. T. Propagation of common-cold virus in tissue cultures, Lancet, **2**:546, 1953.

Andrewes, who had previously failed to grow cold virus in cultures, now claimed success by using explants of human embryonic lung in roller tubes modified from the method of J. Enders ("Bovine amniotic fluid as tissue culture medium in cultivation of poliomyelitis and other viruses," Proc. Soc. Exper. Biol. & Med., **82**:100, 1953). By testing the culture material on human volunteers, "evidence is adduced that the common-cold virus has been propagated through ten serial cultures of embryonic human lung."

22. HUEBNER, R. J., ROWE, W. P., WARD, T. G., PARROTT, R. H., and BELL, J. A. Adenoidal-pharyngeal-conjunctival agents: a newly recognized group of common viruses of the respiratory system, New England J. Med., **251**:1077, 1954.

Using the newer methods of tissue culture, the writers summarize work of their own and of others in which more than a hundred strains of virus have been demonstrated in material obtained from various mild acute diseases of the upper air passages as well as from surgically removed tonsils and adenoids. This work is extremely complex and as yet in an early stage. The agents fall into various immunologically separable groups. "All types grow readily, producing similar and unique cytopathogenic effects, in human epithelial cells and in HeLa cells available commercially. They are resistant to ether and antibiotics—all types cause frequent infections in man, beginning at an early age." On administration of these agents to volunteers, no clinical disease was produced, but in most of them there was a sharp rise in complement-fixing and neutralizing antibody levels and the appearance of virus in nasopharyngeal secretions 3–6 days after inoculation. These methods open a new field in the study of viruses of the respiratory passages; the exact relation of all this to the true common cold is not yet clear.

Bacteriology	Ref. 16
Blood in measles	Ref. 9
Culture of virus	Refs. 20, 21, 25
Electron microscopy of virus	Ref. 24
Epidemiology	Refs. 3, 4
General	Refs. 1, 2, 5, 6, 26
Immunity in measles	Ref. 18
Koplik's spots	Ref. 7
Nervous complications	Ref. 19
Pathology	Ref. 12
Pneumonia in measles	Ref. 14
Prophylaxis with convalescent serum	Refs. 11, 15
Prophylaxis with gamma globulin	Ref. 23
Transmission to animals	Refs. 8, 13, 17, 22
Transmission to man	Refs. 10, 22

Section 24

MEASLES

AN EXCELLENT historical account of measles, with bibliography, is to be found in J. D. Rolleston's book on the *History of the Acute Exanthemata* (London: William Heinemann, 1937), while the modern literature to 1931 is well covered in the "References to Literature" appended to the monograph of David Thomson and Robert Thomson on *Measles* ("Annals of the Pickett-Thomson Research Laboratory," Vol. 7 [London: Baillière, Tindall & Cox, 1931]), page 193. The most recent literature is reviewed in Babbott and Gordon's *Modern Measles* (Ref. 26). Sydenham is usually given credit for distinguishing between measles, scarlet fever, and smallpox, and, although his accounts were more realistic than the earlier ones, they are far from giving a really finished picture of the disease.

What impresses one most in the older descriptions of measles is the somewhat different character of the disease from that now seen. Whereas there were mild cases, there were also many severe outbreaks with high mortality, especially from overwhelming bronchopneumonias, probably with bacteremia, and from gangrene of the face or other structures. It is not too hard to see how these fulminating forms with hemorrhagic skin rashes could be confused with similar violent types of scarlet fever and smallpox.

1. WILLAN, Robert. On cutaneous diseases, **1**:214. London: J. Johnson, 1808.

In this monumental book on cutaneous disorders, measles is discussed as a skin disease under the chapter on exanthemata. The account is vivid in some respects but definitely oriented to the past—to Sydenham and even to the Arabian writers. "On the third, fourth or fifth day of the fever, when there is oppression with anxiety, heaving of the lungs, and a labouring pulse, most practitioners recommend bloodletting," etc. It is evident that early in the century the disease often occurred in very severe form, with rapid death from pneumonia or even gangrene.

2. GREGORY, George. Lectures on the eruptive fevers, chapter vi, "Rubeola, or measles." London: H. Renshaw, 1843.

Gregory's account is of interest because it is transitional between Sydenham and the moderns. An excellent description with consideration of incubation period, prodromes, eruption, and complications is given. He distinguishes measles from scarlet fever: "1. By the character and duration of the eruptive fever, 2. by the character and general aspect of the eruption, 3. by the state of the throat." As to therapy—"On the appearance of the eruption, your object is simply to avoid occasions of aggravation. Let the patient be confined to bed, take occasionally some castor oil, and a simple saline draught, with syrup of tolu and some antimonial wine, every four hours." Gregory goes on with suggestions of mustard plasters, leeches, and bleeding if "mischief is brewing" in the lungs. Of the same general character is the excellent account in F. Rilliet and E. Barthez (*Traité clinique et pratique des maladies des enfants* [Paris: Gearner Baillière, 1843], **2**:671). A. Trousseau (*Clinique médicale de l'Hôtel*

Dieu de Paris [Paris: J.-B. Baillière et fils], **1**:42), the master clinician, gives a good account also, but none of these writers was clear as to the duration of the incubation period, and none described the enanthem precisely. They recognized bronchopneumonia and gangrene as frequent and dreaded complications.

3. PANUM, P. L. Iagttagelser, anstillede under maeslinge-epidemien paa Faeroerne i Aaret, 1846, Bibl. laeger, **1**:270, 1847. (English translation: Observations made during the epidemic of measles on the Faroe Islands in the year 1846, M. Classics, **3**:829, 1939.)

At the age of only twenty-six, Panum was sent to the Faroe Islands by the Danish government to investigate a tremendous epidemic of measles, during which approximately six thousand of the eight thousand inhabitants were affected. The introduction of the disease was brought about by a man who, shortly before, had been in contact with a measles patient in Copenhagen and who did not become ill until he arrived at Thorshaven, the main port of the Faroes. His two closest associates then came down, after which the epidemic spread throughout the islands. Panum's main contribution was epidemiological; he traced the spread of the disease through isolated villages and concluded that there was a latent period between exposure and the outbreak of the rash of exactly 14 (occasionally 13) days. The prodromal period varied from 2 to 6 days. Panum concluded that the disease was definitely communicable, that it was not due to miasm or to spontaneous generation, and that it was most contagious at about the time the rash appeared and not during desquamation, as usually supposed. He found that isolation was effective in stopping the spread of the disease, and he thought that he had evidence that it could be disseminated by fomites (clothes) as well as by direct contact. Panum also made the interesting observation that old people who had had measles in the previous epidemic in 1781 were not affected. The paper begins with an interesting account of the geography, climate, and natural history of the Faroe Islands.

Numerous other epidemics of measles have been described; the earlier literature is reviewed in A. Hirsch, *Handbook of Geographic and Historical Pathology* (London: New Sydenham Society, 1883), **1**:154, and in Charles Leighton, *A History of Epidemics in Britain* (Cambridge, 1894), **2**:632. Quite recently there is a comprehensive study of an outbreak in Greenland, where there had never before been a case of measles (P. E. Christensen, H. Schmidt, O. Jenson, H. O. Bang, V. Andersen, and B. Jordal, "An epidemic of measles in southern Greenland, 1951," Acta med. skandinav., **144**:313, 430, 450, 1952). Almost everyone, young and old, was affected. The incubation period was not so fixed as that found by Panum; in one case it was definitely prolonged to 19 days, and in several others it was as short as 6–10 days. Among 4,257 patients, 77 deaths occurred. An excellent modern discussion of the epidemiology of measles and of specific epidemics is that of J. A. H. Brincker, "A historical, epidemiological and aetiological study of measles," Proc. Roy. Soc. Med., **31**:807, 1938.

4. LAVERAN, [Alphonse]. Des influences nosocomiales sur la marche et la gravité de la rougeole, Gaz. hebd. de méd., Paris, **8**:20, 51, 1861.

Although measles is usually thought of as a childhood disease, it becomes widespread and serious in adults under conditions of assembly of large numbers of soldiers, especially of young men from various districts where measles has not been prevalent. Laveran, who was later to discover the malarial parasite, gives a penetrating analysis of measles among troops concentrated in various barracks in France and points out the high incidence of infection in certain years and the high mortality. In 1860, for example, among 1,000 deaths, 116 were due to measles. F. Printzing (*Epidemics Resulting from Wars* [Oxford: Clarendon Press, 1916]) states that during the American Civil War about 75,000 troops contracted measles, of whom about 5,000 died (p. 179). Printzing also mentions the high incidence of measles even in old men in the concentration camps during the Boer War (p. 293). L. Colin ("Note sur la rougeole observée dans l'armée de Paris pendant le mois de décembre 1870," Bull. Acad. de méd., Paris, **36**:6, 1871) refers to an outbreak in the Army of Paris in which nearly half of those affected died, obviously of secondary bronchopneumonia. W. Kinnear ("Epidemic of measles in the Highland Division at Bedford, 1914–15," Edinburgh M.J., **30**:593, 1923) describes a violent outbreak of measles among recruits from the remoter Highlands; in one group there were 139 cases, with 21 deaths. Measles was also common in the American cantonments during World War I (A. W. Sellards and E. Sturm, "The occurrence of the Pfeiffer bacillus in measles," Bull. Johns Hopkins Hosp., **30**:331, 1919; E. L. Opie, F. G. Blake, J. C. Small, and T. M. Rivers, *Epidemic Respiratory Disease* [St. Louis: C. V. Mosby Co., 1921], chaps. v and vi, pp. 282, 334).

5. THOMAS, [L.] Masern, *in* H. Curschmann, W. Zuelzer, W. Hertz, and H. von Ziemssen, Handbuch der acuten Infectionskrankheiten, Part II. Leipzig: F. C. W. Vogel, 1874.

A detailed discussion, modern in tone, of every aspect of measles, which leaves little to be added. The primary disease is clearly distinguished from secondary bronchopneumonia; there is full discussion of complications and sequelae such as encephalitis. There is an extensive bibliography. Thomas also has an excellent description of what were doubtless Koplik's spots (p. 66).

6. JÜRGENSEN, Theodor. Masern, *in* H. Nothnagel, Specielle Pathologie und Therapie, Vol. **4**, Part 2. Vienna: Alfred Hölder, 1895.

An authoritative comprehensive discussion of all phases of the disease.

7. KOPLIK, Henry. The diagnosis of the invasion of measles from a study of the exanthema as it appears on the buccal mucous membrane, Arch. Pediat., **13**:918, 1896.

In this paper Koplik describes the lesion which bears his name. "On the buccal mucous membrane and the inside of the lips we invariably see a distinct eruption. It consists of small irregular spots of a bright red color. In the centre of each spot there is noted, in strong daylight, a minute bluish white speck." Koplik points out that these spots are best seen *before* the eruption and insists that they "are absolutely pathognomonic of beginning measles" and, when seen, can be relied upon as the forerunner of the skin eruption. In a subsequent article ("The new diagnostic spots of measles on the buccal and labial mucous membrane," M. News, **74**:673, 1899) Koplik complains that his sign has not been adequately recognized in America, and he again describes the spots in detail, with a beautiful colored plate to illustrate them. Meanwhile, Slawyk confirmed the occurrence and value of Koplik's spots ("Ueber das von Koplik als Frühsymptom der Masern beschriebene Schleimhautexanthem," Deutsche med. Wchnschr., 24:269, 1898). W. R. Bett ("Some paediatric eponyms. III. Koplik's spots," Brit. J. Child. Dis., 28:127, 1931) critically reviewed the subject and pointed out that others had mentioned the spots but not with the fulness, accuracy, and tone of conviction of Koplik. Alois Monti ("Studien über das Verhalten der Schleimhaüte bei den acuten Exanthemen," Jahrb. f. Kinderh., 6:20, 1872) in a comprehensive discussion of the mucous membranes in measles reviews the earlier literature and describes his own careful observations. He agrees with previous writers that there is an enanthem, usually appearing before the skin rash and affecting diffusely the pharynx, larynx, palate, and buccal cavity. He probably saw the same spots as Koplik, which he describes as follows: "As to the efflorescences on the gums, they are either irregular, variously shaped, pinhead-sized or larger, isolated or confluent, red spots or varied-sized elevated red papules." He goes on with various details of their appearance. Koplik, however, certainly deserves full credit for forcing the spots on everyone's attention and emphasizing their value in diagnosis before the skin eruption has appeared.

8. JOSIAS, Albert. Recherches expérimentales sur la transmissibilité de la rougeole aux animaux, Méd. mod., 9:153, 1898.

Josias questions the spontaneous occurrence of measles in animals, as well as the previous attempts of Behla to transmit the disease to pigs. Josias first swabbed the noses and throats of young pigs with mucus freshly obtained from human cases of measles. "I will not fatigue the Academy with the details of ten experiments; I will limit myself to saying they were all negative." He then turned to monkeys, who were treated in similar fashion, using in all eight animals. Four "macaques" unaffected; a "sajou capuchin" and two "sajou robustus" monkeys, at intervals of 11–13 days after the swabbing, developed fever, catarrhal symptoms, and a measles-like eruption. However, the descriptions are not altogether convincing, as there seemed to be diffuse erythemas not followed by desquamation. Our verdict from reading this article is that Josias probably, but not certainly, produced measles in his monkeys, although he is generally credited with having actually accomplished this feat.

9. TILISTON, Wilder. The blood in measles, J. Infect. Dis., 1:551, 1904.

Although it was noted many years ago that there was absence of leukocytosis in measles, in contrast to scarlet fever, and, indeed, actually a leukopenia (S. Felsenthal, "Haematologische Mittheilungen," Arch. f. Kinderh., 15:78, 1893), the paper by Tiliston, after a review of the literature, gives comprehensive studies in twenty-eight cases. Tiliston pointed out the now well-known drop in polymorphonuclear leukocytes toward defervescence with increase of lymphocytes. However, the careful and comprehensive counts of B. Benjamin and S. M. Ward ("Leucocytic response to measles," Am. J. Dis. Child., 44:921, 1932) seem definitive. In addition to the hematological findings, they point out changes in the lymph nodes.

10. HEKTOEN, Ludvig. Experimental measles, J. Infect. Dis., 2:238, 1905.

Hektoen reviews the literature on attempts deliberately to transmit measles to man and points out that this was tried for the most part not for scientific reasons but as a practical attempt to produce an immunity to the disease by transmitting a mild attack, after the manner of smallpox inoculation. Practically all these attempts are to be criticized because either the disease produced was atypical and doubtful or because spontaneous infection was not excluded. Nasal secretions, blood, and skin scrapings were all tried as a source of "virus," and inoculations were usually made into skin cuts or occasionally into the upper air passages. Hektoen reports two transmission experiments of his own which he considers successful. In his second case blood was drawn from a patient with measles about 30 hours after appearance of the rash and was incubated in flasks of ascites broth. After 24 hours, 5 cc. were injected subcutaneously into a twenty-eight-year-old man in whom spontaneous infection was definitely excluded. On the eleventh day the temperature began rising and reached 103° F. on the thirteenth day, with the appearance of a typical rubeolous rash. Hektoen later again comprehensively reviewed the subject ("Experimental measles," J.A.M.A., **72**:177, 1919).

    11. CENCI, F. Alcune esperienze di sieroimmunizzazione e sieroterapia nel morbillo, Riv. clin. pediat., **5**:1017, 1907.

Cenci was apparently the first to report on the use of convalescent measles serum as a prophylactic against the disease. None of four children who received injections contracted measles, although repeatedly exposed. However, these children, over a year later when exposed again, took the disease, which showed that the passive protection is brief.

    In spite of these definite observations of Cenci, credit for introducing passive prophylaxis is usually given to Nicolle and Conseil (Ref. 15).

    12. EWING, James. The epithelial cell changes in measles, J. Infect. Dis., **6**:1, 1909.

Ewing reviews the early and confused reports on the histology of measles lesions and describes his own results with material obtained at post mortem and in tissues taken from three patients during life. Ewing concludes that the "widespread occurrence of very acute degeneration and necrosis of epithelial cells, all suggest that measles is referable to infection by a bacterium." Today the changes described would undoubtedly be thought characteristic of a virus. F. B. Mallory and E. M. Medlar ("The skin lesion in measles," J.M. Research, **41**:327, 1920) made a thorough histological study of bits of skin excised during measles. The absence of the polymorphonuclear reaction was striking; there was proliferation of endothelial cells in the capillaries and necrosis of epithelium. Obscure bodies are described in the swollen endothelial cells lining the capillaries which may have been "inclusion bodies," athough the authors do not make this suggestion but regard them as phagocyted cocci in various stages of dissolution. Still later, Warthin (Aldred Scott Warthin, "Occurrence of numerous large giant cells in the tonsil and pharyngeal mucosa in the prodromal stages of measles," Arch. Path., **11**:864, 1931) described a lesion which he regarded as specific of measles, "a subepithelial infiltration of multinucleate syncitial giant cells, lymphocytes and monocytes." W. Finkeldey ("Ueber Riesenzellbefunde in den Gaummenmandeln, zugleich ein Beitrag zur Histopathologie der Mandelveränderungen im Masernincubationsstadium," Virchows Arch. f. path. Anat., **281**:321, 1931) described similar giant cells.

13. ANDERSON, John F., and GOLDBERGER, Joseph. Experimental measles in the monkey: a preliminary note, Pub. Health Rep., **26**:847, 1911.

The writers were apparently not familiar at first with the previous work of Josias (Ref. 8). They used blood drawn from measles patients to inoculate (route not stated) rhesus monkeys. Slight rises in temperature were obtained after incubation periods of 8–10 days with variable maculopapular eruptions over face and body, lasting a few days. In a later paper ("Experimental measles in the monkey: a supplemental note," *ibid.*, p. 887) the writers give details of their experiments. The blood drawn from the donors early in the disease was defibrinated and from 0.5 to 10 cc. were injected intraperitoneally in monkeys. In two instances intracerebral injections were given. The results as to both incubation period and eruption are suggestive. They also thought that they had produced measles with blood drawn from inoculated monkeys. Anderson and Goldberger reported that only two of nine monkeys gave a clearly marked reaction, which they thought was due to "a low degree of susceptibility of the monkey." In another paper ("The period of infectivity of the blood in measles," J.A.M.A., **57**:113, 1911) the same authors found that blood drawn before and early in the exanthem gave positive reactions in monkeys, whereas blood drawn after first appearance of the rash gave no reaction. Soon after, Goldberger and Anderson ("An experimental demonstration of the presence of the virus of measles in the mixed buccal and nasal secretions," *ibid.*, p. 476) turned their attention to the secretions of the upper air passages as a source of infection. They first exposed a young Java monkey to monkeys with "experimental" measles. After a time he developed a fever and an eruption. Subsequently, mixed buccal and nasal secretions from patients in the early stages of measles were swabbed in the throats of monkeys and also given subcutaneously. In some cases it was thought that measles was produced. Still later, Goldberger and Anderson ("The nature of the virus of measles," *ibid.*, p. 971) reported on the characteristics of the virus which they thought passed a Berkefeld filter, resisted desiccation for 25½ hours, and lost its infectivity after heating at 55° C. for 15 minutes. A scrutiny of all these experiments shows results so irregular in time and in the clinical phenomena that one is forced to believe that, while the writers possibly produced measles, one cannot be absolutely certain; for example, in one animal the "eruption" appeared 21 days after inoculation, in others there were febrile reactions without rash, etc.

Meanwhile, Albert S. Grünbaum ("Some experiments on enterica, scarlet fever and measles in the chimpanzee," Brit. M.J., **1**:817, 1904), in two experiments admittedly incomplete, did not succeed in transmitting measles by swabbing nasal secretions in the nose and throat of the monkey. But Ch. Nicolle and E. Conseil ("Reproduction expérimentale de la rougeole chez le Bonnet chinois. Virulence du sang des malades 24 heures avant le début de l'éruption," Compt. rend. Acad. d. sc., **153**:1522, 1911) accepted Anderson and Goldberger's work and reported an experiment of their own. They introduced intraperitoneally into a *Macacus sinicus* 6 cc. of blood drawn from a child 24 hours before the eruption appeared. The monkey developed a fever on the sixth day, which slowly rose until the twelfth day and then receded. No mention is made of an eruption. Ludvig Hektoen and E. H. Eggers ("Experi-

mental measles in the monkey with special reference to the leukocytes,"
J.A.M.A., **57**:1833, 1911) also thought that they had confirmed Anderson and
Goldberger's work and, furthermore, described changes in the blood leukocyte
count which seemed analogous to those of human measles. W. P. Lucas and E.
L. Rizer ("An experimental study of measles in monkeys," J.M. Research,
26:181, 1912) in transmission experiments to monkeys (rhesus) obtained findings similar to those of previous workers, including leukopenia, but they also
described Koplik's spots in the experimental disease. They passed the "disease"
through several monkeys. Finally, Hektoen ("Experimental measles," J.A.M.A.,
72:177, 1919) reviewed the entire subject to date in thorough fashion. He concluded that the disease had been reproduced in monkeys only, but that it was
usually mild and atypical, although definite. "The results in monkeys show that
the cause of measles is present in the naso-pharyngeal secretions and the blood
at least twenty-four hours before the rash as well as for a day or two afterward."

One of the few voices which have questioned the validity of these transmission experiments was that of Sellards, whose critique is well worth reading even
today, when experimental transmission is unquestioned (A. W. Sellards, "A review of investigations concerning the etiology of measles," Medicine, **3**:99,
1924).

14. COLE, Rufus, and MacCALLUM, W. G. Pneumonia at a base hospital,
J.A.M.A., **70**:1146, 1918.

Classical studies of pneumonia following measles at a base hospital. MacCallum
gives a clear description of interstitial (viral) pneumonia but attributes it to
S. *hemolyticus*, which was surely a secondary invader.

15. NICOLLE, Charles, and CONSEIL, E. Pouvoir préventif du sérum
d'un malade convalescent de rougeole, Bull. et mém. Soc. Méd. d. hôp.
de Paris, **2**:336, 1918.

Three of four children in a family had successively come down with measles.
The fourth received an injection of serum from a convalescent brother. He remained well, thus confirming the work of Cenci (Ref. 11). Shortly thereafter,
D. L. Richardson and Hilary Connor ("Immunization against measles,"
J.A.M.A., **72**:1046, 1919) attempted immunization by injections of convalescent serum and by injection of serum together with "virus." By the latter procedure they treated three children, in only one of whom was there a slight reaction, featured by a transient rise in temperature and an atypical rash. Rudolf
Degwitz ("Ueber Versuche mit Masernrekonvaleszentenserum," Ztschr. f.
Kinderh., **25**:134, 1920) treated a considerable number of children with prophylactic injections of convalescent measles serum; none developed measles,
whereas uninjected controls came down. Degwitz soon elaborated these studies
("Ueber Masern-Reconvaleszentenserum," *ibid.*, **27**:171, 1920) and pointed
out that, to confer secure protection, the serum must be given by the sixth day
of the incubation period. A little later Rietschel ("Zur Masernprophylaxie nach
Degwitz, Ztschr. f. Kinderh., **29**:127, 1921) pointed out that serum from the
mother, i.e., from any adult who had had measles, was effective in protecting.
M. Stillerman, H. H. Marks, and W. Thalhimer ("Prophylaxis of measles with
convalescent serum," Am. J. Dis. Child., **67**:1, 1944) reviewed the whole subject to date. Finally, C. F. McKhann and Fu Tang Chu ("Use of placental ex-

tract in prevention and modification of measles," Am. J. Dis. Child., **45**:475, 1933), noting reports on prophylaxis of measles with blood from umbilical cord and placenta, prepared a placental extract which, given intramuscularly early in the incubation period, conferred protection against, or at least attenuation of, the attack of measles.

16. HEKTOEN, Ludvig. The bacteriology of measles, J.A.M.A., **71**:1201, 1918.

Measles, as well as most other infectious diseases, was at one time or another blamed on all sorts of bacteria. The numerous claims are critically reviewed by Hektoen. Although he does not fully clarify the situation, there is an attempt to separate secondary invaders from the primary cause. The subject is also critically reviewed by J. E. McCartney, "A review of recent work on measles," Lancet, **1**:93, 1927.

17. BLAKE, Francis G., and TRASK, James D., Jr. Studies on measles. I. Susceptibility of monkeys to the virus of measles, J. Exper. Med., **33**:385, 1921.

After questioning previous work on transmission of measles to monkeys, Blake and Trask reported experiments of their own in which nasopharyngeal washings from patients were instilled intratracheally into monkeys (*Macacus rhesus*). They concluded that they had produced measles and had transmitted the disease from monkey to monkey. In a second paper ("Studies on measles. II. Symptomatology and pathology in monkeys experimentally infected," *ibid.*, p. 413) Blake and Trask described the clinical course and the microscopic lesions. "The symptoms and course of this reaction closely parallel those of human measles." The lesions of the skin and buccal mucous membranes "are essentially identical with the corresponding lesions of measles in man."

18. HERRMANN, Charles. The relative immunity of infants under five months of age to infection with measles, Arch. Pediat., **40**:678, 1923.

The writer gives statistics showing that infants up to two months old are immune to measles, that they possess a partial resistance up to six or seven months, and that thereafter practically all acquire the disease if exposed. This resistance Herrmann believes due to protective substances transmitted from the mother via the placental circulation.

19. FORD, F. R. The nervous complications of measles, Bull. Johns Hopkins Hosp., **43**:140, 1928.

This is an elaborate and definitive article on the nervous complications of measles. Ford abstracts reports of 113 cases from the literature and adds 12 of his own. The onset is usually on the fourth to sixth day, and the great variety of neurological symptoms is emphasized. The spinal fluid cell count may reach 200 or more. The pathological-anatomical process is that of a toxic-degenerative rather than an inflammatory process. Only about 10 per cent of all patients die, but about 65 per cent of those who survive show residual symptoms. The literature is reviewed.

20. PLOTZ, Harry. Culture "in vitro" du virus de la rogueole, Bull. Acad. d. méd., Paris, **119**:598, 1938.

Plotz placed blood from a patient with measles in flasks of a special medium containing chick embryo hash. Five cubic centimeters of this material from the tenth passage injected subcutaneously produced frank measles in a monkey. "We think, then, that we can conclude that we have grown the measles virus in culture." G. Rake, M. F. Shaffer, and H. P. Jones ("Studies on measles. III. The use of tissue culture in the propagation of measles virus," J. Infect. Dis., **69**:65, 1941) review the attempts at tissue culture by various workers and repeat and confirm Plotz's work.

21. RAKE, Geoffrey, and SHAFFER, Morris F. Studies on measles. I. The use of the chorio-allantois of the developing chicken embryo, J. Immunol., **38**:177, 1940.

The writers criticize previous attempts to grow measles virus in fertile hen's egg, such as those of G. K. Wenckebach and H. Kunert ("Die Züchtung des Masernvirus," Deutsche med. Wchnschr., **63**:1006, 1937), and report experiments of their own. "The agent of measles, obtained from the blood or pharyngeal washings of human cases, has been propagated by serial passage on the chorio-allantois of the fertile hen's egg in the absence of . . . macroscopic lesions. The presence of the agent has been demonstrated by the inoculation of pooled chorio-allantois and viscera of the chick embryos into monkeys (*Macacus mulatto*) with the production of a disease indistinguishable from that brought about by the injection of material obtained from cases of human measles. From monkeys infected with material from either source, measles virus can . . . again be propagated in the fertile hen's egg."

22. SHAFFER, Morris F., RAKE, Geoffrey, STOKES, Joseph, Jr., and O'NEIL, Gerald C. Studies on measles. II. Experimental disease in man and monkeys, J. Immunol., **41**:241, 1941.

The writers try to resolve the doubts of some that the experimental disease is really measles. They simultaneously inoculated some children and monkeys subcutaneously with pooled blood from measles cases and others with chicken embryo-passage virus. In both children and monkeys enough reactions, consisting of fever, coryza, Koplik's spots, leukopenia, and rash, occurred to convince them that the disease was actually measles. However, only four of thirty-six children who received the egg-passage virus developed "mild but definite" measles. J. Stokes, Jr., G. C. O'Neil, M. F. Shaffer, G. Rake, and E. P. Maris ("Studies in measles. IV. Results following inoculations of children with egg-passage measles virus," J. Pediat., **22**:1, 1943) continued these studies. They inoculated a large number of children with egg-passage virus and produced measles, but in a mild, attenuated form in the majority. Human passage did not restore the virulence of the virus. Forty of forty-six children who had had the experimental disease were immune on exposure or reinoculation, which suggested to the writers that active immunization with the mild experimental disease might be useful as prophylaxis of severe measles ("Studies on measles. V. The results of chance and planned exposure to unmodified measles virus in children previously inoculated with egg-passage measles virus," *ibid.*, p. 17). Rake ("Experimental investigations of measles," J. Pediat., **23**:376, 1943) later summarized all his experiments.

23. STOKES, J., Jr., MARIS, E. P., and GELLIS, S. S. XI. The use of concentrated normal human serum gamma globulin (human immune serum globulin) in the prophylaxis and treatment of measles, J. Clin. Investigation, **23**:531, 1944.

These were the first workers to report on the use of "gamma globulin" in measles. Exposed children who received the serum were almost always protected, whereas in those to whom it was given after Koplik's spots or rash were present the disease seemed to be modified in a considerable number. At the same time, C. W. Ordman, C. G. Jennings, Jr., and C. H. Janeway ("XII. The use of concentrated normal human serum gamma globulin [human immune serum globulin] in the prevention and attenuation of measles," J. Clin. Investigation, **23**:541, 1944) found that in an exposed group gamma globulin injections afforded a rate of 71 per cent protection, 27 per cent modification, and only 2 per cent failure among sixty-two inoculated children. A dose of 0.1 cc. per pound of body weight within the first 5 days after exposure appeared adequate as a rule.

24. REAGAN, R. L., HARMON, M., DAY, W., and BRUECKNER, A. L. Electron microscope studies of the virus of measles (Morbilli), Texas Rep. Biol. & Med., **10**:655, 1952.

"Studies by electron microscopy of serum of monkeys infected with the virus of measles show the virus to be round. . . . The virus particles have a diameter of 90 to 100 mμ. These bodies could not be demonstrated in normal monkey serum subjected to the same procedure. . . . The virus in concentrated material was infectious for susceptible monkeys but had no effect on monkeys previously immunized against measles with immune serum globulin." There is an illustration of the virus particle ×130,000.

25. ENDERS, John F., and PEEBLES, Thomas C. Propagation in tissue cultures of cytopathogenic agent from patients with measles, Proc. Soc. Exper. Biol. & Med., **86**:277, 1954.

Since the work of Rake, there had been little progress in isolation of measles virus. Rake's infected tissue cultures showed no visible changes and had to be tested by the awkward method of monkey inoculation. Enders and Peebles apparently succeeded in isolating a virus in cultures of human or monkey kidney cells which produced visible cytopathogenic effects. "Primarily these changes consist in the formation of syncitial giant cells" not unlike those described in man by Warthin (Ref. 12). These effects could be inhibited by convalescent measles sera. "Antigen appears during cultivation *in vitro* of the measles agent that reacts specifically in complement fixation tests with convalescent phase measles sera."

26. BABBOTT, Frank L., Jr., and GORDON, John E. Modern measles, Am. J.M. Sc., **228**:334, 1954.

An extensive critical review, with literature, of all phases of the disease.

SMALLPOX

Clinical	Ref. 2
Complement fixation	Ref. 8
Diagnostic procedures	Refs. 8, 9, 13
General	Ref. 1
Growth of virus in chick embryo	Ref. 12
Guarnieri bodies	Ref. 3
Immunity	Ref. 14
Leukocytes	Ref. 4
Paschen bodies	Ref. 7
Pathology	Ref. 5
Paul test	Ref. 9
Smallpox inoculation	Ref. 1
Smallpox in the monkey	Ref. 6
Statistics	Ref. 11
Viremia	Ref. 14

Section 25

SMALLPOX

BIBLIOGRAPHIES of smallpox are to be found in G. Jochmann's *Pocken und Vaccinationslehre* (Vienna: Alfred Hölder, 1913); in F. R. Blaxall's valuable article on smallpox in *A System of Bacteriology in Relation to Medicine* (London: His Majesty's Stationery Office, 1930), 7:84 ff.; following the article on smallpox in *Virus Diseases of Man* by C. E. Van Rooyen and A. J. Rhodes (New York: Thomas Nelson & Sons, 1948), pages 404 ff.; in the article by J. E. Smadel in T. M. Rivers, *Virus and Rickettsial Infections of Man* (2d ed.; Philadelphia: J. B. Lippincott & Co., 1952), page 414; and in the recent book by Harvey Blank and Geoffrey Rake, *Viral and Rickettsial Diseases of the Skin, Eye and Mucous Membranes of Man* (Boston: Little, Brown & Co., 1955). All these reference lists deal with both smallpox and vaccinia, but the present section of this bibliography is limited to consideration of smallpox; vaccinia will be dealt with separately.

The superficial manifestations of smallpox are so picturesque that it is small wonder that the disease is one of great antiquity associated with popular legend and folklore. Nonetheless, smallpox appears often to have been confused with other disorders, especially measles, perhaps for the following reasons: The early erythematous lesions may be difficult to interpret, and in many severe cases a hemorrhagic rash was associated with death before the typical eruption appeared. This in turn was at times masked by secondary infection, with general sepsis and pneumonia. Neglect and unhygienic surroundings might further modify the picture. To Sydenham is often ascribed the first clear definition of the smallpox, but, while his account is recognizable, it is so buried under an accretion of inconsequential material and humoral doctrine as to be of little more than historical interest. "This sort comes forth sometimes like an erysipelas; sometimes like the measles; and as to outward appearance, they cannot be distinguish'd by any but those that are very conversant in this Disease . . ." (Thomas Sydenham, *The Whole Works*, etc. [4th ed.; London: R. Wellington, 1705], p. 82). Nearly one hundred years later, Huxham, a great authority, seems even more primitive: "For first, when the variolous Contagion attacks a Person of strong tense Fibres, and a rich dense Blood, commonly a smart inflammatory Fever comes; in which sometimes the Lungs, sometimes the Brain, the Throat and other Parts are greatly inflamed, and on Bleeding you have a very thick inflammatory Blood" (John Huxham, *An Essay on Fevers* [4th ed.; London: J. Hinton, 1794], p. 126). By 1811, E. G. Clarke (*The New London Practice of Physic* [7th ed.; London: Longman, Hurst, Rees & Orme, 1811], p. 71) was able to give an excellent account, although his discussion of therapy, dominated by the doctrine of humors, is still primitive: ". . . If the disease should seize people whose constitution labours under an inflammatory diathesis, and has the symptoms of an old inflammatory fever, copious bleeding . . . is necessary," etc.

The history of smallpox has been elaborately dealt with, and those wishing to pursue it further are referred to the following works: James Moore, *The History of the Small-Pox* (London: Longman, Hurst, Rees & Orme, 1815);

444

Charles Creighton, *A History of Epidemics in Great Britain* (Cambridge: Cambridge University Press, 1891), Vol. 1, chap. ix, and Vol. 2, chap. iv; J. D. Rolleston, *The History of the Acute Exanthemata* (London: William Heinemann, 1937); August Hirsch, *Handbuch der historisch-geographischen Pathologie* (2d ed.; Stuttgart; Ferdinand Enke, 1881), 1:88 ff. (in English translation [London: New Sydenham Society, 1883], 1:123). That smallpox was communicable was known at least in the seventeenth century and probably earlier. It was this knowledge and the belief that one attack conveyed immunity that led to the practice of purposeful inoculation with material from smallpox lesions, in order to confer protection by producing what one hoped would be a mild form of the disease. The history of this phase of the subject is of immense interest but does not seem appropriate to this bibliography, since inoculation was generally abandoned in the early part of the nineteenth century. There was, however, a bitter controversy between those who continued to favor inoculation rather than Jennerian vaccination (cowpox), to which appropriate allusion will be made. The history of inoculation with reference to original sources is comprehensively given in Edward J. Edwardes' *A Concise History of Small Pox and Vaccination in Europe* (London: H. K. Lewis, 1902), page 24, and in Crookshank's elaborate *History and Pathology of Vaccination* (London: H. K. Lewis, 1889), Vol. 1, chaps. 1–3. An especially readable account is to be found in Sir James Moore's book (*op. cit.,* chap. viii, pp. 218 ff.). The procedure was evidently one of great antiquity in the Orient. The Chinese are said to have taken "a few dried Small Pox crusts, as if they were seeds, and planted them in the nose" (p. 219); "with the vain hope of mitigating their acrimony, they were sometimes kept in closed jars for years" (p. 219). "But at the beginning of the eighteenth century, there was communicated to the Royal Society of London, a discovery to which the Faculty can lay no claim; and as it was first brought to England from Constantinople, it was at first named the Byzantine operation, although certainly not invented there" (p. 218). "The operation was variously performed and on different parts of the body . . . but it always consisted in scratching or puncturing the skin and inserting into the wound variolous matter" (p. 224). Although several physicians wrote about the practice in English as early as 1715, "no Englishman ever thought of trying it. But soon afterward it accidentally happened that Lady Mary Wortley Montague, then blooming in beauty, traveled into Turkey with her husband, the ambassador to the Ottoman Court in her train." Lady Mary in one of the celebrated letters which she wrote home (*Letters of the Right Honourable Lady M——y W——y M——e: Written during Her Travels in Europe, Asia, and Africa,* Letter XXXI [various eds.])[1] tells about the practice by which the children were hardly made ill and "there was no example of any one dying." She therefore had her own son successfully "ingrafted." On her return to England, her daughter was inoculated by Mr. Maitland with good results. Lady Mary "actually effected a complete revolution in the practice of Small Pox all over Europe."

Caroline, princess of Wales, was now desirous of having her children receive the new treatment. "But not venturing to rely solely upon the medical skill of Lady Mary Wortley Montague, Her Royal Highness obtained from George

---

[1] This letter has so often been reprinted that we shall not take space to do so here.

the First, that six condemned felons should be pardoned, for the good of the public, on condition of their submitting to be inoculated" (p. 229). "Neither the legality nor the morality of this unprecedented act were questioned, and still less did the criminals demur; but an unlooked for obstacle occurred; the surgeon refused to perform the operation, for notwithstanding his former success, he dreaded a failure; and of being stigmatized for doing the work of the executioner." However, the felons were finally inoculated, five contracted smallpox, and all escaped hanging. This success encouraged Mr. Maitland to treat still others. The Princess of Wales was now eager to begin, but, before going ahead, the procedure was tried on eleven charity children of St. James Parish, who all did well. Sir Hans Sloane was now consulted on the propriety of treating the princesses; but he was cautious about taking responsibility, and a long argument ensued. Finally, the two princesses, Amelia and Carolina, were inoculated; and the smallpox "proved of a benign sort."

For the next hundred years the merits of inoculation were hotly debated; not uncommonly, severe or fatal smallpox was produced, and a number of epidemics were initiated. However, it was Jennerian vaccination which finally supplanted inoculation, although much was learned about smallpox and about immunity from the practice. A vast amount was early written on the subject; there may be mentioned as especially interesting the book of Baron T. Dimsdale, *Tracts on Inoculation, Written and Published at St. Petersburg in the Year 1768, by Command of Her Imperial Majesty the Empress of All the Russias* (London: James Phillips, 1781), and the little treatise of Alexander Munro, *An Account of the Inoculation of Small-Pox in Scotland* (Edinburgh: Drummond, 1765), which contains valuable mortality statistics of the procedure. It is of interest that one of the standard arguments against inoculation was that one was flying in the face of providence by interfering with the natural course of disease.

1. TROUSSEAU, A. Clinique médicale de l'Hôtel-Dieu de Paris, 1:60, article "Variole." Paris: J.-B. Baillière et fils, 1861.

It is next to impossible to decide who wrote the first adequate description of smallpox. At any rate, the detailed and graphic account by the master clinician Trousseau, based on accurate personal observation of patients, has been, we believe, surpassed by no one. He divides smallpox into the "discrete" cases, usually benign, and the confluent cases, often fatal. Of the former he says: "The periods which it runs through are easy to distinguish. They are: the period of invasion, the period of eruption, the period of maturation or of suppuration, the period of desiccation." The manifestations of the disease "are precisely characterized, and it is not possible to confuse them even with those of chicken-pox, an essentially different disease. . . . It is important, above all, to distinguish the two principal forms, because the discrete smallpox is ordinarily exempt from danger. Confluent smallpox, on the other hand, is a terrible disease, and everyone knows how rarely it spares those whom it strikes down."

There follows a vivid and precise description of the various stages, often illustrated by examples of individual cases. "You will recall in this connection the patient whom you saw in Bed No. 9 in the St. Agnes Ward, etc."

In connection with the severe confluent forms, secondary infection is emphasized. "What is terrible about small-pox is not only that it kills in the acute phase but that it kills even when it, so to speak, has made its retreat and when the danger seems to have passed; it kills by the severe suppurations of which we have spoken, suppurations invading the tissues of the limbs, the serous membranes, pneumonia which goes on quickly to suppuration." Anasarca, albuminuria, and hematuria are discussed as complications of the confluent forms.

That Trousseau wrote in a modern critical spirit is nowhere better shown than in the remarks on treatment: "This paragraph will necessarily be brief because with the eruptive fevers there is rarely a chance for medicine to intervene effectively. These diseases run a natural course . . . one will be content to prescribe refreshing drinks" and general nursing care. This is in sharp contrast to the "eye of newt and toe of frog" prescriptions of a generation previously.

Of an excellence comparable to Trousseau's is the account by J. F. Marson in Reynolds' *System of Medicine* (Philadelphia: J. B. Lippincott & Co., 1866), 1: 223. The best modern description, comprehensive and precise, is that of Jochmann in his textbook of infectious disease (G. Jochmann, *Lehrbuch der Infectionskrankheiten* [Berlin: Julius Springer, 1914], p. 799) and also that in his larger treatise, *Pocken und Vaccinationslehre*. The article by Smadel in Rivers' *Viral and Rickettsial Infections of Man,* page 414, places emphasis not only on clinical description but on modern aspects of smallpox virus, as does the account in the book by C. E. Van Rooyen and A. J. Rhodes (*op. cit.*).

2. GUARNIERI, G. Recerche sulla pathogenesi ed etiologia dell'infezione vaccinica e variolosa, Arch. per. le sc. med., 16:403, 1893. (German abstract: Ueber die Parasiten der Variola und der Vaccine, Centralbl. f. Bact., 16:299, 1894.)

In histological studies of smallpox Guarnieri described the inclusion bodies which bear his name and are well known today. A less clearly remembered facet of the story is that Guarnieri regarded these bodies as parasites which were the cause of the disease, and he assigned to them the name of *Cytoryctes vacciniae* resp. *variolae*. To these "organisms" he ascribed an ameboid movement when observed in hanging-drop preparations of material from smallpox vesicles, and he also convinced himself that he saw them undergo multiplication. Guarnieri was evidently strongly influenced by the studies on malarial Protozoa which were then being actively pursued in Italy. Guarnieri, interestingly enough, was almost universally believed, and a huge literature of confirmatory reports grew up, with only a few dissenting voices.[2] It would serve no purpose to review the literature, as this has been thoroughly done by Councilman, Magrath, and Brinckerhoff (Ref. 4). It is of interest that as astute and careful an observer as Councilman fully accepted Guarnieri's views ten years later. In a brief paper (W. T. Councilman, G. B. Magrath, and W. R. Brinckerhoff, "A preliminary communication on the etiology of variola," J.M.

---

[2] But see, for example, P. Mühlens and M. Hartmann ("Zur Kentniss des Vaccineerregers," Centralbl. f. Bact., 41:41, 203, 338, 435, 1906), who after an elaborate study conclude: "The Guarnieri bodies are products of a regressive metamorphosis of the nuclear substance of the epithelial cells."

Research, **9**:372, 1903) it is stated: "The bodies in the cells we regard as living organisms, and the gradual growth and final segmentation as a cycle in its life history. At the period of segmentation . . . small round or oval ring-like bodies appear in the nucleus. . . ." Dr. Tyzzer, working with inoculated rabbits and calves, found similar bodies, and "the complete cycle of this organism which corresponds to the primary cycle of the smallpox organism, has been traced. . . . In variola the entire process of development of the parasite is concluded with the formation of the young vesicle. The spores are present in the contents." The bodies are beautifully pictured in Councilman's longer article (Ref. 4) and by Gary Calkins ("The life history of Cytoryctes variolae Guarnieri," J.M. Research, **11**:136, 1904), who traces in detail and elaborately illustrates the cycle of the supposed parasite.

Thus we have the counterpart of what has happened in the history of nearly every infectious disease: the *Bacillus malariae* of Klebs and Tommasi-Crudeli, the globoid bodies of poliomyelitis, Noguchi's leptospira of yellow fever, and innumerable others all had their vogue as the cause of one or another disease. In Osler's *Principles and Practice of Medicine,* smallpox is still classified under diseases of doubtful etiology in the twelfth edition (1935), and under the heading "Nature of the infection" it is still stated that "Protozoön-like bodies were described in the skin lesions by Guarnieri-Cytoryctes variolae." It was not until the thirteenth edition (1938) that smallpox was classified under virus diseases, although the statement about *Cytoryctes variolae* is still preserved.

3. MAGRATH, G. B., BRINCKERHOFF, W. R., and BANCROFT, I. R.
   The leucocyte reaction in variola, J.M. Research, **11**:247, 1904.

The writers review the early literature and find that the first adequate observations on the subject were those of Jules Courmont and V. Montgard ("La Leukocytose dans la variole," J. de physiol. et de path. gén., **2**:557, 1900), who in a comprehensive study found that there was always a leukocytosis, beginning early before vesiculation and consisting of an increase in "mononuclears," whereas polymorphonuclears were relatively diminished. Alexander R. Ferguson ("The leucocytosis of variola," J. Path. & Bact., **8**:411, 1903) reported similar findings. He made daily counts and found the peak of the leukocytosis on or about the ninth day of the disease. Magrath and his associates elaborated these studies still further. They concluded that the leukocytosis of variola owed its characteristic feature "to the failure of the haematopoietic organs to produce the adult cells called for." They found "degenerative phenomena" in the polymorphonuclears in severe cases which they regarded as due to accentuation of the process of leukocyte destruction. Finally, Kano Ikeda ("The blood in purpuric small-pox," J.A.M.A., **84**:1807, 1925) in twelve cases of purpuric smallpox found, in addition to the changes in the leukocytes, a marked thrombocytopenia.

As to the bone marrow, this seems first to have been studied by C. Golgi ("Sulla alterazioni del midollo delle ossa nel vajuolo," Osservatore, Torino, **9**:161, 1873). Golgi found that in hemorrhagic variola, aside from hemorrhages, there was diminution in the number of leukocytes and increase in nucleated red cells, whereas with pustular variola there was an increase in leukocytes and "giant cells." H. Chiari ("Ueber Osteomyelitis variolosa,"

Beitr. z. path. Anat. u. z. allg. Path., **13**:13, 1893) described what he thought was a specific variolous lesion in the bone marrow in the form of disseminated focal lesions. H. Roger, O. Josué, and Émile Weil ("La Moelle osseuse dans la variole," Arch. de méd. expér. et d'anat. path., **12**:545, 1900) later correlated the appearance of the bone marrow with the peripheral blood count.

4. COUNCILMAN, W. T., MAGRATH, G. B., and BRINCKERHOFF, W. R. The pathological anatomy and histology of variola, J.M. Research, **11**:12, 1904.

Councilman and his associates in the Boston epidemic of smallpox of 1901–2 made meticulous gross and microscopic examination of smallpox lesions in fifty-four autopsies. In reviewing the literature, they attributed the first adequate anatomical studies to Carl Weigert (*Anatomische Beiträge zur Lehre von den Pocken* [Breslau: Max Cohen & Weigert, 1874]). Weigert, basing his studies on two hundred cases examined during the Breslau epidemic of 1871–72, confined his description to the skin lesions (*die Pocken-Effloreszenten der aüsseren Haut*). He concluded that the changes were neurotic and irritative and that the bacteria regularly seen were either the carriers of the infectious material or the material itself. Weigert published reproductions of the histological changes. A little later P. G. Unna ("Ueber den Sitz der Pocken in der Epidermis und die ersten Studien des Pockenprocess," Virchows Arch. f. path. Anat., **69**:409, 1877) gave a careful description of the skin lesions, with illustrative plates. Councilman's monograph is, however, in a sense definitive. He and his associates described not only the skin lesions but those of the mucous membranes and of the various viscera. They give numerous beautiful plates of the histological changes, and they conclude that "the specific [skin] lesion of variola is a focal degeneration of stratified epithelium, vacuolar in character, and accompanied by serous exudation and the formation of a reticulum. The fully developed product of these processes is a characteristic multilocular pock or pustule." The visceral lesions, on the other hand, seemed largely non-specific, although all sorts of degenerative changes are described, as, for example, those in the liver (H. Roger and M. Garnier, "Étude anatomique et chimique du foie dans la variole," Arch. méd. expér., **13**:661, 1901). In summary, Councilman divided the lesions into (A) the specific, limited to stratified epithelium of skin and of the mucous membranes of the soft palate, the pharynx, and the esophagus; (B) associated lesions of indeterminate specificity, such as degenerative and cellular infiltrative with mononuclear basophilic elements; and (C) associated lesions, bacterial in origin. It is of interest that Councilman mentioned interstitial changes in the bronchopneumonic pulmonary lesions.

5. MAGRATH, G. B., and BRINCKERHOFF, W. R. On experimental variola in the monkey, J.M. Research, **11**:230, 1904.

The writers attribute the first report of successful monkey inoculation to W. Zuelzer ("Zur Aetiologie der Variola," Centralbl. f. d. med. Wissensch., **12**:82, 1874). An inspection of this article leaves one in doubt, however, as to whether Zuelzer was really successful. Magrath and Brinckerhoff produced the typical disease in monkeys by inoculation of virus into the skin; the reaction, however, was very mild. They concluded that "variola virus can be transferred from a man to a monkey, from the monkey to the rabbit's cornea through four generations, and, when then inoculated on the monkey, can produce a protopustule followed by a general exanthem."

6. PASCHEN, E. Was wissen wir über den Vakzineerreger? München. med. Wchnschr., **53**:2391, 1906.

Guarnieri bodies are to be sharply differentiated from those to which Paschen's name has become attached. The latter are minute granules demonstrable in material from vaccinia, variola, and alastrim. It has been claimed that they were first described by J. B. Buist ("The life-history of the microorganisms associated with variola and vaccina," Proc. Roy. Soc. Edinburgh, **13**:603, 1886), but study of his report leaves one doubtful as to what he actually saw, and credit is usually given to Paschen for discovering them. Convinced that the organisms of smallpox must be present in huge numbers in the lymph of vesicles, Paschen studied smears of diluted material with all sorts of stains: "Microscopic examination of these preparations showed a surprisingly large number of uniformly stained very small bodies." These he divided into four types or stages. "Are we dealing with developmental stages; or with a strange organism or with simple nuclear precipitates? . . . I simply record these findings without drawing any conclusions." The paper is a landmark and includes a careful review of previous work on experimental vaccinia and on previous attempts to demonstrate the etiological agent. It is now believed that the Paschen bodies are identical with the elementary bodies known to be the virus of smallpox.

For an authoritative review of the subject to date, the reader is referred to the article by J. E. Smadel and C. L. Hoagland, "Elementary bodies of vaccinia," Bact. Rev., **6**:79, 1942, as well as chapter 29, "The variola-vaccinia virus: elementary and inclusion bodies," in Van Rooyen and Rhodes, *op. cit.* C. E. Van Rooyen and R. S. Illingworth ("A laboratory test for diagnosis of small pox," Brit. M.J., **2**:526, 1944), impressed by the need of an early diagnostic test for smallpox, utilized the fact that the "elementary bodies" of variola are larger than those of varicella. Scrapings from the base of early lesions were stained by special techniques. The laboratory and clinical findings corresponded in 96 per cent of the cases.

7. GORDON, M. H. Studies of the viruses of vaccinia and variola, p. 108. ("Medical Research Council, Special Reports Series," No. 98.) London: His Majesty's Stationery Office, 1925.

Gordon applied the complement-fixation technique to the diagnosis of smallpox, using a suspension of variola scabs as antigen. R. F. Parker and R. S. Muckenfuss ("Complement fixation in vaccinia and in variola," J. Infect. Dis., **53**:44, 1933) critically reviewed the subject and described a technique of their own, using a specific antivaccinial serum and fluid from the pustules. The subject was further developed by Craigie and Wishart (Ref. 11).

8. TOOMY, John A., and GAMMEL, John A. The Paul test in the diagnosis of small-pox, J. Infect. Dis., **41**:29, 1927.

Guarnieri (Ref. 2) inoculated the corneas of rabbits with smallpox material and demonstrated that a lesion resulted. Others, including Juergens ("Description of microscopic preparations," Berl. klin. Wchnschr., **42**:308, 1905), further emphasized the peculiar proliferations of the corneal epithelium which followed inoculation with smallpox material. Gustav Paul ("Eine neue Untersuchungsmethode der variolierten Hornhaut des Kaninchenauges zur objektiven Sicherung der Varioladiagnose," Wien. klin. Wchnschr., **29**:996, 1916), however, first emphasized the possibility of using the appearance of the variolated cornea as a specific diagnostic test for smallpox, by excising the infected eye and fixing it in bichloride, whereby the epithelial nodules were emphasized. Toomy and Gammel review the literature critically and report their own experience with the Paul test, which was positive in 46 per cent of cases.

9. McKINNON, Neil, and DE FRIES, Robert O. The reaction in the skin of the normal rabbit following intradermal injection of material from small-pox lesions: the specificity of this reaction and its application as a diagnostic test, Am. J. Hyg., **8**:93, 1928.

Although it had been shown long before that the rabbit was susceptible to vaccine virus, the effect of smallpox virus had not been clearly demonstrated, according to McKinnon and De Fries. These authors were able to produce in normal rabbits a definite papular lesion by injection of material from smallpox cases. The specificity of the reaction was shown by the failure of subsequent vaccination with vaccine virus to "take." Material from chicken pox failed to elicit a reaction in rabbits. The same writers ("The laboratory diagnosis of small-pox virus utilizing the rabbit," *ibid.*, p. 107) proposed as a diagnostic test for smallpox the injection of suspected material into normal and vaccine-immunized rabbits. The specific lesion should, of course, develop in the former.

10. HEDRICH, A. W. Changes in the incidence and fatality of small-pox in recent decades, Pub. Health Rep., **51**:363, 1936.

There is a popular idea that vaccination has largely eliminated smallpox in the United States as well as elsewhere and that if the disease occurs, it is usually mild. Nothing could be further from the truth. There were nearly 400,000 cases in the United States from 1921 to 1930, and the death rate per 100 cases varied up to 42.3 in British India. All these matters are discussed in detail in Hedrich's paper, including the view that there are distinct mild and severe strains of smallpox virus which account for these variations. It is thought that the mild virus is responsible for such relatively innocuous entities as "alastrim."

11. LAZARUS, A. S., EDDIE, B., and MEYER, K. F. Propagation of variola in the developing egg, Proc. Soc. Exper. Biol. & Med., **36**:7, 1937.

Using material from a smallpox vesicle, the writers inoculated the chorio-allantoic membrane of the developing chick and were able to carry the virus through forty-five passages. Discrete yellowish-white lesions were seen on the membrane several days after inoculation, and impression smears showed typical Paschen bodies (Ref. 6) with Morosow's stain (M. A. Morosow, "Die Färbung der Paschenschen Körperchen durch Versilberung," Centralbl. f. Bakt., **100**:385, 1926). The presence of virus was also confirmed by the complement-fixation test (James Craigie and F. O. Wishart, "The complement-fixation reaction in variola," Canad. J. Pub. Health, **27**:371, 1936). Others, also, were soon successful in growing the virus of smallpox in chick embryos. C. John

Buddingh ("Infection of the chorio-allantois of the chick embryo as a diagnostic test for variola," Am. J. Hyg., **28**:130, 1938) also injected chick embyros with material from smallpox pustules and produced a pock in which Paschen granules were found and also Guarnieri bodies. A. W. Downie and K. K. Dumbell ("The isolation and cultivation of variola virus on the chorio-allantois of chick embryos," J. Path. & Bact., **59**:189, 1947) also described inclusion bodies in chick embryo variola.

12. PARKER, Robert F. Variola and vaccinia *in* Diagnostic procedures for virus and Rickettsial diseases, p. 83. New York: American Public Health Association, 1948.

The early diagnosis of smallpox becomes especially necessary before an epidemic is under way. The disease may be confused with chicken pox, influenza, or other infections. Laboratory diagnosis is therefore very important. Parker summarizes the modern status of the subject in this article. We have alluded to various tests in the course of this bibliography (Refs. 7, 8, 9, 10).

13. DOWNIE, A. W., McCARTHY, K. M., and MACDONALD, Alexander. Viremia in small pox, Lancet, **2**:513, 1950.

Downie and Dumbell (Ref. 11) had isolated virus from the blood of a case of hemorrhagic smallpox on the fifth day. Downie and his colleagues, however, successfully inoculated chick embryos with blood drawn in the very early stages of the disease before the rash was distinctive in four of seven patients. F. O. MacCallum, C. A. McPherson, and D. F. Johnstone ("Laboratory investigation of small-pox patients with particular reference to infectivity in the early stages," Lancet, **2**:514, 1950) were able to recover smallpox virus by egg inoculation with blood drawn the day before and on the day of onset of the rash. They also recovered the virus from throat swabs taken in the early stages of the disease. The viremia of smallpox evidently occurs early and is more likely to be demonstrable in very severe cases. These writers, following others, also suggest that the portal of entry of smallpox virus is by way of the respiratory passages. Downie ("Infection and immunity in smallpox," Lancet, **1**:419, 1951) further studied the development of smallpox in relation to immunity and antibody formation. His concept is as follows: The site of entry of the virus is in the upper respiratory tract. A minimal lesion occurs, and the virus quickly passes to lymphatic glands and by blood stream to internal organs. Increase of virus in these organs takes place during the incubation period. At onset of illness there is an overflow of virus into the blood stream and liberation of the products of cell breakdown. The skin and other tissues are infected with virus at this time, and in most cases the immune response with the formation of antibody follows a few days later. The speed and extent of the antibody formation determines the extent of the rash and the severity of the disease. Antibody persists at a high level for some years after smallpox. Thus the eruption at its height is really an antigen-antibody reaction.

VACCINIA

Section 26

VACCINIA

It HAS been difficult to decide whether one should combine the bibliographies of smallpox and vaccination or keep them separate. The two diseases are so closely related, caused as they are by viruses in many ways identical, that there is necessarily much overlapping in the literature. Although it finally seemed better to have separate bibliographies, the two should obviously be read and studied together. Thus the general and bibliographical references which we have given for smallpox refer also to the literature on vaccination. Cross-references between the two are designated "S." and "V.," respectively.

1. JENNER, Edward. An inquiry into the cause and effects of the variolae vacciniae, a disease discovered in some of the western counties of England, particularly Gloucestershire, and known by the name of the cow pox. London: Printed for the author by Sampson Low, 1798.

This is the famous work in which Jenner claimed that inoculation with material from cowpox conferred protection against smallpox. With the lapse of time, Jenner's contentions have been amply confirmed, as everyone knows, and he stands out in history as a great man and a benefactor of humanity. But this was not always so, and, at the time, both the doctrines and the findings of Jenner were by no means universally accepted. It has been alleged that Jenner was not a critical scientist; indeed, some claim that he was little more than a quack. First of all, it is said that the idea of cowpox conferring protection against smallpox was not novel with Jenner but was currently popular among dairy folk and cow-leeches at the time. It is stated that one B. Jesty, a farmer of Downshay, in the Isle of Purbeck, in 1774 inoculated his wife and two sons from his cows and that subsequently they resisted the most rigorous trials to confer smallpox upon them. It is claimed that cowpox is not really a "pock" disease, that mere resemblance of names—cowpox, smallpox—somewhat irrationally stimulated Jenner to develop his doctrine, and that, aside from the name, there was no more resemblance between the two disorders than there is between a horse chestnut and a chestnut horse. In 1796 or 1797 Jenner drew up a report of one case, that of James Phipps, whom he inoculated with material from a cowpox vesicle on the hand of the dairymaid Sarah Nelmes. The vaccination took, and inoculation with variolous matter later failed to produce disease. This paper was sent informally to the Royal Society, who evidently did not feel that the evidence was conclusive, and it was not until 1798 that Jenner himself published the famous "Inquiry." All these matters are discussed in detail in Charles Creighton's book, *Jenner and Vaccination* (London: Swan Sonnenschein & Co., 1889), which takes a bitterly antagonistic attitude toward Jenner, as well as in Edgar M. Crookshank's *History and Pathology of Vaccination* (London: H. K. Lewis, 1889), which preserves a somewhat more temperate attitude. Edward J. Edwardes, *A Concise History of Small-Pox and Vaccination in Europe* (London: H. K. Lewis, 1902), on the other hand, deals with the same transactions but in a spirit highly favorable to Jenner.

Now as to the "Inquiry" itself. After an introductory paragraph, Jenner turns immediately to discussion of a disease of horses called "the grease." "It is an inflammation and swelling in the heel, from which issues matter possessing properties of a very peculiar kind, which seems capable of generating a disease in the Human Body (after it has undergone the modification which I shall presently speak of) which bears so strong a resemblance to the Small Pox, that I think it highly probable it may be the source of that disease." Jenner goes on to claim, in brief, that milkers may contaminate cows with material from "the grease" which produces cowpox, which, in turn, may be transmitted to the milkmaids. "Thus the disease makes its progress from the Horse to the nipple of the Cow, and from the Cow to the Human Subject . . . but what renders the Cow-Pox virus so extremely singular is, that the person who has been thus affected is forever after secure from the infection of the Small-Pox; neither exposure to the variolous effluvia, nor the insertion of the matter into the skin, producing this distemper." This does seem a somewhat rash claim on Jenner's part, since it was common knowledge at the time that those who were "Cowpoxed" might later have smallpox; even today we know that a successful vaccination does not confer permanent protection but must be repeated every few years. Jenner continues: "In support of so extraordinary a fact, I shall lay before my Reader a great number of instances." At this point Jenner states in a footnote that one must beware of confusion arising from another variety of "pustulous sores" which "frequently appear spontaneously on the nipples of Cows, and instances have occurred, though very rarely, of the hands [of milkers] being affected with sores in consequence, and even of their feeling an indisposition from absorption." This disease is, however, quite different, he claims, from that caused by infection from horse "grease," and infection with material from this sort of spurious cowpox confers no immunity. "But this disease is not to be considered as similar in any respect to that of which I am treating, as it is incapable of producing any specific effect on the human Constitution. However it is of the greatest consequence to point it out here, lest the want of discrimination should occasion an idea of security from the infection of the Small Pox which might prove delusive." There follow twenty-three case reports, some of people who gave a history of having had the cowpox and whom Jenner found resistant to inoculation with variolous material, and some of people whom Jenner inoculated with "Cow Pox" material, produced disease, and then found them resistant. Case IX opens with the following interesting statement: "Although the Cow Pox shields the constitution from the Small Pox . . . yet it appears that the human body is again and again susceptible to the infectious matter of the Cow Pox." William Smith had contracted the disease in 1780. "One of the horses belonging to the farm had sore heels, and it fell to his lot to attend him. By these means the infection was carried to the cows and from the cows it was communicated to Smith. . . . In the year 1791 the Cow Pox broke out at another farm where he then lived as a servant and he became affected with it a second time; and in the year 1794 he was so unfortunate as to catch it again." It must be admitted that case histories of this sort are of little scientific value. The role of the horse "grease" is mentioned in a number of patients, as in Case XV: "Although in the two former instances the system seemed to be secured, or nearly so, from variolous infection, by the absorption of matter from sores produced by the diseased heels of horses, yet the following case decisively proves that this can not be entirely relied upon, until a disease has been generated by morbid matter of the horse on the nipple of the cow, and passed through that medium to the human subject. Mr. Abraham Riddiford in consequence of dressing a mare that had sore feet was affected with lesions regarded as those of Cow Pox but being exposed to small-pox twenty years later contracted the disease." It was on evidence of this sort that Jenner claimed that the original disease of the horse must be "catalyzed" in the cow before true cowpox could be produced. Case XVI is the famous one of Sarah Nelmes, from whose pustulous sore Jenner inoculated the eight-year-old boy (Case XVII) by means of "two superficial incisions, barely penetrating the cutis, each about half an inch long." On the seventh day he developed malaise and dulness and "maturation of the incisions." He was later twice inoculated with variolous matter without developing smallpox. Jenner then described the cases of two farm hands, Haynes and Virgoe, who, in spite of the fact that they had gone through the smallpox from inoculation, developed from a mare with sore heels "sores in their hands followed by inflamed lymphatic glands in the arm and axillae," etc. "Haynes was daily employed as one of the milkers at the farm, and the disease began to shew itself among the cows about ten days after he first assisted in washing the mare's heels. Their nipples became sore in the usual way." Jenner's later cases were inoculated with cowpox and and then did not take smallpox inoculation.

The last half of the "Inquiry" consists of a rather rambling general discourse on the subject. "May it not, then, be reasonably conjectured, that the source of the Small-pox is morbid matter of a peculiar kind, generated by a disease in the horse, and that accidental circumstances may have again and again arisen, still working new changes upon it until it has acquired the contagious and malignant form under which we now commonly see it making its devastations amongst us?"

It seems to us very difficult to evaluate all this. The great fact stands out that Jenner's main thesis has turned out to be correct, but was this a lucky guess, as some have claimed, or does his published evidence really justify his conclusions? Certainly his position with reference to horse "grease" and true and spurious cowpox was weak.

That there followed a long period during which the value of vaccination was variously judged is quite intelligible. First of all, despite Jenner, it was common knowledge that some of those who had had the cowpox *did* later acquire smallpox. Then when we consider that the procedure, source of virus, collection and preservation of it, and mode of inoculation were absolutely unstandardized and haphazard; that supposed cowpox virus was probably often contaminated with smallpox virus; and that the lesions produced by vaccination were almost always infected with secondary invaders, there is small wonder that many were confused.

2. PEARSON, George. An inquiry concerning the history of the cow pox principally with a view to supersede and extinguish the small pox. London: J. Johnson, 1798.

Pearson published in support of Jenner shortly after the "Inquiry" appeared. He collected evidence on all sides from both physicians and laymen as to immunity to smallpox in those who were cowpoxed. He lists Jenner's claims in a series of propositions and adduces evidence in support of all except the one which states that a person may have cowpox over and over again and yet be immune to smallpox. "They [the professional men] are not averse from admitting the evidence that the Cow Pox may affect the same constitution repeatedly; or even that a person, having had this disease, is insusceptible of the Small Pox, but that the constitution having suffered the Cow Pox should still be susceptible of this disease, and not susceptible of the Small Pox is an assertion with regard to which they demur to acquiesce."

3. WOODVILLE, William. Reports of a series of inoculations for the variolae vacciniae or cow pox; with remarks and observations on this disease, considered as a substitute for the small-pox. London: James Phillips & Son, [1799].

Woodville, who was physician to the Smallpox Hospital in London and who had a vast experience in smallpox inoculation, was naturally interested in Jenner's work. This report begins with experiments in which he inoculated the nipples of cows "with matter of the grease of horses" without any effect. Cowpox later broke out in a dairy and was clinically identified by a panel of expert physicians whom Woodville took there to see the lesions. Sarah Rice, a milkmaid, was also affected with a vesicle on her hand similar to those described by Jenner. Woodville inoculated two hundred people with cowpox lymph obtained, fortunately, early in the disease. Many of these inoculations were from person to person. There are detailed notes on the cases and a long table giving the patients' names and the number of pustules produced; a good many had a large number of pustules, several as many as six to seven hundred. There may have been some confusion with smallpox, but, at any rate, Woodville did the first major operation of vaccinating a large number of people, and he supplied lymph to many physicians, including Jenner.

4. JENNER, Edward. Further observations on the variolae vacciniae or cow pox. London: Printed for the author by Sampson Low, 1799.

In order to explain contradictions which were reported on many sides, Jenner here tries to define the genuine cowpox and the specifications for a reliable virus. "I shall proceed to enumerate the sources, or what appear to me as such, of a spurious Cow Pox. 1st. That arising from pustules on the nipples or udder of the cow; which pustules contain no specific virus. 2ndly. From matter (although originally possessing the specific virus) which has suffered a decomposition, either from putrefaction or from any other cause less obvious to the senses. 3dly. From matter taken from an ulcer in an advanced stage, which ulcer arose from a true Cow Pock. 4thly. From matter produced on the human skin from contact with some peculiar morbid matter generated by a horse."

More and more difficulties and contradictions were being encountered, but, through it all, Jenner remained steadfast to his fundamental thesis.

In still another communication Jenner (*A Continuation of Facts and Observations Relative to the Variolae Vacciniae, or Cow Pox* [London: Printed for the author by D. N. Shury, 1801]) replied to Dr. Woodville (Ref. 3), who produced multiple pustules in so many of his vaccinated patients. Jenner believed, probably correctly, that smallpox virus had somehow entered Woodville's vaccine and that the cases with many pustules were instances of smallpox. All this shows how confused the entire situation was at the time.

5. WATERHOUSE, Benjamin. A prospect of exterminating the small-pox; being the history of the variolae vacciniae, or kine-pox, commonly called the cow-pox, as it has appeared in England, with an account of a series of inoculations performed for the kine-pox in Massachusetts. Cambridge: Cambridge Press, William Hilliard, 1800. Also Part II. Cambridge, 1802.

Waterhouse deserves credit for introducing vaccination into the United States. He became interested in vaccination in 1799 when he read Jenner's "Inquiry." In June, 1800, he received some "matter" from England and promptly vaccinated his children. "I commenced the experiment on July 8th, 1800, on my own children, four of whom, with three of my domestics, passed regularly through the distemper; and that they soon after went into the licensed smallpox hospital, in this neighborhood, and all seven of them were inoculated by Dr. Aspinwall with the matter of small-pox without the least trace of infection" (Part II, p. 5). The whole story of Dr. Waterhouse is told by Robert H. Halsey (*How the President, Thomas Jefferson, and Dr. Benjamin Waterhouse Established Vaccination as a Public Health Procedure* [New York: The Author, 1936]). Waterhouse received requests from the southern states for information about vaccination. These led him into correspondence with Thomas Jefferson. "Young and inexperienced practitioners are most forward in their business; yet such can neither excite attention, nor inspire confidence; whereas, if it came from Mr. Jefferson, it would make, like a body falling from a great height, a deep impression" (Part II, p. 25). The President immediately put the matter into the hands of a long-established, judicious, and successful physician, but various lots of vaccine failed to take, perhaps because of the very hot weather. But on August 6, 1801, takes were obtained at Monticello on some of the President's family. Part II deals systematically with the whole subject of "kine-pox" and vaccination.

6. JENNER, Edward. The origin of the vaccine inoculation. London: Printed by D. N. Shury, 1801.

In this brief communication Jenner tells how he became interested in the subject twenty-five years previously. He outlines his work and the arguments in its favor. "A hundred thousand persons, upon the smallest computation have been inoculated in these realms. The number who have partaken of its benefits throughout Europe and other parts of the globe are incalculable; and it now becomes too manifest to admit of controversy, that the annihilation of the Small Pox, the most dreadful scourge of the human species, must be the final result of this practice."

7. BROWN, Thomas. An inquiry into the antivariolous power of vaccination; in which, from the state of the phenomena, and the occurrence of a great variety of cases, the most serious doubts are suggested of the efficacy of the whole practice, and its powers at best proved to be only temporary. From which also will appear, the necessity of, and proper period for again submitting to, inoculation with variolous virus. Edinburgh: Archibald Constable & Co., 1809.

For years after the publication of the "Inquiry" (Ref. 1) the medical, and indeed the civilian, world was in a ferment of argument about the safety and value of Jennerian vaccination. There were the camps of the vaccinationists and the antivaccinationists. Innumerable books and pamphlets appeared attacking or in defense of the practice. Some of the antivaccinationist literature was bitter, unreasonable, and scurrilous and was motivated by envy or hate. But there were other writers who, in cool appraisal of the whole situation, noted weak spots in Jenner's arguments and in the results of practice, even though the pendulum swung wildly in favor of vaccination and the procedure was officially approved by the Royal College.

Brown gives a temperate analysis of the vaccination problem and astutely notes the obvious flaws in Jenner's argument. "The vaccine practice was introduced and recommended to the public by its author, as a perfect antidote and security, against the smallpox, without any exception or reserve; and if properly patronized, capable of banishing variola from the catalogue of human misery." . . . All who have wrote upon the subject have acquiesced with the grand results of its author, and have practised, and patronized it with a zeal hitherto unexampled" (p. 2). He then complains that anyone who has in any sense criticized vaccination is regarded as a backward-looker and obstructionist. "It has been also asserted, that it had to encounter the opposition of designing, and ignorant men. It must be confessed that, at the commencement of the practice, an opposition arose from a few individuals of the profession; but so far from thinking it was inimical to the new practice, I am convinced that it contributed not a little to increase its reputation and to extend its influence" (p. 4). He continues with a critical analysis of the experiences of Jenner and others.

The most important part of the book is, however, a series of case reports of people who had undergone vaccination meeting all the criteria of a successful procedure, who later had smallpox. He maintains the thesis, which, of course, is correct, that vaccination does not confer permanent protection but that revaccination is always necessary after an appropriate period. "To these material considerations we add, that the Royal College of Physicians, and the Royal Jennerian Society, in London, admit, that cases of small-pox have occurred, where sufficient proof has existed of the most perfect vaccination" (p. 276). "To these statements of such respectable public bodies we have to add those cases given" by various others; "such an accumulation of proof is afforded, as not only to abolish all parallel betwixt the two diseases in this respect, but to point out, in the most striking manner, the *temporary* and *feeble* protection afforded by vaccination, against variolous contagion" (p. 277). Interestingly enough, Brown does not advise revaccination at appropriate intervals but urges the abandonment of vaccination altogether and a return to variolation. Brown was correct in his claim that vaccination did not confer permanent protection, but his conclusion was wrong, and fortunately the pendulum continued to swing strongly to vaccination all over the world. It is easy to see, however, how difficult it must have been for honest critical observers to evaluate the whole situation at the time.

Brown's book is of the greatest interest and must be read to grasp its full implications.

8. MOORE, James. The history and practice of vaccination. London: Printed for J. Callow, 1817.

Moore, who was director of the National Vaccine Establishment, devotes the first few chapters of his book to telling the story of Jenner's work and of the early supporters and detractors of vaccination. "The discovery of a mode of preventing the Small Pox is one of those splendid events which reflect lustre on the English nation: and it must be interesting to learn, whether this was stumbled upon by chance, or unfolded by ingenuity" (p. 1), a question perhaps not entirely settled today. Chapter vi is devoted to "The reception of the vaccine with the public in England." Moore points out that in one year vaccination was diffused throughout Europe and, in less than three, reached India and China. "It is remarkable that the opposition to Vaccination was much more violent in England, where it was discovered than in other countries" (p. 115). He even suggests that some doctors may have been hostile to the elimination of a disease which contributed heavily to their practice. However, "Vaccination in the year 1799 acquired the powerful support of the Commander in Chief," the Duke of York, who, "as soon as the Army Medical Board and other competent judges, had given full assurances and complete proofs that this was the case, a general order was issued . . . to vaccinate every soldier who had not had the Small Pox. By this measure the malady was at once extinguished in the army, and many a gallant soldier preserved." . . . After a short time the Lords of the Admiralty imitated this excellent example" (p. 119). "The difficulty in finding a ready supply of lymph was, for a long time, a considerable obstacle to the diffusion of the vaccine" (p. 120). Apparently the lymph was gained mainly from vaccinated patients and was passed around informally by anyone who had a supply. Meanwhile, feelings about vaccination became emotional, if not hysterical; in July, 1800, a declaration was framed in favor of vaccination, signed by laymen and physicians, and to be followed by other such documents. "Some country ladies even ventured to make use of the lancet: and resolutely vaccinated every child, whose parents they could prevail on, by insinuation or entreaties, to confide in their skill" (p. 123).

On March 17, 1802, Jenner presented a petition to the House of Commons for reimbursement of financial outlay and loss in connection with vaccination. "The business was then referred to Committee, of which Admiral Berkeley was appointed chairman." The committee held hearings and gathered elaborate testimony from many physicians and then drew up a report "expressed in as favourable terms towards Dr. Jenner, as the caution and formality of parliamentary language would admit" (p. 159). The interesting debates upon the measure are quoted in detail by Moore. "The House then divided upon the original motion for granting £10,000 which was carried by a small majority of three" (p. 174).

The action of Parliament "enabled the Vaccine to assume a more lofty demeanor"—in other words, it gave both the vaccine and Jenner a "boost." In 1806 Lord Henry Petty again brought the matter before the House of Commons. He quoted favorable statistics on the decline of smallpox (in Vienna, for example, before vaccination about 835 died each year of smallpox, whereas in 1804 there were only 2 deaths from this cause), and he moved that the king direct the Royal College of Physicians to inquire into the state of vaccine inoculation in the United Kingdom. The college made an elaborate investigation and reported favorably. Among 164,381 persons vaccinated, there were only 66 in whom eruptions of the skin followed. Other important colleges made similar reports. The question of a further reward for Dr. Jenner was again taken up by the House and after a lively debate on July 29, 1807, the House divided "upon the question, that twenty thousand pounds should be granted to Dr. Jenner: sixty votes were in favour of this sum and forty-seven against it" (p. 209).

In chapter x Moore discussed vaccine institutions. It had early been perceived that "the extension of the new practice was much retarded by the want of a constant and convenient supply of Vaccine lymph." Jenner resolved to establish a Vaccine Society and "to place the medical department under the direction of the most eminent professional gentlemen in London" (p. 210). "Accordingly in 1803 proposals to that effect were printed and circulated. The plan met with the most distinguished approbation, for the King, Queen and every British Prince and Princess accepted the title of Patrons and Patronesses; and multitudes of the nobility and gentry became members of an Institution which by unanimous consent was denominated the Royal Jennerian Society" (p. 211). But the society had its difficulties with the distribution of lymph and with vaccinating, and in 1808 Parliament created the National Vaccine Establishment. Seven stations were set up in London for vaccinating all who should apply and for collecting and distributing vaccine lymph to those who wished it. "In 1816, 7771 persons were vaccinated by this Establishment alone, and 44,376 charges of lymph were distributed to the public" (p. 223).

The remainder of the book tells how vaccination was introduced within a few years all over Europe and, indeed, all over the world. Lymph was shipped, apparently dried, and was successfully used even as far away as Turkey and the West Indies.

The final chapter is on the "Practice of vaccination." "The instructions of the National Vaccine Establishment of London were founded upon the experience of many [pp. 274 ff.], and improved by successive observations. . . . The first consideration is the time to be chosen for vaccination. The exquisite irritability of a new-born infant, and the uncertainty of its organization being perfect, are sufficient motives for usually deferring the operation until three weeks after birth. . . . But when the Small Pox infection is at hand, this superlative danger overwhelms all other considerations, and every human being susceptible of the poison, without exception should instantly be vaccinated. . . . Lymph for vaccination should only be taken from a vesicle perfectly regular . . . while the vesicle is uninjured and proceeds in its due course, the lymph certainly preserves its specific quality; but should it be irritated and any undue inflammation excited, rendering the secretion purulent, this is to be considered as vitiated and unfit for use. . . . If surgeons could find a constant succession of subjects, pure lymph in its early and most active state should always be employed; and Vaccination performed by transferring the transparent lymph, directly from arm to arm . . . a little is to be taken up on the point of a lancet, and introduced slantingly into the skin of the arm under the cuticle until it touches the cutis. . . . When pointed quills or bits of ivory are well and repeatedly moistened with lymph, they preserve the virtues of the Vaccine for a long time."[1]

"There are several other methods in use for preserving vaccine lymph. A drop is sometimes inclosed between two bits of square glass; or it may be deposited in a small cavity hollowed out of the centre of a piece of ground glass, and covered accurately with a flat piece of the same size. Lymph desiccated on glass is brought to a proper state for use, by mixing it up with a particle of cold water by the point of a lancet." A most important observation was also made by James Bryce, F.R.S. (*Practical Observations on the Inoculation of Cow Pox* [Edinburgh, 1802]), which anticipated Von Pirquet (Ref. 14) by one hundred years. "This gentleman, indeed, tried the effect of revaccination during every period of the progress of a vaccine vesicle. He noticed that when the first operation succeeded, the inflammation excited by the second was accelerated, and as soon as the primary vesicle acquired the areola, the second, however small it might be, also acquired a proportional areola and both dessicated together" (p. 287).

Many more details are given; indeed, we have only touched a few high spots of this invaluable contemporary account of the state of vaccination.

Debate about the merits and safety of vaccination has continued, however, and much has been written even in modern times in defense of the procedure. Ernest Hart, for example, who was chairman of the National Health Society (England), felt it necessary to write a pamphlet, *The Truth about Vaccination: An Examination and Refutation of the Assertions of the Anti-Vaccinators* (London: Smith Elder & Co., 1880), and similar material continues to be published today.

9. CEELY, Robert. Observations on the variolae vacciniae, Tr. Provincial M. & Surg. A., **8**:287, 1840.

Ceely asks a question which had been much in the air practically ever since vaccination was extensively practiced: "Is vaccine lymph, in passing through many individuals with all due care and selection, susceptible, in process of time, of actual degeneration or essential diminution of intensity?" The writer, of course, refers to the usual practice of vaccination by means of lymph derived from people previously vaccinated. Ceely reviews the question, quoting authorities, who judged the question in various ways. The National Vaccine Establishment in a report ordered by the House of Commons to be printed, April 11, 1838 ("Vaccine Institution. Copy of the last report from the National Vaccine Establishment to Her Majesty's Principal Secretary of State for the Home Department," London M. Gaz., **22**:349, 1838), declared: "No, it has not worn out its protecting property." M. J.-B. Bousquet (*Traité de la vaccine* [Paris: J.-B. Baillière, 1833], p. 217) also felt that there had been no diminution of intensity in comparing an old lymph transferred since 1800 with new vaccines.

---

[1] As late as 1900 the writer recalls being vaccinated by means of an ivory "point" with vaccine dried on it, which Dr. B—— produced from his waistcoat pocket.

George Gregory ("Report laid before the General Court of Governors of the Small Pox and Vaccination Hospital, 1st of February 1838," London M. Gaz., 21:860, 1838), on the other hand, stated: "The lymph in use at this hospital had been preserved in uninterrupted descent, for a very long period of time; but for three or four years past, I had noticed that its intensity was diminished. . . ." Many authorities could be collected on both sides, but at any rate it was doubt about much of the current vaccine which led to efforts to restore its potency by again passing it back to the cow. Ceely himself attempted to do so without good success, but retrovaccination, so called, soon became popular and successful. The subject is reviewed in Dr. Edward Ballard's excellent book, *Vaccination* (London: Longmans, Green & Co., 1868). According to Ballard, Negri in Italy had for a long time been successful in transferring the vaccine from calf to calf and using calf lymph for human vaccination. In 1865–66 there were great discussions in France as to the procedure, but M. Depaul ("Discussion sur la vaccination animale," Bull. Acad. de méd., Paris, 32:1024, 1867) seems to have been most instrumental in introducing vaccination from calf lymph. Ballard describes the method of vaccinating the calves as he saw it in Paris. "The operator then proceeds to shave, with a dry razor, the right side of the abdomen, commencing from the udder, and extending over a space of about ten inches long by six or eight broad. The calf which is the vaccinifer, from which the virus is to be taken, is also securely fastened down . . . and the vaccine matter is obtained from the pock by forcible compression of its base with a pair of spring forceps. . . . The animal on the table is vaccinated upon the shaven surface by puncture in sixty or seventy places. . . . Pocks which finally attain the size of large human vaccine pocks, speedily begin to rise, and are used for the vaccination of children from the fourth to the sixth day" (p. 254).

Calf virus seems to have been imported to the United States by Dr. Henry A. Martin in 1870 ("Animal vaccination," Boston M. & S.J., 83:254, 1870). Martin sent an agent to Paris who received from Dr. Depaul virus from calves through which the virus had been transmitted since originally started from a cowpox strain discovered at Beaugency[2] by Depaul in 1866. The virus arrived in this country safely and was successfully propagated and used for vaccination by Dr. Martin. "In a few days I shall have such arrangements completed as will enable me to invite all who may feel an interest in animal vaccination to see the disease in the heifer, to bring patients to be vaccinated therefrom, and to obtain, if it is desired, their supplies directly from the source." The whole subject was thoroughly discussed a few years later by Martin in a long article, "Report on animal vaccination," Tr. Am. M.A., 28:187, 1877.

Several points remain to be made clear. As to definitions, in the contemporary literature "retrovaccination" refers to virus from a vaccinated human being which is reimplanted in the heifer; animal vaccine, on the other hand, "is the product of natural horse-pox or cow pox which has been cultivated on heifers and has never quitted that soil." It is stated by nearly every contemporary writer, although we have been entirely unable to find the original reports, that

[2] The story of the discovery of this famous case of cowpox is told by M. Depaul ("Cowpox spontané," Bull. Acad. de méd., 31:590, 1866): "It was on a heifer thirty months old, belonging to M. Drouin-Mercier, farmer at Beaugency, that the cow pox arose spontaneously." It was from her that the virus was passed from calf to calf for years to produce Depaul's stock of vaccine.

animal vaccination was extensively practiced in Italy from 1810 on by Galliati and later by his pupil Negri. It is stated that in 1865 Dr. Larroux of Paris made a trip to Naples to view Negri's work and brought home with him a heifer which had been vaccinated, from which vaccinia was passed to other heifers from which physicians were supplied with lymph (Ballard, *op. cit.*, p. 247; E. Warlemont, *A Manual of Animal Vaccination* [Philadelphia: John Wyeth & Bros., 1886], p. 77; Martin, "Report on animal vaccination," p. 200).

The fact that a decline in the immunizing power of vaccine results from lengthy passage through the same vaccinifer has been confirmed in modern times, as, for example, by Blaxall (Ref. 16) and by J. Cunningham ("A note on the degeneration of vaccine lymph on passage through the same vaccinifer," Indian J.M. Research, **15**:373, 1927).

10. RAYNAUD, Maurice. Étude expérimentale sur le rôle du sang dans la transmission de l'immunité vaccinale, Compt. rend. Acad. d. sc., **84**:453, 1877.

Raynaud performed an interesting and early experiment on the immunity of vaccination. A calf which had been vaccinated 6 days previously and was "in full vaccinial eruption" was bled for 200 cc. The blood was immediately transfused into the jugular vein of a three-month-old calf. There was no reaction. After 15 days, sixty inoculations of fresh vaccine were made into the mammary region; all failed to take and did not yield a single pustule. Another calf vaccinated at the same time with the same vaccine broke out 4 days later with a "magnificent vaccinial eruption." Raynaud concluded that under the conditions of his experiment the blood contained a "principle capable of transmitting immunity."

Another early immunological experiment was that of George M. Sternberg ("Practical results of bacteriological researches," Tr. A. Am. Physicians, **7**:68, 1892). He found that vaccine virus mixed with serum from a vaccinated (immune) calf failed to produce a pustule when used to vaccinate a second calf, whereas virus mixed with serum from an untreated calf produced a good "take."

11. KLEBS, E. Der Micrococcus der Variola und Vaccinie, Arch. f. exper. Path. u. Pharmakol., **10**:222, 1879.

It was inevitable that during the early days of the bacteriological era ordinary bacteria should be blamed as the cause of smallpox. Klebs, the great bacteriologist, fell into this error and thought that he found a coccus regularly in smallpox and vaccine lymph. "The essential result of our investigations may be summarized by saying that the organisms of Vaccinia and Variola occur exclusively in the form of micrococci, that they assume no other form in any stage of development than that of tiny spherules."

12. EDWARDES, Edward J. A concise history of smallpox and vaccination in Europe. London: H. K. Lewis, 1902.

There are innumerable statistics on vaccination and smallpox. This little book contains an excellent and comprehensive summary, largely in tabular form, of the dates when vaccination was introduced into various countries, when it was made obligatory, and the number of cases of smallpox in relation to the vaccinated. Rules in force in Britain have been described by Blaxall (Ref. 16) and in the United States by William Fowler ("Principal provisions of smallpox vaccination laws and regulations in the United States," Pub. Health Rep., **56**:1, 1941).

In this connection it is of interest to read the *Memorial of Board of Commissioners of Health of the City of New York on the Subject of Compulsory Vaccination with a View To Exterminate the Small-Pox* (New York: Wm. H. Trafton & Co., 1862), drawn up by Dr. Lewis A. Sayre, resident physician, strongly favoring compulsory vaccination.

13. TYZZER, E. E. The etiology and pathology of vaccinia, J.M. Research, **11**:180, 1904.

Tyzzer made elaborate anatomical studies of vaccinia lesions, including those of the corneas of rabbits and of calves which had been inoculated with vaccine virus. There are beautiful plates of the lesions. Tyzzer, however, like Councilman (Ref. S5), went wrong in concluding that the inclusion bodies were a highly organized parasite.

14. PIRQUET, C. von. Die frühzeitige Reaction bei der Schutzpockenimpfung, Wien. klin. Wchnschr., **19**:855, 1906.

Although Bryce in 1802 (Ref. 8) had described accelerated vaccine reactions, little further interest was taken in the subject until Von Pirquet, the great Viennese pediatrician, conducted his systematic studies. Von Pirquet approached vaccination from the standpoint of allergy. He first carefully noted the time element in the various stages of a vaccination lesion and then studied, in comparison, early and late revaccinations. Theoretically, one would expect a second vaccination to proceed more slowly than the first in an immune or partially immune body. Actually, the reaction is accelerated. "Vaccination produces no absolute immunity, but it alters the reactivity of the body in such a way that it reacts earlier and brings the repeated infection to its conclusion in shorter time." Working along these lines, Von Pirquet made fundamental contributions to the theory of allergy and immunity. Later he ("Ist die vakzinale Frühreaction specifisch?" Wien. klin. Wchnschr., **19**:1407, 1906) answered Kraus's criticism that the accelerated reaction was not specific. He reported careful experiments, from which he concluded: "1. The vaccinal early reaction is a specific reaction between the cowpox lymph and the organism which has been rendered immune (or allergic) to it. . . . 2. The early reaction is quantitatively dependent on the amount of the virus which is introduced and is distinct from a first vaccination, in which the size of the reaction is independent of the amount of infectious material."

Von Pirquet amplified these fundamental studies in a book, *Klinische Studien über Vaccination und vaccinale Allergie* (Leipzig and Vienna: Franz Deuticke, 1907).

15. NOGUCHI, Hideyo. Pure cultivation in vivo of vaccine virus free from bacteria, J. Exper. Med., **22**:539, 1915.

Although it had been shown (for literature see Ref. S5) that the virus of smallpox may localize in various organs, less was known about the circumstances in connection with vaccine virus. Noguchi succeeded in adapting a strain of vaccine virus to testicular growth by passage through testes of rabbits and bulls.

"The multiplication of the virus within the testicle is maximum on the fourth or fifth day after inoculation; the quantity of virus remains about stationary until the eighth day when diminution begins. At the expiration of five weeks no more virus could be detected." This pure virus produces typical vaccine "takes" in human beings. Further characteristics of this virus are described in another paper by Noguchi ("Further studies on the properties of pure vaccine virus cultivated in vivo," J. Exper. Med., **27**:425, 1918). T. P. Hughes, R. F. Parker, and T. M. Rivers ("Immunological and chemical investigations of vaccine virus," J. Exper. Med., **62**:349, 1935) were able to obtain appreciable amounts of elementary bodies of vaccinia in a relatively pure state. This material contained components similar to those found in bacteria and other substances of protoplasmic origin.

A. Marie ("De l'inoculation intracérébrale de la vaccine," Compt. rend. Soc. de biol., **83**:476, 1920) produced an encephalitis by introcerebral inoculation of rabbits with vaccine virus. He was able to transmit the disease in series, although C. Levaditi, P. Harvieu, and S. Nicolau ("Affinités neurotropes du virus de la vaccine," Compt. rend. Soc. de biol., **85**:345, 1921) had less complete success.

At any rate, the principle is brought out that vaccine virus may become adapted so that it has a special affinity for various tissues (for further discussion see Van Rooyen and Rhodes, *loc. cit.*).

16. BLAXALL, F. R. Some notes in connexion with the preparation of vaccine lymph at the Government Lymph Establishment, Proc. Roy. Soc. Med., **15**:1, 1921. (Sec. of Epidemiology and State Medicine.)

Numerous accounts have been given through the years of the technique of preparing vaccine lymph. An authoritative and detailed description is given by Blaxall, including the details of selection of animals, housing, inoculation, collection of virus, etc. Blaxall points out that vaccine may be derived from smallpox direct, from cowpox, or from retrovaccination with lymph from the human arm. He recommends passage of lymph through rabbits from time to time in order to "renew the stock," i.e., to preserve potency. The subject was dealt with at length by a committee of the League of Nations in 1928 (*Report of Commission on Smallpox and Vaccination* [C.H. 739] [Geneva]). A good summary of the practical aspects of vaccination is given in Van Rooyen and Rhodes (*op. cit.*, pp. 874 ff.).

17. MacCALLUM, W. G., and OPPENHEIMER, Ella Hutzler. Differential centrifugalization: a method for the study of filtrable viruses as applied to vaccinia, J.A.M.A., **78**:410, 1922.

Although granules (Paschen bodies, Ref. S7) had been seen for years in vaccine lymph, MacCallum and Oppenheimer opened a new era with their attempts to concentrate the effective virus. By differential centrifugation of commercial vaccine virus in fluids of varying specific gravity, they found that it "floated" in a fluid of specific gravity 1.14, while it "sank" in a fluid of 1.11. "Its own specific gravity is probably about 1.12 or 1.13." Virus was tested for by inoculating samples of the centrifugates from various levels on the cornea of the rabbit. "Examination of a drop of the virulent top layer under the microscope with dark field illumination disclosed myriads of minute granules very much smaller than streptococci or staphylococci." There seems little doubt that these were the elementary bodies. MacCallum promised further work on the subject, but none appeared.

J. C. G. Ledingham ("The aetiological importance of the elementary bodies in vaccinia and fowl-pox," Lancet, **2**:525, 1931) concentrated elementary bodies by a somewhat similar procedure but went a step further in showing that they were specifically agglutinated by immune sera. Further development of the subject is well documented in the review by J. E. Smadel and C. L. Hoagland (Ref. 24).

18. TURNBULL, Hubert M., and McINTOSH, James. Encephalo-myelitis following vaccination, Brit. J. Exper. Path., **7**:181, 1926.

J. Comby in a general article ("L'Encéphalite aigue chez les enfants," Arch. de méd. d. enf., **10**:577, 1907) makes the statement that encephalitis may follow vaccination but reports no specific case. Turnbull and McIntosh were the first to write systematically on the subject. They give careful autopsy reports of seven cases, and they conclude that the histological changes were allied to those of poliomyelitis and encephalitis lethargica but showed characteristic differences. The virus demonstrated experimentally in brain or cord was a vaccinial virus. They also summarize the literature on the specific encephalomyelitis of variola. The subject of vaccinal encephalitis is dealt with in detail in the *Report of the Committee on Vaccination, Ministry of Health* (London: His Majesty's Stationery Office, 1928) and in a *Further Report* (1930) and by Van Rooyen and Rhodes (*op. cit.,* pp. 393 ff.). The latter conclude: "It must be realized that postvaccinal encephalitis is only one of a number of diseases which all present a comparable histological appearance, demyelinization being the main feature." They did not believe that the mechanism was fully understood.

19. GINS, H. A. Impfschäden, Zentralbl. f. d. ges. Kinderh., **24**:145, 1930.

The question of untoward reactions in connection with vaccination is of interest and importance. The idea, prevalent in the early days of vaccination, that the introduction of animal substance into the human might have a "brutalizing effect" is only of historical interest, and the outbreaks of syphilis which were described in connection with vaccination do not, of course, occur with calf lymph.

Generalized vaccinia is an eruption of pustules, blood-borne, which occurs several days after vaccination; it is not due to local transfer of virus from the point of inoculation. It is a serious complication but fortunately very rare, so that from 1920 to 1928 Gins was able to collect only thirteen cases. However, four were fatal. As recently as 1882, however, W. A. Hardaway in his book *Essentials of Vaccination* (Chicago: Jansen, McClurg & Co., 1882) questions the occurrence of general vaccinia (p. 56). J. Henry Dible and Humphrey H. Gleave ("Histological and experimental observations upon generalized vaccinia in man," J. Path. & Bact., **38**:29, 1934) estimate that this complication occurs about once in a million vaccinations. They report a fatal case.

Gins systematically describes the various complications of vaccination.

20. LEDINGHAM, J. C. G. The aetiological importance of the elementary bodies in vaccinia and fowl-pox, Lancet, **2**:525, 1931.

Ledingham brought forward strong evidence that the Paschen bodies represent the actual virus of vaccinia. He found that suspensions of the elementary bodies were specifically agglutinated by convalescent or hyperimmune rabbit sera. Normal sera had no effect.

21. GOODPASTURE, E. W., WOODRUFF, Alice M., and BUDDINGH, G. S. Vaccinal infection of the chorio-allantoic membrane of the chick embryo, Am. J. Path., **8**:271, 1932.

Goodpasture and his associates were the first to grow vaccine virus in the chick embryo. Growth with glycerinated (commercial) material was uncertain, and better results were obtained if virus from fresh infected rabbit's testis was used. The technique of inoculating the eggs is described, as well as the appearance of the lesions. "Guarnieri bodies have been demonstrated for the first time in mesodermal cells (endothelium and fibroblasts). Evidence has been presented that the Guarnieri bodies are composed in part of Paschen corpuscles."

22. PARKER, R. F., and RIVERS, T. M. Immunological and chemical investigations of vaccine virus. IV. Statistical studies of elementary bodies in relation to infection and agglutination, J. Exper. Med., **64**:438, 1936.

Although it was generally believed that the relation of the elementary bodies (Ref. S7) to infection was a close one, these bodies had not been proved to be the actual infectious units; Parker and Rivers developed a method for counting the number of elementary bodies in suspensions which were used to infect rabbits and believed that they showed a direct correlation between the number of elementary bodies and the number of infectious units of virus present in a given suspension. Parker ("Statistical studies of the nature of the infectious unit of vaccine virus," J. Exper. Med., **67**:725, 1938) continued these studies and concluded that the unit of vaccinial virus was particulate and that with certain strains, when properly introduced into the skin of the rabbit, a single particle was capable of infecting. Further work is summarized in Smadel and Hoagland's review (Ref. 25).

23. BLAND, T. O. W., and ROBINOW, C. F. The inclusion bodies of vaccinia and their relationship to the elementary bodies studied in cultures of the rabbit's cornea, J. Path. & Bact., **48**:381, 1938.

Bland and Robinow's work was directed at the problem of the exact nature of Guarnieri's (Ref. S3) inclusion bodies. These authors were able to study the development of vaccine virus grown in epithelial cells of the rabbit's cornea in vitro and found that there was a regular sequence of events. "We conclude that the inclusion bodies are an obligatory stage in the multiplication of the virus and are colonies of the elementary bodies enveloped in a matrix."

24. TWISTON-DAVIES, J. H., JAMES, L. R., and DOWNIE, A. W. Cowpox infections in farm workers, Lancet, **2**:1534, 1938.

Cowpox has been a somewhat apocryphal disorder, and its real relation to human infection and to smallpox has been debated. In this study with modern methods the writers describe an outbreak of "spontaneous" cowpox in cows and three human cases clearly contracted from the infected cows. Interesting immunological observations are reported, and the modern literature is reviewed.

"The evidence indicates that infection was contracted from lesions on the teats of cattle during the process of milking," just as Jenner had claimed (Ref. 1). Some of the patients showed a good antibody response, more active against cowpox virus obtained from one of the cases than against a stock strain of virus.

To show, however, how complicated the whole situation is, A. W. Downie and D. W. Haddock ("A variant of cowpox virus," Lancet, **1**:1049, 1952) were able to isolate on the chorio-allantois of chick embryos a white variant of a cowpox strain which did not produce hemolysis either in the chick embryo or when inoculated into the skin of rabbits. The variant bred true.

25. SMADEL, J. E., and HOAGLAND, C. L. Elementary bodies of vaccinia, Bact. Rev., **6**:79, 1942.

An authoritative review, by experts in the field, of modern work on the elementary bodies. Their identification, physical properties, morphology, chemical nature, antigen, etc., are all discussed.

26. NAGLER, F. P. O., and RAKE, Geoffrey. The use of the electron microscope in diagnosis of variola, vaccinia, and varicella, J. Bact., **55**:45, 1948.

The writers present electron micrographs of the viruses of variola, generalized vaccinia, and varicella. "Virus particles of variola and vaccinia . . . resemble each other very closely in their morphological structure. They are undistinguishable from elementary bodies of these viruses derived from the chorio-allantois of the chick embryo." The average size of the elementary bodies of variola or vaccinia was 238 mμ, whereas the bodies of varicella were somewhat smaller (210 mμ). All are roughly square or brick-shaped. William H. Gaylord and Joseph L. Melnick ("Intracellular forms of pox viruses as shown by the electron microscope [vaccinia, ectromelia, molluscum contagiosum]," J. Exper. Med., **98**:157, 1953) studied with the electron microscope the intracellular development of vaccinia virus, and they believe that a process of maturation proceeds through definite stages. They think that inclusion bodies are made up of particles in the developmental stage imbedded in a matrix (see Ref. 22).

For further details on electron microscopy and size measurement of vaccinia virus see Smadel in Rivers, *op. cit.,* pages 429 ff.

Clinical	Refs. 1, 2, 5
Control	Ref. 26
Epidemiology	Refs. 1, 2
Experimental	Refs. 6, 7, 8
General	Refs. 1, 2
Immunity	Refs. 8, 12, 20
Negri bodies	Ref. 14
Prophylaxis, non-specific	Refs. 3, 4
Prophylaxis, specific	Refs. 9, 10, 11, 17, 25
Rabies and the central nervous system	Refs. 7, 8, 13, 15, 18, 19
Transmission by saliva	Refs. 1, 16
Virus, cultivation in chick embryo	Ref. 24
Virus, size	Ref. 23
Virus, tissue culture	Ref. 22
Virus carriers	Ref. 21

THERE are innumerable monographs and books dealing with rabies; unfortunately, most of these are inaccessible. However, among the earlier ones we may mention those of Zinke (Ref. 1) and of Krügelstein (Ref. 2) and somewhat later that of George Fleming (*Rabies and Hydrophobia* [London: Chapman & Hall, 1872]). Standard older general articles are those of Bollinger ("Die Wuthkrankheit" in H. von Ziemssen, *Handbuch der speciellen Pathologie und Therapie* (Leipzig: F. C. W. Vogel, 1874), **3**:503; and of A. Högyes, *Lyssa* (Vienna: Alfred Hölder, 1897), in both of which there are extensive bibliographies. These articles have sections on the history of the disease, and a comprehensive and readable discussion of this phase of the subject is also to be found in Fleming's book (*op. cit.*, pp. 7–68). Krügelstein's monograph (Ref. 2) contains a most interesting and comprehensive bibliography of the literature before the nineteenth century. There is an excellent modern discussion of rabies with a good bibliography by Harold N. Johnson in T. M. Rivers, *Viral and Rickettsial Infections of Man* (2d ed.; Philadelphia: J. B. Lippincott Co., 1952), page 267; and a thorough discussion of the virology of rabies is to be found in C. E. Van Rooyen and A. J. Rhodes, *Virus Diseases of Man* (New York: Thomas Nelson & Sons, 1948), pages 792 ff. A good introduction to the whole subject is the little book by L. T. Webster, *Rabies* (New York: Macmillan Co., 1942).

Finally, one should mention the authoritative reviews of P. Lépine ("Rage—virus rabique," in C. Levaditi and P. Lépine, *Les Ultravirus des maladies humaines* [Paris: Librairie Maloine, 1938], p. 395), by J. Koch ("Lyssa," in W. Kolle and A. von Wassermann, *Handbuch der pathogenen Mikroorganismen* [3d ed.; Jena: Gustav Fischer, 1930], **8**, Part I, 547), and by R. Kraus and F. Schweinburg ("Ueber die experimentellen Grundlagen der Schutzimpfung gegen Hundswuth, Methoden der Schutzimpfung und ihre Resultäte," in Kolle and Wassermann, *op. cit.*, p. 695). The article by Koch has a very extensive bibliography.

1. ZINKE, Georg Gottfried. Neue Ansichten der Hundswuth, ihrer Ursachen und Folgen, nebst einer sichern Behandlungsart der von toller Thieren gebissenen Menschen. Jena: Christian Ernst Gabler, 1804.

Zinke is universally given credit for first transmitting rabies by means of saliva. His experiments are crude, however, and not entirely convincing. Experiment No. 1 is perhaps the best: "I took saliva from a mad dog . . . as soon as he had been killed, by means of a little paint brush. On the same day I made incisions in the forelegs of a one-year-old dachshund . . . and then painted over the wounds as much saliva as the paint brush would hold. . . . The dog remained lively and ate and drank until the seventh day; on the eighth he ignored his food, did not drink, was sad and crawled into the corner of his cage, and by the tenth day had overt rabies. He was therefore killed and buried in the ground."

Zinke's little book contains much more, however, than these experiments. Beginning with an introduction about dogs in general, he goes on with a detailed description of canine rabies. The second section is on rabies and hydrophobia (*Wasserscheu*) in man. After a thorough discussion of contagion, he concludes that the disease is transmitted by the bite of a mad dog but denies that the saliva of a non-rabid animal can contain the rabies-producing substance or that its bite can cause rabies. He has no idea, however, of a *contagium vivum*. There follows a description of the disease in man and a speculative discussion of the mechanism of hydrophobia. Among various theories is mentioned that which claims an unnatural (*widernatürliche*) increase of nerve action and sensitiveness, especially of the organs of deglutition (p. 124). He himself regarded hydrophobia as a psychotic phenomenon—a peculiar kind of mania (p. 125). As prophylaxis, he advised excision of the wound, cauterization with a red-hot iron, or burning out the wound with gunpowder (p. 143). He described the special methods of various authorities for treating the wound as, for example, "Schmucker's method" or "Haygarth's method." Schumucker made incisions into the wound, rubbed in Spanish fly (Cantharides), and then applied a large plaster of Spanish fly. After 12 hours he opened the blisters so as to increase the suppuration, etc. (p. 146). Haygarth, on the other hand, advised irrigating the wound with warm water for several hours, whereas Desault and Sauvages suggested rubbing in quicksilver. In Persia, according to travelers, they made punctures around the wound into which onions were rubbed (p. 156). Recently galvanism came into fashion. As to internal remedies there are sections on June bugs, Spanish fly, volatile alkali, belladonna, baldrian, opium, taxus, quicksilver, and copper, with references to the advocates of each (p. 158).

The book concludes with an admonition that one take care not to be injured by the patient with rabies or to be sprinkled (*bezudelt*) with his saliva and that one be careful not to touch with bare hands objects which have been in his mouth. Everything in contact with the patient should be thrown into the fire or buried deep in the ground (p. 211).

Thus this little book is a curious mixture of ancient superstition and sound modern ideas.

Hugo Alt-Graf zu Salm-Reifferschied ("Beyträge zu einer Geschichte der Hundswuth," Allg. Anzeiger, 1:2, 1813), a little later, attempted to transmit rabies from a rabid dog which at autopsy showed an inflamed pharynx and lungs congested with blood. Other dogs ate food which had been smeared with saliva obtained during life from the rabid dog or were "vaccinated" ("einimpfung") with liquid or dry saliva; one animal, finally, ate flesh of the dead rabid dog which was cooked with its food. All developed rabies. On the average, the disease was manifest by the eighth to tenth day. One dog was "cured by cherry wine, water, belladonna, cherries and potassium sulfate [*blausäuren Kali*]." Rabid dogs ate well as long as the food was steaming hot; as it cooled, they ceased to eat. We are unable to interpret these observations with finality; the interesting point is that the experimenter was convinced that the saliva contained the causal agent and that the disease was communicable.

2. KRÜGELSTEIN, Franz Christian Karl. Die Geschichte der Hundswuth und der Wasserscheu und deren Behandlung. Gotha: In der Hennings'-schen Buchhandlung, 1826.

This book of 640 pages, on every phase of rabies, seems to have been a land-mark in its time. It opens with a bibliography of some three hundred titles going back to the classical writers and coming up to date. Since the same general plan is followed as in Zinke's book (Ref. 1), we shall not analyze it in detail. Krügelstein thought that there was a rabies-producing poison in the sputum, but he believed that it originated *de novo* under various conditions. Neither he nor Zinke had any idea of a living agent. On the other hand, he says (p. 332): "Rabies or hydrophobia is without doubt a disease of the nervous system. If any nerve ending is infected by the saliva poison, it sickens locally and sends the poison along until, by way of the sympathetic nerves, it reaches the coeliac plexus and thence affects the entire nervous system. From there it spreads by way of the spinal cord, and in the involvement of the centers of 'mood' [*Stimm-nerven*] the disease reaches its acme." Thus Krügelstein clearly insisted on transfer by way of the peripheral nerves to the central nervous system. He sought diligently for pathological changes in the central nervous system but with his primitive methods saw only congestion.

As to the treatment, the variety and type of procedures and medicines show a strong bond with medieval mysticism. They vary all the way from blood-letting to a drink of blood, galvanism, magnetism, and pressure on the carotids (p. 511). There is given a list of some sixty medicaments of every conceivable sort, with directions in "cookbook" style on how to use them.

3. EKSTROM. Rabies epidemic at Stockholm in 1824, London M. Gaz., 6:689, 1830.

Cauterization of rabid dog bites has played such a prominent part in the history of treatment that this note is of considerable interest. "The treatment adopted consisted in making deep incisions in the wound and surrounding parts, in different directions; these were then diligently washed for several minutes either with water or with diluted muriatic acid, or a solution of muriate of lime: the wound being thoroughly cleansed, was then dried, and any remaining blood removed, after which a hot iron or potassa fusa, or in a few instances strong muriatic acid, was applied, always taking care to touch every point of the bottom of the wound and incisions, so that a large eschar was formed." "Of the entire number" who "applied on being bitten only one afterwards suffered from the disease." Ekstrom thought that "the local primary treatment" was "calculated to eliminate or to destroy the poison as soon as possible." Confidence in the method was shaken by the alleged cure of a patient with overt hydrophobia by excision and cauterization of the scar of the bite. Follen Cabot ("Rabies and its preventive treatment: an analysis of cases," M. News, 74:321, 1899) appears to have introduced cauterization (under an anesthetic) of the bite with nitric acid, following some favorable experiments on guinea pigs. Although cauterization with nitric acid was still used, Webster (*op. cit.*, p. 88) concluded: "What nitric acid does to rabies virus when applied to a wound inflicted by a rabid dog is not certainly known." H. J. Shaughnessy and J. Zichis ("Prevention of experimental rabies," J.A.M.A., 123:528, 1943) later explored the subject thoroughly and concluded: "In experiments in which treatment of wounds contaminated with rabies virus was initiated within thirty minutes, only 11 per cent of those treated with fuming nitric acid and only 6 per cent of those treated with soap solution [20 per cent solution of soft soap] became infected, compared with about 63 per cent of untreated controls." The application of treatment after 6 hours was definitely less effective than when it was given within 30 minutes.

4. BOUCHARDAT, [A.]. Rapport général fait à la demande: 1. de M. le ministre de l'intérieur, de l'agriculture et du commerce; 2. de M. le ministre de l'instruction publique et des cultes; 3. de M. le ministre d'état, par la commission permanent des remèdes secrets et nouveaux, sur divers remèdes proposés pour prévenir ou pour combattre la rage, Bull. Acad. de méd., **18**:6, 1852; **20**:714, 1854.

Rabies was a very live subject in France during the middle of the nineteenth century. Innumerable reports and discussions are recorded in the transactions of the various academies. Bouchardat was commissioned to look into the questions of therapeutic claims, and this long paper listed innumerable prescriptions for preventing or curing rabies. Most of these are obviously fanciful, such as the famous "cabalistic omelette"—eggs with ammonia served on oyster shells. Bouchardat concluded: "You will pardon this long and sterile enumeration, but it is important to establish that in all of these claims there is nothing new and nothing useful. . . . We believe that we have shown that these formulas have lost their traditional prestige and that there remains nothing but ridiculous assertions without proof." Thus Bouchardat did a useful job and made a real advance over the days of Zinke (Ref. 1) and Krügelstein (Ref. 2).

5. TROUSSEAU, A. Clinique médicale de l'Hôtel-Dieu de Paris, Vol. **2**: De la rage, p. 342. 2d ed. Paris: J.-B. Baillière et fils, 1865.

The masterly clinical descriptions of Trousseau cannot be surpassed. The following is from his lecture on rabies (p. 357): "During the incubation period, there is no apparent departure from health, and, according to Van Swieten, those who will later become rabid may contract the most diverse maladies, such as smallpox, without the progress of the rabies being in any way modified. When the period of incubation has lasted 2 or 3 months, the man who has been bitten suddenly shows an unaccountable sadness. The patient, who usually does not suspect the nature of his trouble, seeks diversion away from home, but, wherever he may be, his sleep is unquiet, agitated, often he wakes with a start; restlessness is continuous, he draws long sighs, he flees the friends who try to distract or to console him, he takes pleasure in solitude, and begs that no noise be made near him; ministrations increase his restlessness and agitation.

"Aggravation of these symptoms marks the beginning of the second period of the malady, and at the same time other phenomena develop. The patient complains of precordial distress, respiration becomes sighing, the pulse irregular. These troubles with respiration and with circulation, as well as the melancholy and agitation, are the expression of an already considerable implication of the nervous system. This situation becomes worse when the patients are taken with chills or veritable convulsions of all the muscles of the body. Finally, there appears a symptom practically constant in established rabies in man, *the horror of water.*

"The sight of this liquid often suffices to bring on a general tremor; but it is, above all, when the patient wishes to bring water to his lips that this special horror comes on, those convulsions of the face and of the entire body which make such a vivid impression on those who witness an attack. The rabid man completely preserves his reason; he is thirsty; he wishes to drink, he bids his hand carry to his lips the vessel filled with liquid, but no sooner does it touch him than the unhappy creature withdraws terrified, sometimes he cries out that he cannot drink; his face shows agony, his eyes are fixed, his features contracted; then his limbs shake, and his body quivers. This crisis lasts several seconds, gradually calm seems to return, but the least contact, even a breath of air, suffices to start a new crisis, such is the hypersensitivity of the skin. He cannot wash hands or face or comb his hair without being menaced by convulsions. . . . Some with hydrophobia are taken with abrupt terrors, they turn suddenly, thinking they hear someone talking to them. They have indeed hallucinations of sight and hearing.

"In the third, that is to say the last, stage other symptoms are added to those already present in increasing severity; as the thirst becomes more acute and the impossibility of satisfying it more marked, one observes a hoarseness of the voice, first intermittent, later constant; this is probably the consequence of a spasm or of paralysis of some of the laryngeal muscles. In the last hours of life, the patient's mouth often fills with a white froth which is constantly ejected by coughing. Meanwhile . . . the convulsions become more and more frequent; they no longer require anything to precipitate them, but recur spontaneously several times an hour. The end of each convulsive bout is marked by a spasm of the respiratory muscles, with all the signs of an obstacle to breathing. This spasm is prolonged with a final access, and the rabid man dies of asphyxia, *mors convulsiva cum summa in respirando angustia.*"

Trousseau insisted that there was a specific virus in the saliva of the rabid animal which was the only means of transmitting the disease. With the methods available, he found no special anatomical lesions. As to treatment, he advised cauterization with a hot iron (*fer rougi*), raised the question of whether *curare* injected into the vein would help the spasm, and finally gives a formula which the Chinese regard as infallible:

> Musc. . . . . .16 grammes
> Cinabre natif }
> Cinabre factice } . . .aa 20—

6. GALTIER, V. Études sur la rage, Compt. rend. Acad. d. sc., **89**:444, 1879.

Galtier reports that rabies is transmissible to the rabbit, which acts as a harmless test object to tell whether saliva or other liquids come from a rabid animal. He states that rabies is transmissible from rabbit to rabbit but does not give the method of inoculation. The symptoms are paralysis and convulsions. The average incubation period is 18 days.

This appears to have been the first report on transmission to rabbits, unfortunately without much needed detail. The work of Pasteur (Ref. 7) was, on the other hand, definitive. A little later Maurice Raynaud ("Sur la transmissibilité de la rage de l'homme au lapin," Compt. rend. Acad. d. sc., **89**:714, 1879) reported an observation in which saliva from a rabies patient was injected subcutaneously into a rabbit's ear. Four days later the rabbit was seized with a sort of "accès de fureur" and died the following night. Fragments of submaxillary gland introduced into other rabbits subcutaneously are said to have reproduced rabies, as they died on the fifth and sixth days. Autopsy showed only congestion of the lungs.

These observations are not convincing. They are mentioned because often cited as definitive, for example, "Raymond [*sic*] transmitted human rabies to rabbits" (Webster, *op. cit.*, p. 46; Högyes, *op. cit.*, p. 35).

7. PASTEUR, L., avec la collaboration de MM. CHAMBERLAND, ROUX, et THUILLIER. Sur la rage, Compt. rend. Acad. d. sc., **92**:1259, 1881.

At about this time many attempts were being made in France to transmit rabies from man to animal and from animal to animal, and Pasteur's important studies began with this report. His original paper ("Sur une maladie nouvelle, provoquée par la salive d'un enfant mort de la rage," Compt. rend. Acad. d. sc., **92**:159, 1881), describing the injection into rabbits of saliva from a child dead of rabies, clearly dealt with the production of pneumococcus septicemia (see "Pneumococcal Pneumonia," Ref. 11) and not with rabies. So, too, the observations of Raynaud and Lannelongue ("Recherches expérimentales sur la transmission du virus rabique de l'homme au lapin," Bull. Acad. de méd., **10**:61, 1881) probably concerned "sputum septicemia" rather than rabies, since the rabbits all died within 48 hours and there is no description of lesions. Indeed, in the discussion of this paper Pasteur himself insisted that a bacterial infection had been produced. Galtier, on the other hand ("Observations à l'occasion du procès verbal," Bull. Acad. de méd., **10**:90, 1881), may have transmitted rabies from dog to rabbit, since the incubation period is reported as 12–18 days; he also claims to have transmitted the disease from rabbit to rabbit and from rabbit to sheep, but he was unable to produce rabies by injections of material from the central nervous system.

Pasteur, with his extraordinary acumen and experimental ability, resolved the question in this report. Both the symptoms and the histologic changes led Pasteur to the conclusion that "the central nervous system and especially the bulb which joins the spinal cord to the brain are particularly concerned and active in the development of the disease." He then reported success in producing rabies by injection of central nervous system material and spinal fluid. "The seat of rabies virus is not then solely in the saliva. The brain contains it in virulence at least equal to that which it possesses in saliva." Pasteur was bothered by the experimental difficulties of the very long incubation period. He soon found that, by injecting cerebral substance from rabid animals directly into the brains of dogs, the incubation period was shortened to 1 or 2 or, at the most, 3 weeks. This was a radical advance in experimental rabies studies.

8. PASTEUR, L., avec la collaboration de MM. CHAMBERLAND, ROUX, et THUILLIER. Nouveaux faits pour servir à la connaissance de la rage, Compt. rend. Acad. d. sc., **95**:1187, 1882.

Pasteur reported further on his fundamental studies. He pointed out that saliva was not a satisfactory source of virus for experimental work, since its effects were uncertain and the incubation period might be very long. He again referred to the certainty and rapidity with which rabies could be produced by direct intracerebral injections of central nervous system material from rabid animals. He pointed out that virus was found not only in the lower centers of the brain but in the spinal cord as well. He differentiated "dumb" rabies (*rage mue*), featured by paralysis, and "furious" rabies (*rage furieuse*).[1] He found that inoculation into the blood stream first affected the spinal cord and was likely to produce the "dumb" type rather than the "furious." He showed that an animal which recovered after early symptoms of rabies was immune to later inoculations and that some dogs seemed to have a natural resistance. Finally, he produced rabies by intracerebral injection of all parts of the brain of a cow dead of rabies.

> 9. PASTEUR, [L.], avec la collaboration de MM. CHAMBERLAND et ROUX. Nouvelle communication sur la rage, Compt. rend. Acad. d. sc., **98**:457, 1884.

Pasteur now made a more definitive report. Intravenous injection, as previously stated, usually produced a paralytic type of rabies, and dogs sacrified at the first symptom of paralysis showed spinal cords containing virus when there was no evidence as yet of any in the bulb. He also demonstrated virus in the pneumogastric and sciatic nerves and in the salivary glands. "The entire nervous system from center to periphery is then susceptible." Virus preserved its virulence in spinal cords kept at 0°–12° C. Pasteur was unable to cultivate any bacteria from the nervous system or the spinal fluid, but he stated that "one is tempted to believe that a microbe of infinite smallness, having the form neither of a bacillus nor of a micrococcus is the cause." He reported observations to show that the clinical type of rabies produced depended somewhat on the dose of infective material, and he believed that injections of very small amounts of virus did not produce immunity. He discussed the hypothesis of the passage of virus from the periphery to the central nervous system via the nerves, as against the distribution of virus by the blood stream, and, whether or not the former was correct, he regarded the latter as proved. Finally and most important, he discussed the theoretical basis of immunizing injections and made a general statement that he had already achieved some success. A little later, Pasteur (avec la collaboration de MM. Chamberland et Roux, "Sur la rage," *ibid.*, p. 1229) made another communication to the academy, dealing primarily with the problem of attenuation of virus. If one passed rabies virus from dog to monkey and then from monkey to monkey, the virulence of the virus fell off at each passage. If the virus was then returned to dog, rabbit, or guinea pig, it remained attenuated. It did not immediately resume the virulence of street virus (*la rage des rues*) in the dog. Even intracerebral inoculation might not produce the disease, although it established, nonetheless, "a state refractory to rabies." But if virus was passed from rabbit to rabbit, the virulence became exalted, so that, if passed back to the dog, it was much more virulent than street virus and, inoculated into the blood stream, it always caused fatal rabies. By using a series of injections of attenuated virus, he made dogs, as stated, immune or at least refractory. He alluded in a general way to some favorable observations on immunization of man, taking advantage of the

---

[1] Krügelstein (Ref. 2) gives the classifications of older writers: "The Englishman Mayerne describes seven forms of rabies"—the hod madness, the running madness, the fallen madness, the sleepy madness, etc.

long incubation period. He outlined plans for further experiments along these lines.

10. PASTEUR, L. Méthode pour prévenir la rage après morsure, Compt. rend. Acad. d. sc., **101**:765, 1885.

Although Pasteur had alluded to his method of prophylaxis of rabies in previous papers, he here first gave a detailed and comprehensive account. The first step was the intracerebral inoculation of street virus into a rabbit and the passage through successive rabbits. The incubation period gradually became shorter, until it reached a fixed time of seven days. The cords of rabbits of this sort contained virus throughout their extent, which gradually diminished in virulence as the cords were "suspended in dry air." The actual immunization was carried out by injecting into a dog subcutaneously a Pravaz syringe of broth to which was added a tiny bit of rabbit cord, beginning with one dried long enough to be entirely avirulent and successively using more virulent material until "finally one reaches a last very virulent cord." The dog was by this time refractory to rabies, as demonstrated in fifty animals. At about this time there arrived from Alsace a boy of nine years, Joseph Meister, who had been bitten fourteen times by a rabid dog. Drs. Vulpian and Grancher examined the boy and thought that he surely had received a fatal inoculation with rabies. "The death of this child seemed inevitable, and I decided, not without lively and cruel doubts, as one can believe, to try in Joseph Meister the method which had been constantly successful with dogs. . . . Consequently, on July 6 at 8 in the evening, 60 hours after the bites, in the presence of Drs. Vulpian and Grancher, we inoculated under a skin fold in the right hypochondrium of the little Meister a half-syringe of the cord of a rabid rabbit preserved in a flask of dry air for 15 days." Thirteen successive inoculations were made with cords of increasing virulence. The little boy never developed rabies during a period of 3 months and 3 weeks.

Pasteur, with the penetrating curiosity which was so characteristic of him, was not satisfied with practical results but wished to understand the mechanism of his method. He concluded that the dried cords contained fewer and fewer live virus particles, which were not, however, attenuated in individual virulence. Thus the method consisted in essence of injecting larger and larger quantities of virus each day.

An interesting discussion followed the paper. Vulpian said: "Rabies, that terrible malady against which all therapeutic attempts have so far failed, has finally found its remedy." Others expressed themselves with equal enthusiasm, and Pasteur closed the meeting with gracious acknowledgment of what had been said.

A little later Pasteur ("Résultats de l'application de la méthode pour prévenir la rage après morsure," Compt. rend. Acad. d. sc., **102**:459, 1886) reported results of the treatment in three hundred and fifty cases. Only one person developed rabies, a child bitten on the third of October and not brought for treatment until November 9. According to contemporary statistics, rabies should have developed in one-sixth of those bitten. In no case did the injections produce local inflammation, abscess, or other untoward effect. Pasteur concluded: "The prophylaxis of rabies after bite is established. It is time to create a center for vaccination against rabies." A commission was appointed by the academy to help implement Pasteur's proposal. The commission proposed that an establishment, to be called the Pasteur Institute (*Institut Pasteur*), be founded for the treatment of both the French people and foreigners.

Pasteur made further progress reports ("Note complémentaire sur les résultats de l'application de la méthode de prophylaxie de la rage après morsure," *ibid.*, 102:835, 1886). Over seven hundred people had now been treated, including thirty-eight Russians bitten by rabid wolves. Three of this group died, and Pasteur points out the great virulence of wolf bite compared to that of the dog.

> 11. PASTEUR, Louis. Nouvelle communication sur la rage, Compt. rend. Acad. d. sc., **103**:777, 1886.

By this time the Pasteur treatment had become highly standardized. There were ten daily injections of rabbit cord, beginning with material dried for 14 days and concluding with the "5-day cord." Among seventeen hundred patients, the treatment was ineffective in ten. Although this figure was much lower than in untreated cases, Pasteur was a little unhappy. He noted that most of the fatal cases were children bitten about the face. He was not sure that the treatment was adequate for this type of case. He decided to modify the procedure to make it more rapid and more effective. He gave more injections, three, for example, on the first day, and continued treatments over a longer period of days. The important point is that Pasteur himself now recognized that the treatment was not infallible.

Detailed reports appeared each year from the Pasteur Institute. In 1898, for example (H. Pottevin, "Les Vaccinations antirabiques à l'Institut Pasteur," Ann. Inst. Pasteur, **12**:301, 1898), there were reported a total of 20,166 persons treated, with 96 deaths, or a mortality of 0.46 per cent. Högyes (*op. cit.*, p. 237) gives an interesting list of reports from various treatment centers (Pasteur institutes) the world over.

> 12. ROUX, E. Note sur un moyen de conserver les moelles rabiques avec leur virulence, Ann. Inst. Pasteur, **1**:87, 1887.

Roux found that specimens from rabid animals sent in for examination were often putrid. It occurred to him to place the fresh material in glycerine, in which the virus was not destroyed, and he found that substance from the nervous system could be kept for 4 weeks at room temperature and still be virulent. A. Calmette, following this suggestion ("Notes sur la rage en Indo-Chine et sur les vaccinations antirabique pratiquées à Saigon du 14 avril au 1er août 1891," Ann. Inst. Pasteur, **8**:633, 1891) was able to keep a supply of desiccated cords preserved in glycerine on hand so as to be prepared at all times to give antirabic treatment. Various other methods of "attenuating" rabies virus for vaccine have been devised, such as that of G. P. Alivisatos ("Die Schutzimpfung gegen Lyssa durch das mit Aether behandelte Virus fixe," Deutsche med. Wchnschr., **48**:295, 1922), who treated brain containing virus with ether with satisfactory results. (See also Fermi, Ref. 17.)

> 13. DI VESTEA, A., and ZAGARI, G. Sur la transmission de la rage par voie nerveuse, Ann. Inst. Pasteur, **3**:237, 1889.

There have been two main views as to the route whereby rabies virus reaches the nervous system: (1) by the blood stream and (2) by the nerves. Pasteur had shown (Refs. 7, 8) that inoculation by blood stream and intracerebral inoculation were effective. Di Vestea and Zagari ("Compte rendu d'une année d'observations et d'expériences sur la rage, et sur la méthode de traitement préventif de Pasteur," Ann. Inst. Pasteur, **1**:492, 1887) brought forward clinical and experimental evidence that rabies virus was spread from the bite to the central nervous system by passage along nerves. They had shown, for example, that inoculation of fixed virus into the sciatic nerve of a rabbit and of a dog caused death with the same symptoms as those of intracerebral inoculation. Furthermore, disease could be prevented by cutting and cauterization of the nerve after injection. Finally, the type of clinical phenomenon produced seemed to depend on the location of the inoculated nerve and where it entered the central nervous system. Bardach ("Nouvelles recherches sur la rage," Ann. Inst. Pasteur, **2**:9, 1888) came to similar conclusions. E. Roux ("Notes de laboratoire sur la présence du virus rabique dans les nerfs," Ann. Inst. Pasteur, **2**:18, 1888) agreed with these views but held certain reservations. "One sees, then, that inoculation into the nerves does not always produce rabies with the certainty of inoculation by trepanation." Meanwhile, Nocard and Roux ("Expériences sur la vaccination des ruminants contre la rage, par injections intraveineuses de virus rabique," Ann. Inst. Pasteur, **2**:341, 1888) showed that large intravenous injections of rabid spinal cord could be given with impunity to sheep and goats, although immunity was conferred. C. Helman ("Action du virus rabique," Ann. Inst. Pasteur, **3**:15, 1889) concluded that rabies virus produced infection on inoculation only "if introduced directly into the nerve cells, although, if introduced into subcutaneous tissue, it could give immunity." In the present paper Di Vestea and Zagari studied the subject further and concluded that "all cases of human rabies in which the symptoms are in accord with the site of the bite bear witness in favor of absorption of virus by the nervous route." All this shows how exceedingly complex and confused the subject was. Recently Webster (Epidemiologic and immunologic experiments on rabies," New England J. Med., **217**:187, 1937) found that virus injected under the skin of Swiss mice is first detected 5 or 6 days later in the central nervous system at the site in direct connection with the inoculated areas. This finding is consistent with "the view that the virus does travel by way of the nerves." But "virus cannot actually be detected in the peripheral nerves until it has been demonstrated in brain or cord. In the mouse, therefore, we do not know just how the virus travels from the surface to the cord or brain."

14. NEGRI, A. Beitrag zum Studium der Aetiologie der Tollwuth, Ztschr. f. Hyg. u. Infectionskr., **43**:507, 1903. ("Contributo allo studio dell' eziologia della rabbia," Boll. della Soc. med. chir. di Pavia, **3**:88, 1903.)

It is small wonder that Negri, working in the laboratory of Golgi in Pavia, where studies of malaria were being intensively pursued, should regard the bodies which bear his name as living parasites. "The finding, to which I especially wish to draw attention, is the occurrence of a specific micro-organism in the nervous system of rabid animals; everything leads us to the conclusion that it should be included among the Protozoa." These alleged parasites were seen especially in the dog; Negri observed them also in one human case. "The site of predilection of the micro-organism is the horn of Ammon. In this region, especially in the larger nerve cells, the parasites are present in large numbers. . . . They exhibit the form of small, sharply outlined structures." They were also found in spinal ganglia and in the spinal cords of dogs, in which rabies occurred naturally or experimentally, and in rabbits experimentally inoculated. The bodies are of various size, from 1 μ up to 10, 12, or 15 μ or even as large as 27 μ by 5 μ. They are stained best with eosin–methylene blue. Four to six parasites may be found in one cell. Negri thought that he saw evidences of multiplication of these bodies. The many elaborate details of structure must be read in the original paper, which also contains colored microphotographs of the bodies. In another paper Negri ("Zur Aetiologie der Tollwuth. Die Diagnose der Tollwuth auf Grund der neuen Befunde," Ztschr. f. Hyg. u. Infectionskr., **44**:519, 1903) used the presence of "Negri bodies" as a practical diagnostic test for a rabid animal and laid the ground for the method still regularly used today.

The story of events leading to the discovery of the causal agent of rabies is one of great interest. Pasteur himself (Ref. 7) had speculated that the agent was a minute one, unlike ordinary bacteria. V. Babes ("Studien über die Wuthkrankheit," Virchows Arch. f. path. Anat., **110**:562, 1887) reviewed various claims of a bacterial agent and himself isolated several organisms from the nervous systems of rabid animals, with cultures of which he claimed to reproduce rabies; but, interestingly enough, he thought that the causal agent was a minute body perhaps carried in the bacteria. Babes later ("Les Corpuscules de Negri et le parasite de la rage," Presse méd., **14**:669, 1906) confirmed the presence of Negri bodies in rabies but concluded that they represented a reaction to infection and were not parasites, although they might contain them. The causal agent, Babes thought, must be more widespread in the nervous system. He concluded that it was a minute, though visible, body which could be stained as a "dust" and which was found in degenerated cells through the nervous system. These observations were elaborated a little later (V. Babes, "Untersuchungen über die Negrischen Körper und ihre Beziehung zu dem virus der Wutkrankheit," Ztschr. f. Hyg. u. Infectionskr., **56**:435, 1907). Two years later Negri ("Über die Morphologie und den Entwicklungszyclus des Parasiten der Tollwut," Ztschr. f. Hyg. u. Infectionskr., **63**:421, 1909) elaborately redescribed his bodies, still insisting that they were parasites and pointing out that Calkins had named them *Neurocytes hydrophobiae*. Calkins, it should be remembered, worked on the Guarnieri bodies of smallpox (see "Smallpox," Ref. 3) and concluded that they, too, were living parasites. Meanwhile, P. Remlinger ("Isolement de virus rabique par filtration," Compt. rend. Soc. de biol., **55**:1433, 1903) claimed to have produced rabies in rabbits with Berkefelt V filtrates of "putrefied" central nervous system material from rabid dogs and rabbits. Finally, J. Koch and P. Rissling ("Studien zur Aetiologie der Tollwut," Ztschr. f. Hyg. u. Infectionskr., **65**:85, 1910) described "small coccus-like bodies" in the gray matter of the central nervous systems of rabid dogs which they thought might be of etiological significance. Like Babes, they did not accept the Negri bodies as parasites. Later confirmation of the filtrability of rabies virus, of course, rules out the bodies of Negri and of Koch as causal agents, whatever diagnostic value they may have. The subject of the

Negri bodies is critically reviewed by P. Frosch ("Lyssa," in W. Kolle and A. Wassermann, *Handbuch der pathogenen Microorganismen*, Vol. 1, Ergänzungsband [1907], p. 626). The nodules described by Babes ("Sur certains caractères des lésions histologiques de la rage," Ann. Inst. Pasteur, **6**:209, 1892), which seem to be leukocytic accumulations in relation to blood vessels, are now thought to be common to neurotropic virus infections. Indeed, the Negri body is perhaps the only absolutely specific anatomical change. T. F. Sellers ("A new method for staining Negri bodies of rabies," Am. J. Pub. Health, **17**:1080, 1927) developed a useful method of demonstrating Negri bodies by impression preparations of brain tissue specially stained.

15. REMLINGER, P. Accidents paralytiques au cours du traitement antirabique, Ann. Inst. Pasteur, **19**:625, 1905.

This is the first comprehensive discussion of the paralyses occurring in connection with antirabic therapy. Remlinger gives abstracts of all the reported cases—26 in number—beginning in 1888. He analyzes the whole problem and discusses various explanations, including the introduction of non-viral toxic substances. He finally leans toward a "rabic toxin" as the explanation (see also Ref. 19).

16. FERMI, Claudio. Ueber die Virulenz des Speichels und der Speicheldrüsen wutkranker Tiere, Centralbl. f. Bakt., **44**:26, 1907.

Although Zinke (Ref. 1) a century earlier had given evidence that rabies virus is present in saliva, it is amazingly difficult to demonstrate it experimentally. Fermi discusses the discordant results of various investigators and reports extensive observations of his own on the intracerebral and subcutaneous injection of saliva from all sorts of rabid animals into test subjects. In a huge number of experiments, rabies was never produced. E. Bartarelli ("Ueber die Wege auf denen das Wutvirus zu den Speicheldrüsen des Hundes gelangt," Centralbl. f. Bakt., **37**:213, 1904), on the other hand, seemed to show that virus reached the salivary glands in rabid dogs by peripheral travel along nerves. His demonstration consisted in severing first the nervous and then the vascular connections of the parotid gland, after which the animal was inoculated with rabies virus emulsion. The glands from animals in which the nervous, but not the vascular, connections were preserved produced rabies in other animals. Meanwhile, Roux and Nocard ("A quel moment le virus rabique apparaît-il dans la bave des animaux enragés?" Ann. Inst. Pasteur, **4**:163, 1890) showed that rabies virus could be found in the saliva of rabid dogs 2 or 3 days before the least clinical symptoms. J. Nicholas later ("Apparition de la virulence dans la salive mixte des animaux rabiques," Compt. rend. Soc. de biol., **60**:625, 1906) found saliva virulent as long as 6 days before the animal showed any recognizable clinical signs of rabies.

17. FERMI, Claudio. Ueber die Immunizierung gegen Wutkrankheit, Ztschr. f. Hyg. u. Infectionskr., **58**:232, 1908.

Fermi reviews comprehensively the previous methods of vaccination, including Pasteur's, and points out various defects. He introduced a new method in which the vaccine was treated with carbolic acid. One hundred per cent of test animals were saved, whereas 100 per cent of untreated controls died. He mentions, as advantageous, "uniformity of the vaccine and simplicity of preparation instead of the complicated and useless Pasteur method of attenuation." This vaccine can be preserved and sent anywhere so as to be always available. Later in a masterful article on the practical aspects of rabies, Sir David Semple ("On the nature of rabies and antirabic treatment," Brit. M.J., **2**:333, 371, 1919) described a method for preparing a dead carbolized vaccine and reported the cases of 2,009 Europeans in India who were treated, with only 0.19 per cent of failures. If immunization is complete before the virus traveling along peripheral nerves reaches the central nervous system, the patient survives; otherwise he dies. Hence mild bites at the periphery with a long incubation period are more favorable for immunization than severe bites on the face with a brief incubation. L. T. Webster ("The immunizing potency of antirabies vaccines: a critical review," Am. J. Hyg., **30**:113, 1939) gives an elaborate review of all the reported laboratory experiences in rabies vaccination. He concludes: "All workers save Fermi, have failed to demonstrate a significant protective effect of vaccination *following* experimental exposure to rabies virus by any route." On the other hand, vaccine, virulent or non-virulent, given *before* exposure has been found effective under limited conditions. These rather gloomy conclusions do not seem in harmony with reports of human vaccination (Ref. 25).

18. STUART, G., and KRIKORIAN, K. S. The neuro-paralytic accidents of anti-rabies treatment, Ann. Trop. Med., **22**:326, 1928.

That paralysis occurred in a certain number of instances during or following antirabic vaccination was an unquestioned fact (Ref. 15). A debate went on for years as to whether these accidents represented rabies from the bites of the rabid animal or whether, in cases where the animal turned out not to be rabid, atypical rabies was produced by rabies virus in the vaccine.

E. Centanni ("Sui prodotti tossici secondarii nelle infezioni," Riforma med., **3**:637, 1898) and A. Aujeszky ("Ueber Immunisierung gegen Wut mit normaler Nervensubstanz," Centralbl. f. Bakt., **27**:5, 1900) thought that it might be possible to produce immunity to rabies by injections of *normal* nervous system material. They found the animals did badly, lost weight, developed skin abscesses, and sometimes died, but no paralytic accidents are mentioned. Eduard Müller ("Ueber acute Paraplegien nach Wutschutzimpfungen," Deutsche Ztschr. f. Nervenh., **34**:252, 1908) in the course of a masterful description of paralytic accidents following rabies vaccine stated: "A further possibility . . . is the fact that in the Pasteur treatment not insignificant amounts of foreign and diseased spinal cord substance are introduced subcutaneously into the human body." He did not, however, make any experimental observations. P. Remlinger ("Accidents paralytiques d'origine médullaire provoqués chez le lapin par des inoculations de substance nerveuse normale homologue," Compt. rend. Soc. de biol., **83**:171, 1920) first produced paralysis in a healthy rabbit by injections of brain from a normal rabbit. He points out the rarity of this finding but notes: "This fact is interesting from the point of view of the paralyses which sometimes occur in man in connection with Pasteur therapy." Fritz Schweinburg ("Klinische und experimentelle Beobachtungen über Lähmungen nach Wutschutzimpfung," Wien. klin. Wchnschr., **37**:797, 1924) reported similar findings. Stuart and Krikorian in an article definitive to date concluded that "in the basic nerve substance of all antirabic vaccines there seems to exist some deleterious component which . . . is capable . . . of producing neuro-paralytic disorders." They then actually showed that "paralytic accidents can be produced experimentally by the repeated inoculation of nerve substance, normal or rabid, homologous or heterologous." Later T. M. Rivers, D. H. Sprunt, and G. P. Berry ("Observations on attempts to produce acute disseminated encephalomyelitis in monkeys," J. Exper. Med., **58**:39, 1933) showed that repeated intramuscular injections of brain extracts and emulsions into monkeys might be followed by an inflammatory reaction, with demyelinization. Similar findings were described by E. A. Kabat, A. Wolf, and A. E. Bezer ("The rapid production of acute disseminated encephalomyelitis in rhesus monkeys by injection of heterologous and homologous brain tissue with adjuvants," J. Exper. Med., **85**:117, 1947) and by Isabel M. Morgan ("Allergic encephalomyelitis in monkeys in response to injection of normal monkey nervous tissue," J. Exper. Med., **85**:131, 1947). A good modern summary of the subject is that of L. Weinstein and M. Goldfield ("Reactions to rabies vaccine, with a report of two cases of encephalomyelitis," Boston M. Quart., **4**:7, 1953). Statistics are given in the paper by E. Appelbaum, M. Greenberg, and J. Nelson ("Neurological complications following antirabies vaccination," J.A.M.A., **151**:188, 1953) and in McKendrick's review (Ref. 25).

Recently J. F. Bell, J. T. Wright, and K. Habel ("Rabies vaccine freed of the factor causing allergic encephalitis," Proc. Soc. Exper. Biol. & Med., **70**:457, 1949) have tried to reduce the danger of neurological accidents by removing from vaccine the encephalitis-causing factor.

19. REMLINGER, P. La Rage de laboratoire, Bull. Acad. de méd., Paris, **113**:836, 1935.

It had long been noted that various "paralytic" accidents were associated with antirabic therapy. There might be a Landry-like ascending paralysis, signs of a lumbodorsal myelitis, or peripheral palsy of the seventh or fifth cranial nerve. It had been assumed that these accidents were true rabies of a type different from the spontaneous disease—laboratory rabies (*la rage de laboratoire*). This term was first used by Chauveau in a discussion of Peters' paper ("Inoculations antirabiques intensives et mort par la rage," Bull. Acad. de méd., Paris, **17**:16, 1887), in which he questioned the value of antirabic vaccination (Pasteur) and created a violent discussion which went on for months in the academy (*ibid.*, pp. 28, 72). Remlinger in this paper discusses the question of whether these accidents of therapy are actually rabies, especially the mild non-fatal ones. No final answer was reached, although he concluded that "with the exception of certain paralyses following dead vaccine, the accidents of antirabic therapy are largely due to fixed virus." (But see also Ref. 15.)

20. WEBSTER, L. T., and DAWSON, J. R., Jr. Early diagnosis of rabies by mouse inoculation. Measurement of humoral immunity to rabies by mouse protection test, Proc. Soc. Exper. Biol. & Med., **32**:570, 1935.

The early literature on infection of mice with rabic virus is reviewed by A. Hoyt and C. W. Jungeblut ("Experimental rabies in white mice and attempted chemotherapy," J. Infect. Dis., **47**:418, 1930); but, to obtain useful results, Webster and Dawson found it necessary to breed mice specially for high susceptibility to neurotropic viruses. Using such animals, they found that rabies was readily produced by intracerebral inoculation of fresh dog brain containing Negri bodies. "This brief experience suggests . . . that rabies may be diagnosed within 7 days." They also developed a mouse protection test for the quantitative measurement of protective antibodies against rabies. Webster soon elaborated this material in another paper ("Diagnostic and immunologic tests of rabies in mice," Am. J. Pub. Health, 26:1207, 1936), and, finally ("A mouse test for measuring the immunizing potency of antirabic vaccines," J. Exper. Med., 70:87, 1939), Webster, using the mouse test, was able to appraise the potency of vaccines, showing that "virulent virus, injected intraperitoneally as a vaccine, immunized mice within 10 days and for a period of at least 9 months. Demonstrable neutralizing antibodies accompanied this immunity. Virus subcutaneously failed to immunize as effectively." Commercial vaccines containing virulent virus gave results similar to those obtained with laboratory virus, but commercial vaccine inactivated with phenol generally failed to immunize mice. It is interesting that various commercial vaccines varied greatly in their immunizing potency. Similar results were obtained in dogs (L. T. Webster and J. Casals, "A dog test for measurng the immunizing potency of antirabies vaccines," J. Exper. Med., 71:719, 1940). Confirmatory experiments were also reported by R. W. G. Wyckoff and C. E. Beck ("The potency of anti-rabic vaccines," J. Immunol., 39:17, 1940). Charles N. Leach ("Comparative methods of diagnosis of rabies in animals," Am. J. Pub. Health, 28:162, 1938) confirmed the practical value of Webster's mouse test and, indeed, found it positive in 12 per cent of brains reported negative for Negri bodies (Ref. 14), whereas only 3 specimens among 338 reported positive gave a negative mouse test. K. Habel and J. T. Wright ("Some factors influencing the mouse potency test for rabies vaccine," Pub. Health Rep., 63:44, 1948) developed a test for the immunizing potency of commercial vaccine.

21. PAWAN, J. L. Rabies in the vampire bat of Trinidad, with special reference to the clinical course and the latency of infection, Ann. Trop. Med., 30:401, 1936.

A carrier state is so common with viral infections that one naturally inquires whether there are asymptomatic carriers of rabies virus. The vampire bat of Trinidad has definitely been shown to be such a carrier. The earlier phases of this interesting story are told by E. W. Hurst and J. L. Pawan ("An outbreak of rabies in Trinidad, without history of bites, and with the symptoms of acute ascending myelitis," Lancet, 221:622, 1931; "A further account of the Trinidad outbreak of acute rabic myelitis; histology of the experimental disease," J. Path. & Bact., 35:301, 1932). In 1936 Pawan ("The transmission of paralytic rabies in Trinidad by the vampire bat [*Desmodius rotundus murinus,* Wagner, 1840]," Ann. Trop. Med., 30:101, 1936) first showed that human beings bitten by vampire bats develop sensory symptoms at the bitten site, followed by paralysis and death, and that the bats were definitely infected. Finally, in the present paper Pawan demonstrated that vampire bats might become carriers of rabies after "recovery" from the furious form of the disease. In this state, while apparently well, they may remain capable of spreading infection by their bites for prolonged periods.

22. WEBSTER, L. T., and CLOW, A. D. Propagation of rabies virus in tissue culture and the successful use of culture virus as an antirabic vaccine, Science, **84**:487, 1936.

Webster and Clow first succeeded in growing rabies virus in tissue culture. The medium consisted of Tyrode solution containing normal monkey serum plus a suspension of minced mouse embryo brain. The inoculum consisted of brain from a mouse prostrate on the seventh or eighth day following an intracerebral injection of rabies virus. Material was passed through such culture medium as often as 88 times, and the supernatant was still found to be virulent unless neutralized by sera from persons given Semple antirabic vaccine. In order to get away from the adverse effects of injection of brain or cord material implicit in the older vaccine, the supernatant culture fluid was used and was found highly effective when injected intraperitoneally, making the mouse resistant to 100 intracerebral fatal doses of street virus. Webster and Clow soon published a more elaborate account of these studies ("Propagation of rabies virus in tissue culture," J. Exper. Med., **66**:125, 1937).

23. GALLOWAY, I. A., and ELFORD, W. J. The size of the virus of rabies ("fixed" strain) by ultrafiltration analysis, J. Hyg., **36**:532, 1936.

Remlinger (Ref. 14) made early studies on the filtrability of rabies virus. Later, Galloway and Elford, using graded collodion membranes, assigned a diameter of 100–150 mμ to the virus of rabies. Thus it falls among the larger viruses, poliomyelitis particles, for example, being one-fifth as large.

24. BERNKOPF, H., and KLIGLER, I. Characteristics of a fixed rabies virus cultivated on developing chick embryos, Proc. Soc. Exper. Biol. & Med., **45**:332, 1940.

Two groups of workers (I. J. Kligler and H. Bernkopf, "Cultivation of rabies virus in developing chick embryo," Nature, **143**:899; J. R. Dawson, Jr., "Infection of chicks and chick embryos with rabies," Science, **89**:300, 1939) succeeded at about the same time in growing rabies virus in the chick embryo. Kligler and Bernkopf inoculated the chorio-allantois, Dawson the brain, of the embryo. In this paper Bernkopf and Kligler describe their work more in detail and point out that the chick embryo virus after many passages showed greatly reduced virulence for rabbits. Dawson ("A study of chick-embryo-adapted rabies virus," Am. J. Path., **17**:177, 1941) also found the virulence reduced for the rabbit and pointed out other interesting implications from the standpoint of rabies infection and immunity. H. Koprowski and H. R. Cox ("Studies on chick embryo adapted rabies virus. I. Culture characteristics and pathogenicity," J. Immunol., **60**:533, 1948), among others, developed this subject further.

25. McKENDRICK, A. G. A ninth analytical review of reports from Pasteur institutes on the results of anti-rabies treatment, League of Nations, Bull. World Health Organ., **9**:31, 1940–41.

As rabies is, up to the present, an incurable disease, there has been tremendous emphasis on preventive measures. The early work of Pasteur and others has already been mentioned (Ref. 10). McKendrick gives a definitive review of the various methods of prophylactic therapy; he lists the methods, which can be divided into injections of "attenuated" live virus (Pasteur) or of virus "killed" by phenolization or some other method. Among 1,062,707 persons treated, there was an over-all mortality of 0.33 per cent. Every conceivable factor was taken into account in the breakdown of the figures, such as severity of the bite, position, intervention of clothing, and delay in commencing treatment. Paralytic accidents with various methods are discussed. In general, there seems little choice between most of the methods, although after wolf bites the mortality is 6.78 as against 0.26 with dog bites. Deep bites as against superficial, bites on head as against leg, and delay in starting treatment are all unfavorable factors. However, all this complicated material must be consulted in the original. Webster (*Rabies*, p. 100) gives a penetrating analysis of McKendrick's figures and concludes that they do not definitely answer the question of whether vaccine does or does not protect against rabies. In practice, however, he feels strongly that antirabic therapy should be used in certain groups of cases, such as those bitten through the skin by a dog proved rabid.

G. Proca and S. Bobes ("Anti-rabic immunization; living vaccines and killed vaccines," League of Nations, Bull. World Health Organ., **9**:79, 1940–41) further analyze the problem. They point out that "the harmlessness of live vaccines [Pasteur] is not a rule with no exceptions." On the other hand, Fermi's carbolized vaccine (Ref. 17) behaves like an avirulent chemical vaccine when injected subcutaneously. Moreover, intracerebral inoculation of rabbits with larger doses may occasionally still produce rabies, so that, clearly, every virus particle is not definitely killed. The authors incline to the use of chemical vaccines as being safer but feel that the final word is not yet said. The problem seems similar to that of the Salk vaccine for poliomyelitis; it is a question whether a completely killed vaccine retains full immunizing power.

26. KOPROWSKI, Hilary. Experimental studies on rabies virus, Canad. J. Pub. Health, **40**:60, 1949.

It is not possible in this bibliography to go into all the details of control measures against rabies—muzzling, quarantining, etc. These are fully discussed in the general references given at the beginning of this article. We shall refer, however, to the question of protecting dogs by immunization. S. Umeno and Y. Doi ("Antirabic inoculation of dogs and results of its protective application," Kitasato Arch. Exper. Med., **4**:89, 1921) first prepared such a vaccine, which was used with success in dogs in single doses. H. Koprowski has recently reviewed the subject. He tried to produce a "single-injection" method for immunization of dogs by means of an egg-passage virus. Potent antirabies serum was also obtained from rabbits which Koprowski believed useful in both animal and human rabies as a supplement to vaccination. Later Koprowski with J. Van der Scheer and C. E. and J. Black ("Use of hyperimmune antirabies concentrates in experimental rabies," Am. J. Med., **8**:412, 1950) found that one injection of hyperimmune antiserum protected small animals which had been infected 24 hours previously with street virus. In contrast, 14 injections of rabies vaccine begun 24 hours after exposure failed in all instances to protect. They believe that antiserum plus vaccine should be applied in all cases of exposure to rabies.

YELLOW FEVER

It SEEMS natural that so dramatic and picturesque a disease as yellow fever, and one for a long time so puzzling, should have been much written about. The history of the subject is well covered in Henry Rose Carter's scholarly book, *Yellow Fever* (Baltimore: Williams & Wilkins Co., 1931), to which is appended an extensive bibliography. George Augustin's huge volume, *History of Yellow Fever* (New Orleans: Searcy & Pfaff, Ltd., 1909), also contains much interesting, though undocumented, material. Extensive historical bibliographies are to be found in the works of La Roche (Ref. 3) and of Hirsch (Ref. 5), and the recent literature is well covered in Strode's monograph (Ref. 29). There is an immense number of books dealing, often dramatically, with individual epidemics, in some of which are listed in ghoulish detail the names of the many hundreds who died of the disease, for example, J. M. Keating, *The Yellow Fever Epidemic of 1878 in Memphis, Tennessee* (Memphis: Printed for the Howard Association, 1879). Of special interest is the book edited by Chauncey D. Leake, *Yellow Fever in Galveston, Republic of Texas, 1839* (Austin: University of Texas Press, 1951), which contains admirable brief "stories of the men who conquered yellow fever," and, finally, there is a readable account of the whole subject in H. Harold Scott, *A History of Tropical Medicine* (Baltimore: Williams & Wilkins Co., 1939), Vol. 1, chap. vii, "Yellow Fever," page 279.

1. RUSH, Benjamin. An account of the bilious remitting yellow fever as it appeared in the city of Philadelphia in the year 1793. 2d ed. Philadelphia: Thomas Dobson, 1794.

We may well open this bibliography with an account of yellow fever by one of the outstanding physicians of the time. However, Rush's thinking and description are definitely oriented to the eighteenth century and actually are of little value except as historical material. "The causes which induced indirect debility were, 1. Fatigue of body or mind induced by labour. . . . It was labour which excited the disease so universally among the lower class of people. . . . A hard trotting horse brought it on two of my patients. . . . A fall excited it in a girl. . . . 2. Heat from every cause but more especially heat of the sun was a very common exciting cause of the disorder. . . ." In addition, intemperance, fear, grief, cold, etc., were assigned as precipitating causes (pp. 29 ff.). The clinical description is based on the humoral theory of disease: "The blood vessels are the 'seat and throne' of this as well as of all other fevers. I have publickly taught for several years, that a fever is occasioned by a convulsion in the arterial system" (p. 40). Rush goes on to describe in great detail the pulse and other features of the disease, without, of course, any adequate physical examination. "There were for several weeks two sources of infection viz. exhalation and contagion. The exhalation infected at a distance of three and four hundred yards; while the contagion infected only across the streets" (p. 104). As to the causes which checked the disorder: "On the fifteenth of October it pleased God to alter the state of the air. The clouds at last dropped health in showers of rain. . . . The appearance of this rain was like a dove with an olive branch in its mouth, to the whole city" (p. 130). The discussion of treatment is fanciful and need not be described in detail (pp. 193 ff.). There are elaborate and controversial arguments about the place in therapy of purging, bloodletting, blisters, etc. Rush came to feel that the disease was not contagious, and in his *Medical Inquiries and Observations* (3d ed.; Philadelphia: Benjamin & Thomas Keith, etc., 1809), 4:235–84, he has a long section, giving his reasons in detail. Of course, the truth of the matter is that yellow fever *is not* contagious, although rapidly transmitted by the mosquito, about which Rush knew nothing at the time.

Rush was undoubtedly a great man and a great physician in his day; but we must think of him as an exponent of eighteenth-century medicine and not of the views developed in France at the turn of the century.

A graphic account of this epidemic is given by W. S. Middleton, "The yellow fever epidemic of 1793 in Philadelphia," Ann. M. Hist., **10**:434, 1928, and by J. H. Powell, *Bring Out Your Dead: The Great Plague of Yellow Fever in Philadelphia in 1793* (Philadelphia: University of Pennsylvania Press, 1949). With regard to Rush and his ideas on yellow fever see C. E. A. Winslow, *The Conquest of Epidemic Disease* (Princeton, N.J.: Princeton University Press, 1943), chap. xi, "The Enigma of Yellow Fever," page 193.

2. LOUIS, P. Ch. A. Anatomical, pathological and therapeutic researches on the yellow fever of Gibraltar of 1828. Translated from the manuscript by G. C. Shattuck, Jr., M.D. Boston: Charles C. Little & James Brown, 1839. (Precedes the French edition.)

Once more, as in the case of his book on typhoid fever, one must pay homage to Louis for his cool objectivity in handling the facts and for his clear analysis of results. Louis was, of course, an outstanding member of the young group of French clinician-pathologists at the beginning of the nineteenth century who revolutionized and modernized the study of disease. Louis with Chervin and Trousseau were sent to Gibraltar as a commission by the French government to study the epidemic of yellow fever then rampant. Louis set out to do autopsies on fatal cases with meticulous care; these were correlated with objective clinical findings. The descriptions are masterpieces of clarity and precision and would do credit to a modern medical service or autopsy room. Anatomically, Louis soon centered his attention on the liver. "But the most remarkable lesion of the liver was the alteration of its color. . . . This alteration consisted in a discoloration, the liver being sometimes the color of fresh butter, sometimes of a straw color, sometimes of the color of coffee and milk . . . etc." (p. 117). Later, in interpreting the lesions: "Lesions, apparently slight, may explain death when they have taken place rapidly, as in the cases now under consideration. And then again, in the present state of science we can not appreciate the nature of the specific lesion of the liver, and consequently we can not determine how far it had anything to do with death" (p. 144). "As then, a strict analysis . . . proves the existence of a cause, unequal in its operation, and of which but one effect is constant, the specific alteration of the liver, and as in a third part of the cases it is directly to this cause that we are obliged to refer death, we naturally ask how does this cause act, through the medium of what system does it exert its influence on the economy?" (p. 164). But the objective Louis speculates no further; he simply assembles evidence and waits. He shows later by extensive statistics that yellow fever confers an immunity to a second attack even after a lapse of many years. As to treatment, he compares that of the English and the Spanish physicians at Gibraltar. "It is true, that, in the army, the ratio of mortality was one in four and a half, and that, in the city, it was only one in six, so that, all other things being equal, it would seem to result from these two principal classes of facts, either that the treatment of the Spanish physicians was very efficacious, or that of the English physicians was very injurious" (p. 330).

The translator in his Introduction says this about Louis: "Some seem to have been misled by the term numerical system, which has been said to be that of M. Louis. They seem to have thought that his peculiarity consists in this merely, that he counts. . . . We call some experienced, scientific. Is it not by comparing individual cases, by adding what they have observed in one to what they have observed in another, by *counting*, that they have become so?" (p. xii).

3. LA ROCHE, R. Yellow fever, considered in its historical, pathological, etiological and therapeutical relations. 2 vols. Philadelphia: Blanchard & Lea, 1855.

This monumental treatise deals with every phase of the subject, which is made vivid by innumerable allusions to the literature and to the opinions and actions of individual physicians as well as commissions, boards of health, etc. It opens with a bibliography of over a thousand titles, presumably definitive to date. The next section of some hundred pages deals with the various Philadelphia outbreaks. Symptoms and clinical features are then discussed in minute detail (pp. 129–383), after which comes a chapter on the pathological anatomy of the disease. As to the liver: "The secreting cells were pale, ill-defined, and less granular than when in the normal state. In the cells with few exceptions, no nucleus could be detected." The incubation period was regarded for the most part as from 3 to 6 days. "Dr. Harrison, of New Orleans, remarks that persons who arrive in that city during an epidemic, from the healthiest regions . . . are subject to attack on the sixth, fifth, fourth, or even as early as the third day after their arrival," a finding which indicates the promptness with which people were likely to be bitten by mosquitoes in an infected area. There is next an analysis of the mortality of yellow fever (pp. 513–46).

Volume 2 deals largely with the questions of etiology and contagion. There was, of course, no idea of a living virus or of any part played by mosquitoes. Among various "circumfusa" which we now know have nothing to do with the disease, such as light, electricity, and atmospheric pressure, the writer was quite clear as to the relation to temperature: "The yellow fever is undeniably a disease of hot climates and hot seasons." As to the immediate cause, "much diversity of opinion has existed . . . relative to the nature of the efficient cause of yellow fever—to the sources whence that cause is derived—as well as to the mode of diffusion of the disease after it has once made its appearance. By one set of physicians . . . the disease is regarded as the offspring of a morbid poison found and elaborated in a diseased body, and is invariably referred to importation from abroad." By others "the fever has been invariably referred to the evolution, under particular circumstances, both terrestrial and meteorological, of a febrile poison originating in molecular changes . . . independent of . . . the arrival of vessels from sickly ports" (**2**:190). The major portion of this volume is then devoted to an intensive discussion of contagion versus non-contagion, to the latter of which the author adheres. He tells how important physicians have changed from contagionists to non-contagionists. "Dr. Rush, who, as we have seen, had originally espoused the cause of contagion . . . at last relinquished his former views. Not satisfied with doing so silently . . . this eminent physician published a formal recantation"[1] (**2**:253). However, there was a common belief that the disease arose by "infection" with a "miasma," and, interestingly enough, many analogies with malaria were noted. "It is, like other miasmal diseases, under the influence of atmospheric vicissitudes. . . . It is limited in the sphere of its prevalence, never extending beyond certain boundaries, attacking those who venture within those boundaries, even in the absence of the sick, and sparing those who keep aloof. To these limits it may be restricted by a cessation of intercourse; while the disease is arrested in its progress by the dispersion of the inhabitants of the infected localities, and by preventing further access to these by artificial means" (p. 595). Under the subject of prophylaxis, "it is necessary to effect the removal of all local nuisances before the accession of hot weather . . . whereas, docks or other localities liable to be visited by the disease, courts, yards, gutters, cellars should be left perfectly clear; all accumulations of filth and stagnant water should be carefully removed; streets, courts, and alleys should be paved. . . . The holds of vessels must be left clean and pure, and all foul bilge water carefully pumped out" (**2**:732). The author, however, opposed quarantine both because he thought it useless and because of inconvenience to individuals and commercial losses (*ibid.*, p. 737). "Much more useful will it be to obtain at once the complete evacuation of all the inhabitants of infected spots" (*ibid.*, p. 749). Under treatment, a fantastic list of agents is discussed—bleeding, local depletion, emetics, purgatives, mercury, diaphoretics, sedatives, oxide of bismuth, rhatamy, tannin, creosote, adrue, nitrate of silver, lime-water, chloroform, opium, external applications, affusions, drinks, injections, cool air, sinapisms, moxa, actual cautery, Peruvian bark, sulphate of quinia, oil, melambo, charcoal, moral treatment, and diet.

4. MACDONALD, J. Dennis. Yellow fever: a system of medicine, **1**:475. Edited by J. Russell Reynolds. Philadelphia: J. B. Lippincott & Co., 1868.

A standard account of the disease shortly before the bacteriological era shows little recent advance in knowledge. The author states that the infectious nature of yellow fever is now generally admitted. He is unclear, however, as to how the disease is transmitted and goes definitely wrong when he says that "the clothing of infected persons or of healthy persons having communicated with infected places or persons may impart infection to other places or persons."

---

[1] "To prevent recurrence of the fever, I early pointed out the domestic origin. In this opinion I was opposed by nearly the whole College of Physicians, who derived it from a foreign country, and who believed it to be a specific disease. They were followed by nearly all the citizens of Philadelphia" (*The Autobiography of Benjamin Rush*, ed. George W. Corner [Princeton, 1948], p. 97).

The whole question of anticontagionism is thoroughly discussed in Erwin H. Ackerknecht's "Anticontagionism between 1821 and 1867," Bull. Hist. Med., **22**:562, 1948.

Under treatment are mentioned the usual congeries of drugs: "Acetate of ammonia, nitrate of potash, nitrous ether, and tincture of squills and henbane may be combined with lime-juice for a drink."

An authoritative modern discussion of the clinical aspects and diagnosis of yellow fever is that of J. Austin Kerr in Strode (Ref. 29, pp. 381 ff.). In this article the findings of various clinical laboratory tests are also summarized.

> 5. HIRSCH, August. Handbook of geographical and historical pathology, 1:316, chap. viii, "Yellow Fever." Translated from the second German edition. London: New Sydenham Society, 1883.

This is the great storehouse of information about epidemics of yellow fever, which are listed in detail as to time and place. It is pointed out that yellow fever rarely occurs as a pandemic and that epidemic outbreaks never happen suddenly; a series of isolated cases always precedes them. Often the disease remains limited to one quarter of a town. The duration of epidemics varies greatly. Many other circumstances of outbreaks are discussed. Hirsch regards it as shown that yellow fever is communicable; "it is not now a question of whether communication actually takes place but only of how it takes place." Difference of opinion on this point "depends not so much upon conflicting facts, but rather the significance ascribed to them." There is, of course, no mention of the mosquito.

The article is followed by a lengthy bibliography.

> 6. FINLAY, Carlos J. The mosquito hypothetically considered as the agent of transmission of yellow fever. Translated by Dr. Finlay from the Anales de la Academia de ciencias médicas, físicas y naturales de la Habana, 18:147, 1881. *In* Trabajos selectos del Dr. Carlos J. Finlay. Havana: República de Cuba, 1912.

To Finlay seems to belong the credit for first clearly insisting that the mosquito was the vehicle for transmission of yellow fever.[2] "I feel convinced that any theory which attributes the origin and the propagation of yellow fever to atmospheric influences, to miasmatic or meteorological conditions, to filth or to neglect of general hygienic precautions must be considered as utterly indefensible. . . . I shall not concern myself with the nature or form of the morbific cause of yellow fever, beyond postulating the existence of a material, transportable substance, which may be an amorphous virus, a vegetable or animal germ, a bacterium, etc., but at any rate constitutes something tangible which requires to be conveyed from the sick to the healthy before the disease can be propagated." He then enumerated the reasons which made him select the mosquito as the only suitable vector. Finlay postulated that the mosquito carried the virus from

[2] The long rambling article by Josiah C. Nott ("Yellow fever contrasted with bilious fever—reasons for believing it a disease sui generis—its made of propagation—remote cause, probable insect or animalcular origin," New Orleans M. & S.J., 4:563, 1848), to whom credit is often given for first claiming that yellow fever is transmitted by the mosquito, is thus criticized by Ronald Ross (*Memoirs* [London: John Murray, 1923]): "Speculations of this kind are apt to be much overrated by penmen. It is easy for persons to sit in arm-chairs and weave hypotheses; many imagined America before Columbus; but an ocean had to be traversed between the dream and reality. Theorists who do not trouble to verify their own speculations deserve little credit" (p. 424).

one person to another on the mouth-parts. He attempted five inoculations by means of mosquito bites with equivocal results. He concluded: "Should it finally be proven that the mosquito-inoculation not only reproduces the yellow fever, but that it constitutes the regular process through which the disease is propagated, the conditions of existence and of development for that dipterous insect would account for the anomalies hitherto observed in the propagation of yellow fever."

Apparently, Finlay did not stimulate anyone to further investigation at the time, and, of course, his idea that the virus was mechanically transported was incorrect; had he known that the infective period of yellow fever lasts for only 3 or 4 days and that the mosquito must carry the virus for about 12 days before its bite becomes dangerous, he might actually have solved the problem. Nonetheless, he deserves full credit for pushing the idea of mosquito transmission. Later ("Yellow fever: its transmission by means of the Culex mosquito," Am. J.M. Sc., 92:394, 1886) he described in interesting fashion the feeding habits of local mosquitoes and reported more transmission experiments, which again did not seem to convince anyone. But Finlay continued to expose his views, as, for example, in a systematic discussion, "Yellow fever," Edinburgh M.J., 40:35, 1894, and in many papers, some of which are controversial, reprinted in *Selected Papers*.

Finlay's life and work are sympathetically appraised by Carlos E. Finlay, *Carlos Finlay and Yellow Fever* (New York: Oxford University Press, 1940).

7. SANARELLI, J. Étiologie et pathogénie de la fièvre jaune, Ann. Inst. Pasteur, 11:433, 673, 1897.

With the development of the bacteriological era, many physicians became convinced that yellow fever was caused by a living germ. As was the case with almost all infectious diseases, reports poured in of claims for one or another bacterial agent. The early claims are concisely summarized in *Carlos Finlay and Yellow Fever* (Ref. 6), only to be demolished by George M. Sternberg (*Report on the Etiology and Prevention of Yellow Fever* [Washington: Government Printing Office, 1890]), who states in his conclusions: "The specific infectious agent in yellow fever has not been demonstrated. The most approved bacteriological methods fail to demonstrate the constant presence of any particular microorganism in the blood and tissues of yellow fever cadavers" (p. 221). However, Sanarelli's long paper was so emphatic with its report of isolating a specific bacterium, *Bacillus icteroides*, both from living patients and at autopsy, and of the reproduction of lesions compatible with those of yellow fever in small animals that many were convinced for some years. Sodré and Couto, for example, in their authoritative treatise on yellow fever (*Das Gelbfieber* [Vienna: Alfred Hölder, 1901]) accept the organism of Sanarelli without reservation (pp. 63 ff.). An abbreviated translation of Sanarelli's paper also appeared in English ("A lecture on yellow fever," Brit. M.J., 2:7, 1897). But soon thereafter Reed and Carroll of the United States Army undertook to study *B. icteroides*. Reed was particularly well qualified, having worked on hog cholera with Welch at Johns Hopkins. In their first paper (Walter Reed and James Carroll, "Bacillus icteroides and Bacillus cholerae suis: a preliminary note," M. News, 74:513, 1899) they gave cultural and experimental data for considering Sanarelli's organism as simply a variety of the hog-cholera bacillus. Sanarelli unfortunately took this report as a personal affront and in another paper struck back (G. Sanarelli, "Some observations and controversial remarks on the specific cause of yellow fever," M. News, **75**:193, 1899) angrily but feebly. To this Reed and Carroll replied once more ("The specific cause of yellow fever: a reply to Dr. Sanarelli," M. News., **75**:321, 1899): "We pass by, therefore, as unworthy of comment, Sanarelli's insinuation that we could lend ourselves to the support of any personal controversy." They gave many more data and arguments and, finally, in a very comprehensive report ("A comparative study of the biological characters and pathogenesis of Bacillus X [Sternberg], Bacillus icteroides [Sanarelli] and the hog-cholera bacillus [Salmon and Smith]," J. Exper. Med., **5**:215, 1900) laid the ghost of this controversy.

8. CARTER, H. R. A note on the interval between infecting and secondary cases of yellow fever from the records of the yellow fever at Orwood and Taylor, Miss. in 1898, New Orleans M. & S.J., **52**:617, 1900.

That brilliant, if eccentric, student of yellow fever, H. R. Carter, made the important observation (in a rural community where circumstances were such as to make the induction valid) that after the first case of yellow fever appeared in a certain locale at least 2 weeks elapsed before secondary cases arose. Although Carter drew no (written) conclusions as to insect carriage, his work helped to strengthen in Walter Reed's mind the probability that the mosquito was the vector of yellow fever (Ref. 9).

9. REED, Walter, CARROLL, James, AGRAMONTE, A., and LAZEAR, Jesse W. The etiology of yellow fever: a preliminary note, Philadelphia M.J., **6**:790, 1901.

The famous yellow fever commission, consisting of Walter Reed,[3] James Carroll, Jesse W. Lazear, and Aristides Agramonte, had recently been assembled at Havana, where yellow fever had appeared in American troops. This is the first of a series of communications announcing the work of the commission and its conclusions. The report deals first with cultures from yellow fever cadavers with more comments on *B. icteroides* (see Ref. 7). The second part gives a review of Carter's work (Ref. 8). "In view of the foregoing observations we concluded to test the theory of Finlay [Ref. 6] on human beings." Non-immune men were bitten by infected mosquitoes (*Culex fasciatus*). "It will be seen that we record nine negative and two positive results." The two positive cases were bitten by mosquitoes which had fed on yellow fever patients 12 and 10 days previously; the "failures" were bitten by mosquitoes which had fed 2–8 days previously. The two cases reported in detail are Carroll, who survived, and Lazear, who died.

The final conclusion of the paper is this: "The mosquito serves as the intermediate host for the parasite of yellow fever, and it is highly probable that the disease is only propagated through the bite of this insect."

---

[3] By far the best and most accurate account of the yellow fever commission and its work is that of Howard A. Kelly, *Walter Reed and Yellow Fever* (New York: McClure, Phillips & Co., 1906). There is a full bibliography of the papers written by the members. Other books on Walter Reed dealing to some extent with yellow fever are Albert E. Truby, *Memoir of Walter Reed* (New York: Paul B. Hoeber, 1943), and L. N. Wood, *Walter Reed, Doctor in Uniform* (New York: Julian Messner, Inc., 1943).

In the second communication (Walter Reed, James Carroll, and Aristides Agramonte, "The etiology of yellow fever: an additional note," J.A.M.A., **36**:431, 1901) the authors tell first of the establishment of an experimental sanitary station (hospital) under full quarantine for the continuation of their studies. There are then reported the details of further inoculation experiments, from which the following important conclusions are drawn: An interval of about 12 days or more after contamination appears necessary before the mosquito is capable of conveying the infection. The bite of the mosquito at an earlier period does not appear to convey any immunity. Yellow fever can be produced by subcutaneous injection of blood drawn during the first and second days of the disease. The incubation period of the experimental infection varied from 41 hours to 5 days and 17 hours. Yellow fever is not conveyed by fomites. The spread of yellow fever can be most effectively controlled by destroying mosquitoes and protecting susceptible people against mosquito bite. Thus the principal facts of the mode of transmission of yellow fever were definitely established. In a third note Walter Reed, James Carroll, and A. Agramonte, "Experimental yellow fever," Am. Med., **2**:15, 1901), they describe the clinical features of the experimental disease and emphasize the occurrence of mild cases which can be diagnosed only with difficulty. Another paper (Walter Reed and James Carroll, "The prevention of yellow fever," M. Rec., **60**:641, 1901) soon followed, in which the harmful mosquito is described, with its habits of breeding and feeding, and a review is given of preventive measures, including quarantine, which they found requires a longer period than the usual 5 days. Meanwhile, Reed gave an interesting review of all his work (Walter Reed, "The propagation of yellow fever; observations based on recent researches," *ibid.*, p. 201) before the Medical and Chirurgical Faculty of the State of Maryland. Finally, in the last of Reed's early series of papers (Walter Reed and James Carroll, "The etiology of yellow fever: a supplemental note," Am. Med., **3**:301, 1902) he reports the production of yellow fever with serum which has been passed through "a new Berkefeld laboratory-filter." He discusses the possibility of filtrable toxin but concluded that the agent is probably a filtrable virus.

10. REED, Walter. Recent researches concerning the etiology, propagation and prevention of yellow fever, by the United States Army commission, J. Hyg., **2**:101, 1902.

The fruits of the commission's studies were not only an understanding of the transmission of yellow fever but invaluable clues to the control of the disease. In this lecture Reed, after reviewing material already presented in his previous papers, tells how under the efficient management of General Gorgas yellow fever was practically extirpated in Havana in one year. In October, 1900, for example, the epidemic reached a peak of over three hundred cases; in the same month a year later there were only three cases. This amazing result was achieved by quarantine, screening, and mosquito destruction and set the precedent for the final elimination of the disease in civilized communities, as epidemic after epidemic was stamped out and endemic foci were cleared. Gorgas himself (William C. Gorgas, "Sanitation of the tropics with special reference to malaria and yellow fever," J.A.M.A., **52**:1075, 1909) summarized his methods and accomplishments.

A recent authoritative book on all aspects of mosquito control is that of William Brodbeck Herms and Harold Farnsworth Gray, *Mosquito Control* (2d ed.; New York: Commonwealth Foundation, 1944).

11. THOMAS, H. Wolferston. Yellow fever in the chimpanzee, Brit. M.J., **1**:138, 1907.

There was a general belief that man was the only intermediate host of yellow fever; in other words, the cycle was thought to be mosquito—man—mosquito. Thomas was the first to report the infection of a monkey by mosquito bite. A large number of mosquitoes were fed on a yellow fever patient, and 21 days later the survivors were allowed to bite a chimpanzee, who, 27 hours later, developed fever and ran the clinical course of yellow fever. This experiment anticipated the classical studies of Stokes, Bauer, and Hudson (Ref. 15) and also raised the important question of whether animals aside from man could be storehouses of yellow fever virus in nature (Ref. 13). The whole question of various mammalian hosts of yellow fever is discussed in Strode (Ref. 29, pp. 303 ff.).

12. DA ROCHA-LIMA, H. Zur pathologischen Anatomie des Gelbfiebers, Verhandl. d. deutsch. path. Gesellsch., **15**:163, 1912.

Da Rocha-Lima was one of the first to devote a paper exclusively to the anatomical changes of yellow fever. However, as early as 1890, W. T. Councilman, at the instigation of Sternberg, made a report on the histology of yellow fever, with special emphasis on the liver changes (see George M. Sternberg, *Report on the Etiology and Prevention of Yellow Fever* [Washington: Government Printing Office, 1890], p. 151). E. Marchoux and P.-L. Simond ("Études sur la fièvre jaune," Ann. Inst. Pasteur, **20**:161, 1906), among their elaborate studies of yellow fever, have a section on the pathology of the disease, with numerous colored plates. The early studies of Louis (Ref. 2) are also not to be forgotten. For a recent critical discussion of the lesions, with a bibliography, see Strode (Ref. 29, pp. 141 ff.).

13. BALFOUR, Andrew. The wild monkey as a reservoir for the virus of yellow fever, Lancet, **1**:1176, 1914.

Balfour raised the question of whether wild monkeys might not act in some places as a reservoir of yellow fever, on the basis of a story that in a certain part of Trinidad red howler monkeys are said to be found dead and dying in the forest preceding an epidemic of yellow fever. Certain people who went into the woods also acquired yellow fever. Various outbreaks of yellow fever, such as that reported by F. L. Soper, H. Penna, E. Cardoso, J. Serafim, Jr., M. Frobisher, Jr., and J. Pinheiro ("Yellow fever without Aedes aegypti: study of a rural epidemic in the Valle do Chandan, Espírito Santo, Brazil, 1932," Am. J. Hyg., **18**:555, 1933), were obviously not caused by the bite of *Aedes aegypti* and did not occur on the basis of the classical man—mosquito—man cycle. Studies of this sort led to the concept of jungle yellow fever, with a forest or animal—mosquito cycle propagated in remote areas into which man steps only secondarily. It is only in such areas that yellow fever is today endemic. The problem of jungle fever and localities in which foci persist is discussed in detail in Strode (Ref. 29, pp. 463 ff.).

14. NOGUCHI, Hideyo. Etiology of yellow fever. I. Symptomatology and pathological findings of the yellow fever present in Guayaquil, J. Exper. Med., **29**:547, 1919.

The formation of the Rockefeller Foundation Yellow Fever Commission is told in Strode's book (Ref. 29, pp. 14 ff.). Noguchi was a member of the commission, and in this paper and its sequels he announced the cause of yellow fever as a leptospira which he named *Leptospira icteroides*. This claim, of course, turned out to be erroneous, and Noguchi's apologists have stated that he was actually working on Weil's disease, which is easily confused with yellow fever and which is, in fact, caused by a leptospira. A careful scrutiny of the original articles, however, throws doubt on this position. In the present paper, for example, Noguchi describes at length the disease upon which he worked in the Yellow Fever Hospital at Guayaquil; he points out the skill and experience of the personnel, and he lays special stress on the accuracy of the diagnosis. In the second paper ("II. Transmission experiments on yellow fever," *ibid.,* p. 565) he tells how he injected blood from yellow fever patients into many varieties of animals and thought that he had produced a disease analogous to yellow fever in guinea pigs. "In the blood, liver and kidneys of guinea pigs experimentally infected with the blood of yellow fever patients a minute organism was demonstrated. . . . The leptospira obtained from cases of yellow fever has been given the provisional name of Leptospira icteroides." In the next paper ("III. Symptomatology and pathological findings in animals experimentally infected," *ibid.,* p. 585) the experimental disease produced in guinea pigs, dogs, and marmosets by injection of infected material or of pure cultures of the organism is described, but we are not yet told how the pure cultures were obtained. There follow numerous other papers, in which the whole subject becomes more and more confused. In Paper VI ("Cultivation, morphology, virulence and biological properties of Leptospira icteroides," *ibid.,* **30**:13, 1919) isolation of the organism by special culture methods from three of eleven yellow fever patients is reported, and its properties are described. As he found that it passed through Berkefeld filters, Noguchi raised the question of its having a granular phase under certain conditions. Examination of fresh blood from yellow fever patients by the dark-field microscope made in more than 27 cases revealed the presence of *L. icteroides* in three ("VII. Demonstration of Leptospira icteroides in the blood, tissues, and urine of yellow fever patients and of animals experimentally infected with the organism," *ibid.,* p. 87). Finally, in another paper ("IX. Mosquitoes in relation to yellow fever," *ibid.,* p. 401) Noguchi concluded: "The foregoing experiments show that symptoms and lesions closely resembling those of yellow fever in man may be induced in guinea pigs by the bite of female Stegomyias that have previously sucked the blood of a yellow fever patient." Within the next few years more papers by Noguchi appeared, and others also claimed to confirm his work, until Beeuwkes, Stokes, and Bauer and their associates, working on yellow fever in West Africa, completely failed to isolate *Leptospira* from their cases or to reproduce the disease in small animals (Ref. 15). There is an excellent critical review of Noguchi's work in Klotz's De Lamar Lecture (Oscar Klotz, *Yellow Fever in West Africa* [Baltimore: Williams & Wilkins Co., 1928]).

15. STOKES, Adrian, BAUER, J. H., and HUDSON, N. Paul. The transmission of yellow fever to Macacus rhesus: preliminary note, J.A.M.A., **90**:253, 1928.

The authors, working under the West African Yellow Fever Commission of the Rockefeller Foundation, opened the modern era of yellow fever research by showing beyond question that the disease could be regularly transmitted to *M. rhesus* monkeys both by injections of blood from patients and by the bite of infected mosquitoes. The disease could also be passed from monkey to monkey both by blood and by mosquito bite. Mosquitoes were infective 16 days after feeding on an infected animal and remained so until death. Stokes unhappily acquired yellow fever and died before this paper was published.

There shortly appeared by the same authors a full report of their work ("Experimental transmission of yellow fever to laboratory animals," Am. J. Trop. Med., **8**:103, 1928). They showed, in addition, that serum passed through Berkefeld and Seitz filters was infective, although a filtrate of infected mosquitoes macerated in salt solution failed to produce disease. The specific pathological findings in infected monkeys are reported in detail. They also showed that convalescent serum in doses of 0.1 cc. protected monkeys against infection, while 2 cc. of normal human serum failed to protect. Numerous other phases of the subject are discussed.

The circumstances of this epoch-making work are graphically told by Wilbur A. Sawyer, "Recent progress in yellow fever research," Medicine, **10**:509, 1931.

Stokes, Bauer, and Hudson's work was soon confirmed by C. Mathis, A. W. Sellards, and J. Laigret ("Sensibilité du Macacus rhesus au virus de la fièvre jaune," Compt. rend. Acad. d. sc., **186**:604, 1928), who isolated in monkeys at Dakar the famous "French" strain which was much used in later experimental work.

16. BAUER, Johannes H. The transmission of yellow fever by mosquitoes other than Aedes aegypti, Am. J. Trop. Med., **8**:261, 1928.

It had heretofore been thought that *Aedes aegypti* was the only mosquito which could transmit yellow fever. Bauer found in West Africa that "A. luteocephalus and A. africoannulatus transmitted this disease in all respects in the same manner as A. aegypti," thus opening the subject of multiple vectors. A full discussion of the complicated question of arthropod vectors of yellow fever is given in Strode (Ref. 29, pp. 233 ff.).

17. SAWYER, W. A., KITCHEN, S. F., FROBISHER, Martin, Jr., and LLOYD, Wray. The relationship of yellow fever of the Western Hemisphere to that of Africa and to leptospiral jaundice, J. Exper. Med., **51**:493, 1930.

There had been great uncertainty whether "yellow fever" in various localities was the same disease. In South America, for example, Noguchi had isolated a leptospira (Ref. 14) which was not obtainable in West Africa by Stokes and his associates. Sawyer and his associates collected strains of virus from all over the world and, by cross-protection tests, showed that "the yellow fever now in South America, the present yellow fever of Africa and the historic yellow fever of Panama and other American countries are the same disease." They also showed that there was no cross-immunity between yellow fever and leptospiral jaundice.

18. COWDRY, E. C., and KITCHEN, S. F. Intranuclear inclusions in yellow fever, Am. J. Hyg., **11**:227, 1930.

The discovery of intranuclear inclusion bodies of a sort common in diseases due to filtrable viruses was of the greatest importance in the etiologic study of yellow fever. Such bodies were early described by C. M. Torres ("Inclusions nucléaires acidophiles [dégénérescence oxychromatique] dans la foie de Macacus rhesus inoculé avec le virus brésilien de fièvre jaune," Compt. rend. Soc. de biol., **99**:1344, 1928) and by Cowdry and Kitchen ("Intranuclear inclusions in yellow fever," Science, **69**:252, 1929), but the present impressive study is definitive. The inclusions are described in great detail and are illustrated by beautiful plates. They were found both in liver cells of infected monkeys and in human material and are regarded as specific. No signs of any such bodies were found in infected mosquitoes. "In conclusion . . . the nuclear response in yellow fever is of the same general type . . . which occurs in many other virus diseases, especially chickenpox, herpes, virus III disease and submaxillary disease."

19. BAUER, Johannes H., and MAHAFFY, Alexander F. Studies on the filtrability of yellow fever virus, Am. J. Hyg., **12**:175, 1930.

Although Stokes, Bauer, and Hudson (Ref. 15) had reported preliminary experiments on the filtrability of yellow fever virus, their work was incomplete, and Bauer and Mahaffy studied the subject systematically. They found that the virus passed through filters without marked diminution in potency; serum was infective at times in amounts as small as 0.0000001 cc.; the lack of infectivity of a filtrate of mosquitoes ground in salt solution was due to the toxicity of the diluent for the virus; no evidence was found to indicate that virus in blood differed from that in mosquitoes.

20. THEILER, Max. Studies on the action of yellow fever virus in mice, Ann. Trop. Med., **24**:249, 1930.

Although transmission of yellow fever to monkeys was a discovery of the greatest importance, monkeys turned out to be difficult to work with and too costly for extensive use. A smaller animal was necessary. Theiler therefore made a great contribution when he found that yellow fever virus could be established in white mice. It occurred to Theiler to try the intrathecal route; following injection, the animals became sick, and, at autopsy, sections of brain invariably showed an encephalitis and specific nuclear changes. Theiler was able to pass the disease indefinitely through mice in this fashion. Infective mouse brain stored at −8° C. retained its virulence for at least 160 days. He was not able to protect mice successfully by an injection of an immune serum. The mouse virus produced yellow fever in monkeys. Many other details are discussed.

21. BERRY, G. P., and KITCHEN, S. F. Yellow fever accidentally contracted in the laboratory: a study of seven cases, Am. J. Trop. Med., **11**:365, 1931.

In the course of their meticulous studies on "laboratory" yellow fever, Berry and Kitchen, after reviewing the previous literature, report careful counts of the leukocytes. They noted a progressive fall in number from onset to the fifth or sixth day. The counts fell as low as 2,625, the polymorphonuclear neutrophils dropping to levels as low as 500–1,000. From the sixth to eighth days the total leukocyte count increased, soon reaching normal levels.

22. SAWYER, W. A., and LLOYD, Wray. The use of mice in tests of immunity against yellow fever, J. Exper. Med., 54:533, 1931.

The need of a test for immunity to yellow fever had become obvious. Following Theiler, Sawyer and Lloyd developed a workable and reliable protection test in mice. The unknown serum to be tested for its protective power was mixed with yellow fever virus, fixed for mice, and injected intraperitoneally into mice which had been prepared by an intracerebral injection of starch solution. If the serum was protective, the mice remained well; if not, the virus localized in the brain at the site of the starch injection. This test has turned out to be of great value both in research and in epidemiological studies.

23. SAWYER, W. A., KITCHEN, S. F., and LLOYD, Wray. Vaccination against yellow fever with immune serum and virus fixed for mice, J. Exper. Med., 55:945, 1932.

"The method here presented for vaccination against yellow fever was devised primarily to interrupt the long series of accidental infections of persons making laboratory investigations." The writers first review previous unsatisfactory attempts at vaccination and then describe their own method. "After preliminary experiments on monkeys, 15 persons were actively immunized by a single injection of a dried mixture of living yellow fever virus, fixed for mice, and human immune serum, with separate injections of enough additional serum to make up the amount required for protection. . . . Immunity rose in a few weeks to a height comparable to that reached after an attack of yellow fever and remained there through an observation period of 2 months."

24. LLOYD, Wray, THEILER, Max, and RICCI, N. J. Modification of the virulence of yellow fever virus by cultivation in tissues in vitro, Tr. Roy. Soc. Trop. Med. & Hyg., 29:481, 1936.

Although E. Haagen and M. Theiler ("Untersuchungen über das Verhalten des Gelbfiebervirus in der Gewebecultur," Centralbl. f. Bakt., 125:145, 1952) had successfully grown a neurotropic strain of yellow fever virus in a medium of minced chicken embryo tissue and serum-Tyrode solution, no one had succeeded in growing an unmodified pantropic strain. This the authors succeeded in doing during a period of 21 months and through more than 150 subcultures. The complicated technique is described, as well as various antigenic characteristics of the virus and the immunological reactions. A little later Hugh H. Smith and Max Theiler ("The adaptation of unmodified strains of yellow fever virus to cultivation in vitro," J. Exper. Med., 65:801, 1937) succeeded in cultivating yellow fever virus in a medium containing mouse embryo brain tissue.

25. ELMENDORF, John E., Jr., and SMITH, Hugh H. Multiplication of yellow fever virus in the developing chick embryo, Proc. Soc. Exper. Biol. & Med., 36:171, 1937.

The writers were the first successfully to cultivate yellow fever virus in the developing chick embryo. John P. Fox and Hugo W. Laennert, Jr. ("The cultivation of yellow fever virus. II. Observations on the infection of developing chick embryos," Am. J. Hyg., 46:21, 1947), elaborated these observations. With reference to human vaccination they showed that prolonged passage of the 17 D strain did not apparently alter the virus and did not increase neurotropic virulence for monkeys or man.

26. WHITMAN, Loring. The multiplication of the virus of yellow fever in Aëdes aegypti, J. Exper. Med., 66:133, 1937.

After reviewing some older and inconclusive work, the authors showed that, "following an incubation period, titers of virus can be recovered from mosquitoes which are significantly higher than at any preceding time." They concluded that "Aëdes aegypti have been shown to be capable of multiplying the Asibi strain of yellow fever virus in their bodies. Following the ingestion of infected blood, the content of virus falls for several days, reaching a minimum during the first week. It then increases rapidly until quantities of virus greater than those previously encountered can be demonstrated." At about the same time L. Whitman and P. C. A. Antunes ("Studies on Aëdes aegypti infected in the larval stage with the virus of yellow fever," Proc. Soc. Exper. Biol. & Med., 37:664, 1938) showed that "Aëdes aegypti can be infected in the larval stage with the virus of yellow fever, providing they are exposed to large quantities of virus. The resultant adults, both male and female, are infected."

27. THEILER, Max, and SMITH, Hugh H. The use of yellow fever virus modified by in vitro cultivation for human immunization, J. Exper. Med., 65:787, 1937.

Using a strain of yellow fever virus modified by prolonged cultivation, the authors vaccinated human beings without the simultaneous injection of immune serum. Eight normal persons were used, with minimal reactions, and their sera 2–4 weeks after inoculation showed the presence of yellow fever antibodies. H. H. Smith, H. A. Penna, and A. Paoliella ("Yellow fever vaccination with cultured virus [17 D] without immune serum," Am. J. Trop. Med., 18:437, 1938) grew the virus in chick embryos and prepared a vaccine which they used on a large scale with good results. G. M. Findlay and F. O. MacCallum ("Note on acute hepatitis and yellow fever immunization," Tr. Roy. Soc. Trop. Med. & Hyg., 31:297, 1937) were the first to report a considerable number of instances of acute hepatitis following yellow fever vaccine; they came to no definite conclusions as to cause. With the occurrence of many cases of acute hepatitis following mass vaccination in the United States Army, W. A. Sawyer, K. F. Meyer, M. D. Eaton, J. H. Bauer, Persis Putnam, and F. F. Schwentker ("Jaundice in army personnel in the western region of the United States and its relation to vaccination against yellow fever," Am. J. Hyg., 39:337, 1944; 40:35, 1945) took up the subject in earnest and issued a report on their elaborate studies: "The most plausible hypothesis as to the source and nature of the icterogenic agent was that it had been introduced into the vaccine in human blood serum secured from supposedly normal donors and used in manufacture of the vaccine, that the agent was most probably an unknown filtrable virus capable of causing disease in man."

The whole story of induced immunity to yellow fever is told in Strode (Ref. 29, pp. 203 ff.).

28. PICKELS, Edward G., and BAUER, Johannes H. Ultrafiltration studies of yellow fever virus, J. Exper. Med., **71**:703, 1940.

The writers already knew the approximate size of the virus particles from observations made in previous ultrafiltration studies (J. H. Bauer and T. P. Hughes, "Ultrafiltration studies with yellow fever virus," Am. J. Hyg., **21**:101, 1935). In the present study they observed, in the ultracentrifuge by optical methods, the behavior of yellow fever virus particles directly in the unaltered serum from infected monkeys and were able to estimate the size of the particles to be between 12 and 19 mμ. For a detailed discussion of the physical and chemical properties of the virus see Strode (Ref. 29, pp. 46 ff.).

29. STRODE, George K. (ed.). Yellow fever. New York: McGraw-Hill Book Co., 1951.

An impressive compilation dealing with all phases of yellow fever, with a comprehensive bibliography. An invaluable reference book.

HERPES ZOSTER

HERPES ZOSTER

MUCH of the bibliography of herpes zoster is concerned with the relation of the disease to other vesicular dermatoses, especially chickenpox. This puzzling question is not yet entirely settled, although it appears from the literature that there must be a close relation between, if not an identity of, the causal agents. Thorough modern discussions of the whole problem of chickenpox and zoster with bibliography are to be found in the recent book by Harvey Blank and Geoffrey Rake, *Viral and Rickettsial Diseases of the Skin, Eye and Mucous Membranes of Man* (Boston: Little, Brown & Co., 1955) (p. 71), and in the article by J. Stokes, "Varicella–herpes zoster group" in T. M. Rivers (ed.), *Viral and Rickettsial Infections of Man* (2d ed.; Philadelphia: J. B. Lippincott Co., 1952) (p. 506). R. Doerr's review ("Ergebnisse der neueren experimentellen Forschungen über die Ätiologie des Herpes simplex und des Zoster," Zentralbl. f. Haut- u. Geschlechtskr., **15**:1, 1924) covers the experimental side to date, whereas the monumental review by W. Schönfeld ("Zoster," in *Handbuch der Haut und Geschlechtskrankheiten* [1928], Vol. **7**, Part I) reviews the entire literature to 1928, including a section on the history of the disease.

1. CHARCOT. Note sur quelques cas d'affection de la peau dépendent d'une influence du système nerveux. Obs. III. Névralgie consécutive à une lésion traumatique et accompagnée d'une éruption de vésicules d'herpes, J. de physiol. de l'homme et des animaux, **2**:111, 1859.

There is a huge literature on "secondary" herpes: herpes following the use of certain drugs such as arsenic, following fevers, with lymphatic leukemia, with malignancy of various sorts, and following trauma. Charcot reports an early case after an injury. There has been in the modern literature, which is reviewed by J. Klauder ("Herpes zoster appearing after trauma," J.A.M.A., **134**:245, 1947), much dispute as to the relation of trauma to viral infection in certain cases of zoster.

2. VON BÄRENSPRUNG, [Felix]. Die Gürtelkrankheit, Ann. d. Charité-Krankenhaus, **9**:40, 1861.

The modern study of herpes zoster may be said to begin with this classical paper, or rather monograph, since it occupies ninety pages. After a historical introduction and an account of the origin of the term "herpes," Von Bärensprung gives a systematic discussion of the topography of the lesions based on cases he had actually observed. "From the beginning of my medical studies I have noted all cases which I have seen and have sketched many of them." He insists on the unilateral occurrence of the eruption and gives detailed case reports with graphic sketches of the areas involved. These are followed by a clinical analysis. Fever was noted in only 5 of 65 cases. The eruption is described as a sequence of erythema, papule, and vesicle. "The slightly alkaline content of the vesicles is a light serum without solids; later it becomes milky as the white cellular layer becomes emulsified in it; very rarely it becomes purulent. Scab formation between the fifth and eighth days . . . after the separation

of scabs red scars remain which later become pale and usually leave no trace."
In most cases the disorder is painless except for slight burning. But sometimes
"the patients complain of severe burning which they liken to red-hoat coals; it
increases with warmth, prevents sleep, and the slightest touch causes pain."
Von Bärensprung remarks that the pain may be severe, with a very small area
of eruption, and in other cases the pain spreads not only through the affected
area but through "neighboring nerve domains." Pain often precedes the eruption by a shorter or longer time and remains with great severity long after healing. As to etiology: "Zoster is an inflammation of the skin of typical form and
course, the essential peculiarity of which is that it appears to be confined to the
peripheral domain of cerebral and spinal nerves or their branches. . . . The
eruption has a noteworthy correspondence with the distribution of the nerves
of the skin: these facts justify the conclusion that the cause of the inflammation
is not carried in from the surface or by way of the blood, but rather through
the nerves themselves." The distribution of the eruption rules out a central
source. By exclusion, he finally settled on the posterior nerve roots as the source
of the disease, or, more specifically, the posterior root ganglia, in which he
thought that sympathetic fibers coursed. Of the exact nature of the irritation of
the ganglia and nerves which led to zoster Von Bärensprung had no idea. Treatment stood much the same as today; there was no effective remedy, but he
emphasized the importance of protecting and not interfering with the vesicles.

This monograph is a model of good organization, accurate description, and
keen reasoning; with few exceptions, what is said stands today. Von Bärensprung's paper excited great interest in the subject, and descriptions of cases
seen by others and reported to him are detailed in another paper ("Fernere
Beiträge zur Kentniss des Zoster," *ibid.*, **10**:37, 1862).

3. VON BÄRENSPRUNG. Beiträge zur Kenntniss des Zoster (Dritte Folge),
   Ann. d. Charité-Krankenhaus, **11**:96, 1863.

Von Bärensprung reiterated his views that the posterior root ganglia were the
site of the initial trouble in herpes zoster. He went wrong, however, in thinking
that the ganglia had a system of special nerve fibers of their own which had no
connection with the fibers of the posterior root and of the peripheral nerve. An
autopsy on a baby with herpes who died of pulmonary tuberculosis confirmed
Von Bärensprung's ideas about the site of the disease. "One was struck by the
increased thickness and redness of the sixth, seventh, and eighth nerves, especially the seventh, which seemed to depend on swelling, with dilated and tortu-
ous vessels running through the neurilemma. . . . The spinal ganglia belonging
to these three nerves were adherent to the wall of the intervertebral canal; the
connective tissue here also was reddened and thickened so that the volume of
the ganglion seemed increased. . . . The microscope also disclosed indubitable
residuals of inflammation. . . . The autopsy showed then what we expected in
advance, that in zoster one was not concerned with a destructive process but
with a mild reversible change. . . . It seems of special interest that the inflammation of the ganglion does not extend along the posterior root to the cord, but
only in the peripheral direction." Thus he thought the findings indicated an inflammation in the substance of the ganglion and not just in the neurilemma.
While his interpretation was not altogether correct, he deserves credit for first
clearly stating the relation of the eruption to the spinal ganglia.

4. HUTCHINSON, Jonathan. A clinical report on herpes zoster frontalis seu ophthalmicus (shingles affecting the forehead and nose), Ophthal. Hosp. Rep., **5**:191, 1866.

Hutchinson refers to a few previous isolated case reports, but he was the first to deal systematically with the subject. The disease is thought to be rare and is probably often misdiagnosed erysipelas. "Herpes frontalis is always limited to one side, never transgresses the median line of the forehead and nose. It never affects the cheek, although there may be some sympathetic edema of the part. There can be little doubt that the local processes of inflammation in the skin and eyes are produced directly through the medium of the nerves, in this instance of the ophthalmic division of the fifth." There are eighteen detailed case reports.

5. [LANDOUZY]. Fièvre zoster et exanthèmes zostériformes (leçon receuillie par M. le docteur H. Jonas, chef de clinique), Semaine méd., **3**:245, 1883.

Landouzy seems to have been the first to insist in emphatic terms on the infectious nature of zoster. Aside from fever and occurrence in epidemics, he stressed the fact that only infectious diseases confer immunity against further attacks. He concludes: "(*a*) zoster is an acute disease, almost cyclic, infectious, conferring immunity, a generalized disease . . . an infectious neuropathy with secondary cutaneous dystrophy; (*b*) zoster is a generalized disease like scarlatina. There is a zoster fever as there is a scarlatinal fever, zosteriform eruptions as there are scarlatiniform exanthems."

6. HEAD, Henry, and CAMPBELL, A. W. The pathology of herpes zoster and its bearing on sensory localization, Brain, **23**:353, 1900.

This is the classical article in which, on the basis of herpetic eruptions, the peripheral distribution of the sensory roots was worked out by Head and Campbell; the diagrams here first published are the ones familiar to every student in his textbooks for the next fifty years. Head and Campbell first review the literature on the pathology of zoster and point out that since Von Bärensprung (Ref. 3) there had been only five adequately reported autopsies. To these Head and Campbell added twenty-one.

Next is a general discussion of the pathology of zoster. It is pointed out that, at the height of the eruption, "the affected ganglion will be found to be in a condition of profound inflammation. The interstitial tissue will be crowded with small round cells which stain deeply with methylene blue and other nuclear dyes. . . . If these foci of inflammatory cells are examined in several sections they will occasionally be found to be situated around extravasated blood. . . . In the centre of these haemorrhagic foci the ganglion cells are absolutely destroyed . . . ultimately the focus of inflammation becomes converted into fibrous tissue and the density and extent of this scar depend on the severity and extent of the original inflammation." Corresponding to the affection of the ganglia, Head and Campbell demonstrated degeneration in the posterior roots, "and it is probable that this degeneration begins to make its appearance ten days after the appearance of the eruption." The changes consisted of "an acute degeneration followed by a greater or less amount of secondary sclerosis according to the severity of the acute destruction. The anterior root was in all cases normal." There were also degenerative changes in the fibers that entered the posterior root ganglia, as well as acute degeneration in the posterior columns of the spinal cord. These lesions are all beautifully pictured in colored drawings, micro-photographs, and diagrams. Special sections are devoted to zoster of the trigeminal nerve, zoster secondary to implication of the ganglion in general disease processes, and zoster arising in the course of diseases of the nervous system. As to changes in the skin, "Sections through an unruptured vesicle of herpes zoster show a cavity, the floor of which is formed of naked papillae. These papillae are in a condition of profound inflammation and are infiltrated with masses of small round cells which stain deeply. . . . The vesicle is split into incomplete cavities by septa extending from the roof to the floor. These septa are evidently the remains of incompletely-raised epithelial layers that retain their attachment to the roof and to the floor of the vesicle . . . microscopic examination of the fluid and careful staining of the sections of the skin failed to reveal any sign of micro-organisms. . . . The lymphatic glands enlarge and frequently become tender very early in the disease." Head and Campbell regarded zoster as an acute specific disease, analogous to lobar pneumonia. They commented on its occurrence at times in epidemics, the rarity of second attacks, and the analogy to anterior poliomyelitis. "Of the nature of the agent which is responsible for this process we are completely ignorant. Microscopically, we have not been able to find any signs of bacterial infection. . . . The unknown agent responsible for the inflammation in the ganglion not only shows a specific attraction for the posterior root ganglia but commonly attacks one ganglion only. This selection of one group of cells is also partly characteristic of the poison that causes anterior poliomyelitis. . . . But if the case be seen before the rash appears it is sometimes possible to map out the area subsequently occupied by the eruption by means of the hyperalgesia that is present. This hyperalgesia . . . is followed by erythema. Then, on the erythematous surface, vesicles appear."

The remainder of the study consists of meticulous comparisons of the skin areas involved with the lesions in the dorsal roots at autopsy. On the basis of these observations were mapped the classical "Head's zones," which are illustrated by detailed diagrams.

7. CHAUFFARD, A., and FROIN, G. Nature, évolution et durée de la réaction méningée dans la zona, Bull. et mém. Soc. méd. d. hôp. de Paris, **19**:994, 1902.

Although changes in the spinal fluid in herpes zoster had been noted before, Chauffard and Froin seem to have been the first to recognize them as indicative of an encephalitis. "One must admit that there is a toxi-infectious impregnation of the entire neuraxis when one sees an ophthalmic zona accompanied by such an intense lymphocytosis in the spinal fluid; it is quite comparable in its morphology to that which gives rise to the most characteristic spinal infectious processes such as tuberculous meningitis, tabes, or general paralysis." Later C. I. Schiff and W. Russell Brain ("Acute meningo-encephalitis associated with herpes zoster," Lancet, **2**:70, 1930) reviewed the literature and reported a fatal case of their own. He not only died of acute meningoencephalitis but showed aberrant herpes vesicles and apparently transmitted varicella to his son.

8. HUNT, J. Ramsay. On herpetic inflammations of the geniculate ganglion: a new syndrome and its complications; J. Nerv. & Ment. Dis., **34**:73, 1907.

P. Strübing ("Herpes zoster und Lähmungen motorischer Nerven," Deutsches Arch. f. klin. Med., **37**:513, 1885) reviews the older literature and reports a case in which herpes was associated with facial paralysis. O. Körner ("Ueber den Herpes zoster oticus [Herpes an der Ohrmusckel mit Lähmung des Nervus acusticus und des Nervus facialis]," München. med. Wchnschr., **51**:6, 1904) carried the subject further, but Hunt is generally recognized as having written definitively insofar as he related the cases to lesions of the geniculate ganglion. He divided the clinical syndrome into three groups: "(1) Herpes zoster auricularis. (2) Herpes zoster in any of the zoster zones of the cephalic extremity (herpes auricularis, herpes facialis, and herpes occipito-collaris) with facial palsy. (3) Herpes zoster of the cephalic extremity with facial palsy and auditory symptoms (tinnitus, deafness, vertigo, vomiting, nystagmus, and disturbances of equilibrium)."

9. WEBER, F. Parkes. Two cases of herpes zoster associated with a generalized eruption of varicella-like spots: one of the cases followed by oculomotor paresis, mydriasis, and frontal anesthesia, Brit. J. Dermat., **28**:13, 1916.

Parkes Weber, that master of the reporting of rare cases, discusses the whole subject of generalized vesicular eruptions with herpes zoster, with a thorough review of the literature. It appears that the question of generalized eruptions as a modified form of varicella did not arise until after Von Bókay's paper (Ref. 11). At any rate, leukemia seems to predispose both to local herpes and to generalized eruptions.

10. LIPSCHÜTZ, B. Untersuchungen über die Aetiologie der Krankheiten der Herpesgruppe (Herpes zoster, Herpes genitalis, Herpes febrilis), Arch. f. Dermat. u. Syph., **136**:428, 1921.

Lipschütz seems to have been the first to demonstrate, by special stains, inclusion bodies in the cells at the site of the eruption of herpes. He concluded that these bodies were derived from "autochthonous nuclear substance" and were the expression of a specific cellular or nuclear reaction to the virus of herpes zoster. He thus definitely departed from previous views that such bodies were parasites. He inclined to a filtrable virus as the cause and quoted Rist as saying as long ago as 1904: "Perhaps we are concerned with one of those microbes called invisible which have been demonstrated in molluscum contagiosum, etc."[1] In four of seven attempts he produced a keratitis in the rabbit cornea with material from herpes zoster, with characteristic inclusion bodies. He later stated that herpes zoster could be transmitted only "occasionally," in contrast to herpes genitalis and herpes labialis which would "take" on the rabbit cornea in approximately 100 per cent of the cases. Lipschütz felt that he had demonstrated that the "infection" was not only in the central nervous system but in the skin lesions, which many had thought were "trophic" in nature. R. Cole and A. Kuttner ("The problem of the etiology of herpes zoster," J. Exper. Med.,

---

[1] E. Rist in article "Zona" in E. Besnier, L. Brocq, and L. Jacquet, *La Pratique dermatologique* (Paris: Masson et Cie, 1904), **4**:920.

42:799, 1925) critically analyze the literature, pro and con, on transmission of herpes to animals and come up with a verdict of "not proved." Their own carefully performed experiments, in which they repeated Lipschütz' inoculation of the rabbit's cornea, all turned out negative. Nor were they able to produce evidence of herpes in monkeys. Direct inoculation into the central nervous system was negative, and so was intra-testicular inoculation of rabbits. S. Seidenberg ("Untersuchungen über das Herpes- und Zostervirus," Ztschr. f. Hyg. u. Infectionskr., **112**:134, 1931), using modern techniques, was also unable to produce a reaction in the rabbit's cornea with material from zoster vesicles, although corneas treated in this way did not become immune to inoculation with herpes simplex material. W. J. Cheatham ("The relation of heretofore unreported lesions to pathogenesis of herpes zoster," Am. J. Path., **29**:401, 1953) later described inclusion bodies in the dorsal root ganglia and elsewhere scattered widely through the body.

11. V. BÓKAY, Johann. Ueber die Herpes-zoster-Varizellen-Frage, Jahrb. f. Kinderh., **105**:8, 1924.

Von Bókay tells how in 1888 he saw a child who had typical herpes zoster, and 10 days later another child in the family developed chickenpox. Soon after, he saw a similar sequence of events in another family. These observations so strongly suggested a relation between chickenpox and herpes that, in a paper written in 1909 (J. V. Bókay, "Ueber den ätiologischen Zusammenhang der Varizellen mit gewisser Fällen von Herpes zoster," Wien. klin. Wchnschr., **22**:1323, 1909), he said: "Varicella virus as a result of unknown circumstances can call forth, instead of a general eruption, a typical zoster, and, from the zoster, varicella is transferred to other individuals." Suggestive observations by others are also reviewed. He added (1924): "Naturally I invoked the varicella etiology only in a portion of the zoster cases." He later saw varicella occur in a patient with zoster, and now (1924) he analyzed the whole literature in a somewhat nostalgic way and reported further relationships. He concluded: "I described the fundamentals of the clinical picture of Herpes zoster varicellosis 35 years ago at the beginning of my career, and I feel happy now in old age that in the course of time the disease picture built up by me has been accepted by the 'specialists' at home and abroad. Furthermore, our previous concepts of zoster have not been altered by the Zoster varicellosis described by me, since it has, of course, been known for a long time that zoster does not comprise an etiologically uniform disease." Von Bókay's thesis received support by Bruusgaard's inoculation experiments (Ref. 12) and by the work of E. Paschen ("2. Elmentarkörperchen im Bläscheninhalt bei Herpes zoster und Varizellen," Centralbl. f. Bakt., **130**:190, 1933), who demonstrated, in the vesicle fluid of zoster, elementary bodies similar in appearance to those found in varicella. Paschen's observations were confirmed by C. R. Amies ("The elementary bodies of zoster and the serological relationship to those of varicella," Brit. J. Exper. Path., **15**:314, 1934), who showed that "pure suspensions of these bodies prepared by high-speed centrifugalization of zoster vesicle fluid, are specifically agglutinated by zoster convalescent sera" and that "attempts to demonstrate the relationship of zoster and varicella by means of cross agglutination tests have met with a fair measure of success." The final link is perhaps forged by the similarity in appearance of the viruses of chickenpox and herpes in the electron microscope (Ref. 14). H. Blank and G. Rake (*op. cit.*, p. 71) sum the matter up, by saying: "It is believed that there is now sufficient evidence to consider chickenpox (varicella) and zoster (herpes zoster, shingles, zona) as different clinical manifestations of infections with the same virus." However, certain discrepancies still exist which are analyzed by J. Stokes in his article, "Varicella–herpes zoster group," in Rivers (*op. cit.*, pp. 509 ff.). It has been pointed out, for example, that zoster is non-contagious, whereas varicella is highly communicable; that a leukopenia with relative mononucleosis is the rule in chickenpox but not in zoster; that both chickenpox and zoster confer immunity against a second attack of the same disease but not against each other. Useful epidemiological observations in the relation of the two diseases are given in the report of the School Epidemics Committee, *Epidemics in Schools* ("Medical Research Council Special Report Series," No. 227 [1938]), page 181.

12. KUNDRATITZ, Karl. Experimentelle Übertragungen von Herpes zoster auf Menschen und die Beziehungen von Herpes zoster zu Varicellen, Ztschr. f. Kinderh., **39**:379, 1925.

Kundratitz points out that no one so far has succeeded in transmitting herpes zoster to man. He inoculated fluid from herpes vesicles into the arms of children by scarification, and concluded: "The inoculation of herpes zoster vesicle fluid from person to person in childhood up to 5 years of age has definitely been successful. Thereby the infectiousness of herpes zoster for man and the presence of the virus in the vesicle fluid has been unimpeachably demonstrated." Detailed protocols are given. At the point of vaccination, after about 9 or 10 days, small vesicles appeared which had the apperance of chickenpox vesicles. Vaccinations of children who had had chickenpox did not take. He interpreted these findings as in favor of the identity of the viruses of herpes and varicella. Kundratitz' work was confirmed by E. Bruusgaard ("The mutual relation between zoster and varicella," Brit. J. Dermat., **44**:1, 1932), who succeeded in producing a varicella-like eruption in children by vaccination with fluid from herpes vesicles.

13. GOODPASTURE, Ernest W., and ANDERSON, Katherine. Infection of human skin, grafted on the chorioallantois of chick embryos, with the virus of herpes zoster, Am. J. Path., **20**:447, 1944.

E. W. Goodpasture, B. Douglas, and K. Anderson ("A study of human skin grafted upon the chorioallantois of chick embryos," J. Exper. Med., **68**:891, 1938) had previously developed a method of transplanting human skin into chick embryos. Such transplants were now inoculated with fluid from zoster vesicles and "were successfully infected with the virus of herpes zoster. The experimental lesions did not vesiculate grossly but became pustular, and otherwise remembled those in the natural disease, including the presence of intranuclear acidophilic inclusions, first described by Lipschütz [Ref. 10] in the affected epithelial cells." This work was confirmed by H. Blank, L. L. Coriell, and T. F. McN. Scott ("Human skin grafted upon the chorioallantois of the chick embryo for virus cultivation," Proc. Soc. Exper. Biol. & Med., **69**:341,

1948). They used human prepuce as a source of epidermis and added penicillin and streptomycin to obviate most bacterial contaminations. Chicken embryo tissues themselves seemed non-susceptible.

14. RAKE, G., BLANK, H., CORIELL, L. L., NAGLER, F. P. O., and SCOTT, T. F. McN. The relationship of varicella and herpes zoster: electron microscope studies, J. Bact., **56**:293, 1948.

In zoster vesicle fluid collected 24–144 hours after the first appearance of the vesicle the authors found it hard to demonstrate viral bodies by means of the electron microscope. However, in a specimen withdrawn only 12 hours after the appearance of the vesicles, elementary bodies were plentiful, although 48 hours later most of the particles had disappeared. The bodies closely resembled those previously described by F. P. O. Nagler and G. Rake ("The use of the electron microscope in diagnosis of variola, vaccinia and varicella," J. Bact., **55**:45, 1948) in varicella. Average measurement was 196 by 218 mμ, about 8 per cent smaller than those seen in chickenpox. In another case of zoster, fluid was examined that apparently initiated an outbreak of varicella. Scanty but characteristic brick-shaped bodies were found in both the zoster and the varicella fluids. Here, then, is further evidence of the relationship of zoster and varicella viruses.

15. CARTER, A. Barbeau. Investigation into the effects of aureomycin and chloramphenicol in herpes zoster, Brit. M.J., **1**:987, 1951.

Carter made a systematic study of the spinal fluid in zoster in 44 cases; the fluid was abnormal in 14, of which 10 were of the ophthalmic type. The protein was as high as 210 mg., and the cells as many as 62 soon after the eruption; in some cases the fluid was still abnormal after 3 weeks or more. These observations were made in the course of a study of antibiotics in zoster, which, incidentally, yielded no beneficial effects. However, as long ago as 1901, Brissaud and Sicard ("Cytologie du liquide céphalo-rachidien au cours du zona thoracique," Bull. et mém. Soc. méd. d. hôp. de Paris, **18**:260, 1901) found in two cases of zoster an increase in mononuclear cells in the fluid. The entire literature to 1928 is reviewed in Schönfeld (*op. cit.*, p. 30). All observers agreed that changes in the fluid did not occur in every case of zoster. "They are to be looked upon as secondary, that is, as expressions of the extension of the inflammatory process to surrounding areas (*ibid.*).

Clinical	Refs. 1, 2, 4
Complement-fixation tests	Ref. 14
Epidemiology	Refs. 2, 8, 13
Experimental mumps	Refs. 7, 10, 11
General	Refs. 1, 2, 4
Immunity	Refs. 11, 14
Incubation period	Ref. 3
Neurological complications	Refs. 1, 6
Orchitis	Ref. 5
Pancreatitis	Ref. 9
Pathology	Refs. 5, 12, 21
Prophylaxis	Refs. 15, 17
Virus, cultivation, measurement, etc.	Refs. 16, 18, 19, 21

ALTHOUGH mumps is thought of as a relatively insignificant disease, it boasts of a surprisingly prolific literature. Until the 1930's, clinical and epidemiological questions were especially pursued, but, following the work of Johnson and Goodpasture (Refs. 10, 11, 12) and the development of modern technical methods, mumps has served as a topic for endless study along virological lines.

As to general accounts and bibliographies, the book of Comby is to be specially mentioned.[1] Perhaps the best comprehensive treatise is the one by H. Schottmüller, *Parotitis epidemica* (Vienna: Alfred Hölder, 1904), which deals with every phase of the disease to date and contains a selected bibliography of 176 titles. C. Wesselhoeft's discussion ("Mumps: its glandular and neurologic manifestations," in J. E. Gordon *et al.*, *Virus and Rickettsial Diseases* [Cambridge, Mass.: Harvard University Press, 1940], p. 309) carries the subject further with a more modern bibliography, and John F. Enders' authoritative article on "Mumps" in T. M. Rivers, *Viral and Rickettsial Infections of Man* (2d ed.; Philadelphia: J. B. Lippincott Co., 1952), page 512, brings the subject up to date. An excellent chapter on mumps, with special emphasis on recent virological and immunological work, is to be found in C. E. Van Rooyen and A. J. Rhodes, *Virus Diseases of Man* (New York: Thomas Nelson & Sons, 1948).

1. HAMILTON, Robert. An account of a distemper by the common people of England vulgarly called the mumps, Trans. Roy. Soc. Edinburgh, 2:59, 1790.

Hamilton is much quoted as early insisting on the contagiousness of the mumps. In this account, however, he makes no direct claim but simply says: "The mumps made its appearance in an epidemic form at Lynn in 1758. . . . Two companies of the Norfolk regiment of militia were quartered here. . . . It raged more among these soldiers in proportion to their numbers than amongst the inhabitants of the town." However, Hamilton refers to a work by Dr. Russel, who "thinks it contagious," and he also states that "people are not liable to have this disease more than once."

Hamilton gives a detailed and brilliant description of the clinical features: "A lassitude, a heaviness, a general restless uneasiness, not easily described, are perceived several days before the swelling which characterises the disease, begins to appear. These disagreeable feelings are attended with gentle rigors, and some degree of fever, which being slight, is commonly disregarded. Then a stiffness, with obtuse pain, is felt in one or both sides of the articulation of the lower jaw, impeding its motion and of course mastication; which symptoms

---

[1] J. Comby, *Les Oreillons* (Paris, 1893). We have been unable to see a copy of this much-quoted book. It is not in the Lane Medical Library, the copy in the Army Medical Library is unavailable, nor is it among the holdings of the New York Academy of Medicine.

increasing, a swelling appears upon the parts the following day, and quickly extends to the parotid glands, the neighboring skin, and cellular membrane. Here, in some, it stops without discolouring the skin; and, by keeping the parts moderately warm, and cautiously avoiding the cold external air, the patient is soon freed from it, without any medical assistance. But, when this is not the case, the parts affected generally redden the next day, the tumor becomes more diffused, and sometimes increases so suddenly in size, that, on the third day from its first appearance, it occupies the salivary glands and surrounding cellular membrane on that side; and, if both sides are affected, the parts are so much swelled, and the tumor descends so low, that the countenance is rendered of a frightful enormous magnitude; and now deglutition becomes more or less impeded. All this is frequently without much pain; but most commonly there is now a great deal, and a considerable degree of fever. When this happens, the countenance appears florid, and a dusky erysipelatous inflammation covers the tumor, which is deepest in colour where there is the greatest hardness, viz. on the parotid and maxillary glands. In many subjects here it ends. And it seems probable from the natural resolution of the disease, which now immediately follows, that the tumor has attained its greatest magnitude, and the distemper its acmé; for, about the morning of the fourth day from the first appearance of the swelling, a discharge begins from the emunctories behind the ears; a dew-like sweat, frequently in large drops, issues from every pore of the extended surface of the tumor; a gentle diaphoresis covers the body, if in bed; the inflammation abates, the swelling gradually lessens, and, with these favourable circumstances, the fever goes off, and the distemper totally disappears about the fifth day, if nature is not interrupted in her business. But if the tumor subsides suddenly about the fourth day, and one or both testicles begin to swell, sometimes with much pain, heat, inflammation, new rigors, and a fresh exacerbation of fever, much is to be apprehended from this new morbid appearance, and much circumspection is required in the treatment of it. For the means employed by nature to promote the resolution of the tumified testes, are exactly similar to those which take place in the termination of the tumors below the ears; a spontaneous discharge issues from the skin of the parts affected, and, if this is copious and continued, and accompanied with a free perspiration from the surface of the whole body in bed, the disease ends happily without farther trouble; but if it is scanty, partial, or interrupted by accidental cold or imprudent treatment, the tumors of the testicles subside suddenly, the patient becomes restless, a fresh exacerbation of fever insues, the head is affected, delirium follows, with convulsions and other dreadful symptoms, and sometimes death closes the scene."

Hamilton observed swelling of the testicles followed by atrophy, but it is a question whether or not he described true neurological complications. "On the day following this, the testicles were found lessened in size, and the patient was become restless, delirious, and with much fever." He gradually recovered. Another case, a man of twenty-two, is mentioned: "The catastrophe was dreadful: For the swelled testicles subsided suddenly the next day, the patient was seized with a most frantic delirium, the nervous system was shattered with strong convulsions, and he died raving mad the third day after."

2. DUNCAN, Andrew. Report presented to the Royal College of Physicians of Edinburgh respecting the contagious epidemic diseases which have prevailed in that city and its neighborhood during the year 1810, etc., Edinburgh M.J., 7:431, 1811.

That mumps was long recognized as occurring in epidemics is clear from the name "epidemic parotitis." Hirsch ("Parotitis polymorpha" in *Handbuch der historisch-geographischen Pathologie* [Erlangen: Ferdinand Enke, 1862], p. 182) has done us the service of collecting in tabular form references to a great number of outbreaks from 1714 to 1859. One or two of these may be mentioned as examples. Duncan reports on an epidemic in Edinburgh in 1810: "About the beginning of the year, the most remarkable epidemic which I saw . . . was the cynanche parotidea of Dr. Cullen; a disease which . . . is generally known in England by the name of mumps. . . . That this disease arises only from a peculiar and specific contagion . . . can, I think, admit of no doubt. This was clearly demonstrated during the present epidemic. For after it was introduced into some schools, it affected almost all the children attending them." He noted that in this epidemic the disease was confined to children, and he observed no instance of the swelling of the neck "being accompanied or followed by swelling of the testis."

But by no means everyone considered the disease contagious. Andrew Hammersley ("Observations on cynanche parotidea, as it occurred in the New-York State Prison during the winters of 1821 and 1822," M. Repository, N.S., 7:413, 1822), the resident physician at the prison, for example, described a sudden outbreak of eighty cases between December 8, 1821, and February 5, 1822. These cases were, of course, in adults and in eleven instances the salivary gland swelling was accompanied or succeeded by an affection of one or both testes and in six more cases one or both testes were involved "independent of any stiffness or tumour of the jaw. . . . Thus were it not that these cases occurred during the rage of this epidemic . . . and a recollection of this so common metastasis, we should have been without the diagnostic mark of the complaint." As to contagion, he concluded: "Indeed, from a survey of every thing connected with this interesting malady as it occurred at the State Prison, the idea of specific contagion can hardly be entertained."

These two reports illustrate the common occurrence of mumps in closed institutions, such as schools, jails, and military installations (see also Ref. 8).

3. LEITZEN, E. Angina parotidea, J. d. pract. Heilk., 86:101, 1838.

In describing an outbreak of mumps in an orphan asylum, it was noted that six cases appeared in the last four days of April. Among some students who were in contact with these patients, the first case of mumps did not appear until May 16, after an interval of about 18 days, which corresponds well with modern average estimates of the incubation period (Ref. 13). F. Roth ("Ueber die Incubation und Uebertragbarkeit der Parotitis epidemica," München. med. Wchnschr., 33:345, 1886) reviews the older reports on the incubation period and describes a case in which a doctor in contact with mumps made daily visits to a patient who came down after 18 days with the disease, although the doctor himself remained well. Roth reports this as a case of indirect transmission. As to the period of contagion of mumps, Rendu ("De la période de contagiosité des oreillons," Bull. et mém. Soc. méd. d. hôp. de Paris, **10**:107, 1893) was fortunate enough to observe two patients with mumps whose only exposure to others was in the 48 hours before the onset of clinical symptoms. Antony ("Oreillons: quelques considérations sur leur contagiosité et leur évolution, Bull. et mém. Soc. méd. d. hôp. de Paris, **10**: 150, 1893) from a study of mumps in an army camp also concluded that the disease was most communicable during the incubation period, although it was also "transmissible after healing for an as yet indeterminate period."

4. TROUSSEAU, A. Clinique médicale de l'Hôtel-Dieu de Paris, **1**:218, "Mumps (oreillons)." Paris: J.-B. Baillière et fils, 1861.

Trousseau describes the disease in his usual precise and masterful fashion. He differentiates mumps from "parotiditis": "They are essentially different affections. One is an inflammation of the gland, of the cellular tissue which is a component of it, and this inflammation, which occurs during the course of severe fevers in general, may and does frequently go on to suppuration. The other . . . never terminated with suppuration. Furthermore while parotiditis generally affects only one side, in mumps the two sides are implicated, one, it is true, a little before the other." Thus he clearly differentiated mumps from suppurative parotitis, a condition common at the time and often confused with mumps. "Mumps are a specific disease with many resemblances to the eruptive fevers. Like them specific, like them actively contagious, they attack usually the young, although they attack at times adults or the aged." Then comes a brief vivid description of the familiar clinical features, with a discussion of metastases in men to testes, epididymis, and tunica vaginalis; in females to the breast or sometimes the labia. "Mumps are then characterized by a swelling of the parotid glands; I will add of the salivary glands in general because the submaxillary and sublingual are often affected. They manifest themselves by a bruise-like pain which the patient refers to the parotid region, by difficulty in chewing partly from pain and partly from suppression of salivary secretion, which obliges him to drink incessantly while eating. The swelling of the affected parts is more or less considerable; sometimes it extends to the neck, invades the face in a manner to disfigure the patient, at other times the swelling extends to the tonsils and adjacent regions and leads to difficulty in swallowing."

Another excellent early description of the disease is that of Gustav Joseph ("Bemerkungen über die vom Januar bis März 1864 epidemischen genuinen Ohrspeicheldrüsenerkrankungen," Berl. klin. Wchnschr., **1**:297, 1864). He concluded that, on the whole, the disease was contagious, although he was puzzled by the fact that no mumps occurred in children when, "after examination of the oral cavity, he examined the mouths of other healthy children without washing the fingers which were introduced." He thought that the opening of Steno's duct was the portal of entry.

5. LAVERAN, A. Du diagnostic et de la prophylaxie des oreillons chez l'adulte et en particulier de l'orchite ourlienne, Bull. et mém. Soc. méd. d. hôp. de Paris, **15**:61, 1879 (Séance de 10 mai 1878).

Although the occurrence of orchitis with mumps had been known since Hippocrates, this article by Laveran is one of the first modern accounts. Laveran reviews the older literature on the frequency and incidence of mumps orchitis, discusses the nature of the condition, and describes cases beginning with orchitis without overt parotitis. "The swellings of the salivary glands and of the testicles develop under the influence of the same causes, under the influence of the same morbid principle which spares sometimes the testicles and sometimes the salivary glands, which finally can act on other glandular tissues such as the breast, ovary, and prostate. Orchitis is a manifestation of mumps of the same category as the swelling of the salivary glands." Final proof of this statement had to wait until fifty years later, when E. W. Hook, Jr., S. O. Poole, and W. F. Friedewald ("Virus isolation and serological studies on patients with clinical mumps," J. Infect. Dis., **84**:236, 1949) isolated the virus of mumps from material obtained by orchidotomy inoculated into the amniotic sac of eight-day-old embryonated hen's eggs. Laveran discussed in detail the question of postorchitic atrophy and believed it usually to be associated with loss of libido and potentia. He was convinced that mumps was contagious and, as a preventive measure, advocated immediate isolation of any cases in a special hospital ward.

Further authoritative discussions on mumps orchitis are to be found in Comby (*loc. cit.*) and in Schottmüller (*loc. cit.*). C. Wesselhoeft ("Orchitis in mumps," Boston M. & S.J., **183**:425, 458, 491, 520, 1920) gives a comprehensive review of every phase of the subject, with an extensive bibliography, as does A. Stengel, Jr. ("Mumps orchitis," Am. J.M. Sc., **191**:340, 1936). Stengel gives in tabular form the incidence of orchitis in mumps as set down by various observers. The figures run all the way from 13.9 to 100 per cent. In most of the large series, however, the incidence was not over 20 per cent.

As to the lesion in mumps orchitis, E. A. Gall ("The histopathology of acute mumps orchitis," Am. J. Path., **23**:637, 1947) obtained bits of tissue during the course of orchidotomy in a large number of acute cases, on the basis of which the histopathology is described. Gall found considerable variation in the character and extent of the lesion, but at its height the process consisted of "a diffuse lymphocytic infiltration of the interstitial tissue with focal hemorrhages and pronounced destruction of germinal epithelium." He reviews the few cases reported in the literature, most of which dealt with late lesions appearing in chronic orchitis. However, G. G. Smith ("Two cases of orchitis due to mumps treated by operation," Boston M. & S.J., **167**:323, 1912), as long ago as 1912, obtained biopsy specimens from two patients in the early days of mumps orchitis. Grossly, the testicles were greatly enlarged and appeared intensely inflamed. Histological examination by Dr. S. Burt Wolbach was in accord with that reported by Gall.

6. LANNOIS, M., and LEMOINE, G. Des manifestations méningitiques et cérébrales des oreillons, Arch. de neurol., **11**:1, 1886.

Cerebral manifestations with mumps had long been recognized. Hamilton (Ref. 1) is credited with first reporting a death because of a cerebral accident, but the account leaves one in doubt as to just what happened. Lannois and Lemoine review other early case reports, which are all unsatisfactory because, of course, there was no lumbar puncture nor was there any autopsy. They point out that mumps must be regarded not as a local affection of the parotid but as a generalized infection implicating not only salivary glands but also testes, vulva, breast, joints, heart, eye, and ear. "One would be surprised if under these conditions the brain and its coverings remained protected." They report a number of cases with meningeal symptoms, with paralyses or aphasia, and they regard the lesion as a meningoencephalitis. G. N. Ackers ("Parotitis complicated with meningitis," Am. J. Dis. Child., **6**:399, 1913) reviewed the subject in 1913 and reported 2 cases but had no idea of a viral etiology, nor did R. L. Haden ("The cerebral complications of mumps," Arch. Int. Med., **23**:737, 1919), who observed 9 cases in an army camp among 476 patients admitted to hospital for mumps. E. M. Holden, A. Y. Eagles, and J. E. Stevens ("Mumps involvement of the central nervous system," J.A.M.A., **131**:382, 1946), also from an army camp but in World War II, deliberately sought, by clinical scrutiny and lumbar puncture, for evidence of meningoencephalitis in 100 consecutive cases of mumps. "Thirty-three cases showed clinical signs of meningoencephalitis; 28 of these showed abnormal spinal fluid." J. W. Brown, H. B. Kirkland, and G. E. Hein ("Central nervous system involvement during mumps," Am. J.M. Sc., **215**:434, 1948) obtained similar results and remark: "It seems reasonable to believe that every patient with mumps is subject to the neurotropic effects of this virus." Indeed, L. W. Kane and J. F. Enders ("Immunity in mumps. III. The complement fixation test as an aid in the diagnosis of mumps meningoencephalitis," J. Exper. Med., **81**:137, 1945) have shown that acute aseptic meningoencephalitis in patients with no clinical evidence of mumps may be due to the specific agent of mumps. Earlier literature on this point is summarized by Wesselhoeft (*op. cit.*, p. 324). C. B. McKaig and H. W. Woltman ("Neurologic complication of epidemic parotitis," Arch. Neurol. & Psychiat., **31**:794, 1934) in a useful paper summarize, with literature, the various types of lesion which may occur; these they classify as myelitis, psychiatric disorders, meningitis, encephalitis, neuritis, neuro-ophthalmic complications, and complications affecting the eighth nerve. As to lesions, V. de Lavergne, P. Kissel, and H. Accoyer ("Les Bases anatomopathologiques de la névraxite ourlienne," Ann. méd., **42**:327, 1937) were able to find autopsy reports of only 12 fatal cases with cerebral complications of mumps. No uniform lesion was described. These authors thought that they were able to produce cerebral lesions in rabbits, as did M. Wollstein ("Experimental mumps meningitis," J. Exper. Med., **34**:537, 1921). Wollstein injected filtered mouth washings from children with mumps into the subarachnoid space of cats and obtained a transient reaction, with evidences of inflammation and an increase of *polynuclear* cells and globulin. One is not convinced of a true mumps encephalitis. W. L. Donohue ("The pathology of mumps encephalitis," J. Pediat., **19**:42, 1941) again reviewed the subject and reported a case. He concluded that the fundamental lesion was a perivascular demyelinization similar to that seen in other postinfection encephalitides. Mumps virus was first claimed to be isolated from spinal fluid through monkey inoculation by A. Swan and J. Mawson ("Experimental mumps: transmission of the disease to monkeys; attempts to propagate the virus in developing hen's eggs," Australian M.J., **1**:411, 1943) and by G. Henle and C. L. McDougall ("Mumps meningo-encephalitis. Isolation in chick embryos of virus from spinal fluid of a patient," Proc. Soc. Exper. Biol. & Med., **66**:209, 1947) through egg culture. Recent literature on the subject is reviewed by Gordon and Kilham (Ref. 13).

7. WOLLSTEIN, Martha. An experimental study of mumps. J. Exper. Med., **23**:353, 1916.

As was the case with most viral infections, they were at first attributed to ordinary bacteria. Wollstein refers to the early bacteriological studies in mumps and to the claims made for various cocci which different observers isolated from mumps cases. As recently as 1919, Russell Haden, a careful worker ("The bacteriology of mumps: report of findings at Camp Lee," Am. J.M. Sc., **158**:698, 1919), concluded that "mumps is probably caused by a gram-positive diplococcus and not by a filterable virus." He had isolated this coccus from blood, spinal fluid, and lymph nodes of patients with mumps and had produced orchitis in rabbits by injection of cultures. And yet his conclusions are now shown to be erroneous. S. Granata ("Sulle etiologia degli orecchioni da virus filtrable," Med. ital. Napoli, **6**:647, 672, 1908) seems to have been the first to consider seriously a filtrable agent as the cause of mumps, but his experiments on rabbits with filtrates of saliva seem inconclusive. C. Nicolle and E. Conseil ("Essai de réproduction expérimentale des oreillons chez le singe," Compt. rend. Acad. d. sc., **157**:340, 1913) inoculated material aspirated from the parotid glands of patients with mumps into the parotids of three monkeys. They produced a reaction, but "the disease is ordinarily reduced in the animal to a fever of 4 to 7 days' duration, the general symptoms are slight or absent, and swelling of the parotid is usually undetectable." Wollstein was then the first to make a serious systematic study of the effects of filtrates. Mouth washings from patients with mumps were filtered through Berkefeld candles and injected into the parotid glands and testes of cats. After 6 or 7 days, tenderness and swelling appeared in the inoculated areas, lasting in the parotid 2–5 days, in the testis 10–14 days. The leukocytes rose markedly. Wollstein was also able to transmit the disease from cat to cat. Control experiments were negative. Histologically, "the most marked changes appeared coincidently with the third and fourth transfers. In some examples, the glands showed infiltration of the interlobular connective tissue with mononuclear and a few polynuclear cells in addition to the edema. . . . The epithelium of the acini was swollen and cloudy in these instances." There were also constant changes in the testis. Wollstein did not claim in this paper, however, that she had reproduced mumps but said: "Whether this active material is a microorganism and if so whether it is the specific microbic cause of parotitis or mumps, remains to be ascertained." In a later paper ("A further study of epidemic parotitis," J. Exper. Med., **28**:377, 1918) Wollstein used material from adults (soldiers) and obtained the same results. "The 'virus' of parotitis was detected most readily in the saliva during the first 3 days of the disease, less easily on the 6th day, and not at all on the 9th day. It was detected also in the blood of patients who showed marked constitutional symptoms, and in the saliva of a case of recurrent mumps at the period of enlargement of the parotid glands. . . . It was not detected in the cerebrospinal fluid." Finally, Wollstein published a summary of all her work ("An experimental study of parotitis," J.A.M.A., **71**:639, 1918).

8. RADIN, M. J. The epidemic of mumps at Camp Wheeler, October 1917–March 1918, Arch. Int. Med., **22**:354, 1918.

We have already alluded to outbreaks of mumps in closed groups (Ref. 2), but this tendency was exquisitely shown during World War I by the tremendous epidemics which occurred in recruits assembled at some of the army cantonments. In the outbreak here described, among approximately 18,000 men there were 5,756 cases, an incidence of 32 per cent. At the peak of the epidemic, as many as 140 soldiers with mumps were admitted to hospital on one day. The writer and his associates made many important observations. Suppuration occurred in only one case, and that was questionable. Among 4,397 cases there were 611, or 13.91 per cent, with orchitis. Fourteen cases of a symptom complex of nausea and anorexia with pain and tenderness in the epigastrium were interpreted as pancreatitis. It is of interest that in this huge series no cases of encephalitis are mentioned. The writer failed to grow an organism from puncture material of the parotid gland. Interesting statistics of all sorts are presented. In World War II also there was trouble with mumps (H. C. McGuiness and E. A. Gall, "Mumps at army camps in 1943," War Med., **5**:95, 1944), and the subject is also reviewed by C. Wesselhoeft and C. F. Walcott ("Mumps as a military disease and its control," War Med., **2**:213, 1942).

9. SIMONIN. La Pancréatite ourlienne: étude clinique, Bull. et mém. Soc. méd. d. hôp. de Paris, **20**:928, 1903.

Pancreatitis in association with mumps had been vaguely talked about from the beginning of the nineteenth century, and the early papers with possible bearing on the subject are listed by L. W. Farnam ("Pancreatitis following mumps: report of a case with operation," Am. J.M. Sc., **163**:859, 1922). Cuche ("Localisation de l'infection ourlienne sur le pancréas," Bull. et mém. Soc. méd. d. hôp. de Paris, **14**:340, 1897) is given credit for arousing modern interest in the subject, but his paper is simply a brief note stating that he had observed tenderness on pressure in the epigastrium 20 times in 26 cases of mumps. Simonin goes further and reports in detail 10 cases of mumps with severe epigastric pain (*douleur pancréatique*) and tenderness, often with fever and prostration, which he interpreted, not unreasonably, as pancreatitis. G. H. Lemoine and F. Lapasset ("Un cas de pancréatite ourlienne avec autopsie," Bull. et mém. Soc. méd. d. hôp. de Paris, **22**:640, 1905) report a case in which pancreatitis was confirmed at autopsy, and in Farnam's patients pancreatitis was found at laparotomy. The whole subject is reviewed by Wesselhoeft (*op. cit.*, p. 321).

10. JOHNSON, Claud D., and GOODPASTURE, Ernest W. An investigation of the etiology of mumps, J. Exper. Med., **59**:1, 1934.

Johnson and Goodpasture review the literature on attempts to establish the etiology of mumps (see Ref. 7), and they conclude: "One gains no conviction that anyone has unquestionably succeeded in inducing mumps experimentally or has demonstrated the true etiological agent of this disease." They then describe their own, now classical, experiments, in which they definitely reproduced mumps in monkeys by injection of unfiltered saliva from mumps patients in the early stages directly into the parotid ducts. "The infectious agent which we have obtained from the saliva of patients in the early stages of mumps presents characteristics of a filterable, cytotropic virus having a predilection for the parenchymal cells of the parotid glands of *rhesus* monkeys. The virus is free of demonstrable micro-organisms; it is filterable and resistant to drying and glycerination; it causes a lesion which is primarily a degeneration and necrosis of the parenchymal cells of the parotid; and it confers immunity to reinoculation. . . . There is good evidence, we consider, that this virus is the cause of mumps. . . . The clinical disease induced in *M. rhesus* monkeys . . . is analogous to mumps in the human being. The histology of the parotitis of human mumps is as yet undetermined, but the lesions of the experimental disease are quite comparable to those found in the specific orchitis of mumps." In order to prove the matter "to the hilt," Johnson and Goodpasture ("The etiology of mumps," Am. J. Hyg., **21**:46, 1935) attempted to produce the disease in human volunteers by introducing into the buccal cavity virus which had been carried through fourteen successive generations in monkeys. "The success of the experiment recorded in this paper in inducing typical clinical mumps in six, and questionable mumps in three, out of a total of 13 presumably susceptible persons is to us conclusive evidence that we are dealing with the true causative agent. . . . The incubation period varied from 18 days, which is the average incubation period . . . to 33 days. . . . The disease was characterized by the unilateral or bilateral enlargement of the parotid glands with pain and swelling of the face over the gland, and a mild fever. The saliva from a typical case was recovered, and with it the experimental disease in monkeys was reproduced. . . . The secret of success seems to have been the injection of large amounts of material directly into Stenson's duct."

G. M. Findlay and L. P. Clarke ("The experimental production of mumps in monkeys," Brit. J. Exper. Path., **15**:309, 1934) soon confirmed this work and found that injection of the virus into the tunica vaginalis of monkeys caused a non-suppurative orchitis. Mice, rats, and guinea pigs inoculated intracerebrally did not develop any symptoms. C. Levaditi, R. Martin, A. Bonnefoi, and R. Schoen reported similar results ("Contribution à l'étude étiologique des oreillons," Bull. Acad. de méd., Paris, **114**:251, 1935).

11. JOHNSON, Claud D., and GOODPASTURE, Ernest W. Experimental immunity to the virus of mumps in monkeys, Am. J. Hyg., **23**:329, 1936.

A. F. Hess ("A protective therapy for mumps," Am. J. Dis. Child., **10**:99, 1915) appears to have been the first to attempt the prevention of mumps by passive immunization—the injection into susceptibles of human convalescent serum. Among seventeen "susceptible" children who were exposed to mumps, no case of the disease occurred following 6–8 cc. of whole blood. L. H. Barenberg and J. Ostroff ("Use of human blood in protection against mumps," Am. J. Dis. Child., **42**:1109, 1931) had somewhat less good results—39 per cent incidence among the untreated against 15 per cent among those who received treatment. They also thought that mumps was markedly attenuated by this form of serotherapy. Cambesédès ("L'Emploi du sérum de convalescents dans les oreillons," Ann. d'hyg. pub., N.S., **11**:83, 1933) also reports the use of convalescent serum as a useful prophylactic.

Johnson and Goodpasture subjected the question to more exact experimental trial with mumps produced in monkeys. First of all, they found that "attempts to confer passive immunity to intraparotid infection by injections of serum from persons immune to mumps have with rare exceptions failed." Overt infections, however, seemed to confer an invariable immunity to a second attack. There was also evidence that subclinical infection conferred immunity. All this supports the clinical experience that a definite attack of mumps renders a person resistant to a second attack.

12. JOHNSON, C. D., and GOODPASTURE, E. W. The histopathology of experimental mumps in the monkey, *Macacus rhesus,* Am. J. Path., **12**:495, 1936.

Since patients very rarely die from mumps, there has been little opportunity to study the pathology of the lesions. Johnson and Goodpasture give a critical review of the scattered observations in the literature on the changes in the parotid. They construct a composite picture from these reports of necrosis of glandular epithelium, desquamation of epithelial cells, with serous and cellular infiltration. Next they made careful gross and histological studies of the experimental lesions in monkeys. "The essential lesion is the result of a specific action of mumps virus on acinar epithelial cells in focal areas resulting in degeneration and necrosis of the affected cells. The inflammatory cellular response is secondary to the specific injury and consists of an infiltration of the area by mononuclear phagocytic cells and later by various types of lymphocites. . . . Inclusions are described in the affected epithelial cells, and they are interpreted as specific."

13. GORDON, John E., and HEEREN, Ralph K. The epidemiology of mumps, Am. J.M. Sc., **200**:412, 1940.

In this valuable review, all phases of the subject—pathogenesis, spread of virus, carriers, mode of transmission, portal of entry, period of infectiousness, communicability, immunity, mortality rates, and other matters—are discussed, with bibliography. The subject is brought up to date by a further review (J. E. Gordon and L. Kilham, "Ten years in the epidemiology of mumps," Am. J.M. Sc., **218**:338, 1949), in which special stress is placed on the newer laboratory aids.

14. ENDERS, John F., and COHEN, Sidney. Detection of antibody by complement-fixation in sera of man and monkey convalescent from mumps, Proc. Soc. Exper. Biol. & Med., **50**:180, 1942.

The appearance of outbreaks of mumps in the armed forces in World War II, together with the development of new techniques of virus study, led to a tremendous burst of work on the disease. The huge and, for the most part, highly technical literature on the subject is not suitable for detailed notice in this bibliography. However, we have tried to select papers in which a new development is described or in which an outstanding advance in knowledge is made.

Enders and Cohen were the first to develop a complement-fixation test for mumps. Using Goodpasture's technique, they produced mumps in monkeys. As antigen for complement fixation, they used suspensions of ground-up monkey parotid glands excised at the height of the disease. "It is evident, however, that the extensive application of the test will depend upon the discovery of a more readily available and cheaper source of antigen." Nonetheless, within 3–5 days following the acute stage, a high titer of complement-fixing antibody was present. After a month or so the titer declined but then appeared to remain constant for months. Enders ("Observations on immunity in mumps," Ann. Int. Med., **18**:1015, 1943) described the results of complement-fixation tests in greater detail. In tests of humans, antibody occurred in about 92 per cent of the sera of those giving a positive history of mumps. But 50 per cent of the sera from people who gave no history of mumps was also positive. This the writers interpret as evidence of the frequency of inapparent or "silent" infection. On the other hand, it was concluded that most of those who gave a negative reaction were susceptible.

The significance of the complement-fixation test was further elaborated by E. P. Maris, J. F. Enders, J. F. Stokes, Jr., and L. W. Kane ("Immunity in mumps. IV. The correlation of the presence of complement-fixing antibody and resistance to mumps in human beings," J. Exper. Med., **84**:323, 1946), who showed that "with very rare exceptions individuals giving positive complement fixation tests for mumps are resistant to infection by natural exposure" and that a positive complement fixation indicates previous infection with this virus. The complexity of the subject is revealed, however, by the later work of G. Henle, G. Harris, and W. Henle ("The reactivity of various human sera with mumps complement fixation antigens," J. Exper. Med., **88**:133, 1948), who found that there are two serologically distinct complement-fixing antigens against which antibodies arise at different times.

Using suspensions of infected parotid, Enders also developed a skin test. At the site of injection "in nearly 100 per cent of those giving a history of mumps, an erythematous reaction occurred after 24 to 48 hours. . . . The group giving no history of mumps revealed about equal numbers of negative and positive reactors." Both these tests were subsequently investigated for rapid determination of susceptibility or immunity to mumps, so important in epidemiological problems. Thus details of the significance of the skin test were worked out by J. F. Enders, L. W. Kane, E. P. Maris, and J. Stokes, Jr. ("Immunity in mumps. V. The correlation of the presence of dermal hypersensitivity and resistance to mumps," J. Exper. Med., **84**:341, 1946) and by G. Henle *et al.* ("Studies on the prevention of mumps. I. The determination of susceptibility," J. Immunol., **66**:535, 1951). They showed that clinically inapparent infections were frequent and conferred immunity as well as an overt attack.

An interesting and authoritative review of the immunological problems of mumps is that of J. F. Enders ("Mumps: technique of laboratory diagnosis, tests for susceptibility, and experiments on specific prophylaxis," J. Pediat., **29**:129, 1946).

15. GELLIS, S. S., McGUINNESS, A. C., and PETERS, M. A study on the prevention of mumps orchitis by gamma globulin, Am. J.M. Sc., **210**:661, 1945.

Little, if anything, is available in the way of therapy for established mumps other than symptomatic measures. Gellis and co-workers have obtained suggestive evidence that convalescent human gamma globulin in doses of 20 cc. reduced the incidence of orchitis from 27.4 to 7.8 per cent. Normal serum gamma globulin, however, in 50-cc. doses was not followed by a reduction in incidence.

16. HABEL, Karl. Cultivation of mumps virus in the developing chick embryo and its application to the studies of immunity to mumps in man, Pub. Health Rep., **60**:201, 1945.

Habel, using an emulsion of parotid glands from monkeys infected with mumps (Ref. 10) inoculated the yolk sac, the amniotic sac, and the allantoic sac of chick embryos. He succeeded in growing virus in all these situations, as tested by monkey inoculation, complement-fixation tests, and neutralization tests. The chick embryo virus turned out to be a suitable antigen for complement fixation and for human skin testing. J. H. Levens and J. F. Enders ("The hemagglutinative properties of amniotic fluid from embryonated eggs infected with mumps virus," Science, **102**:117, 1945) soon confirmed Habel's work; they were unable to demonstrate antigen in the yolk sac, although it was present in other tissues. They also showed that the amniotic fluid of infected eggs agglutinated fowl red cells in a manner analogous to influenza and other viruses, a reaction most useful for rapid diagnosis of mumps; thus hemagglutination is inhibited by the sera of man and monkey convalescent from mumps. W. I. B. Beveridge, P. E. Lind, and S. G. Anderson ("Mumps. I. Isolation and cultivation of the virus in the chick embryo," Australian J. Exper. Biol. & M. Sc., **24**:15, 1946) in the following year reported successful growth in the chick embryo after either yolk-sac or amniotic inoculation of human saliva from patients early in the course of mumps. G. R. Leymaster and T. G. Ward ("Direct isolation of mumps virus in chick embryos," Proc. Soc. Exper. Biol. & Med., **65**:346, 1947), using fresh saliva treated with penicillin and streptomycin, were able to infect directly the amniotic sac of chick embryos with material from eight of nine patients with mumps.

Aside from the monkey (Ref. 10), the chick embryo seems to be the only animal which has so far been found susceptible to mumps.

17. STOKES, J., ENDERS, J. F., MARIS, E., and KANE, L. W. Immunity in mumps. VI. Experiments on the vaccination of human beings with formolized mumps virus, J. Exper. Med., **84**:407, 1946.

In certain situations, such as assemblies of young soldiers in camps, or in schools, it seems of the utmost importance to prevent the spread of mumps. To this end the writers experimented with attempts to produce active immunity in susceptible people by vaccination with (killed) formol-inactivated mumps virus. They concluded that this procedure led to increased resistance in about 50 per cent of children. K. Habel ("Vaccination of human beings against mumps; vaccine administered at the start of an epidemic. I. Incidence and severity of mumps in vaccinated and control groups," Am. J. Hyg., **54**:295, 1951; "II. Effect of vaccination upon the epidemic," *ibid.*, p. 312), using formolized infected allantoic fluid, vaccinated a large number of individuals in army camps. He concluded that "vaccination at the beginning of an epidemic in a highly susceptible population caused a reduction in the incidence of mumps." Also the mumps seemed less severe in the vaccinated, and there was less tendency toward orchitis. He also thought that there was evidence that vaccination controlled the severity of an incipient epidemic of mumps. It was found by J. F. Enders *et al.* ("Attenuation of virulence with retention of antigenicity of mumps virus after passage in the embryonated egg," J. Immunol., **54**:283, 1946) that, by repeated passages in the embryonated egg, mumps virus had lost the capacity to produce parotitis in monkeys, although it still immunized the animal against a subsequent inoculation with virulent virus. It also seemed incapable of producing mumps in susceptible humans when sprayed into the oral cavity. G. Henle *et al.* ("Studies on the prevention of mumps. IV. The effect of oral spraying of attenuated virus," J. Immunol., **66**:579, 1951) also felt that oral spraying of children with active attenuated mumps virus probably produced active immunity as measured by the appearance of antibodies and by clinical exposure.

Thus real progress seems to be in the making.

18. WEIL, M. L., BEARD, Dorothy, SHARP, D. G., and BEARD, J. W. Purification and sedimentation and electron micrographic characters of the mumps virus, Proc. Soc. Exper. Biol. & Med., **68**:309, 1948.

The writers measured particle size of mumps virus in the electron microscope. The great variations in size are well shown in their photographs. "The shape of the formolized virus was judged to be spherical and flattened." Electron micrographic images have a diameter of 190 ± 42 mμ. I. M. Dawson and W. J. Elford ("The investigation of influenza and related viruses in the electron microscope, by a new technique," J. Gen. Microbiol., **3**:298, 1949), using a method in which virus is adsorbed on the membranes of laked fowl red cells for examination in the electron microscope, got a value for mumps virus size of 179 ± 28. Thus mumps virus evidently is relatively large.

19. KILHAM, L. Isolation of mumps virus from the blood of a patient, Proc. Soc. Exper. Biol. & Med., **69**:99, 1948.

Kilham was the first to make a plausible claim of having isolated mumps virus from circulating blood. "Virus of mumps was isolated from blood of a patient with bilateral parotid swelling, through cultivation in embryonated eggs. Inhibition of hemagglutination and complement fixation tests confirmed the clinical diagnosis and identified the agent as mumps virus." A very small quantity of plasma sufficed. This finding strongly supports the view that mumps is primarily a general infection, with localization in various situations.

20. MORGAN, H. R., ENDERS, J. F., and WAGLEY, P. F. A hemolysin associated with the mumps virus, J. Exper. Med., **88**:503, 1948.

Levens and Enders in unpublished experiments had noticed hemolysis of suspensions of chicken erythrocytes exposed to amniotic or allantoic fluids derived from chick embryos infected with mumps virus. The present paper gives the results of systematic studies of this hemolytic factor. The hemolysin is specific and is inhibited by serum of man and monkey convalescent from mumps. Many other features are discussed.

21. HENLE, G., DEINHARDT, F., and GUARDI, A. Cytolytic effects of mumps virus in tissue cultures of epithelial cells, Proc. Soc. Exper. Biol. & Med., **87**:386, 1954.

Johnson and Goodpasture (Ref. 12) had noted, years previously, that mumps virus produced necrosis of parotid epithelium. The present writers, using cultures of HeLa or monkey kidney epithelial cells inoculated with mumps virus, produced interesting effects, which they regarded as cytolytic. "Cytolysis was specifically prevented by human mumps convalescent and postvaccination sera."

WHOOPING COUGH

WHOOPING COUGH

IN THE concluding section of Volume 1 of this bibliography, we have taken the liberty of discussing pertussis as a disease of unknown etiology, since there are a number of facts which throw an element of doubt on the Bordet-Gengou organism as the sole cause of the disease. These are as follows: (1) the isolation in tremendous numbers of other organisms from cases of pertussis, as noted by Jochmann and Krause (Ref. 3); (2) Bordet and Gengou's arbitrary dismissal of all other claims (Ref. 5); (3) the confused state of immunity reactions, which apparently concern the Bordet bacillus but do not rule out another agent; (4) the solid immunity and the frequency in early childhood suggest a virus disease; (5) the inclusion bodies of McCordock and others which suggest a virus disease (Ref. 9); (6) the occurrence of interstitial pneumonia and of encephalitis resembling those seen in viral diseases such as influenza and measles; (7) it seems improbable that one hemophilic bacillus (*B. influenzae*) should be a notable secondary invader, whereas another rather similar organism should be a highly specific pathogen; (8) until 1921, equally consistent claims were made for *B. influenzae* as the cause of influenza. F. G. Blake, T. M. Rivers, and J. G. Small ("The etiology of influenza," in *Epidemic Respiratory Disease* [St. Louis: C. V. Mosby, 1921], chap. i), representing general opinion in America, say: "Consideration of all the evidence available makes it seem highly probable that B. influenzae is the specific etiological agent of epidemic influenza." Blake and Cecil (Ref. 6) later thought that they had produced influenza in monkeys by inoculation with the bacillus.

In favor of the Bordet-Gengou bacillus as the cause of whooping cough are (1) its frequent presence in the sputum in large numbers, especially in early cases; (2) its presence among the cilia in the respiratory tract (Ref. 7); (3) the reproduction of a disease apparently identical with pertussis in man in monkeys (Ref. 10); and (4) the protection against the disease conferred by vaccination (Ref. 11).

The reader may make his choice; we have tried to review the literature in an unbiased way.

The classical textbook account of the disease is that of Georg Sticker (*Der Keuchhusten* [Vienna: Alfred Hölder, 1896]), written just before the discovery of the Bordet-Gengou bacillus and containing an extensive bibliography of older references. The standard modern treatise is J. H. Lapin's book *Whooping Cough* (Springfield, Ill.: Charles C Thomas, 1943), which has chapters on every phase of the disease with extensive bibliographies; finally, one should mention the chapter by Louis W. Sauer, "Whooping cough," in Brennemann's *Practice of Pediatrics*, ed. McQuarrie (Hagerstown: W. F. Prior, n.d.), chapter 34, as a good brief review of the subject.

1. WATT, Robert. Treatise on the history, nature and treatment of chin-cough. Glasgow: John Smith & Son, 1813.

While whooping cough has been recognized for hundreds of years, even relatively recent accounts are of little value. Thus as late as 1769, John Millar's account (*Observations on the Asthma and on the Hooping Cough* [London: T. Cadel, 1769]) leans heavily on humoral doctrines, although there is a good clinical description of the disease. Robert Watt wrote one of the first books on the subject, saying in justification: "The disease, in fact, has been very generally abandoned by the profession and left, as Willis observes, to the management of old women and quacks." Watt regarded whooping cough as contagious. "The chincough is a highly infectious disease, and seems always to arise from a specific contagion" (p. 25). Predisposition, immunity to second attacks, and relation to climate and season are next discussed, followed by an accurate and detailed clinical analysis. "There is hardly any disease for which Chincough can be mistaken." As to confusion with asthma, "the one proceeds from a specific contagion, and occurs only once in the same individual. The other is often an hereditary disease, often proceeds from ordinary causes, and when it does appear, it is apt to continue for life. The one is a disease, as we have seen, almost peculiar to the ages below puberty, while the other seldom occurs till manhood, and most generally, indeed, not till the decline of life, and sometimes not till old age" (p. 76). Several cases are reported with autopsies. The first two, Robert Watt and Janet Watt, are evidently the author's children; at autopsy what was clearly bronchopneumonia was the outstanding finding. The long section on therapy is hardly worth reviewing; numerous medicines and treatments are described in contemporary fashion—opium, cantharides, asafoetida, hemlock, castor, oil of amber, etc.

2. EDMONSTONE, Henry. Brief outline of a plan for diminishing the prevalence and fatal tendency of hooping-cough, Edinburgh M. & S.J., **7**:16, 1811.

"The mortality which hooping-cough produces among the children of the country, is a perpetual source of sorrow and anxiety to all classes of the community . . . in many of those who escape the immediate effect [death], it lays the foundation of complaints that prove equally destructive, or it induces a predisposition to pulmonary affections, which otherwise might never have existed. . . . I would therefore propose, that persons affected . . . should wear some conspicuous article of dress, by which they might be easily discerned at a distance, and an opportunity, by that means, offered to all who might be so inclined, of keeping beyond the sphere of contagion. A red hat, cap or ribbon, for example might be worn for this purpose. . . . I appeal, therefore, with confidence, to parents, guardians . . . to give it their support."

3. JOCHMANN, Georg, and KRAUSE, Paul. Zur Aetiologie des Keuchhustens, Ztschr. f. Hyg. u. Infectionskr., **36**:193, 1901.

The writers first review numerous claims for various bacteria as the cause of whooping cough. Those dealing with Protozoa or cocci need not detain us, but, in view of the work of Bordet and Gengou (Ref. 5), some of those dealing with bacilli require analysis. Carl Burger ("Der Keuchhustenpilz," Berl. klin. Wchnschr., **20**:7, 1883) as early as 1883 described the presence of a tiny bacillus in enormous numbers in the sputa of whooping-cough patients. It was not found in other conditions. E. Czaplewski and R. Hensel ("Bacteriologische Untersuchungen bei Keuchhusten," Deutsche med. Wchnschr., **23**:586, 1897) examined fresh sputum brought up during a paroxysm of coughing in early cases of whooping cough in an epidemic at Königsberg. They found small rods with rounded ends in huge numbers in thirty consecutive cases. The bacteria resembled influenza bacilli but grew without addition of blood to the medium. No lesions were produced in animals. "By the constant finding [of these bacilli] we are forced to the conclusion that the bacterium in question is the cause of whooping cough. . . . We believe that Burger described our bacilli." H. Koplik ("The bacteriology of pertussis," Bull. Johns Hopkins Hosp., **9**:79, 1898), in pure culture from the sputa of early cases of whooping cough, also obtained a small bacillus which grew without hemoglobin and produced no lesions in animals. Without making any out-and-out claims as to etiology, Koplik says: "What significance can we attribute to the bacterium which is the theme of this paper? I doubt whether this can be solved except by direct experiment on the human subject." Jochmann and Krause themselves found three varieties of bacteria resembling influenza bacilli in size and shape in the sputa of early whooping-cough cases. One variety, obtained in eighteen cases, was Gram-negative and grew only on blood agar in "dewdrop" colonies. This organism was often present in tremendous (*massenhaften*) numbers in direct smears. In fatal cases the organism was found in pure culture in bronchopneumonic foci. Jochmann and Krause named this organism *Bacillus pertussis* Eppendorf.

Here, then, are a few examples of the findings of various bacteriologists who obtained more or less pure growths of small influenza-like bacilli from whooping cough. Since these were obviously not all the same, the only possible conclusion is that whooping cough paves the way for a tremendous invasion by a group of bacteria which have some resemblances among themselves and all of which are somewhat similar to influenza bacilli. Since it is now known that the influenza bacilli are only secondary invaders in influenza on a soil prepared by a virus infection, the question is naturally raised whether the same state of affairs does not exist in pertussis. This thought is especially pertinent in view of the widespread belief that the bacillus of Bordet and Gengou is the cause of whooping cough (Ref. 5).

4. NEURATH, Rudolph. Die nervösen Komplicationen und Nachkrank-heiten des Keuchhustens, Arb. a. d. neurol. Inst. an d. Wiener Univ., **11**:258, 1904.

This monograph of over a hundred pages deals with every phase of the neuro-logical complications and sequels of whooping cough. Convulsions, meningitis, cerebral palsies, psychic disturbances, sensory disturbances, spinal cord affec-tions, and polyneuritis are all discussed in detail, with an elaborate review of the literature and a long bibliography. The writer thinks that hemorrhage from increased venous pressure is most important, but the perivascular cuffing with round cells described in a number of his own autopsies raises the question of virus encephalitis.

5. BORDET, J., and GENGOU, O. Le Microbe de la coqueluche, Ann. Inst. Pasteur, **20**:731, 1906.

The authors point out that for twenty years others have made claims of having isolated the causal organism of whooping cough. But none of these claims has been confirmed. By paying attention to obtaining material for study early in the disease and expectorated from the depths of the lung during a paroxysm of cough, Bordet and Gengou were able to "find, in considerable quantity the microbe of whooping cough, which, in favorable cases, was present in almost pure culture." If specimens are obtained later in the disease, the specific bacilli are scarce, and there are numerous other banal organisms present.

Bordet and Gengou tell of their first experience in 1900 with a five-month-old infant with whooping cough: "One of us was able to collect from the first crisis of typical cough a bit of whitish exudate unmixed with saliva. Microscopic examination after staining . . . showed that this exudate contained in enormous numbers a little bacterium, ovoid in shape, sometimes slightly elongated, sometimes short to the point of resembling a coccus, but in general rather constant in appearance. . . . Gram stain was negative. . . . The organism was present in such abundance and with a purity so perfect that one could not deny a causal relation between this infection and whooping cough." Bordet and Gengou were at first unable to obtain growth on various artificial media, but later they devised a hemoglobin-containing medium on which they were able to cultivate their organism. They describe the cultural appearance: "These colonies were bluish or grayish, slightly raised in the center, always a little diaphanous, especially toward the borders, almost transparent in the yellow cultures, where they appeared as little rose-colored drops. Under the microscope one saw a very small microbe, not taking the Gram stain. . . . It was easy to establish that we were in the presence of an organism identical with, or very similar to, that found by Pfeiffer in influenza, which other bacteriologists emphasized in whooping cough and even considered as the specific microbe." They refer to the work of Jochmann and Krause (Ref. 3), "who described this organism very exactly, and mentioned the need for hemoglobin." There follows a lengthy but unclear discussion on the actual relation of this microbe to their own. "In brief, this organism [of Jochmann and Krause], so like that described by Pfeiffer as provoking influenza, is not the agent of whooping cough." Bordet and Gengou now (1906) isolated from a baby with whooping cough, as they had in 1900, a similar bacterium which grew with great delicacy on their medium. "The comparison, in culture, of this parasite with the microbe of influenza shows that these two species are essentially different," as shown by comparison of cultures. The authenticity of this microbe as the causal agent of whooping cough "rests largely on serological reactions. . . . The serum of individuals not having had whooping cough does not agglutinate the microbe. The serum of children recently cured of this disease possesses agglutinative power of moderate degree, but it is constant and manifest." Bordet and Gengou employed the method of complement fixation. Emulsions of whooping-cough bacilli were used as antigens. "As for the microbe so like that described in influenza, it behaves with whooping cough serum as if it were in the presence of normal serum. . . . The findings relative to the etiology of whooping cough seem to us thus well established; we hope to make known shortly the results of trials of serotherapy or active immunization." In another paper ("Note complémentaire sur le microbe de la coqueluche," Ann. Inst. Pasteur, **21**:720, 1907) Bordet and Gengou describe their organism further, lay down criteria of differentiation from the influenza bacillus, and discuss agglutination tests. Whereas the organism was regularly clumped by artificial sera (horse), "unhappily the sera of children sick with or convalescent from pertussis are extremely inconstant from the point of view of this property. It often is manifest without being very intense; sometimes it is even absent altogether." Another paper ("L'Endotoxine coqueluíheuse," *ibid.*, 23:445, 1909) deals with endotoxin. They found that cultures injected into the guinea pig's peritoneum were highly toxic, although the bacteria did not multiply, and they felt that death was due to "intoxication." They developed methods for extracting the "endotoxin" from cultures. C. Fraenkel ("Untersuchungen zur Entstehung des Keuchhustens," München. med. Wchnschr., 55:1683, 1908) soon sounded a conservative note. While he isolated and grew the organism of Bordet and Gengou, he found the serological reactions variable and doubtful, and, although he produced a respiratory infection in monkeys, he was not certain it was whooping cough. Fraenkel did not mention the experiments of Klimenko (Ref. 6), and the latter chided him in a second paper (Klimenko, "Zur Aetiologie des Keuchhustens," Deutsche med. Wchnschr., 34:2030, 1908).

What, then, is the significance of the organism of Bordet and Gengou? One should note that they dismiss abruptly all previous work, although, as reviewed by Jochmann and Krause, many workers had found various small bacilli, some resembling influenza bacilli, some Gram-negative, in practically pure culture in whooping cough. Why is the bacillus of Bordet and Gengou entitled to more consideration as a causal agent? Indeed, Bordet and Gengou themselves had trouble differentiating it from other influenza bacillus-like "bacteria." As far as the serological tests by the method of complement fixation are concerned, confirmation of their results has failed (Ref. 5, Fraenkel). Indeed, one wonders at the general acceptance of Bordet and Gengou's claims.

6. KLIMENKO, W. N. Die Aetiologie des Keuchhustens. Experimenteller Keuchhusten, Centralbl. f. Bakt., 48:64, 1908.

Klimenko confirmed the finding of Bordet and Gengou's bacillus in whooping cough, but he concentrated his efforts on trying to reproduce the disease in animals. Injections of cultures into the bodies of rabbits and guinea pigs were without effect. In monkeys, on the other hand, there was some fever, nasal discharge, conjunctivitis, and diarrhea. One monkey died of intercurrent infection, and the Bordet-Gengou bacillus was recovered from the air passages. Six monkeys had a "barking" cough. A female received the contents of an agar slant of culture and developed cough with recovery of the organism; her cage mate developed fever and cough, and the Bordet-Gengou organism was recovered from the nose on the fifth, tenth, and twentieth days. Similar results were obtained in still other animals, although, as a rule, the reaction was "abortive." Three dogs, each receiving the growth from two agar slants, remained perfectly well. In 48 young dogs there was a high incidence of infection by contact, both experimental and spontaneous, featured by fever and catarrhal symptoms. Animals which died or were killed all showed, at autopsy, inflammation in the respiratory passages. The Bordet-Gangou organism was recovered from all these animals.

There seems no doubt that Klimenko produced a disease in dogs. The question is whether it was whooping cough. He says himself: "How shall one designate the disease which the Bordet-Gengou bacillus evokes in animals? I think one can call it an 'infectious catarrh of the air passages'; such a designation certain clinicians . . . also give to whooping cough." He concludes, however, that the Bordet-Gengou bacillus is undoubtedly the cause of whooping cough and that one can reproduce the disease in young dogs and monkeys.

It seems to us, however, that it is not proved that the experimental disease was actually pertussis. One must recall a similar situation with reference to the influenza bacillus, which is now, of course, proved not to be the cause of influenza. Yet F. G. Blake and R. L. Cecil ("The production of an acute respiratory disease in monkeys by inoculation with Bacillus influenzae," J.A.M.A., **74**:170, 1920) concluded that "the disease appears to be identical with influenza in men . . . it seems reasonable to infer that B. influenzae is the specific cause of influenza."

7. MALLORY, F. B., and HORNOR, A. A. Pertussis: the histological lesion in the respiratory tract, J.M. Research, **27**:115, 1913.

Mallory and Hornor emphasized the presence of huge numbers of a small Gram-negative bacillus, presumably similar to the Bordet-Gengou organism, between the cilia of the cells lining the trachea and bronchi. "The location of the organism is apparently characteristic for the disease. Its action seems to be largely mechanical. It interferes by its presence with the normal movements of the cilia and possibly leads to their destruction." The lesion is well pictured. A little later Mallory and Hornor with F. F. Henderson ("The relation of the Bordet-Gengou bacillus to the lesion of pertussis," *ibid.*, p. 391) reported reproducing this "specific" lesion in animals with sputum and with pure cultures of the bacillus. They conclude that they have fulfilled Koch's laws in relating the Bordet bacillus to whooping cough. L. J. Rhea ("The comparative pathology of the tracheal and bronchial lesions produced in man by B. pertussis [whooping cough] and those produced in dogs by B. bronchisepticus [canine distemper]," J.M. Research, **32**:47, 1915), however, questioned the final validity of this position, since he found a similar lesion in dogs infected with *B. bronchisepticus*. He felt that, in addition to histological examination, "B. pertussis must be recovered . . . and completely identified by bacteriological as well as agglutination reactions."

8. CHIEVITZ, I., and MEYER, A. H. Recherches sur la coqueluche, Ann. Inst. Pasteur, **30**:503, 1916.

The writers, dissatisfied with the isolation of Bordet bacilli from pertussis patients, had them cough directly at Petri plates containing appropriate media and were highly successful in obtaining growth of the organisms in question. During the second week of the disease these "cough plates," which later were universally used in diagnosing pertussis, were positive in 89 per cent of cases, a figure which had dropped by the fourth week to 32 per cent and by the seventh week to zero. A similar diagram is to be found in the article on whooping cough by L. W. Sauer (in Brennemann's *Practice of Pediatrics*, Vol. **2**, chap. 34, p. 7). J. J. Miller ("Etiology of whooping cough," J.A.M.A., **100**:681, 1933) refers to the Danish experience with cough plates; he says the method is universally accepted in Scandinavia.

9. McCORDOCK, H. A. Intranuclear inclusions in pertussis, Proc. Soc. Exper. Biol. & Med., **29**:1228, 1932.

Not everyone was willing blindly to accept the Bordet-Gengou bacillus as the cause of whooping cough. F. Freyer in an elaborate study of the pathology of pertussis ("Ueber die pathologische Anatomie der Lungenveränderungen beim Keuchhusten," Frankfurt. Ztschr. f. Path., **35**:213, 1927) described a case with intranuclear inclusions in the lung cells, "signs of the presence of a peculiar virus." McCordock, however, enumerated the points of resemblance between pertussis and known virus infections, namely, the interstitial pneumonia indistinguishable from that seen in influenza and measles and the encephalitis which also occurs following measles and influenza. He pointed out that inclusion bodies are often associated with virus diseases, and he found them in twelve of thirty-five cases of whooping cough. "The presence of intranuclear inclusions in the lungs in such a high percentage of our cases of pertussis and their infrequency in a variety of other childhood diseases . . . suggest that the possible role of a filterable virus must be considered in this disease." Later, at a meeting of the American Association of Pathologists (Am. J. Path., **13**:644, 1937) McCordock stated: "To date we have demonstrated them [intranuclear inclusions in pertussis] both in our St. Louis material and also in sections from other cities in about 30 per cent of all cases of pertussis examined. They cannot be produced by bacteria. This phase of the pertussis problem can never be solved by repeating experiments with hemophilic bacteria." A. R. Rich ("On the etiology and pathogenesis of whooping cough," Bull. Johns Hopkins Hosp., **51**:346, 1932) also analyzes the literature on the bacillus versus a virus etiology and is unconvinced that "the Bordet-Gengou bacillus represents the whole story of the etiology of whooping cough."

10. RICH, A. R., LONG, P. H., BROWN, J. H., BLISS, E. A., and HOLT, L. E., Jr. Experiments upon the cause of whooping cough, Science, **76**:330, 1932.

At about the time that a virus etiology was being pushed by McCordock (Ref. 9), H. MacDonald and E. J. MacDonald ("Experimental pertussis," J. Infect. Dis., **53**:328, 1933), on the basis of the production of whooping cough by inoculation with cultures of the Bordet-Gengou bacillus and failure to produce disease in vaccinated controls or in boys inoculated with filtrates, concluded that "a filter passing virus plays no rôle in the etiology of pertussis. The disease is caused by the bacillus of Bordet and Gengou. Active immunity is conferred by the injection of B. pertussis vaccine." As only a very few subjects were used, there is some question as to the MacDonalds' emphatic and sweeping conclusions. J. M. Frawley ("A study of the virus factor in whooping cough," J. Pediat., **16**:18, 1940) also failed to produce any symptoms "resembling whooping cough" in twelve children given nasal instillations of filtered washings from children with whooping cough.

Rich and his colleagues report the production of a disease in chimpanzees in every way indistinguishable from whooping cough and associated with the presence of the Bordet bacilli in huge numbers in cough plates, following the instillation of Bordet bacilli into the respiratory passages. Filtrates of sputum from early cases of pertussis, on the other hand, produced only mild "febrile upper respiratory catarrhs." G. S. Shibley ("Etiology of whooping cough," Proc. Soc. Exper. Biol. & Med., **31**:576, 1933) inoculated a chimpanzee with a strain of the Bordet bacillus subcultured long enough to rule out the association with a virus and produced in the animal what was regarded as typical whooping cough. At autopsy *H. pertussis* was recovered from bronchi and bronchioles, but Shibley did not demonstrate "H. pertussis-like organisms embedded in cilia."

The numerous transmission experiments recorded in the literature are reviewed by Lapin (*op. cit.*, p. 43). However, in evaluating these experiments, one should remember that washings from influenza, a disease now known to be caused by a virus, have also failed to produce disease in man (M. J. Rosenau, "Experiments to determine mode of spread of influenza," J.A.M.A., 73:311, 1919), whereas reliable workers thought that they had produced influenza with instillations of the influenza bacillus.

11. MILLER, J. J., Jr. The present status of immunization against pertussis, California & West. Med., 53:25, 1940.

Early after the discovery of the Bordet-Gengou bacillus, attempts were made at treatment and prophylaxis by vaccines prepared from these organisms, H. N. Appel and O. I. Bloom ("Whooping cough and its treatment," Arch. Pediat., 39:145, 1922) give a list of the most important reports, beginning in 1909, and show that variable conclusions were drawn. A. H. Meyer, M. Christensen, and E. Sörensen ("Whooping cough vaccination," Acta paediat., 4:21, 1925) in Scandinavia, where much work was done, were in doubt as to the results but thought that further efforts were worthwhile. M. Madsen ("Whooping cough," Boston M. & S.J., 192:50, 1925), the great Danish authority, in his Cutler Lecture at Harvard was also optimistic but uncertain about the effects of vaccine. P. H. Leslie and H. D. Gardner ("The phases of Haemophilus pertussis," J. Hyg., 31:423, 1931) opened a new chapter in the subject when they showed that the antigenic powers of pertussis bacilli were altered by growth on artificial media and implied that organisms freshly isolated on blood agar (in Phase I) were perhaps "the only antigen for the production of active immunity in guinea-pigs." L. Sauer ("Present status of preventive inoculation against whooping cough," Am. J. Dis. Child., 54:979, 1937), an enthusiastic advocate of the vaccine, concludes: "Inoculation with potent antigen confers protection on a high precentage of young children." J. J. Miller, Jr., and H. K. Faber ("Immunization against pertussis," J.A.M.A., 112:1145, 1939), using Phase I vaccine, concluded that good protection was achieved in most cases. "These observations indicate that the vaccine used conferred either complete or partial protection on the great majority of those inoculated." J. J. Miller critically reviews the whole problem. "I think it is self-evident that active immunization against pertussis has been accomplished with certain preparations under certain conditions." Finally, H. M. Felton and C. Y. Willard ("Current status of prophylaxis by Hemophilus pertussis vaccine," J.A.M.A., 126:294, 1944) review the literature to date and conclude that, while the earlier work was doubtful, recently developed vaccines "do confer significant protection as measured by reduction in attack rate and severity of pertussis."

In summary, then, according to published reports, the case seems conclusive in favor of the Bordet-Gengou bacillus as the cause of whooping cough. However, it seems to us that the *final* word as to exclusion of a viral etiology has not yet been said.